CLINICAL NEUROLOGY

FOR PSYCHIATRISTS

CLINICAL NEUROLOGY
FOR PSYCHIATRISTS

DAVID MYLAND KAUFMAN, M.D.
Department of Neurology
Montefiore Medical Center
Albert Einstein College of Medicine
Bronx, New York

W.B. SAUNDERS COMPANY
A Harcourt Health Sciences Company
Philadelphia   London   New York   St. Louis   Sydney   Toronto

W.B. SAUNDERS COMPANY

A Harcourt Health Sciences Company

The Curtis Center
Independence Square West
Philadelphia, Pennsylvania 19106

Library of Congress Cataloging-in-Publication Data

Kaufman, David Myland.
    Clinical neurology for psychiatrists / David Myland Kaufman. — 5th ed.
      p.   cm.
    Includes bibliographical references and index.
    ISBN 0-7216-8995-7
    1. Nervous system—Diseases. 2. Neurology. 3. Psychiatrists.   I. Title.
    [DNLM: 1. Nervous System Diseases—diagnosis 2. Diagnosis, Differential
    3. Psychiatry   WL 141 K21c 2001]
    RC346 .K38   2001
    616.8—dc21

                                     00-063722

CLINICAL NEUROLOGY FOR PSYCHIATRISTS   ISBN 0-7216-8995-7

Printed in the United States of America

Last digit is the print number: 9   8   7   6   5   4   3   2   1

This is dedicated
to the ones I love—
MY FAMILY:

my wife of 30 years, Rita,
and our children,
Rachel and Bob, Jennifer and Sarah

Acknowledgments

I thank Mr. Michael Lipton for his many helpful suggestions, sensitive and meticulous attention to all details and phases of editing, and his congenial work ethic. In addition, Ms. Abbey Rathbone provided helpful, literate suggestions. Dr. Maurice Preter has offered critical editorial guidance, especially as to the relationship of neurology and psychiatry. Ms. Meryl Ranzer, Mr. Barry Morden, and Ms. Ann Mannato captured the sense of neurology in their wonderful illustrations. Mr. David H. Bernstein, a partner in DeBevoise & Plimpton, gave thoughtful, sound counsel. My students, house staff, and colleagues at Montefiore Medical Center, Albert Einstein College of Medicine, have reviewed each chapter and question and answer set. The speakers and syllabus for the course Clinical Neurology for Psychiatrists gave rise to this book.

Notes About References

Most chapters provide specific references from the neurologic and general medical literature. Several standard, well-written textbooks contain appropriate information about many topics:

Adams RD, Victor M, Ropper AH: Principles of Neurology (6th ed.). New York, McGraw-Hill, 1997.

Barclay L (Ed.): Clinical Geriatric Neurology. Lea & Febiger, Philadelphia, 1993.

Berg BO (Ed.): Principles of Child Neurology. New York, McGraw-Hill, 1996.

Coffey CE, Brumback RA (Eds.): Textbook of Pediatric Neuropsychiatry. Washington, D.C., American Psychiatric Press, 1998.

David RB (Ed.): Child and Adolescent Neurology. St. Louis, Mosby, 1998.

Feinberg TE, Farah MJ: Behavioral Neurology and Neuropsychology. New York, McGraw-Hill, 1997.

Fitzgerald MJT: Neuroanatomy: Basic and Clinical. Philadelphia, Baillière Tindal, 1992.

Frank Y: Pediatric Behavioral Neurology. New York, CRC Press, 1996.

Goetz CG, Pappert CJ: Textbook of Clinical Neurology. Philadelphia, WB Saunders, 1999.

Heilman KM, Valenstein E: Clinical Neuropsychology (3rd ed.). New York, Oxford University Press, 1993.

Joynt RJ, Griggs RC (Eds.): Clinical Neurology. Philadelphia, J.B. Lippincott-Raven, 1997.

Kaplan PW (Ed.): Neurologic Disease in Women. New York, Demos, 1998.

Pfeffer CR, Solomon GE, Kaufman DM (Eds.): Neurologic disorders: Developmental and behavioral sequelae. In *Child and Adolescent Psychiatric Clinics of North America*. Philadelphia, W.B. Saunders, October, 1999

Rowland L (Ed.): Merritt's Textbook of Neurology (10th ed.). Philadelphia, Lea & Febiger, 2000.

WEB SITES THAT OFFER INFORMATION ABOUT SEVERAL AREAS

(Sites that pertain to single areas are listed in each chapter's references and in Appendix 1.)

Grateful Med	http://igm.nlm.nih.gov
National Institutes of Health	http://www.nih.gov

Preface

PURPOSE

I have written *Clinical Neurology for Psychiatrists* from my perspective as a neurologist at a major teaching hospital, as a collegial, straightforward guide. In a format combining traditional neuroanatomic correlations with symptom-oriented discussions, the book should help the reader learn about neurologic conditions that are common to psychiatry and neurology, illustrate a basic science principle, and cause or mimic psychiatric symptoms. Having evolved from a course I started in 1971, the book should help readers prepare for specialty and certifying examinations.

Section I reviews classic anatomic neurology and describes how a physician might approach patients with a suspected neurologic disorder, identify central or peripheral nervous system disease, and correlate physical signs. Section II discusses common and otherwise important clinical areas, emphasizing aspects a psychiatrist is likely to encounter. Topics include neurologic illnesses, such as multiple sclerosis, brain tumors, and strokes; common symptoms, such as headaches, chronic pain, and seizures; and conditions with many different manifestations, such as involuntary movement disorders and traumatic brain injury. For each topic, chapters describe the relevant history, neurologic and psychiatric findings, easily performed office and bedside examinations, appropriate laboratory tests, differential diagnosis, and management options.

Many chapters are supplemented with outlines of the relevant history; reproductions of standard bedside tests, such as the Mini-Mental Status Test, hand-held visual acuity card, and Abnormal Involuntary Movement Scale (AIMS); and references to recent articles, reviews, and classic studies. Appendices, which contain information pertaining to most chapters, include Patient and Family Support Groups (Appendix 1); Costs of Various Tests and Treatments (Appendix 2); and Diseases Transmitted by Chromosome Abnormalities, Mitochondria Abnormalities, and Excessive Trinucleotide Repeats (Appendix 3).

The book relies on a visual approach. Each chapter includes abundant illustrations because they help explain the underlying basic science, personify or reinforce clinical descriptions, best describe many disorders, and serve as the basis for question-based learning. Moreover, this approach reflects that the diagnosis of entire categories of neurologic illnesses, such as gait abnormalities, psychogenic neurologic deficits, neurocutaneous disorders, and facial dyskinesias, still relies on observation or "diagnosis by inspection." In fact, highly sophisticated procedures—computed tomography (CT), magnetic resonance imaging (MRI), and electroencephalography (EEG)—are visual records, which are also reproduced.

Clinical Neurology for Psychiatrists complements the text with question-based learning, which is an informative, interactive, and efficient didactic approach adopted by many medical schools. It is not just a quiz or preparation for an examination but an integral part of the book. Most chapters and two review sections are followed by short-answer or case questions. In keeping with the visual emphasis of the book, many of the questions are based on sketches of patients, MRIs, CTs, or other imaging tests. Questions at the end of the chapters refer to material discussed within that chapter. Those in the review sections require that the reader compare neurologic disorders that have appeared in different chapters.

The book also includes frank discussions of the many neurologic conditions that have become subjects of public policy. Psychiatrists should become well-versed in these conditions and their implications because they are liable to be drawn into debates involving their patients or the medical community:

- Amyotrophic lateral sclerosis and multiple sclerosis as the battleground of assisted suicide
- Meningomyelocele with Arnold-Chiari malformation as an indication for late-term abortion and the value of spending limited resources on this fatal or severely limiting condition
- Cancer (malignant) pain as the fulcrum for legalizing marijuana and heroin
- Opioid (narcotic) treatment for chronic benign pain, such as low back pain
- Parkinson's disease treatment with fetal cell transplant
- Persistent vegetative state and continuing life-support technology

CHANGES AND ADDITIONS FOR THE FIFTH EDITION

The first four editions of *Clinical Neurology for Psychiatrists* have enjoyed considerable success in the United States, Canada, and abroad. The book has been translated into Japanese and Italian. In the fifth edition, which was written 5 years after the preceding one, I have clarified my presentations of many neurologic topics, discussed numerous recent developments that have occurred in virtually all areas of neurology, and added computer-generated graphics and clinical-anatomic illustrations.

I have also made some stylistic changes that reflect an increased respect for patients and physicians. I have replaced *"Chief Complaint"* with *"Primary Symptom"* or simply a description of the symptoms that brought the patient to the physician. Race and ethnicity groupings are not included in the initial identifying information. The currently accepted *Asian* has replaced *Oriental*. When such information is relevant, it is included as part of the social history. In assessing a patient's comprehension, "ability to follow *commands*" has been changed to "ability to follow *requests.*" Likewise, in acknowledging the physicians who do the bulk of patient care, *"local medical doctor (LMD),"* *"general practitioner (GP),"* and *"private medical doctor (PMD),"* have been replaced by *"primary care physician (PCP)."* Finally, in an effort to simplify medicine, generally understood words are substituted for technical ones. For example, the vernacular term *"stroke"* has replaced *"cerebrovascular accident."*

Also in keeping with the book's clinical orientation, I have included web sites, as well as the mailing addresses, of patient support groups and the current cost of the diagnostic tests and treatments.

Because the diagnoses of neurologic illnesses, which have not been codified, must be translated into comparable psychiatric terms, this edition introduces the comparable definitions from the *Diagnostic and Statistical Manual of Mental Disorders-IV (DSM-IV)*. Along the same line, it points out the occasional discrepancies and omissions.

The text now includes the addition or expansion of several topics. For didactic purposes, most are included within discussions of the relevant illness rather than as separate subjects:

- Basic science of neurologic illnesses: neuroanatomy, synthesis of neurotransmitters, epidemiology, and genetics
- Normal age-related neurologic changes

- Pathogenesis by apoptosis, excessive trinucleotide repeats, excitotoxicity, ion channel abnormalities, and mitochondrial DNA abnormalities

- Conditions that first become apparent in childhood and persist into adulthood: Klinefelter's syndrome and other sex chromosome disorders; Prader-Willi and Angelman's syndrome, which are examples of genetic imprinting; tic disorders, which recently have been proposed to result from an immunologic disturbance; and child abuse

- Illnesses, in addition to Alzheimer's disease, that cause dementia: diffuse Lewy body disease, frontotemporal dementia, new variant Creutzfeldt-Jakob ("mad cow") disease, and other spongiform encephalopathies

- Neurotransmitters and drug abuse in neurologic disorders

- New treatments for chronic pain, epilepsy, erectile dysfunction, migraines, multiple sclerosis, and Parkinson's disease

One word of caution, *Clinical Neurology for Psychiatrists* is demanding. It asks the reader to follow a rigorous course in order to master difficult material. It assumes the reader is well educated, thoughtful, and hard working. The book, like the practice of neurology, is dense, rich, and fulfilling. Despite the additions, the fifth edition of *Clinical Neurology for Psychiatrists* remains manageable in size, depth, and scope. It is succinct enough to be read and enjoyed from cover to cover.

David Myland Kaufman, M.D.

Physician-Readers, Please Note

Clinical Neurology for Psychiatrists discusses medications, testing, procedures, and other aspects of medical care. Despite purported effectiveness, many of these therapies are fraught with side effects and other adverse outcomes. These discussions are neither recommendations nor medical advice, and they are not intended to apply to individual patients. The physician, who should consult the package insert and the medical literature, is responsible for medications' indications, dosage, contraindications, precautions, side effects, and alternatives, including doing nothing. Some aspects of medical care are widely and successfully used for particular purposes not approved by the Food and Drug Administration (FDA) or other review panel. As regards these unorthodox or "off-label" treatments, as well as conventional ones, this book is merely reporting use by neurologists and other physicians.

David Myland Kaufman, M.D.

Contents

CLASSIC ANATOMIC NEUROLOGY

First Encounter with a Patient: Examination and Formulation

Despite the ready availability of sophisticated tests, the "hands on" neurologic examination remains the fundamental aspect of the specialty. Beloved by neurologists, this examination provides a vivid portrayal of function and illness. When neurologists say they have seen a case of a particular illness, they mean that they have really *seen* it.

When a patient's history suggests a neurologic illness, the neurologic examination unequivocally demonstrates it. Even if they themselves will not actually be examining patients in the physical sense, psychiatrists should appreciate certain neurologic signs and be able to assess a neurologist's conclusion.

Physicians should examine patients systematically. They should test interesting areas in detail during a sequential evaluation of the nervous system's major components. Undeviating adherence to routine is vital to avoid omission, duplication, and ultimately confusion. Despite obvious dysfunction of one part of the nervous system, all areas are evaluated. A physician can complete an initial or screening neurologic examination in about 20 minutes and return to perform special testing of particular areas, such as the mental status.

EXAMINATION

Physicians should note the patient's age, sex, and handedness, and then review the primary symptom, present illness, medical history, family history, and social history. They should include detailed questions about the primary symptom, associated symptoms, and possible etiologic factors. If a patient cannot relate the history, the physician might interrupt the process to look for language, memory, or other cognitive deficits. Many chapters in Section 2 of this book contain outlines of standard questions related to common symptoms.

After obtaining the history, physicians should anticipate the patient's neurologic deficits and be prepared to look for disease, primarily of the central nervous system (CNS) or the peripheral nervous system (PNS). At this point, without yielding to rigid preconceptions, the physician should have developed some feeling for the problem at hand.

Then physicians should look for the site of involvement (i.e., "localize the lesion"). "Localization" is a hallowed goal of the examination and is useful in most cases. However, it is often somewhat of an art, supplanted by imaging or inapplicable to several important neurologic illnesses.

The examination, which overall remains irreplaceable in diagnosis, consists of a functional neuroanatomy demonstration: mental status, cranial nerves, motor system, reflexes, sensation, and cerebellar system (Table 1–1). This format should be followed during every examination. Until it is memorized, a copy should be taken to the patient's bedside to serve both as a reminder and a place to record neurologic findings.

The examination usually starts with an assessment of the mental status because it is the most important neurologic function, and impairments may preclude an accurate assessment of other neurologic functions. The examiner should consider specific intellectual deficits, such as language impairment (see Aphasia, Chapter 8), as well as general intellectual decline (see Dementia, Chapter 7). Tests of cranial nerves may reveal malfunction of nerves either individually or in groups, such as the *ocular motility nerves* (III, IV, and VI) and the *cerebellopontine angle nerves* (V, VII, and VIII) (see Chapter 4).

The examination of the motor system is usually performed more to detect the pattern than the severity of weakness. Whether weakness is mild to moderate *(paresis)* or complete *(plegia)*, the pattern has much more value than severity in localization. Three common important patterns are easy to recognize. If the lower face, arm, and leg on one side of the body are paretic, the pattern is called *hemiparesis* and it indicates damage to the contralateral cerebral hemisphere or brainstem. Both legs being

TABLE 1–1. *Neurologic Examination*

Mental status
   Cooperation
   Orientation (to month, year, place, and any deficits [physical or mental])
   Language
   Memory for immediate, recent, and past events
   Higher intellectual functions: arithmetic, similarities/differences
Cranial nerves
   I—Smell
   II—Visual acuity, visual fields, optic fundi
   III, IV, VI—Pupils' size and reactivity, extraocular motion
   V—Corneal reflex and facial sensation
   VII—Strength of upper and lower facial muscles, taste
   VIII—Hearing
   IX–XI—Articulation, palate movement, gag reflex
   XII—Tongue movement
Motor system
   Limb strength
   Spasticity, flaccidity, or fasciculations
   Abnormal movements (e.g., tremor, chorea)
Reflexes
   DTRs
      Biceps, triceps, brachioradialis, quadriceps, Achilles
   Pathologic reflexes
      Extensor plantar response (Babinski sign), frontal release
Sensation
   Position, vibration, stereognosis
   Pain
Cerebellar system
   Finger-to-nose and heel-to-shin tests
   Rapid alternating movements
   Gait

weak, called *paraparesis,* usually indicates spinal cord damage. Paresis of the distal portion of all the limbs indicates PNS rather than CNS damage.

Eliciting two categories of reflexes assists in determining whether paresis or another neurologic abnormality originates in the CNS or PNS. *Deep tendon reflexes (DTRs)* are normally present with uniform reactivity in all limbs, but neurologic injury often alters their activity or symmetry. In general, with CNS injury that includes corticospinal tract damage, DTRs are hyperactive, whereas with PNS injury, DTRs are hypoactive.

In contrast to DTRs, *pathologic reflexes* are not normally elicitable beyond infancy. If found, they are a sign of CNS damage. The most widely recognized pathologic reflex is the famous *Babinski sign.* Judging from current medical conversations, the terminology regarding this sign must be clarified. After plantar stimulation, the great toe normally moves downward (i.e., it has a flexor response). With brain or spinal cord damage, plantar stimulation typically causes the great toe to move upward (i.e., to have an extensor response). This reflex extensor movement, which is a manifestation of CNS damage, is the Babinski sign (see Fig. 19–3). It and other signs may be "present" or "elicited," but they are never "positive" or "negative." In the same way, a traffic stop sign may be present or absent but never positive or negative.

Frontal release signs, which are other pathologic reflexes, reflect frontal lobe injury. They are helpful in indicating an "organic" basis for a change in personality. In addition, to a limited degree, they are associated with intellectual impairment (see Chapter 7).

The sensory system examination is long and tedious. Moreover, unlike abnormal DTRs and Babinski signs, which are reproducible, objective, and virtually impossible to mimic, the sensory examination relies almost entirely on the patient's report. Its subjective nature has led to the practice of disregarding the sensory examination if it varies from the rest of the evaluation. Under most circumstances, the best approach is to test the major sensory modalities in a clear anatomic order and tentatively accept the patient's report.

Depending on the nature of the suspected disorder, the physician may test sensation of position, vibration, and stereognosis (appreciation of an object's form by touching it)—all of which are carried in the posterior columns of the spinal cord. Pain (pinprick) sensation, which is carried in the lateral columns, should be tested carefully with a nonpenetrating, disposable instrument, such as a Q-Tip cotton swab.

Cerebellar function is evaluated by observing the patient for intention tremor and incoordination during several standard maneuvers that include the *finger-to-nose test* and rapid repetition of *alternating movement test* (see Chapter 2). If at all possible, physicians should watch the patient walk because a normal gait requires intact CNS and PNS motor pathways, coordination, proprioception, and balance. Moreover, all these systems must be well integrated.

When examining a patient's gait, physicians should watch not only for cerebellar-based incoordination *(ataxia),* but for hemiparesis and other signs of corticospinal tract dysfunction, involuntary movement disorders, apraxia (see Table 2–3), and even orthopedic conditions. Keep in mind that gait impairment is not merely a neurologic or orthopedic sign but a condition that routinely leads to fatal falls and permanent incapacity for numerous elderly people each year.

FORMULATION

Although somewhat ritualistic, a succinct and cogent *formulation* remains the basis of neurologic problem solving. The classic formulation is an appraisal of the four aspects of the examination: symptoms, signs, localization, and differential diagnosis. The clinician might also have to support a conclusion that neurologic disease is present or, equally important, absent. For this step, psychogenic signs must be separated, if only tentatively, from neurologic ("organic") ones. Evidence must be demonstrable for a psychogenic or neurologic etiology while acknowledging that neither is a diagnosis of exclusion. Of course, as if to confuse the situation, patients often manifest grossly exaggerated symptoms of a neurologic illness (see Chapter 3).

Localization of neurologic lesions requires the clinician to determine at least whether the illness affects the CNS, PNS, or muscle system (see Chapters 2 through 6). Precise localization of lesions within them is possible and generally expected. The physician must also establish whether the nervous system is affected diffusely or in a discrete area. The site and extent of neurologic damage will indicate certain diseases. A readily apparent example is that cerebrovascular accidents (strokes) and tumors generally involve a discrete area of the brain, but Alzheimer's disease causes widespread, symmetric changes.

Finally, the differential diagnosis is the disease or diseases—up to three—most consistent with the patient's symptoms and signs. When specific diseases cannot be suggested, major categories, such as "structural lesions," should be offered.

A typical formulation might be as follows: "Mr. Jones, a 56-year-old man, has had left-sided headaches for 2 months and a generalized seizure on the day before admission. He is lethargic. He has papilledema, a right hemiparesis with hyperactive DTRs, and a Babinski sign. The lesion seems to be in the left cerebral hemisphere. Most likely, he has a tumor, but a stroke is possible." This formulation briefly recapitulates the crucial symptoms, positive and negative elements of the history, and physical findings. It tacitly assumes that neurologic disease is present because of the obvious, objective physical findings. The localization is based on the history of seizures and the right-sided hemiparesis and abnormal reflexes. The differential diagnosis is based on the high probability of these conditions being caused by a discrete cerebral lesion.

To review, the physician should present a formulation that answers *The Four Questions of Neurology*:

- What are the *symptoms* of *neurologic* disease?
- What are the *signs* of *neurologic* disease?
- *Where* is the lesion?
- *What* is the lesion?

RESPONDING TO CONSULTATIONS

Psychiatry residents in many programs rotate through neurology departments where they are expected to provide neurology consultations solicited by physicians working in the emergency department, medical clinic, and other referring services. When responding to a request for a neurology consultation, the psychiatry resident must work with a variation of the traditional summary-and-formulation format. The response should be primarily or exclusively to answer to the question posed by the referring physician. Moreover, the consultant should not expect to follow the patient throughout the illness, much less establish a long-term physician-patient relationship. Rather, attention should be directed to the referring physician, who is shouldering the burden of primary care and may or may not accept the consultant's suggestions.

Before beginning the consultation, both the referring physician and consultant should be clear on the reason for it. The consultation may concern a single aspect of the case, such as the importance of a neurologic finding, the significance of a computed tomography report, or whether one or another treatment would be best. The consultant should insist on a specific question and ultimately answer that question. Eventually, the differential diagnosis should contain no more than three possible etiologies—starting with the most likely. Even at tertiary-care institutions, common things occur commonly. As an example of the saying that "hoofbeats are usually from horses, not zebras," patients are more likely to have hemiparesis from a stroke than from an unwitnessed seizure.

Consultants should be helpful by ordering routine tests, not by merely suggesting them. On the other hand, consulting psychiatry residents should not suggest hazardous tests or treatments without obtaining a second opinion.

Finally, consultants should avoid overassertiveness by maintaining awareness of the entire situation with its incomplete and conflicting elements. They should also be mindful of the position of the referring physician and patient before responding as a specialist arriving on the scene after the preliminary work has been completed.

Central Nervous System Disorders

Lesions in the two components of the central nervous system (CNS)—the brain and the spinal cord—typically cause paresis, sensory loss, and visual deficits (Table 2–1). In addition, lesions in the cerebral hemispheres (the cerebrum) cause neuropsychologic disorders. Symptoms and signs of CNS disorders must be contrasted to those resulting from peripheral nervous system (PNS) and psychogenic disorders. Neurologists generally tend to rely on the physical rather than mental status evaluation, thereby honoring the belief that "one Babinski sign is worth a thousand words."

SIGNS OF CEREBRAL HEMISPHERE LESIONS

Of the various signs of cerebral hemisphere injury, the most prominent is usually *contralateral hemiparesis* (Table 2–2): weakness of the lower face, trunk, arm, and leg opposite to the side of the lesion. It results from damage to the *corticospinal tract*, which is also called the *pyramidal tract* (Fig. 2–1). During the corticospinal tract's entire path from the cerebral cortex to the anterior horn cells of the spinal cord, it is considered the *upper motor neuron (UMN)* (Fig. 2–2). The anterior horn cells, which are part of the PNS, are the beginning of the *lower motor neuron (LMN)*. The division of the motor system into upper and lower motor neurons is a basic tenet of clinical neurology.

Cerebral lesions that damage the corticospinal tract are characterized by *signs of UMN injury* (Figs. 2–2 to 2–5):

- Paresis with muscle spasticity
- Hyperactive deep tendon reflexes (DTRs)
- Babinski signs

In contrast, peripheral nerve lesions, including anterior horn cell or motor neuron diseases, are associated with *signs of LMN injury:*

- Paresis with muscle flaccidity and atrophy
- Hypoactive DTRs
- No Babinski signs

Cerebral lesions are not the only cause of hemiparesis. Because the corticospinal tract has such a long course (see Fig. 2–1), lesions in the brainstem and spinal cord as well as the cerebrum may produce hemiparesis and other signs of UMN damage. Signs pointing to injury in various regions of the CNS can indicate the origin of hemiparesis.

TABLE 2–1. *Signs of Common CNS Lesions*

Cerebral hemisphere*
    Hemiparesis with hyperactive deep tendon reflexes (DTRs), spasticity, and Babinski sign
    Hemisensory loss
    Homonymous hemianopsia
    Partial seizures
    Aphasia, hemi-inattention, and dementia
    Pseudobulbar palsy
Basal ganglia*
    Movement disorders: parkinsonism, athetosis, chorea, and hemiballismus
Brainstem
    Cranial nerve palsy with contralateral hemiparesis
    Internuclear ophthalmoplegia (MLF syndrome)
    Nystagmus
    Bulbar palsy
Cerebellum
    Tremor on intention[†]
    Impaired rapid alternating movements (dysdiadochokinesia)[†]
    Ataxic gait
    Scanning speech
Spinal cord
    Paraparesis or quadriparesis
    Sensory loss up to a "level"
    Bladder, bowel, sexual dysfunction

MLF, Medial longitudinal fasciculus syndrome.
*Signs contralateral to lesions.
[†]Signs ipsilateral to lesions.

TABLE 2–2. *Signs of Common Cerebral Lesions*

Either hemisphere*
    Hemiparesis with hyperactive DTRs and a Babinski sign
    Hemisensory loss
    Homonymous hemianopsia
    Partial seizures: simple, complex, or secondarily generalized
Dominant hemisphere
    Aphasias: fluent, nonfluent, conduction, isolation
    Gerstmann's syndrome: acalculia, agraphia, finger agnosia, and left-right confusion
    Alexia without agraphia
Nondominant hemisphere
    Hemi-inattention
    Anosognosia
    Constructional apraxia
Both hemispheres
    Dementia
    Pseudobulbar palsy

*Signs contralateral to lesions.

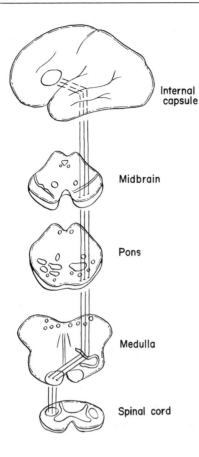

Internal
capsule

Midbrain

Pons

Medulla

Spinal cord

FIGURE 2–1. Each corticospinal tract originates in the cerebral cortex, passes through the internal capsule, and descends into the brainstem. It crosses in the pyramids, which are long protuberances on the inferior portion of the medulla, to descend in the spinal cord as the *lateral corticospinal tract.* It terminates by forming a synapse with the *anterior horn cells* of the spinal cord, which give rise to peripheral nerves. The corticospinal tract is sometimes called the *pyramidal* tract because it crosses in the pyramids. A complementary tract, which originates in the basal ganglia, is called the *extrapyramidal* tract.

Another indication of a cerebral lesion is loss of certain sensory modalities over one half of the body (i.e., *hemisensory loss*) (Fig. 2–6). A patient with a cerebral lesion characteristically loses contralateral position sensation, two-point discrimination, and the ability to identify objects by touch (stereognosis). Loss of those modalities is often called a "cortical" sensory loss.

Pain sensation, a "primary" sense, is perceived in the thalamus. Because the thalamus is the uppermost portion of the brainstem, pain perception is retained with cerebral lesions. For example, patients with cerebral infarctions may be unable to identify a painful area but will still feel the intensity and discomfort of pain. Also, patients in intractable pain did not obtain relief when they underwent experimental surgical resection of the cerebral cortex. The other aspect of the thalamus' role in sensing pain is seen when patients with thalamic infarctions develop spontaneous, disconcerting, burning pains over the contralateral body (i.e., thalamic pain) (see Thalamic Pain, Chapter 14).

Visual loss of the same half-field in each eye, *homonymous hemianopsia* (Fig. 2–7), is a characteristic sign of a contralateral cerebral lesion. Other equally characteristic visual losses are associated with lesions involving the eye, optic nerve, or optic tract (see Chapters 4 and 12). Because they would be situated relatively far from the visual pathway, lesions in the brainstem, cerebellum, or spinal cord do not cause visual field loss.

Another conspicuous sign of a cerebral hemisphere lesion is the development of *partial seizures* (see Chapter 10). The major varieties of partial seizures—elementary, complex, and secondarily generalized—clearly result from cerebral lesions. In fact, about 90% of partial complex seizures originate in the temporal lobe.

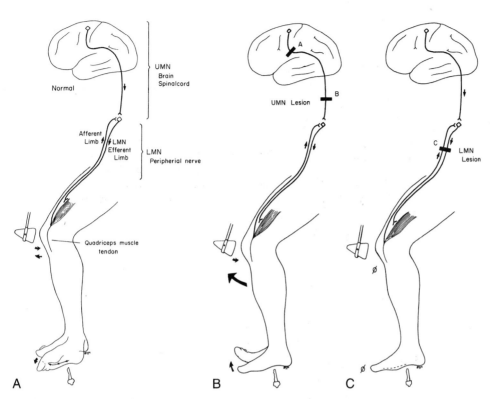

FIGURE 2–2. **A,** Normally, when the quadriceps tendon is struck with the percussion hammer, DTR is elicited. In addition, when the sole of the foot is stroked to elicit a plantar reflex, the big toe bends downward (flexes). **B,** When brain or spinal cord lesions involve the corticospinal tract and cause UMN damage, the DTR is hyperactive, and the plantar reflex is extensor (i.e., a Babinski sign is present). **C,** When peripheral nerve injury causes lower motor neuron *(LMN)* damage, the DTR is hypoactive and the plantar reflex is absent.

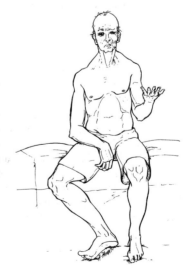

FIGURE 2–3. This patient with severe right hemiparesis typically has weakness of the right lower face, arm, and leg. The right-sided facial weakness causes the widened palpebral fissure and flat nasolabial fold; however, the forehead muscles are normal (see Chapter 4 regarding this discrepancy). The right arm is limp, and the elbow, wrist, and fingers are flexed. The right hemiparesis also causes the right leg to be externally rotated and the hip and knee to be flexed.

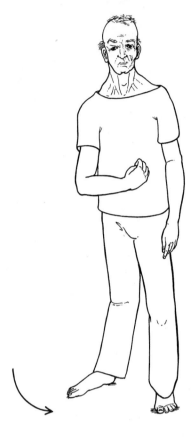

FIGURE 2–4. When the patient stands up, his weakened arm retains its flexed posture. His right leg remains externally rotated, but he can walk by swinging it in a circular path. This is an effective maneuver that results in *circumduction* or a *hemiparetic gait*.

Although hemiparesis, hemisensory loss, homonymous hemianopsia, and partial seizures may result from lesions of either cerebral hemisphere, several neuropsychologic deficits are referable specifically to either the dominant or nondominant hemisphere. Because approximately 95% of people are right-handed, unless physicians know otherwise about an individual patient, they should assume that the left hemisphere is always the dominant hemisphere. Lesions of the dominant hemisphere usually cause language impairment, *aphasia* (see Chapter 8). Moreover, because the

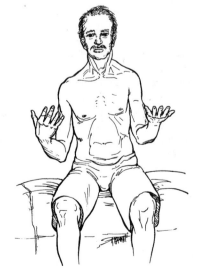

FIGURE 2–5. Mild hemiparesis may not be obvious. To exaggerate a subtle hemiparesis, the physician has asked this patient to extend both arms with his palms held upright, as though holding a water glass on his outstretched hand. After a minute, the weakened arm slowly sinks (drifts), and the palm turns inward (pronate). The imaginary water glass would spill inward, falling off the right palm. This arm's drift and pronation represent a *forme fruste* of the posture seen with severe paresis (see Fig. 2–3).

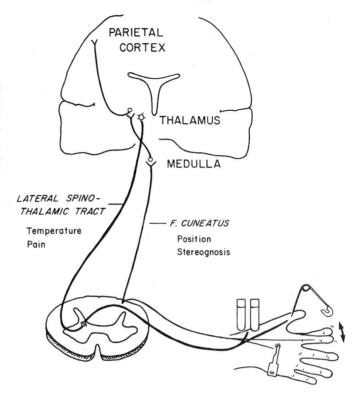

FIGURE 2–6. Pain and temperature sensations are carried to the spinal cord where, after a synapse, these sensations cross and ascend in the *contralateral lateral spinothalamic tract.* For practical purposes, pain tracts terminate in the thalamus. Position sense (tested by movement of the distal finger joint) and stereognosis (tested by tactile identification of common objects) are carried in the *ipsilateral f. cuneatus* and *f. gracilis,* which together constitute the *posterior columns* (see Fig. 2–14). These tracts cross, synapse in the thalamus, and terminate in the cortex of the contralateral parietal lobe. (When testing pain, to avoid spreading blood-borne illnesses, examiners should not use a pin but a cotton stick.)

language centers are adjacent to the corticospinal tract (see Fig. 8–1), such lesions typically produce an accompanying right hemiparesis.

When the *non*dominant parietal lobe is injured, patients typically have *hemi-inattention,* a constellation of disorders in which patients neglect left-sided visual and tactile stimuli (see Chapter 8). Patients may not even acknowledge their (left) hemiparesis—a condition known as *anosognosia.* With *constructional apraxia,* patients cannot arrange matchsticks into certain patterns or copy simple forms (Fig. 2–8).

All signs discussed so far are referable to one cerebral hemisphere (i.e., unilateral damage). Bilateral cerebral hemisphere damage produces several disturbances, including *pseudobulbar palsy.* This condition, best known for its emotional lability, results from damage to the *corticobulbar tract.* This is a UMN tract that innervates the brainstem motor nuclei and their nerves that supply the head and neck muscles (see Chapter 4). The corticobulbar tract is the cranial counterpart of the corticospinal tract, which innervates the spinal motor neurons and their nerves that supply the trunk and limb muscles.

Dementia also indicates that both cerebral hemispheres are damaged. Alzheimer's disease, multiple infarctions, alcohol-related damage, or other *diffuse* structural or metabolic injuries usually cause it (see Chapter 7). Because such CNS damage is usually extensive, dementia is associated with bilateral hyperactive DTRs, Babinski signs, and frontal lobe release reflexes, although not necessarily with hemiparesis or other

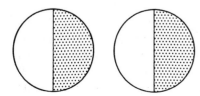

FIGURE 2–7. In homonymous hemianopsia, the same half of the visual field is lost in each eye. In this case, a right homonymous hemianopsia is attributable to damage to the left cerebral hemisphere.

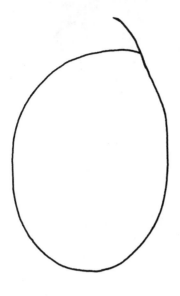

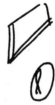

FIGURE 2–8. With constructional apraxia from a right parietal lobe infarction, a 68-year-old woman was hardly able to complete a circle *(top figure)*. She could not draw a square on request *(second highest figure)* or even copy one *(third highest figure)*. She spontaneously tried to draw a circle and began to retrace it *(bottom figure)*. Her constructional apraxia is seen in the rotation of the forms, perseveration of certain lines, and the incompleteness of the second and lowest figures. In addition, the figures tend toward the right-hand side of the page, which indicates that she is ignoring or has neglect of the left-hand side of the page.

lateralized findings. Whenever possible, a diagnosis of dementia should be buttressed by a description of physical abnormalities.

In general, in acute care hospitals the five conditions most likely to cause discrete unilateral or bilateral cerebral lesions are cerebral infarctions and other cerebrovascular accidents ("strokes"), primary or metastatic brain tumors, trauma, complications of acquired immune deficiency syndrome (AIDS), and multiple sclerosis (MS). (Section 2 offers detailed discussions of these conditions.)

SIGNS OF BASAL GANGLIA LESIONS

The basal ganglia, located subcortically in the cerebrum, are composed of the globus pallidus, the putamen, the substantia nigra, and the subthalamic nucleus (corpus of Luysii) (see Fig. 18–1). They give rise to the *extrapyramidal* tract, which modulates the corticospinal (pyramidal) tract. This tract controls muscle tone, regulates motor activity, and generates the postural reflexes through its efferent fibers that

TABLE 2–3. *Gait Abnormalities Associated with CNS Disorders*

Gait	Associated Illness	Figure
Apraxia	Normal pressure hydrocephalus	7–7
Astasia-abasia	Hysteria	3–3
Ataxia	Cerebellar damage	2–13
Festinating (*marche à petits pas*)	Parkinson's disease	18–9
Hemiparetic	Cerebrovascular accidents	
Circumduction		2–4
Spastic hemiparesis		13–3
Steppage	Tabes dorsalis (CNS syphilis)	2–18
	Peripheral neuropathies	

play on the cerebral cortex, thalamus, and other CNS structures. However, the extrapyramidal tract's efferent fibers are confined to the brain and do not act directly on the spinal cord or LMNs.

The characteristic feature of basal ganglia injury is a group of fascinating, often dramatic, *involuntary movement disorders* (see Chapter 18):

- *Parkinsonism* is the combination of resting tremor, rigidity, bradykinesia (slowness of movement) or akinesia (absence of movement), and postural abnormalities. Minor features include micrographia and festinating gait (Table 2–3). Parkinsonism is associated with damage to the substantia nigra from degeneration (Parkinson's disease), antipsychotic medications, or toxins.

- *Athetosis* is the slow, continuous, writhing movement of the fingers, hands, face, and throat. Kernicterus or other perinatal brain injury usually causes it.

- *Chorea* is intermittent jerking of limbs and trunk. The infamous hereditary condition, *Huntington's disease*, is associated with caudate nucleus atrophy.

- *Hemiballismus* is the intermittent flinging of the arm and leg on one side of the body. It is classically associated with small infarctions of the contralateral subthalamic nucleus, but similar lesions in other basal ganglia may be responsible.

In general, when damage is restricted to the extrapyramidal tract, as in many cases of hemiballismus and athetosis, patients have no paresis, DTR abnormalities, or Babinski signs—signs of corticospinal (pyramidal) tract damage. More important, in many of these cases, patients have no neuropsychologic abnormality. On the other hand, several involuntary movement disorders in which the cerebrum is affected are notoriously associated with dementia, depression, or psychosis. The most noteworthy are Huntington's disease, Wilson's disease, and advanced Parkinson's disease (see Table 18–4).

Unlike illnesses that affect the cerebrum, most basal ganglia diseases are slowly progressive, cause bilateral damage, and result from biochemical abnormalities rather than discrete structural lesions. When there is unilateral basal ganglia damage, the signs are found contralateral to the lesion. For example, hemiballismus results from infarction of the contralateral subthalamic nucleus, and unilateral parkinsonism ("hemiparkinsonism") results from degeneration of the contralateral substantia nigra.

SIGNS OF BRAINSTEM LESIONS

The brainstem contains the cranial nerve nuclei, the corticospinal tracts and other "long tracts" that travel between the cerebral hemispheres and the limbs, and several self-contained systems. Combinations of cranial nerve and long tract signs indicate the presence and location of a brainstem lesion. The localization should be supported by the *absence* of visual field cuts, neuropsychologic deficits, and other signs of cerebral injury. For example, brainstem injuries cause *diplopia* (double vision) because of cranial nerve impairment, but visual acuity and visual fields remain normal because the visual pathways, which pass from the optic chiasm to the cerebral hemispheres, do not travel within the brainstem (see Fig. 4–1). Similarly, a right hemiparesis associated with a left third cranial nerve palsy indicates that the lesion is in the brainstem and that aphasia will not be present.

Massive brainstem injuries, such as extensive infarctions or barbiturate overdoses, cause coma, but otherwise brainstem injuries do not impair mentation. Few illnesses simultaneously damage the brainstem and the cerebrum.

Several brainstem syndromes are important because they illustrate critical anatomic relationships, such as the location of the cranial nerve nuclei or the course of the corticospinal tract, but none of them involves neuropsychologic abnormalities. Although each syndrome has an eponym, for practical purposes it is only necessary to identify them as the result of a lesion in the brainstem or, if possible, in one of the *three divisions of the brainstem: midbrain, pons, or medulla* (Fig. 2–9). Most lesions are caused by an infarction in small branches of the basilar or vertebral arteries.

In the midbrain, where the oculomotor (third cranial) nerve passes through the descending corticospinal tract, both pathways can be damaged by a single small infarction. Patients with oculomotor nerve paralysis and contralateral hemiparesis typically have a midbrain lesion ipsilateral to the paretic eye (see Fig. 4–8).

Patients with abducens (sixth cranial) nerve paralysis and contralateral hemiparesis likewise have a pons lesion that is ipsilateral to the paretic eye (see Fig. 4–10).

Lateral medullary infarctions create a classic but complex picture. Patients have paralysis of the ipsilateral palate because of damage to cranial nerves IX through XI; ipsilateral facial hypalgesia because of damage to cranial nerve V, with contralateral anesthesia of the body *(alternating hypalgesia)* because of ascending spinothalamic tract damage; and ipsilateral ataxia because of ipsilateral cerebellar dysfunction. Fortunately, it is unnecessary to recall all the features of this syndrome: physicians primarily need to realize that those cranial nerve palsies and the alternating hypalgesia are characteristic of a lower brainstem (medullary) lesion (Fig. 2–10).

Although these particular brainstem syndromes are distinctive, the most frequently observed sign of brainstem dysfunction, which is nonspecific, is *nystagmus* (repetitive jerk-like eye movements). Resulting from any injury of the brainstem's large vestibular nuclei, nystagmus is usually a manifestation of one of the following disorders: intoxication with alcohol, phenytoin (Dilantin), or barbiturates; ischemia of the vertebrobasilar artery system; MS; Wernicke-Korsakoff syndrome; or viral labyrinthitis. It may also be associated with *internuclear ophthalmoplegia,* a disorder of ocular motility in which the brainstem's medial longitudinal fasciculus (MLF) is damaged by MS or an infarction (see Chapters 4 and 15).

SIGNS OF CEREBELLAR LESIONS

The cerebellum is composed of two hemispheres and a central portion, the *vermis.* Each hemisphere controls motor coordination of the ipsilateral limbs, and the vermis controls coordination of "midline structures," which are the head, neck, and trunk. The control of coordination of the limbs on the *same side of the body* gives the cerebellum a unique quality captured by the aphorism, "Everything in the brain, except for the cerebellum, is backward." Another unique feature of the cerebellum is

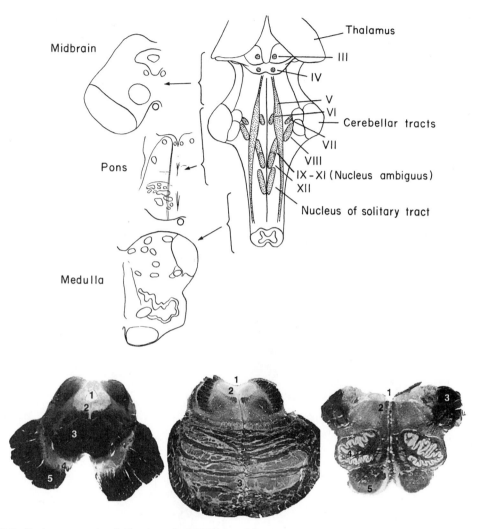

FIGURE 2–9. *Top,* In cross-section *(left)* and overview *(right),* the midbrain contains the nuclei of cranial nerves III and IV; the pons, nuclei V through VIII; and the medulla, nuclei IX through XII. The brainstem also contains the long tracts that pass from the cerebellum and cerebrum to the spinal cord. In addition, several other tracts, including the medial longitudinal fasciculus *(MLF)* and the reticular activating system, are contained and act solely within the brainstem. *Bottom, left,* A photograph of a myelin-stained midbrain, which has a distinctive outline, designates the (1) aqueduct of Sylvius, which is surrounded by the periaqueductal gray matter; (2) oculomotor nerve nucleus, and the termination of the medial longitudinal fasciculus *(MLF);* (3) red nucleus; (4) substantia nigra, which is unstained in this preparation; and (5) cerebral peduncle (crus cerebri), which is deeply stained, inferior to the substantia nigra, and contains the corticospinal tract. This photograph of the midbrain should be compared with a functional drawing (see Fig. 4–8), a computer-generated rendition (see Fig. 18–2), and a sketch (see Fig. 21–1). *Middle,* A photograph of the pons designates the (1) fourth ventricle, (2) abducens nerve nucleus, and (3) basis pontis or the "basilar portion of the pons," which contains the cerebellar outflow tract as well as the corticospinal tract. This photograph of the pons should be compared with a functional drawing (see Fig. 4–6) and an idealized sketch (see Fig. 21–2). *Right,* A photograph of the medulla designates the (1) fourth ventricle, (2) hypoglossal nerve nucleus, (3) inferior cerebellar peduncle (restiform body), (4) scallop-shaped inferior olivary nucleus, and (5) pyramid, which contains the corticospinal tract that is crossing. This photograph of the medulla should be compared with a functional drawing (see Fig. 2–10).

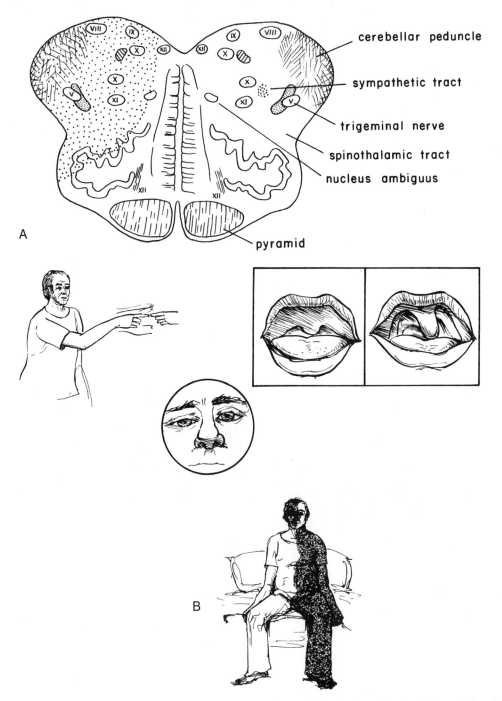

FIGURE 2–10. A, Whenever the posterior inferior cerebellar artery *(PICA)* is occluded, the lateral portion of the medulla suffers infarction. This infarction damages important structures: the cerebellar peduncle, the nucleus of the trigeminal nerve, the spinothalamic tract, the nucleus ambiguus (motor nuclei of cranial nerves IX to XI), and poorly delineated sympathetic fibers. Medial structures that escape damage are the corticospinal tract, hypoglossal nerve, and the medial longitudinal fasciculus *(MLF)*. The stippled area represents the lateral medulla, which suffers infarction when the right PICA or its parent artery, the vertebral artery, is occluded. **B,** This patient, who sustained an infarction of the right lateral medulla, has a right-sided Wallenberg syndrome. He has a right-sided Horner's syndrome (ptosis and miosis) because of damage to the sympathetic fibers (also see Fig. 12–15, *B*). He has right-sided ataxia because of damage to the ipsilateral cerebellar tracts. He has an alternating hypalgesia: diminished pain sensation on the *right* side of his face, accompanied by loss of pain sensation on the *left* trunk and extremities. Finally, he has hoarseness and paresis of the right soft palate because of damage to the right nucleus ambiguus: on voluntary phonation or in response to the gag reflex, the palate deviates upward toward his left because the right side of the palate is weak.

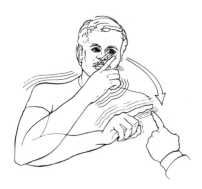

FIGURE 2–11. This young man, who has an MS plaque in the right cerebellar hemisphere, has an *intention tremor.* During repetitive *finger-to-nose* movements, as his finger approaches his own nose and then the examiner's finger, it develops a coarse and irregular path. The irregular rhythm is called *dysmetria.*

that when one hemisphere is damaged, the other will eventually be able to perform almost all the functions for both. Thus, although loss of one cerebellar hemisphere will cause incapacitating ipsilateral incoordination, the disability improves as the remaining hemisphere compensates almost in full.

Cerebellar lesions characteristically cause ipsilateral incoordination but not paresis or significant reflex abnormality. Moreover, with the cerebellum being isolated from the cerebral hemispheres, even its total destruction does not cause neuropsychologic deficits. A good example is the normal intellect of children who have undergone resection of a cerebellar hemisphere for removal of a cerebellar astrocytoma (see Chapter 19).

The characteristic sign of a cerebellar lesion is *intention tremor,* which is elicited during the finger-to-nose (Fig. 2–11) and heel-to-shin tests (Fig. 2–12). It is present when the patient moves willfully but absent when the patient rests. In a classic contrast, Parkinson's disease causes a *resting tremor* that is present when the patient is sitting quietly and is reduced or even abolished during movement (see Chapter 18).

Another sign of a cerebellar lesion is impaired ability to perform rapid alternating movements, *dysdiadochokinesia.* When asked to slap the palm and then the back of the hand rapidly and alternately on his or her own knee, for example, a patient with dysdiadochokinesia will use uneven force, move irregularly, and lose the alternating pattern.

Damage to either the entire cerebellum or the vermis alone causes incoordination of the trunk (i.e., *truncal ataxia*). It forces patients to place their feet widely apart when standing and produces a lurching, unsteady, and wide-based pattern of walking known as an *ataxic gait* (Table 2–3 and Fig. 2–13). This gait abnormality is dramatically apparent in the staggering and reeling of people who are intoxicated with alcohol.

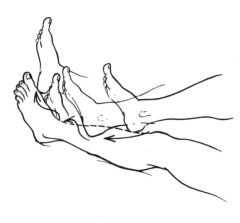

FIGURE 2–12. In the *heel-to-shin test,* the patient with the right-sided cerebellar lesion in Fig. 2–11 displays limb *ataxia* or *tremor on intention* as his right heel wobbles when he moves it along the crest of his left shin.

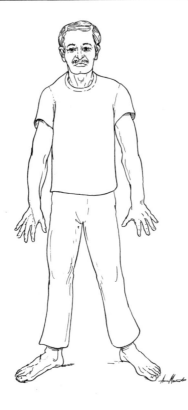

FIGURE 2–13. This man, a chronic alcoholic, has diffuse cerebellar degeneration. He has a typical *ataxic gait:* broad-based, unsteady, and uncoordinated. He stands with his feet pointed outward to widen and thus steady his stance.

With extensive cerebellar damage, poor modulation, irregular cadence, inability to separate adjacent sounds, and prolonged pauses between syllables impair voice production. This variety of speech disorder *(dysarthria)* is called *scanning speech*. Dysarthria—from cerebellar injury, bulbar and pseudobulbar palsy, and other CNS conditions—should be distinguishable from aphasia, which is a language disorder that includes writing problems (see Chapter 8). (The nomenclature of dysdiadochokinesia, dysarthria, and dysmetria suggests that cerebellar disease gives rise to the *"dys"* words, from Greek for *bad* or *difficult*.) Finally, a subtle sign of cerebellar disease is that muscle tone is hypotonic and DTRs are pendular.

The illnesses that are responsible for most *cerebral* lesions—strokes, tumors, trauma, AIDS, and MS—also cause most *cerebellar* lesions. The cerebellum also seems particularly vulnerable to toxins and deficiencies. In an almost unique situation, alcoholism or taking certain medications, such as phenytoin, leads primarily or exclusively to damage to the vermis. In the infamous Wernicke-Korsakoff syndrome, poor nutrition, which is usually but not necessarily related to alcoholism, leads to cognitive impairment characterized by memory loss (amnesia), as well as ataxia and nystagmus. (Any patient even suspected of having Wernicke-Korsakoff syndrome should immediately receive thiamine 50 mg intravenously to prevent serious brain injury.) Deficiency of vitamin E, a fat-soluble antioxidant, which may result from a genetic disorder, also leads to cerebellar dysfunction.

Cerebellar injury also results from a group of progressive neurodegenerative disorders that are inherited in an autosomal dominant fashion. Because these disorders also typically involve the spinal cord, they have been referred to as the *spinocerebellar degenerations*. Their hallmark is an ataxic gait often accompanied by other signs of cerebellar degeneration, such as progressively severe incoordination of their limbs and scanning speech. Depending on the particular spinocerebellar degeneration, patients may also have signs that other systems are degenerating, such as grossly impaired sensation, spasticity, and ocular motility problems. However, despite widespread CNS dysfunction, spinocerebellar degenerations do not cause dementia.

With use of a genetic classification, the disparate spinocerebellar degenerations have been consolidated into several relatively well-established and clinical homogeneous *types* of *spinocerebellar ataxia (SCA)*. The SCAs result from expansions of a trinucleotide repeat sequence (see Chapter 6), each in a different chromosome (Appendix 3D).

Cerebellar dysfunction has been suspected in autism because some magnetic resonance imaging and autopsy studies have detected cerebellar hemisphere hypoplasia and a reduction of more than 50% in one of its characteristic elements, the Purkinje cells. However, most abnormalities are inconsistent, do not correlate with the clinical findings, and are found in other conditions. In addition, children who have undergone removal of a cerebellar hemisphere do not manifest significant serious neuropsychologic deficits.

SIGNS OF SPINAL CORD LESIONS

At the spinal cord's center is a broad H-shaped, gray matter structure composed largely of neurons that transmit nerve impulses in a horizontal plane. White matter, composed of myelinated tracts conveying information in a vertical direction, surrounds the gray matter (Fig. 2–14). Because most signs of spinal cord injury are due to interruption of the myelinated tracts, spinal cord injury is often called "myelopathy." The arrangement of the spinal cord anatomy—gray matter on the inside with white outside—is the opposite of that of the cerebrum.

The major descending pathway is the *lateral corticospinal tract.*

The major ascending pathways, which are virtually all sensory, include the following:

- *Posterior columns,* which carry position and vibration sensations to the thalamus

- *Lateral spinothalamic tracts,* which carry temperature and pain sensations to the thalamus

- *Anterior spinothalamic tracts,* which carry light touch sensation to the thalamus

- *Spinocerebellar tracts,* which carry joint position and movement sensations to the cerebellum.

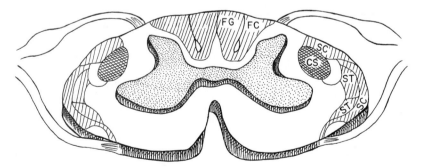

FIGURE 2–14. In this drawing of the spinal cord, the centrally located gray matter is stippled. The surrounding white matter contains myelin-coated tracts that ascend and descend within the spinal cord. Clinically important ascending tracts are the spinocerebellar tracts *(SC)*, the lateral spinothalamic tract *(ST)*, and the posterior column (fasciculus cuneatus *[FC]*, from the upper limbs, and fasciculus gracilis *[FG]*, from the lower limbs). The most important descending tract is the lateral corticospinal *(CS)* tract.

Discrete Injuries

The site of a spinal cord injury—cervical, thoracic, or lumbosacral—determines the nature of the motor and sensory deficits. A cervical spinal cord injury causes the loss of motor function and sensation below the neck. The arms and legs will have paralysis *(quadriparesis)* and, after 1 to 2 weeks, spasticity, hyperactive DTRs, and Babinski signs. In addition, limb and trunk sensations will be interrupted. Similarly, a midthoracic spinal cord injury will lead to leg paralysis *(paraparesis)*, reflex changes, and sensory loss of the legs and trunk below the nipples (Fig. 2–15). In general, spinal cord injuries disrupt bladder control and sexual function, which rely on delicate and intricate systems (see Chapter 16).

Even with devastating spinal cord injury, however, cerebral function is preserved. In an admittedly tragic example, patients with a penetrating gunshot wound of the cervical spinal cord, although quadriplegic, retain intellectual, visual, and verbal facilities. Patients surviving spinal cord injuries are often beset with depression from isolation, lack of social support, and physical impairment. They have a high divorce rate. Their suicide rate is about five times greater than the general population's. In addition, several patients with quadriplegia have requested withdrawal of life support not only immediately after the injury, when their plans may be attributed to depression, but also several years later when they are clearheaded and not overtly depressed.

Of the various spinal cord lesions, the most instructive is the *Brown-Séquard syndrome*. This classic disturbance results from an injury that transects the lateral half of the spinal cord (Fig. 2–16). It is characterized by corticospinal tract damage that causes paralysis of the ipsilateral limb(s) and by lateral spinothalamic tract damage that causes pain loss *(hypalgesia)* in the contralateral limb(s). Simply put, one leg is weak and the other is numb.

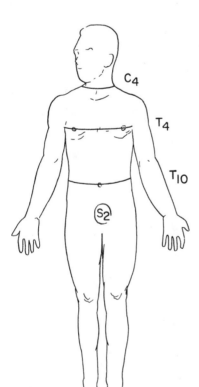

FIGURE 2–15. In a patient with a spinal cord injury, the "level" of hypalgesia will indicate the site of the damage: C4 injuries cause hypalgesia below the neck; T4 injuries, hypalgesia below the nipples; T10 injuries, hypalgesia below the umbilicus.

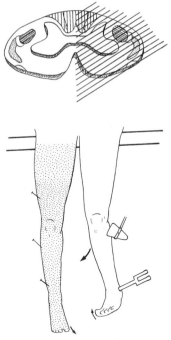

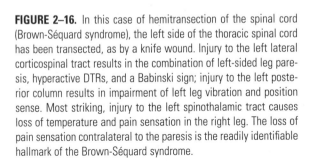

FIGURE 2–16. In this case of hemitransection of the spinal cord (Brown-Séquard syndrome), the left side of the thoracic spinal cord has been transected, as by a knife wound. Injury to the left lateral corticospinal tract results in the combination of left-sided leg paresis, hyperactive DTRs, and a Babinski sign; injury to the left posterior column results in impairment of left leg vibration and position sense. Most striking, injury to the left spinothalamic tract causes loss of temperature and pain sensation in the right leg. The loss of pain sensation contralateral to the paresis is the readily identifiable hallmark of the Brown-Séquard syndrome.

The cervical region of the spinal cord is particularly susceptible to common nonpenetrating trauma because in most accidents hyperextension of the neck crushes the cervical vertebrae. Approximately 50% of civilian spinal cord injuries result from motor vehicle crashes, 20% from falls, 15% from gunshot wounds and other violence, and 15% from sports injuries, mostly diving accidents. The other dangerous sports are football, skiing, surfing, trampoline work, and horseback riding. Hanging by the

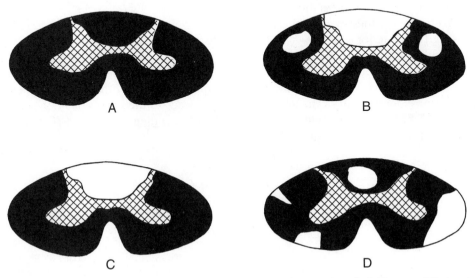

FIGURE 2–17. **A,** A standard spinal cord histologic preparation stains normal myelin (white matter) black and leaves the central H-shaped column gray. **B,** In combined system disease (vitamin B_{12} deficiency), posterior column and corticospinal tract damage causes their demyelination and lack of stain. **C,** In tabes dorsalis (syphilis), damage to the posterior column leaves them unstained. **D,** MS, however, leads to asymmetric, irregular, demyelinated plaques.

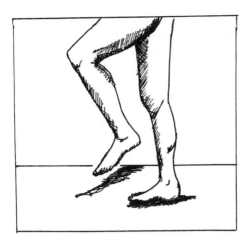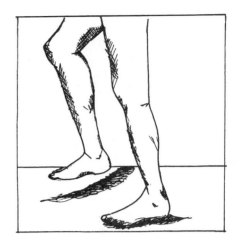

FIGURE 2–18. The steppage gait consists of each knee being excessively raised when walking to compensate for a loss of position sense. This maneuver elevates the feet to ensure that they will clear the ground, stairs, and other obstacles. It is a classic sign of posterior column spinal cord damage from tabes dorsalis; however, peripheral neuropathies more commonly impair position sense and cause this gait impairment.

neck fractures or dislocates cervical vertebrae, which crushes the cervical spinal cord and cuts off the air supply. Survivors are likely to be quadriplegic as well as brain damaged.

Neurologic Illnesses

MS, which is the most common disabling neurologic illness of North American and Northern European young and middle-aged adults, typically causes myelopathy alone or in combination with cerebellar, optic nerve, or brainstem damage (see Chapter 15). Tumors of the lung, breast, and other organs that spread to the vertebral bodies often compress the spinal cord.

With several illnesses, only specific tracts of the spinal cord may be affected (Fig. 2–17). The posterior columns—*fasciculus gracilis* and *f. cuneatus*—seem to be particularly vulnerable. For example, in tabes dorsalis (syphilis), combined system disease (B_{12} deficiency, see Chapter 5), and the SCAs and their variant, Friedreich's ataxia, the posterior columns are damaged alone or in combination with other tracts. In these conditions, impairment of the posterior columns leads to the loss of position sense that prohibits affected people from standing erect with their eyes closed *(Romberg's sign)* and produces a *steppage gait* (Fig. 2–18).

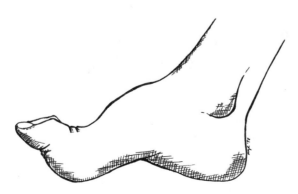

FIGURE 2–19. The *pes cavus* foot deformity consists of a high arch, elevation of the dorsum, and retraction of the first metatarsal. When it occurs in families with ataxia and posterior column sensory deficits that begin in late childhood, pes cavus is virtually pathognomonic of Friedreich's ataxia.

Friedreich's ataxia represents an interesting contrast to the SCAs. Like them, it is a progressive neurodegenerative disorder that causes ataxia, loss of posterior column sensation, and usually no cognitive impairment. Although both the SCAs and Friedreich's ataxia result from excessive trinucleotide repeats, Friedreich's ataxia is inherited as an autosomal *recessive* disorder (see Appendix 3D). Another distinction is that patients with Friedreich's ataxia often have prominent nonneurologic manifestations, including cardiomyopathy and the classic *pes cavus* foot deformity (Fig. 2–19).

Most importantly, in several illnesses myelopathy is associated with dementia because of concomitant cerebral damage. Examples of this association are tabes dorsalis, combined system disease, AIDS, and MS, when it is disseminated throughout the entire CNS.

3

Psychogenic Neurologic Deficits

Classic studies of hysteria, conversion reactions, and related conditions included patients who had only rudimentary physical examinations and minimal, if any, laboratory testing. Studies that re-evaluated the same patients after many years reported that as many as 20% of them eventually had specific neurologic conditions, such as movement disorders, multiple sclerosis (MS), or seizures, that probably had been responsible for the original symptoms. In addition, some patients had systemic illnesses such as anemia or congestive heart failure that could have at least contributed to their symptoms. Another interesting aspect of these studies is that many illnesses assumed to be entirely "psychogenic" in the first two-thirds of the twentieth century are now acknowledged to be "neurologic," such as Tourette's syndrome, writer's cramp, and other focal dystonias, migraines, and trigeminal neuralgia.

Although today's physicians still fail to reach 100% accuracy in diagnosis, they readily and skillfully diagnose psychogenic deficits. Their greater accuracy does not mean that they are inherently more astute than their classic counterparts. Rather, they usually have been trained in a formal program; subsequently have been given continual education through journals, conferences, and teaching videotapes; and have had to apply specific, relatively strict diagnostic criteria. When uncertain, they have colleagues readily available to provide second opinions. Moreover, they commonly have at their disposal an arsenal of high-tech testing facilities, including computed tomography (CT), magnetic resonance imaging (MRI), and closed circuit television (CCTV) monitoring.

THE NEUROLOGISTS' ROLE

Nevertheless, even in the face of flagrant psychogenic signs, neurologists have the burden of confirming the absence of neurologic disease. They generally test for most neurologic conditions that could explain symptoms, particularly for those that would be serious or life threatening. In addition, although the course of the illness regularly proves to be the best test to determine its origin, neurologists tend to request extensive testing or investigations during the initial evaluation to obtain objective evidence of disease or its absence.

Neurologists typically disregard specific psychiatric diagnoses, such as somatization disorder and conversion disorder (somatoform disorders), in which patients have "pseudoneurologic" symptoms. They also disregard the distinction between somatoform disorders, which are not under voluntary control, and factitious disorders and malingering, which are under voluntary control. In addition, neurologists typically include gross exaggerations of a neurologic deficit, *embellishment*, as psychogenic. For various reasons, they merge all these psychiatric diagnoses into the category "psychogenic disturbance."

Within the context of this potentially oversimplified designation, neurologists routinely and reliably diagnose psychogenic seizures (see Chapter 10), diplopia and other visual problems (see Chapter 12), and tremors and other movement disorders (see Chapter 18). In addition, they acknowledge the psychogenic aspects of pain (see Chapter 14), sexual dysfunction (see Chapter 16), and posttraumatic headaches and whiplash injuries (see Chapter 22). They realize that unrecognized mental illnesses, such as somatization disorders, often form the basis of chronic medical disabilities.

In dealing with patients who have been shown to have a psychogenic disturbance, neurologists usually offer reassurances, strong suggestions that the deficits will resolve by a certain date, and a referral for psychiatric consultation. Sometimes they allow patients acceptable exits by prescribing placebos or nonspecific treatment, such as physical therapy. They avoid ordering invasive diagnostic procedures, surgery, and medications, especially habit-forming or otherwise potentially dangerous ones.

Patients often have mixtures of neurologic and psychogenic deficits, disproportionate posttraumatic disabilities, and minor neurologic illnesses that preoccupy them. As long as serious, progressive physical illness has been excluded, physicians can consider some symptoms to be chronic illnesses. For example, chronic low back pain can be treated as a "pain syndrome" with empiric combinations of antidepressant medications, analgesics, rehabilitation, and psychotherapy, without expecting either to cure the pain or determine its exact cause (see Chapter 14).

PSYCHOGENIC SIGNS

What clues prompt a neurologist to suspect a psychogenic disturbance? When a deficit violates the *laws of neuroanatomy*, neurologists almost always deduce that it has a psychogenic origin. For example, if temperature sensation is preserved but pain perception is "lost," the deficit is *nonanatomic* and therefore likely to be psychogenic. Likewise, tunnel vision, which clearly violates these laws, is a classic psychogenic disturbance (see Fig. 12–8).

Also, when a deficit changes, neurologists conclude that it is likely to be psychogenic. For example, someone with psychogenic paralysis might either walk when unaware of being observed or walk despite seeming to have paraplegia while in bed. Another noted example occurs when someone with a psychogenic seizure momentarily "awakens" and stops convulsive activity but resumes it when assured of being observed. The psychogenic nature of a deficit can be confirmed if it is reversed during an interview under hypnosis or barbiturate infusion.

Motor Signs

One indication of psychogenic weakness is a nonanatomic distribution, such as loss of vision in one eye, hearing in one ear, and strength in the arm and leg—all on the same side of the body. Another indication is the absence of functional impairment despite claims of profound weakness.

Intermittent paresis is evident in a "give-way" effort, in which the patient has a brief (several seconds) exertion before returning to an apparent paretic position. Intermittent paresis is also demonstrable by use of the *face-hand test*, in which the patient momentarily exerts sufficient strength to deflect a falling hand from hitting the face (Fig. 3–1).

An indication of unilateral psychogenic leg weakness is *Hoover's sign* (Fig. 3–2). Normally, when someone attempts to raise a genuinely paretic leg, the other leg

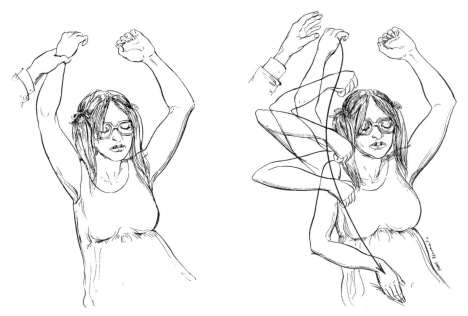

FIGURE 3–1. In the face-hand test, a young woman with psychogenic right hemiparesis inadvertently demonstrates her preserved strength by deflecting her falling "paretic" arm from striking her face as it is dropped by the examiner.

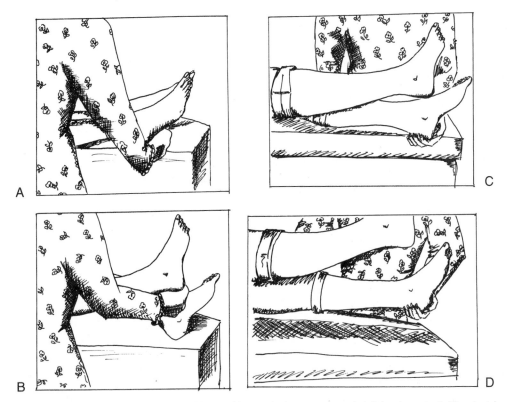

FIGURE 3–2. Hoover's sign is demonstrated in a 23-year-old man who has a psychogenic left hemiparesis. **A,** The physician asks him to raise his left leg as she holds her hand under his right heel. **B,** Revealing his lack of effort, the patient exerts so little downward force with his right leg that she easily raises it. **C,** When she asks him to raise his right leg while cupping his left heel, the patient reveals his intact strength as he unconsciously forces his left, "paretic" leg downward—the Hoover sign. **D,** As if to carry the example to the extreme, the patient forces his left leg downward with enough force to allow her to use his left leg as a lever to raise his lower torso.

presses down. The examiner can feel the downward force at the patient's normal heel and can use the straightened leg, as a lever, to raise the entire leg and lower body. In contrast, Hoover's sign consists of the patient unconsciously pressing down with a "paretic" leg when attempting to raise the unaffected leg and failing to press down with the unaffected leg when attempting to raise the "paretic" leg.

A similar test involves adduction of the legs (bringing the legs together). Normally, when asked to adduct their legs, people squeeze both knees together. Someone with psychogenic weakness who is asked to adduct both legs against resistance might unconsciously adduct the "paretic" leg or fail to adduct the normal leg.

Gait Impairment

Many psychogenic gait impairments closely mimic neurologic disturbances, such as tremors in the legs, ataxia, or weakness of one or both legs. The most readily identifiable and psychogenic gait impairment is *astasia-abasia*. In this disturbance, patients stagger, balance momentarily, and appear to be in great danger of falling; however, by grabbing hold of railings, furniture, and even the examiner, they never actually injury themselves (Fig. 3–3).

Another blatant psychogenic gait impairment occurs when patients drag a "weak" leg, as though it were a totally lifeless object apart from their body. In contrast, patients with a true hemiparetic gait (as previously discussed [see Fig. 2–4]), swing their leg outward with a circular motion (i.e., "circumduct" their leg).

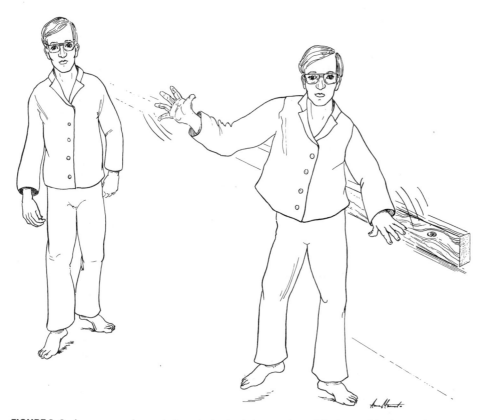

FIGURE 3–3. A young man demonstrates astasia-abasia by seeming to fall when walking but catching himself by balancing carefully. He even staggers the width of the room to grasp the rail. He sometimes grasps physicians and pulls them toward himself and then drags them toward the ground. While dramatizing his purported impairment, he actually displays good strength, balance, and coordination.

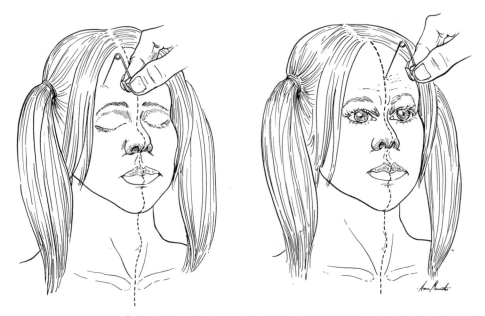

FIGURE 3–4. A young woman with psychogenic right hemisensory loss appears not to feel a pinprick until the pin reaches the midline of her forehead, face, neck, or sternum (i.e., she splits the midline). When the pin is moved across the midline, she appears to feel a sharp stick. (The pin in this sketch is used for teaching purposes only.)

Sensory Deficits

Although the sensory examination is the least reliable portion of the neurologic examination, several sensory abnormalities indicate a psychogenic basis. For example, loss of sensation to pinprick* that stops abruptly at the middle of the face and body is the classic *splitting the midline*. This finding suggests a psychogenic loss because the sensory nerve fibers of the skin normally spread across the midline (Fig. 3–4). Likewise, because vibrations naturally spread across bony structures, loss of vibration sensation over half the forehead, jaw, sternum, or spine strongly suggests a psychogenic disturbance.

A similar abnormality is loss of sensation of the entire face but not the scalp. This pattern is inconsistent with the anatomic distribution of the trigeminal nerve, which innervates the face and scalp anterior to the vertex but not the angle of the jaw (see Fig. 4–11).

A psychogenic sensory loss, as already mentioned, can be a discrepancy between pain and temperature sensations, which are normally carried together by the peripheral nerves and then the lateral spinothalamic tracts. (Discrepancy between pain and *position* sensations in the fingers, in contrast, is indicative of syringomyelia: in this condition the central fibers of the spinal cord, which carry pain sensation, are ripped apart by the expanding central canal.) A maneuver designed to expose a psychogenic sensory loss in the limbs is testing for sensory loss when the arms are twisted, placed out of sight behind the patient's back, or seen in a mirror.

Finally, because sensory loss impairs function, patients with genuine sensory loss in their feet or hands cannot perform many tasks if their eyes are closed. In contrast

---

*Neurologists now use pins cautiously, if at all, to avoid blood-borne infections. Testing for pain is performed with nonpenetrating, disposable instruments, such as cotton sticks.

to this expectation, patients with psychogenic sensory loss, with their eyes closed, can still generally button their shirts, walk short distances, and stand with their feet together and their eyes closed. People with a true sensory loss in both feet who keep their eyes closed when standing erect tend to fall (i.e., they have *Romberg's sign*). Similarly, people with injury of the posterior columns of their spinal cord, usually from tabes dorsalis, MS, or vitamin B_{12} deficiency, have Romberg's sign (see Chapter 2).

Special Senses

Blindness, tunnel vision, and diplopia are also commonly diagnosed as psychogenic disturbances when they violate the laws of neuroanatomy. In this case, the laws stem in large part from the standard laws of optics. Psychogenic and neurologic visual disorders may thus be readily separated (see Chapter 12).

A patient with psychogenic deafness usually responds to unexpected noises or words. Unilateral hearing loss in the ear ipsilateral to a hemiparesis is highly suggestive of a psychogenic etiology because extensive auditory tract synapses in the pons ensure that some tracts reach the upper brainstem and cerebrum despite central nervous system lesions (see Fig. 4–15). If doubts about hearing loss remain, audiometry, brainstem auditory-evoked responses, and other technical procedures can be performed.

Patients can genuinely lose the sense of smell (anosmia) from a head injury (see Chapter 22) or advanced age; however, these patients can usually perceive noxious volatile substances, such as ammonia or alcohol, because these chemicals irritate the nasal mucosa endings of the trigeminal nerve rather than the olfactory nerve. This distinction is usually unknown to individuals with psychogenic anosmia, who typically claim not to be able to smell any substance.

Miscellaneous Conditions

A distinct but common psychogenic disturbance, the *hyperventilation syndrome,* occurs in people with an underlying anxiety disorder, including panic disorder. It leads to lightheadedness and paresthesias around the mouth, fingers, and toes, and, in severe cases, to *carpopedal spasm* (Fig. 3–5). Although the disorder seems distinctive, physicians should be cautious before diagnosing it because partial complex seizures and transient ischemic attacks (TIAs) produce similar symptoms.

In this syndrome, hyperventilation first causes a fall in carbon dioxide tension that leads to respiratory alkalosis. The rise in blood pH from the alkalosis produces hypocalcemia, which produces the tetany of muscles and paresthesias. To demonstrate to the patient that the symptoms are from hyperventilation, physicians might re-create them by having a patient hyperventilate. This procedure may induce giddiness, anxiety, or confusion. If so, the physician should abort it by having the patient continually rebreathe expired air from a paper bag cupped around the mouth.

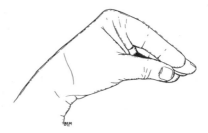

FIGURE 3–5. Carpopedal spasm, which is the characteristic neurologic manifestation of hyperventilation, consists of flexion of the wrist and proximal thumb and finger joints. Also, although the thumb and fingers remain extended, they are drawn together and tend to overlap.

POTENTIAL PITFALLS

The neurologic examination of a patient suspected of having a psychogenic deficit requires particular sensitivity. It can be undertaken in conjunction with a psychiatric evaluation, need not follow the conventional format, and can be completed in two or more sessions. A threatening, embarrassing, or otherwise inept evaluation might obscure the diagnosis, harden the patient's resolve, or precipitate a catastrophic reaction.

Despite their general usefulness, guidelines are fallible. Patients may display psychogenic signs because of pain, fatigue, or desire to please the examiner or to exaggerate a neurologic deficit. Change or lack of change in affect and similar indications of a deficit being psychogenic are unreliable. In particular, one famous psychiatric sign, *la belle indifférence,* is found in hemi-inattention, Anton's syndrome, frontal lobe injury, MS, and other neurologic problems.

Although the neurologic examination itself seems rational and reliable, it contains many potentially misleading findings. For example, many anxious or "ticklish" individuals, with or without psychogenic hemiparesis, have brisk deep tendon reflexes and extensor plantar reflexes—as they would with cerebral or spinal cord damage. Another potentially misleading finding is a right hemiparesis unaccompanied by aphasia. In fact, a stroke might cause this situation if the patient were left-handed, or if the stroke were small and located in the internal capsule or upper brainstem (i.e., a subcortical motor stroke).

Neurologists tend to misdiagnose several types of disorders as psychogenic when they are unique or bizarre or when their severity is greater than expected. This error may simply reflect an individual neurologist's lack of experience. Neurologists also misdiagnose disorders as psychogenic when a patient has no accompanying objective physical abnormalities. This determination might be faulty in illnesses where objective signs are often transient or subtle, such as in MS, partial complex seizures, and small strokes. With an incomplete history, neurologists may not appreciate transient neurologic conditions, such as transient hemiparesis induced by migraines, postictal paresis, or TIAs and transient mental status aberrations induced by alcohol, medications, seizures, or other conditions (see Table 9–4).

Another potential pitfall is dismissing an entire case because a patient is grossly exaggerating a deficit. Patients may be seeking attention for a problem by overstating or overreacting to it. In addition, the prospect of having developed a neurologic disorder may trigger overwhelming anxiety.

Possibly the single most common error is failure to recognize MS because its early signs may be evanescent, exclusively sensory, or so disparate as to appear to violate *several* laws of neuroanatomy. The correct diagnosis can now usually be made early and reliably with MRIs, visual evoked response testing, and cerebrospinal fluid analysis (see Chapter 15). On the other hand, trivial sensory or motor symptoms that are accompanied by normal variations in these highly sensitive tests might lead to some false-positive diagnoses of MS.

Neurologists are also prone to err in diagnosing involuntary movement disorders as psychogenic. These disorders, in fact, have some stigmata of psychogenic illness (see Chapter 18): they can be bizarre, precipitated or exacerbated by anxiety, or apparently relieved by tricks, such as when a dystonic gait can be alleviated by walking backward. Also, involuntary movements will usually be reduced or even abolished during an interview under a barbiturate. Because laboratory tests are not available for many disorders—chorea, tics, tremors, and focal and generalized dystonia—the diagnosis rests on the neurologist's clinical evaluation. As a general rule, movement disorders should first be considered neurologic (see Chapter 18).

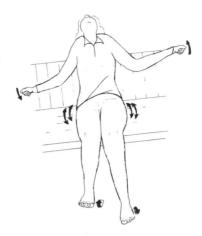

FIGURE 3–6. This young woman, who is screaming during an entire 30-second episode, is having a psychogenic seizure. Its nonneurologic nature is revealed in several typical features. In addition to verbalizing throughout the episode rather than only at its onset (as in an epileptic cry), she maintains her body tone, which is required to keep her sitting upright. She has alternating flailing limb movements rather than organized bilateral clonic jerks. She has subtle but suggestive pelvic thrusting. After psychogenic seizures patients are fully alert, oriented, and able to recall events immediately preceding and possibly during the episode, rather than being lethargic, dull, and amnestic.

Epileptic and psychogenic seizures are often misdiagnosed in both directions (see Chapter 10). In general, psychogenic seizures are clonic and unaccompanied by incontinence, tongue biting, or loss of body tone (Fig. 3–6). Immediately afterward, patients regain awareness and have no retrograde amnesia. However, numerous exceptions exist. Frontal lobe seizures and mixtures of epileptic and psychogenic seizures notoriously mimic psychogenic seizures. CCTV monitoring of episodes and any associated electroencephalographic changes has become the standard diagnostic test.

In the past, individuals with changes in their mental status have often been misdiagnosed—often by default—as having a psychogenic disturbance. Some of them were eventually found to be harboring meningiomas or other tumors in the frontal lobe. These tumors notoriously escape early detection because they can produce affective or thought disorders without accompanying physical defects. Now, with the ready availability of CT and MRI, physicians rarely overlook any tumor.

REFERENCES

Baker GA, Hanley JR, Jackson HF, et al: Detecting the faking of amnesia: Performance differences between simulators and patients with memory impairments. J Clin Exp Neuropsychol 15: 668–684, 1993

Baker JHE, Silver JR: Hysterical paraplegia. J Neurol Neurosurg Psychiatry 50: 375–382, 1987

Caplan LR, Nadelson T: Multiple sclerosis and hysteria: Lessons learned from their association. JAMA 243: 2418–2421, 1980

Feldman MD, Eisendrath SJ: *The spectrum of factitious disorders.* Washington, D.C., American Psychiatric Press, 1996

Fishbain DA, Goldberg M: The misdiagnosis of conversion disorder in a psychiatric emergency service. Gen Hosp Psychiatry 13: 177–181, 1991

Glatt SL, Kennedy D, Barter R, et al: Conversion hysteria: A study of prognosis with long-term follow-up. Neurology 41 (Suppl 1): 120, 1991

Hayes MW, Graham S, Heldorf P, et al: A video review of the diagnosis of psychogenic gait. Move Disord 14: 914–921, 1999

Hurst LC: What was wrong with Anna O? J R Soc Med 75: 129–131, 1982

Mace CJ, Trimble MR: Ten-year prognosis of conversion disorder. Br J Psychiatry 169: 282–288, 1996

Maloney MJ: Diagnosing hysterical conversion reactions in children. J Pediatr 97: 1016–1020, 1980

Matas M: Psychogenic voice disorders. Can J Psychiatry 36: 363–365, 1991

Reich P, Gottfried LA: Factitious disorders in a teaching hospital. Ann Intern Med 99: 240–247, 1983

Richtsmeier AJ: Pitfalls in diagnosis of unexplained symptoms. Psychosomatics 25: 253–255, 1984

Therapeutics and Technology Assessment Subcommittee, American Academy of Neurology: Assessment: Neuropsychological testing of adults. Neurology 47: 592–599, 1996

Wolf M, Birger M, Ben Shoshan J, et al: Conversion deafness. Ann Otol Rhinol Laryngol 102: 349–352, 1993

4

Cranial Nerve Impairments

Individually, in pairs, or in groups, the cranial nerves are vulnerable to numerous conditions. Moreover, when a nerve seems to be impaired, the problem might not be damage to the cranial nerve itself but rather an underlying cerebral injury or psychogenic disturbance. Following custom, this chapter uses the 12 cranial nerves' Roman numeral designations that can be recalled with the old mnemonic device, "On old Olympus' towering top, a Finn and German viewed some hops."

I	Olfactory	VII	Facial
II	Optic	VIII	Acoustic
III	Oculomotor	IX	Glossopharyngeal
IV	Trochlear	X	Vagus
V	Trigeminal	XI	Spinal accessory
VI	Abducens	XII	Hypoglossal

OLFACTORY (FIRST)

Olfactory nerves transmit the sensation of smell to the brain. From sensory receptors within each nasal cavity, branches of the pair of olfactory nerves pass upward through the multiple holes in the cribriform plate of the skull to several areas of the brain. They terminate mostly on the undersurface of the frontal cortex, which is the home of the olfactory sensory areas, but some terminate more deeply in the hypothalamus and amygdala, the cornerstones of the limbic system (see Fig. 16–5). The olfactory nerves' input into the limbic system, at least in part, accounts for the influence of smell on psychosexual behavior and memory.

When both olfactory nerves are impaired, patients, who are then said to have *anosmia*, cannot perceive smells or appreciate the aroma of food. Sometimes anosmia has life-threatening consequences, as when people cannot smell escaping gas. More commonly, food without a perceptible aroma is virtually tasteless. Thus, people with anosmia, to whom food is completely bland, tend to have a decreased appetite.

To test the olfactory nerve, the patient is asked to identify certain substances by smelling through one nostril while the examiner compresses the other nostril. Testing must be done with readily identifiable and odoriferous but innocuous substances, such as coffee. A set of "scratch and sniff" odors has been manufactured for detailed testing. Volatile and irritative substances, such as ammonia and alcohol, are not suitable because they may trigger intranasal trigeminal nerve receptors and bypass a (possibly damaged) olfactory nerve.

Unilateral anosmia may result from tumors adjacent to the olfactory nerve, such as olfactory groove meningiomas (see Fig. 20–5). In the classic Foster-Kennedy syndrome, anosmia is associated with optic atrophy when these tumors compress the nearby optic nerve as well as the olfactory nerve. If the tumors grow into the frontal lobe, personality changes, dementia, seizures, or hemiparesis accompanies anosmia.

Anosmia may of course be psychogenic. A psychogenic origin can be revealed when a patient is apparently equally unable to "smell" either irritative or innocuous aromatic substances. Such a complete sensory loss would be possible only if both trigeminal and both olfactory nerves were obliterated.

Olfactory hallucinations may be a manifestation of partial complex seizures that originate in the medial-inferior surface of the temporal lobe, the *uncus*. Formerly called "uncinate fits" that began with an unpleasant smell, these seizures consist of episodes lasting only several seconds in which ill-defined, but often sweet or otherwise pleasant smells are superimposed on impaired consciousness and behavioral disturbances (see Chapter 10).

Also, olfactory hallucinations can be purely psychogenic. In contrast to smells induced by uncinate seizures, psychogenic "odors" are almost always foul smelling, continuous, and not associated with impaired consciousness.

Although these neurologic and psychogenic disturbances may be tantalizing, most disturbances of smell are mundane. Some individuals have a genetically based anosmia to one of several hundred perceptible smells. In older people, normal age-related neuronal degeneration causes anosmia: more than 50% of individuals older than 65 years and 75% of those older than 80 years have an impaired sense of smell. In Alzheimer's disease, patients have a high incidence of anosmia, which is thought to be another manifestation of neurodegeneration.

Anosmia is also found in anyone with nasal congestion. In addition, because the olfactory nerve can be sheared off as it passes through the cribriform plate, even minor head trauma from almost any direction can cause anosmia (see Head Trauma, Chapter 22). Similarly, most abnormal smells, which are characteristically putrid, originate in sinusitis and other head and neck infections.

OPTIC (SECOND)

The optic nerves and their tracts have two main functions in transmitting light. They convey visual information from the eye to the cerebral cortex and light intensity status from the eye to the brainstem. The optic nerves and a small portion of the acoustic nerve, unlike other cranial nerves, are actual myelin-coated projections of the brain, which makes them part of the central nervous system (CNS). Thus, the optic nerves are susceptible to CNS illnesses, particularly childhood-onset metabolic storage diseases, migraines (see Chapter 9), and multiple sclerosis–induced optic neuritis (see Chapter 15).

The optic *nerves'* receptors are in the retinas. At the optic chiasm, their nasal fibers cross while the temporal fibers continue uncrossed (Fig. 4–1). Temporal fibers of one eye join nasal fibers of the other to form the optic *tracts*. The tracts pass through the temporal and parietal lobes to terminate in the calcarine cortex of the occipital lobe. Thus, each occipital lobe receives visual information from the contralateral visual field.

In their other function, the optic nerves and tracts form the afferent limb of the *light reflex* by sending small branches containing information about light intensity to the midbrain. After a single synapse, the oculomotor nerves (the third cranial nerves) form the efferent limb. The light reflex adjusts pupil size to the brightness of light that strikes the retina. This reflex constricts the pupils in response to increased light. A similar mechanism, the *accommodation reflex*, constricts the pupils when gaze is moved from a distant to a close object.

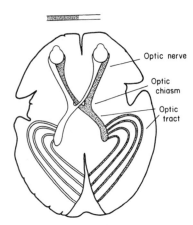

FIGURE 4–1. The optic nerves extend from the retinas to the optic chiasm, where they divide to form the optic tracts. The primary effect of this system is that the impulses from each visual field are brought to the cortex of the contralateral occipital lobe.

Routine testing of the optic nerve includes examination of (1) visual acuity (see Fig. 12–2), (2) visual fields (Fig. 4–2), and (3) the ocular fundi (Fig. 4–3). Because the visual system is important, complex, and subject to numerous ocular, neurologic, iatrogenic, and psychogenic disturbances, those visual disturbances particularly relevant to psychiatry are given an entire chapter (see Chapter 12).

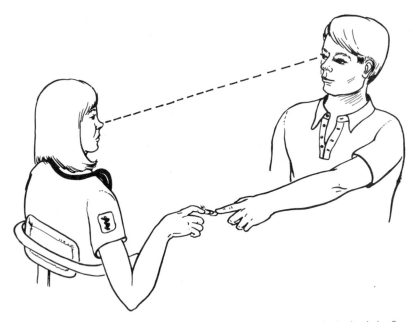

FIGURE 4–2. In testing visual fields by the confrontation method, this physician wiggles her index finger as the patient points to it without diverting his eyes from her nose. Each eye must be tested individually, and the four quadrants of each eye's visual field must be tested. (Only in this way will the examiner detect a bitemporal quadrantanopia, which is a characteristic of pituitary adenomas.) Young children and others unable to comply with this testing method may be examined in a more superficial but still meaningful manner. The physician assesses the response to an attention-catching object introduced to each visual field. If a dollar bill, toy, or glass of water fails to capture the patient's attention, visual field deficit(s) may be present.

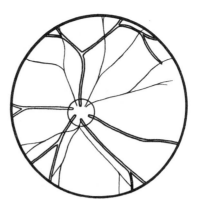

FIGURE 4–3. The normal optic fundus or disk is yellow, flat, and clearly demarcated from the surrounding red retina. The retinal veins, as everywhere else in the body, are larger than their corresponding arteries. The retinal veins can normally be seen to pulsate except when intracranial pressure is elevated.

OCULOMOTOR, TROCHLEAR, ABDUCENS (THIRD, FOURTH, SIXTH)

The oculomotor, trochlear, and abducens nerves are considered as a group because they move the eyes in unison to provide normal *conjugate gaze.* The oculomotor nerves (third cranial nerves) originate in the midbrain (Fig. 4–4) and eventually supply the pupil constrictor, eyelid, and adductor and elevator muscles of each eye (medial rectus, inferior oblique, inferior rectus, and superior rectus). Oculomotor nerve impairment, which is common, leads to a distinctive constellation: a dilated pupil, ptosis, and outward deviation (abduction) of the eye (Fig. 4–5).

The trochlear nerves (fourth cranial nerves) also originate in the midbrain. They supply only the superior oblique muscle, which is responsible for depression of the eye when it is adducted (turned inward). To compensate for an injured trochlear nerve, patients tilt their head away from the affected side. Unless the physician sees a patient with diplopia perform this maneuver, a trochlear nerve injury is difficult to diagnose.

The abducens nerves (sixth cranial nerves), unlike the third and fourth cranial nerves, originate in the pons (Fig. 4–6 and see Fig. 2–9). They too have only a single function—abduction—for which they innervate only a single muscle—the lateral rectus. Abducens nerve impairment, which is relatively common, causes inward devia-

MIDBRAIN

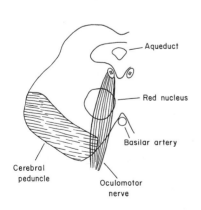

Aqueduct

Red nucleus

Basilar artery

Cerebral peduncle

Oculomotor nerve

FIGURE 4–4. The oculomotor (third cranial) nerves arise from nuclei in the dorsal portion of the midbrain (see Fig. 2–9). Each descends through the red nucleus, which carries cerebellar outflow fibers to the contralateral limbs. Then each passes through the cerebral peduncle, which carries the corticospinal tract destined to innervate the contralateral limbs.

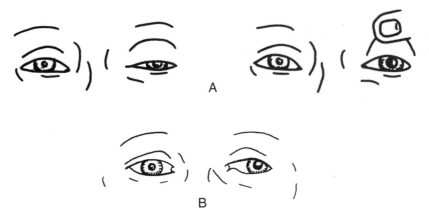

FIGURE 4–5. **A,** The patient with paresis of the left oculomotor nerve has ptosis and lateral deviation of the left eye, which has a dilated and unreactive pupil. **B,** In a milder case, close inspection reveals subtle ptosis, lateral deviation of the eye, and dilation of the pupil. In both cases, patients have diplopia that increases when adducting the left eye because looking to the right requires increased reliance on the paretic left medial rectus muscle (also see Fig. 12–13).

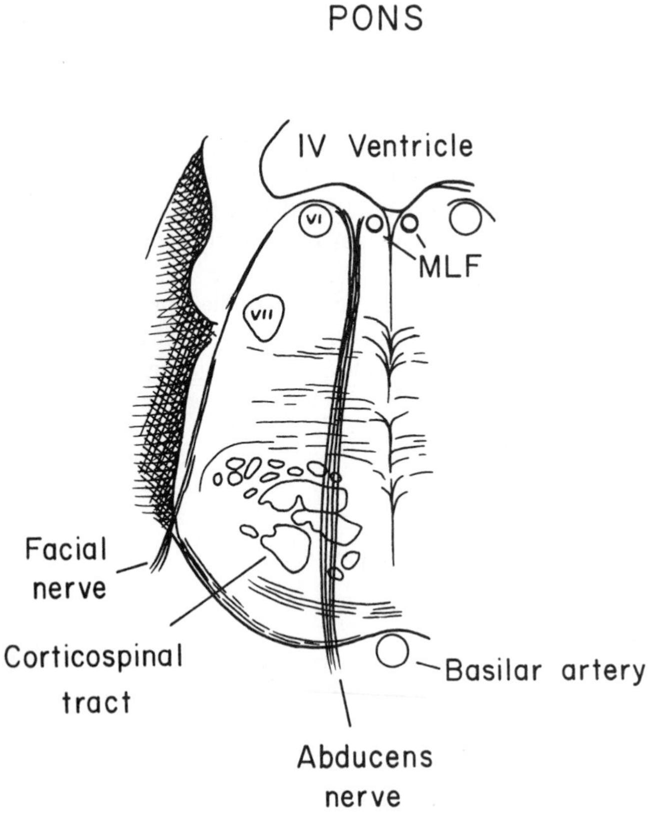

PONS

FIGURE 4–6. The abducens (sixth cranial) arise from nuclei located in the dorsal portion of the pons. These nuclei are adjacent to the medial longitudinal fasciculus (*MLF,* see Fig. 15–3). As the abducens nerves descend, they pass medial to the facial nerves and then penetrate the corticospinal tract.

FIGURE 4–7. The patient with paresis of the left abducens nerve has medial deviation of the left eye. There will be diplopia on looking ahead and toward the left but not when looking to the right (see Fig. 12–14).

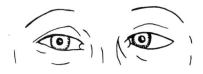

tion (adduction) of the eye, but no ptosis or pupil changes (Fig. 4–7). In summary, the lateral rectus muscle is innervated by the sixth cranial (abducens) nerve, the superior oblique by the (trochlear) fourth, and all the rest by the (oculomotor) third. The mnemonic device LR_6SO_4 captures this relationship.

To produce conjugate eye movements, the oculomotor nerve on one side is complementary to the abducens nerve on the other. For example, when one looks to the left, the left sixth nerve and right third nerve innervate their respective muscles to produce conjugate leftward eye movement. Complementary innervation is essential for conjugate gaze. If both third nerves were simultaneously innervated, the eyes would look toward the nose; if both sixth nerves were simultaneously innervated, the eyes would look toward opposite walls.

Dysconjugate gaze results in diplopia (double vision). Diplopia is most often attributable to a lesion in the oculomotor nerve on one side or the abducens nerve on the other. For example, if a patient has diplopia when looking to the left, then either the left abducens nerve or the right oculomotor nerve is paretic. Diplopia on right gaze, of course, suggests a paresis of either the right abducens or left oculomotor nerve. Although elaborate diagnostic tests may be performed, the presence or absence of other signs of oculomotor nerve palsy (a dilated pupil and ptosis) usually indicates whether that nerve is responsible.

The ocular cranial nerves may be damaged by lesions in the brainstem, in the nerves' course from the brainstem to the ocular muscles, or in their neuromuscular junctions but not in the cerebral hemispheres (the cerebrum). Because cerebral lesions do not injure these cranial nerves, conjugate gaze is preserved. Thus, patients with advanced Alzheimer's disease and those who have sustained cerebral anoxia have devastating cerebral lesions but normal, full conjugate ocular motility. These patients typically maintain a persistent vegetative state while retaining normal eye movements.

Brainstem lesions, which routinely damage cranial nerves, produce combinations of injuries of the ocular nerves and the adjacent corticospinal (pyramidal) tract or red nucleus, which carries cerebellar outflow to the contralateral limbs. These lesions cause diplopia and contralateral hemiparesis or ataxia. Almost all cases result from brainstem infarctions caused by occlusion of a small branch of the basilar artery (see Chapter 11).

Despite producing complex neurologic deficits, brainstem lesions generally do not impair cognitive function. However, *Wernicke's encephalopathy,* one well-known exception, consists of memory impairments (amnesia) accompanied by nystagmus and oculomotor or abducens nerve impairment (see Chapter 7). Another exception is *transtentorial herniation,* in which a cerebral mass lesion, such as a subdural hematoma, squeezes the temporal lobe through the tentorial notch. In this situation, the mass compresses the oculomotor nerve and brainstem to cause coma and a dilated pupil (see Fig. 19–3).

With a right-sided midbrain infarction—a typical brainstem lesion—a patient would have a right oculomotor nerve palsy, which would cause right ptosis, a dilated pupil, and diplopia, accompanied by left hemiparesis (Fig. 4–8). With a slightly different right-sided midbrain infarction, a patient might have right oculomotor nerve palsy and left tremor (Fig. 4–9). A right-sided pontine lesion translates into a right

MIDBRAIN

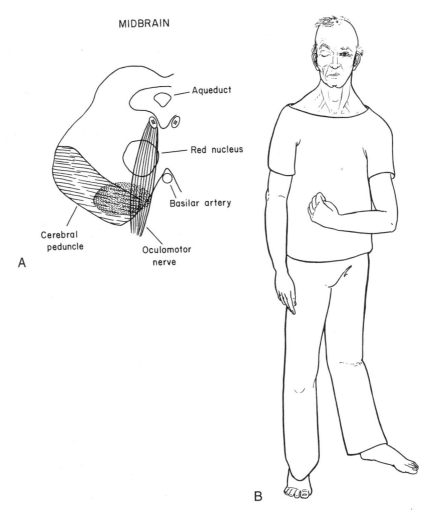

FIGURE 4–8. **A,** A right midbrain infarction damages the oculomotor nerve that supplies the ipsilateral eye and the adjacent cerebral peduncle, which contains the corticospinal tract that subsequently crosses in the medulla, ultimately supplying the contralateral arm and leg. **B,** The patient has right-sided ptosis from the right oculomotor nerve palsy and left hemiparesis from the corticospinal tract injury. Also note that the ptosis elicits a compensatory unconscious elevation of the eyebrow to uncover the eye. (Similar eyebrow elevations can be seen in other conditions that cause ptosis, including cluster headache, myasthenia gravis, and lateral medullary syndrome.)

abducens nerve paresis and left hemiparesis (Fig. 4–10). Notably, in each of these brainstem injuries, mental status is normal because the cerebrum is unscathed.

Another common site of brainstem injury that affects the ocular nerves is the *medial longitudinal fasciculus (MLF)*. This structure is the heavily myelinated midline tract that links the nuclei of the oculomotor and abducens nerves (see Figs. 2–9, 4–10, 15–3, and 15–4). Its interruption produces the *MLF syndrome*, which is often called *internuclear ophthalmoplegia (INO)*. This syndrome, which is characteristic of multiple sclerosis, consists of nystagmus of the abducting eye and failure of the adducting eye to cross the midline.

Lesions occur more frequently in the long paths of the oculomotor or abducens nerves, between the brainstem and the ocular muscles, than in the brainstem. These lesions produce simple, readily identifiable clinical pictures: nerve damage without hemiparesis, ataxia, or mental status impairment. *Diabetic infarction,* the most frequently occurring lesion of the oculomotor nerves, produces a sharp headache and paresis of the affected muscles that lasts several months. Although otherwise typical, diabetic oculomotor nerve infarctions characteristically spare the pupil: in other words, ptosis and ocular abduction occur, but the pupil remains normal in size.

The oculomotor nerve, just as it exits from the midbrain, may also be injured by ruptured aneurysms of the posterior communicating artery. In this case, oculomotor nerve palsy—which would be the least of the patient's problems—is one component of a subarachnoid hemorrhage that usually renders patients prostrate with a severe headache. Children occasionally have migraine headaches that cause temporary oculomotor nerve paresis (see Chapter 9, ophthalmoplegic migraine). In contrast, in the motor neuron diseases, amyotrophic lateral sclerosis (ALS) and poliomyelitis, the oculomotor and abducens nerves are normal despite destruction of large numbers of motor neurons. Patients may have full, conjugate eye movements despite being unable to breathe, lift their limbs, or move their heads.

Disorders of the neuromuscular junction—the nervous system's furthest extent—also produce oculomotor or abducens nerve paresis. In myasthenia gravis (see Fig. 6–3) and botulism, for example, impairment of acetylcholine transmission leads to combinations of ocular and other cranial nerve paresis. These deficits may be perplexing to physicians because the muscle weakness is subtle and variable in severity and pattern. These disorders are always important, especially in their extremes. Respiratory impairment may ensue in severe cases, and mild cases may be overlooked or misdiagnosed as psychogenic.

In a related condition, people with congenital dysconjugate or "crossed" eyes, *strabismus,* do not have double vision. Their brain suppresses one of the images. If uncorrected in childhood, strabismus leads to blindness of the deviated eye, *amblyopia.*

People can usually feign ocular muscle weakness only by staring inward, as if looking at the tip of their nose. Children often do this playfully; however, adults with their eyes in such a position are easily recognized as displaying voluntary, bizarre activity. Another disturbance, found mostly in health care workers, comes from surrepti-

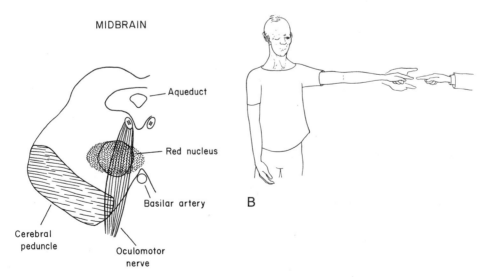

FIGURE 4–9. **A,** A right midbrain infarction damages the oculomotor nerve and *red nucleus,* which conveys left cerebellar hemisphere outflow to the left arm and leg by a "double-cross." **B,** This patient has right ptosis from the oculomotor nerve palsy and left arm ataxia from the damage to the cerebellar outflow tract.

PONS

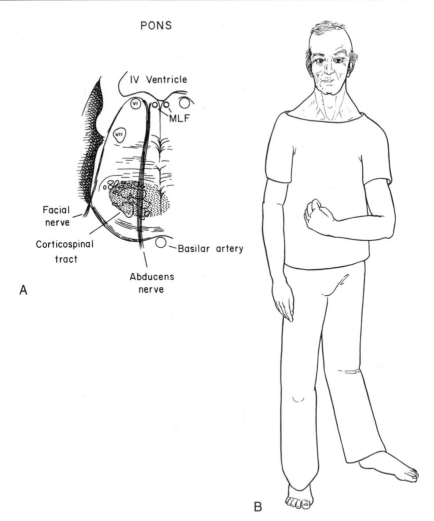

A

B

FIGURE 4–10. **A,** A right pontine infarction damages the abducens nerve, which supplies the ipsilateral eye, and the adjacent corticospinal tract, which supplies the contralateral limbs. (This situation is analogous to midbrain infarctions, see Fig. 4–8.) **B,** The patient has inward deviation of the right eye from paresis of the right abducens nerve and left hemiparesis from right corticospinal tract damage.

tiously instilling eye drops that dilate the pupil to mimic ophthalmologic or neurologic disorders.

TRIGEMINAL (FIFTH)

The trigeminal nerves' main jobs are to convey sensation from the face and innervate the large, powerful muscles that protrude and close the jaw. Because these muscles' main function is to chew, they are often called the "muscles of mastication." The motor nucleus of each nerve is situated in the pons, but its sensory nucleus extends from the midbrain through the medulla (see Fig. 2–9). The nerves leave the brainstem at the side of the pons, together with the facial and acoustic nerves, to become the three cranial nerves—V, VII, and VIII—that pass through the cerebellopontine angle.

Examination of the trigeminal nerve begins by testing sensation in its three sensory divisions (Fig. 4–11). The examiner touches the side of the patient's forehead,

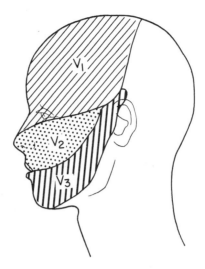

FIGURE 4–11. The three divisions of the trigeminal nerve convey sensory innervation of the face. The first division (V_1) supplies the forehead, the cornea, and the scalp up to the vertex; the second (V_2) supplies the malar area; and the third (V_3) supplies the lower jaw except for the angle. These distributions have more than academic importance. These dermatomes may be mapped by *herpes zoster* infections ("shingles"), trigeminal neuralgia (see Chapter 9), and facial angioma in the Sturge-Weber syndrome (see Fig. 13–7) but not respected in psychogenic facial sensory loss.

cheek, and jaw. Areas of reduced sensation, *hypalgesia,* should conform to anatomic outlines.

Assessing the *corneal reflex* is useful, especially in examining patients whose sensory loss does not conform to neurologic expectations. The corneal reflex is a "superficial reflex" that is basically independent of upper motor neuron (UMN) status. It begins with stimulation of the cornea by a wisp of cotton or a breath of air that triggers the trigeminal nerve's V_1 division, which forms the afferent limb. A brainstem synapse stimulus innervates both facial (seventh cranial) nerves, the efferent limb, which innervate both sets of orbicularis oculi muscles. If the cotton tip is first applied to the right cornea and neither eye blinks, and then to the left cornea and both eyes blink, the right trigeminal nerve (afferent limb) is impaired. If cotton on the right cornea fails to provide a right eye blink but succeeds in provoking a left eye blink, the right facial nerve (efferent limb) is impaired.

Testing jaw muscle strength is done by asking the patient to clench and then protrude the jaw. The *jaw jerk reflex,* which is similar to a deep tendon reflex, consists of a prompt but not overly forceful closing after a tap (Fig. 4–12). A hyperactive response indicates a UMN (corticobulbar tract) lesion, and a hypoactive response in-

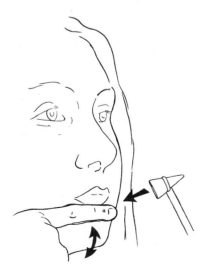

FIGURE 4–12. Tapping the normal, open, relaxed jaw will move it slightly downward. The jaw jerk reflex is the soft rebound. Abnormalities are mostly a matter of rapidity and strength. In a hypoactive reflex, as found in bulbar palsy and other LMN injuries, there is little or no rebound. In a hyperactive reflex, as in pseudobulbar palsy and other UMN (corticobulbar tract) lesions, there is a quick and forceful rebound.

dicates a lower motor neuron (LMN) or cranial nerve lesion. The physician should test the jaw jerk in patients with dysarthria, dysphagia, and emotional lability—mostly to assess the likelihood of pseudobulbar palsy (see below).

Injury of a trigeminal nerve causes facial hypalgesia, afferent corneal reflex impairment, jaw jerk hypoactivity, and deviation of the jaw toward the side of the lesion. Such damage may be caused by nasopharyngeal tumors, gunshot wounds, and tumors of the cerebellopontine angle, such as acoustic neuromas.

In the opposite situation, *trigeminal neuralgia* (tic douloureux) results from trigeminal nerve irritation by an aberrant vessel or other lesion in the cerebellopontine angle. Instead of having hypalgesia, patients with trigeminal neuralgia have bursts of lancinating face pain in the distribution of the third or other division of the nerve (see Chapter 9). Another common trigeminal nerve problem is *herpes zoster* infection, which causes a rash followed by excruciating pain *(postherpetic neuralgia)* in one division of the nerve (see Chapter 14).

Finally, a psychogenic sensory loss involving the face will usually encompass the entire face or be included in a sensory loss of one half the body. In almost all cases, the following three nonanatomic features will be present: (1) the sensory loss will not involve the scalp (although the portion anterior to the vertex is supplied by the trigeminal nerve), (2) the corneal reflex will remain intact, and (3) when only one half the face is affected, sensation will be lost sharply rather than gradually at the midline (i.e., the midline will be split) (see Fig. 3–4).

FACIAL (SEVENTH)

The facial nerves' major functions, like the trigeminal nerves' major functions, are sensory and motor: to convey taste sensation and to innervate the facial muscles. Moreover, just as the trigeminal nerves supply the muscles of mastication, the facial nerves supply the "muscles of facial expression." Their motor and sensory nuclei are in the pons, and the nerves exit through the side of the brainstem with the other cerebellopontine angle nerves.

In a unique and potentially confusing arrangement in neuroanatomy, cerebral impulses innervate both the contralateral and ipsilateral facial nerve motor nuclei. Each facial nerve supplies its ipsilateral temporalis, orbicularis oculi, and orbicularis oris muscles—those responsible for a frown, raised eyebrows, wink, smile, and grimace. In the classic explanation, because of their crossed and uncrossed supply, the upper facial muscles are ultimately innervated by both cerebral hemispheres, whereas the lower facial muscles are innervated by only the contralateral cerebral hemisphere (Fig. 4–13). In an alternative explanation, interneurons link the facial nerve nuclei. This theory postulates that the "crossing" takes place in the brainstem rather than the cerebrum.

Taste sensation is more straightforward. The facial nerves convey impulses from taste receptors of the anterior two thirds of the tongue, and the glossopharyngeal nerves (the ninth cranial nerve) convey those from the posterior third. A remarkable aspect of this sensation is that, despite the extraordinary variety of foods, taste perceptions are normally quite limited. Taste receptors detect only four fundamental sensations: bitter, sweet, sour, and salty. Food actually derives most of its flavor from its aroma, which is detected by the olfactory nerve. Moreover, the olfactory nerve, not the facial nerve, has extensive connections with the frontal lobe and limbic system.

Routine facial nerve testing involves examining the strength of the facial muscles and, at certain times, assessing taste. An examiner observes the patient's face, first at rest and then during a succession of maneuvers that use various facial muscles: look-

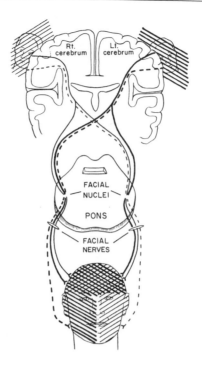

FIGURE 4–13. In the classic portrayal, corticobulbar tracts originating in the ipsilateral, as well as in the contralateral, cerebral hemisphere supply each facial nerve nucleus. Each facial nerve supplies the ipsilateral muscles of facial expression. Because the upper half of the face receives cortical innervation from both hemispheres, cerebral injuries lead to paresis only of the lower half of the contralateral face. In contrast, facial nerve injuries lead to paresis of both the upper and lower half of the ipsilateral side of the face.

ing upward, closing the eyes, and smiling. When weakness is detected, the examiner should try to ascertain whether it involves both the upper and lower or only the lower facial muscles. Upper and lower paresis suggests a lesion of the facial nerve itself. In this case, taste is also likely to be impaired.

With unilateral or even bilateral facial nerve injuries, of course, patients have no mental changes. In contrast, paresis of only the lower facial muscles suggests a lesion of the contralateral cerebral hemisphere, which may be associated with mental changes and also ipsilateral hemiparesis. In addition, with weakness of the right lower face, aphasia may be present. In these cases, taste sensation will be preserved.

To test taste, the examiner applies either a dilute salt or sugar solution to the anterior portion of each side of the tongue, which must remain protruded to prevent the solution from spreading. A patient will normally be able to identify the fundamental taste sensations but not those "tastes" that depend on aroma, such as onion and garlic.

Facial nerve damage produces paresis of the ipsilateral upper and lower face muscles with or without loss of taste sensation. Most such injuries, labeled *Bell's palsy,* have traditionally been attributed to an idiopathic inflammatory condition (Fig. 4–14). In some of these cases, however, the culprit has been an infection by *herpes simplex* virus or *Borrelia burgdorferi,* a relatively common infectious spirochete in several regions of the United States that causes *Lyme disease* (see Chapters 5 and 7). Destructive injuries include lacerations and cerebellopontine angle tumors.

Lesions that stimulate the nerve have the opposite effect. As in trigeminal neuralgia, aberrant vessels in the cerebellopontine angle irritate the facial nerve. Intermittent facial nerve stimulation produces involuntary contractions of the muscles of the ipsilateral side of the face. This condition, *hemifacial spasm* (see Chapter 18), is the facial nerve's counterpart of trigeminal neuralgia.

People cannot mimic unilateral facial paresis. Some people who refuse to be examined, particularly children, might forcefully close their eyelids and mouth. The willful nature of this maneuver is evident when the examiner finds resistance on

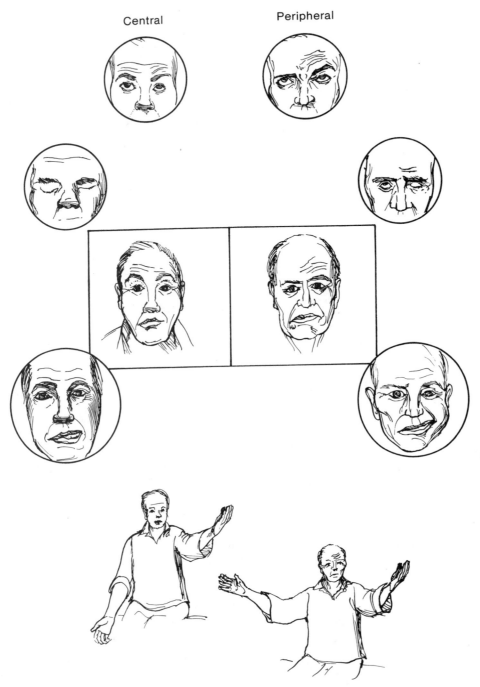

FIGURE 4–14. The patient on the left has weakness of his right lower face from thrombosis of the left middle cerebral artery. He might be said to have a "central" (CNS) facial paralysis. The patient on the right has right-sided weakness of both his upper and lower face from a right facial nerve injury (Bell's palsy). He might be said to have a "peripheral" facial (cranial nerve) paralysis. In the *center boxed sketches,* the man with the central palsy *(left)* has flattening of the right nasolabial fold and sagging of the mouth downward to the right. This pattern of weakness indicates paresis of only the lower facial muscles. The man with the peripheral palsy *(right),* however, has right-sided loss of the normal forehead furrows in addition to flattening of his nasolabial fold. This pattern of weakness indicates paresis of the upper as well as the lower facial muscles. In the *circled sketches at the top,* the patients have been asked to look upward—a maneuver that would exaggerate upper facial weakness. The man with central weakness has normal upward movement of the eyebrows and furrowing of the forehead. The man with peripheral weakness has no eyebrow or forehead movement, and the forehead skin remains flat.   *Legend continued on opposite page*

opening the eyelids and jaw, and sees, when the eyelids are pried open, that the eyeballs retrovert (Bell's phenomena).

ACOUSTIC (EIGHTH)

The acoustic nerves, like the optic nerves, are at least partially covered with myelin produced by the CNS. Their covering contrasts with the other cranial nerves' covering that is myelin produced, as in the peripheral nervous system (PNS), by Schwann cells. Each acoustic nerve is actually composed of two divisions with separate courses and functions: hearing and balance. The *cochlear nerve*, one of the two nerves, transmits auditory impulses from the middle and inner ear mechanisms to the superior temporal gyri of both cerebral hemispheres (Fig. 4–15). This bilateral cortical representation of sound explains the fact that damage to the acoustic nerve or ear itself may cause deafness in that ear, but unilateral lesions of the brainstem or cerebral hemisphere—CNS damage—will not cause hearing impairment. Cerebral lesions that spare hearing occur in patients whose extensive cerebrovascular accidents (strokes) or tumors cause aphasia without impairing their (nonspecific) response to sounds. Although patients with Alzheimer's disease often have hearing loss, that impairment results from age-related nerve and inner ear changes.

During the routine examination, hearing is tested initially by the examiner whispering into each of the patient's ears while covering the other. Acoustic nerve injury may result from medications, such as aspirin or streptomycin; by skull fractures severing the nerve; or by cerebellopontine angle tumors, particularly acoustic neuromas associated with neurofibromatosis. Congenital deafness, as well as mental retardation, commonly results from in utero rubella infections or kernicterus (see Chapter 13).

On the other hand, when patients seem to mimic deafness, the examiner may attempt to startle them with a loud sound or may watch for an *auditory-ocular reflex* (observing whether they look involuntarily toward a noise). The diagnosis of psychogenic hearing loss may be confirmed by testing brainstem auditory-evoked responses (BAERs, see Chapter 15).

About 25% of people older than 65 years have hearing impairments from degeneration of the acoustic nerve or the cochlea and other middle ear structures. This hearing loss associated with older age *(presbycusis)* typically begins with loss of high-tone hearing and eventually includes all frequencies. Speech discrimination, especially in crowded rooms, is usually the first and generally always the most troublesome symptom.

Presbycusis thus carries the potential for inattention and feelings of isolation. In addition, when visual and hearing impairments are superimposed on a marginal cognitive capacity, the sensory deprivation may precipitate hallucinations. As a gen-

---

In the *circled sketches second from the top,* the men have been asked to close their eyes—a maneuver that also would exaggerate upper facial weakness. The man with the central weakness has widening of the palpebral fissure, but he is able to close his eyelids and cover the eyeball. The man with the peripheral weakness is unable to close the affected eyelids, although his genuine effort is made apparent by the retroversion of the eyeball (Bell's phenomenon). In the *lowest circled sketches,* the men have been asked to smile—a maneuver that would exaggerate lower facial weakness. Both men have strength only of the left side of the mouth, and thus it deviates to the left. If tested, the man with Bell's palsy would have loss of taste on the anterior two thirds of his tongue on the affected side. The *bottom sketches* show the response when both men are asked to elevate their arms. The man with the central facial weakness also has paresis of the adjacent arm, but the man with the peripheral weakness has no arm paresis. In summary, the man on the left with the left middle cerebral artery occlusion has paresis of his right lower face and arm. The man on the right with right Bell's palsy has paresis of his right upper and lower face and loss of taste.

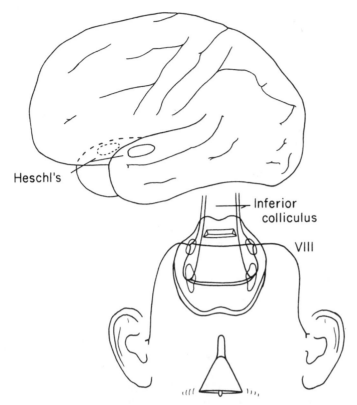

Heschl's

Inferior
colliculus

VIII

FIGURE 4–15. The cochlear division of the acoustic nerve synapses extensively in the pons. Crossed and uncrossed fibers pass upward through the brainstem to terminate in the auditory (Heschl's gyrus) cortex of both temporal lobes. In each hemisphere, the Heschl's gyrus is symmetric and located adjacent to the planum temporale. Both gyri receive auditory stimuli predominantly from the contralateral ear. In addition, Heschl's gyrus in the dominant hemisphere, which is adjacent to Wernicke's language area (see Fig. 8–1), may also have a role in language function.

eral rule, in treating the elderly, physicians should dispense hearing aids readily and even on a trial basis.

Another common problem among the elderly is a persistent ringing or whistling sound, *tinnitus*. Although it may be caused by medications that damage the inner ear, tinnitus is most often caused by ischemia from atherosclerotic cerebrovascular disease. An audible heartbeat, while often the result of heightened sensitivity, may also be a manifestation of atherosclerosis because a rigid arterial tree transmits undampened cardiac contractions all the way to the small vessels of the inner ear.

Auditory evaluations are necessary in patients suspected of having a psychogenic hearing impairment; children with autism, cerebral palsy, mental retardation, speech impediments, and poor school performance; and most older adults.

The other division, the *vestibular nerve*, transmits impulses from the labyrinth governing equilibrium, orientation, and change in position. The most characteristic symptom of vestibular nerve damage is *vertigo*, a sensation that one is spinning within the environment or that the environment is itself spinning. Unfortunately, patients casually say "dizziness" when they mean lightheadedness, anxiety, weakness, or unsteadiness, rather than vertigo. The most common cause of vertigo is vestibular injury, such as viral infections of the inner ear, *labyrinthitis,* or ischemia. When the vertigo is induced by an otherwise normal patient placing the head in certain positions or merely changing positions, the disorder is called *benign positional vertigo.* One theory suggests that this disorder, which is relatively common among middle-aged and older individuals, is caused by free-floating debris in the semicircular canals ("otoliths"). In any case, exercises that place the head in certain positions alleviate the symptom in some individuals, presumably by securing the debris in innocuous places.

Ménière's disease, which deserves special attention, is a relatively common chronic vestibular disorder of unknown etiology that causes attacks of unequivocal vertigo, unilateral tinnitus, and nystagmus. Developing in women more often than in men, it also leads to progressive hearing loss. Although most attacks of Ménière's disease are obvious, they may be indistinguishable from basilar artery transient ischemic attacks (TIAs), basilar artery migraines, and mild hyperventilation.

BULBAR: GLOSSOPHARYNGEAL, VAGUS, SPINAL ACCESSORY NERVES (NINTH, TENTH, ELEVENTH)

The *bulbar* cranial nerves (IX through XII)—the last of the three cranial nerve groups—arise from nuclei in the brainstem caudal to the ocular (III, IV, and VI) and the cerebellopontine (V, VII, and VIII) cranial nerve groups. The bulb is technically equivalent to the medulla; however, clinically it also includes the pons.

Besides containing the nuclei and initial portions of cranial nerves IX through XII, the bulb contains the descending corticospinal, ascending sensory, and sympathetic nervous system tracts. The cranial nerves innervate the muscles of the soft palate, pharynx, larynx, and tongue. They implement speaking and swallowing. Lateral medullary infarction, the most common brainstem stroke, has already illustrated the bulbar cranial nerves' relationship to certain CNS tracts and signs of their injury (see Wallenberg syndrome, Fig. 2–10).

Although the bulbar cranial nerves originate in the lower end of the brainstem, which is nowhere near the cerebral cortex, and their functions are simple and mechanical, they are involved in several neurologic illnesses that have psychiatric aspects. Their impairment often leads to *bulbar palsy*, which has received most attention when contrasted with the infamous *pseudo*bulbar palsy that appears to induce overwhelming emotional changes (see below). Likewise, the *locked-in syndrome*, which is important itself, may be contrasted with the persistent vegetative state (for both, see Chapter 11), in which cognitive function is obliterated but vegetative functions—respiration, sleeping, and swallowing—persist. Finally, bulbar nerve overactivity leads to certain seemingly bizarre disorders, such as spasmodic dysphonia and spasmodic torticollis, that until recently have been considered psychogenic and untreatable (see Chapter 18).

Bulbar Palsy

Bulbar cranial nerve injury within the brainstem or along the course of the nerves leads to bulbar palsy. This commonly occurring disorder is characterized by *dysarthria* (speech impairment), *dysphagia* (swallowing impairment), and a hypoactive jaw and gag reflexes (Table 4–1).

To assess bulbar nerve function, the examiner should listen to the patient's spontaneous speech during casual conversation and while eliciting the history. The patient should be asked to repeat syllables that require lingual ("la"), labial ("pa"), and guttural ("ga") speech mechanisms. Most patients with bulbar palsy speak with a thick, nasal intonation. Some are mute. Even if a patient's speech is not strikingly abnormal during casual conversation, repetition of the guttural consonant, "ga . . . ga . . . ga . . . ," will usually evoke typically thickened, nasal sounds, uttered "gna . . . gna . . . gna. . . ." In addition, when saying "ah," a patient with bulbar palsy will have little or no palate elevation because of paresis.

In contrast, the speech of patients with cerebellar dysfunction is characterized by an irregular rhythm (scanning speech), which is akin to ataxia (see Chapter 2). The speech of patients with spasmodic dysphonia has a "strained and strangled" quality, often with a superimposed tremor (see Chapter 18). Unlike aphasic patients (see Chapter 8), those with bulbar palsy have normal comprehension and can express themselves in writing.

TABLE 4–1. *Comparison of Bulbar and Pseudobulbar Palsy*

	Bulbar	Pseudobulbar
Dysarthria	Yes	Yes
Dysphagia	Yes	Yes
Movement of palate		
Voluntary	No	No
Reflex	No	Yes
Respiratory impairment	Yes	No
Jaw jerk	Hypoactive	Hyperactive
Emotional lability	No	Yes
Intellectual impairment	No	Yes

In addition to causing dysarthria, impaired palatal and pharyngeal movement in bulbar palsy causes dysphagia. Food tends to lodge in the trachea or go into the nasopharyngeal cavity. Liquids tend to be regurgitated through the nose. Impairment of palate sensation or movement also leads to the characteristic loss of the gag reflex (Fig. 4–16). Finally, extensive bulbar damage will injure the medullary respiratory center or the nerves that innervate respiratory muscles. For example, the bulbar form of poliomyelitis ("polio") forced its childhood victims into "iron lungs" to support their respiration. Even today, many patients with bulbar palsy from Guillain-Barré syndrome, myasthenia gravis, and similar conditions must undergo tracheostomy for respiratory support.

Depending on its cause, bulbar palsy is associated with still other physical findings. When the jaw muscles are involved, the jaw jerk reflex will be depressed (see Fig. 4–12). If a brainstem lesion also damages the corticospinal tract, patients may have hyperactive deep tendon reflexes (DTRs) and Babinski signs. However, as in other conditions with exclusive brainstem damage, bulbar palsy is not associated with cognitive impairment or emotional abnormalities.

Conditions that commonly cause bulbar palsy by damaging the nerves within the brainstem are ALS, poliomyelitis, and infarctions, such as lateral medullary infarction. Diseases that damage the cranial nerves after they have emerged from the brainstem are Guillain-Barré syndrome, chronic meningitis, and tumors that grow along the base of the skull or within the adjacent meninges. Myasthenia gravis and botulism cause bulbar palsy by impairing neuromuscular junction transmission (see Chapter 6). Most important, none of these conditions *directly* changes the mental status because the damage does not involve the cerebrum.

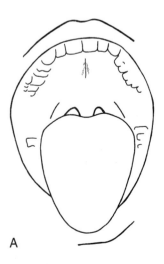

A

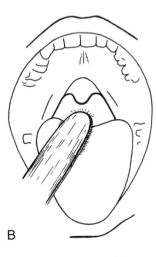

B

FIGURE 4–16. A, The soft palate normally forms an arch from which the uvula seems to hang. **B,** When the pharynx is stimulated, the gag reflex elicits pharyngeal muscle contraction; the soft palate rises with the uvula remaining in the midline. With bulbar nerve injury (bulbar palsy)—LMN injury—the palate has little, no, or asymmetric movement. With corticobulbar tract injury (pseudobulbar palsy)—UMN injury—the reaction is brisk and forceful. It often precipitates retching, coughing, or crying.

PSEUDOBULBAR PALSY

When dysarthria and dysphagia result from frontal lobe damage, the condition is termed pseudobulbar palsy. Better known than bulbar palsy, it is typically associated with dementia, aphasia, and unprovoked and fragile emotions that overshadow physical changes.

Dysarthria in pseudobulbar palsy is characterized by variable rhythm and intensity and is often said to have an "explosive" cadence. For example, when asked to repeat the consonant "ga," patients might blurt out "GA . . . GA . . . GA . . . ga . . . ga . . . ga." The dysphagia often results in inadequate nutrition and aspiration. Although these complications might be circumvented by surgical placement of gastrotomy tubes, installing these mechanical devices has created almost as much controversy as the use of respirators in artificially prolonging life.

From an admittedly narrow neurologic perspective, an important distinguishing characteristic of pseudobulbar palsy is hyperactivity of certain reflexes because of damage to the UMN corticobulbar tracts (Fig. 4–17): thus, it is sometimes called "suprabulbar" palsy. As in bulbar palsy, patients with pseudobulbar palsy have little or no palatal or pharyngeal movement in response to voluntary effort, as when attempting to say "ah." However, when the gag reflex is tested, these patients have brisk elevation of the palate and contraction of the pharynx, often overreacting with coughing, crying, and retching (see Fig. 4–16). Likewise, the jaw jerk reflex, depressed in bulbar palsy, is hyperactive in pseudobulbar palsy because of UMN corticobulbar tract damage. In addition, in pseudobulbar palsy, damage to the frontal lobes is so common that it almost always leads to signs of bilateral corticospinal tract damage, such as hyperactive DTRs and Babinski signs. Frontal lobe damage also leads to corticobulbar tract damage that makes the face sag and impairs expression (Fig. 4–18).

The most notorious feature of pseudobulbar palsy is "emotional lability," a tendency to cry or, less often, laugh in response to minimal provocation. With their affect appearing to alternate unexpectedly between euphoria and depression, patients often describe themselves as being awash with emotions. Amitriptyline, given in relatively low doses (e.g., 75 mg or less daily), may suppress the unwarranted *pathologic laughing* and *crying*, apart from its antidepressant effect.

Although pseudobulbar palsy has become the commonly accepted explanation for unwarranted emotional states in people with brain damage, tearfulness should not always be ascribed to brain damage. A great deal of true sadness can be expected with neurologic illness.

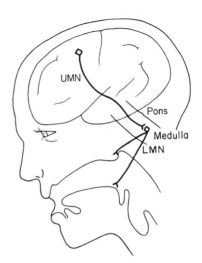

FIGURE 4–17. Damage to the bulbar cranial nerves (bulbar palsy) abolishes the jaw jerk and gag reflexes, which are characteristic of LMN injury (see Fig. 2–2, *C*). Although mental changes may be the most conspicuous feature of pseudobulbar palsy, corticobulbar tract damage leads to hyperactive reflexes, which are characteristic of UMN injury (see Fig. 2–2, *B*).

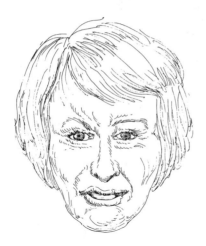

FIGURE 4–18. Patients with pseudobulbar palsy, such as this woman who has sustained multiple cerebral infarctions, often sit with a slack jaw, furrowed forehead, and vacant stare.

Pseudobulbar palsy is associated with dementia as well as emotional lability because extensive cerebral damage usually underlies it. Likewise, when the left cerebral hemisphere is heavily damaged, pseudobulbar palsy may be associated with aphasia, usually nonfluent (see Chapter 8). This association also might account for aphasic patients crying at minimal provocation, even in frustration at naming objects. In any case, patients with pseudobulbar palsy should be evaluated for dementia and aphasia.

Damage to both frontal lobes or, more often, the entire cerebrum by any of a wide variety of degenerative, structural, or metabolic disturbances causes pseudobulbar palsy. Its most common causes are Alzheimer's disease, multiple cerebral infarctions, head trauma, and multiple sclerosis. Congenital cerebral damage (i.e., cerebral palsy) causes pseudobulbar palsy along with bilateral spasticity and choreoathetotic movement disorders. Finally, because ALS causes both UMN and LMN damage, it leads to a mixture of bulbar and pseudobulbar palsy; however, because ALS is exclusively a motor neuron disorder, it is not associated with either dementia or aphasia (see Chapter 5).

HYPOGLOSSAL (TWELFTH)

The hypoglossal nerves originate from paired nuclei near the midline of the medulla and descend through the base of the medulla (see Fig. 2–9). They pass through the base of the skull and travel through the neck to innervate the tongue

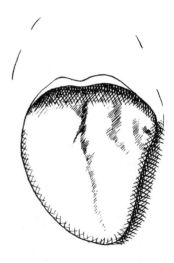

FIGURE 4–19. With (left) hypoglossal nerve damage, the tongue deviates toward the weaker side and its affected (left) side undergoes atrophy.

muscles. Each nerve innervates the ipsilateral tongue muscles. These muscles move the tongue within the mouth, protrude it when people eat and speak, and push it contralateral. Because the pressure on each side is balanced, the tongue protrudes in the midline.

If one hypoglossal nerve is injured, that side of the tongue will become weak and, with time, atrophic. When protruded, the tongue will deviate toward the weakened side (Fig. 4–19), which illustrates the adage, "the tongue points toward the side of the lesion." If both nerves are injured, as in bulbar palsy, the tongue will become immobile. Patients with ALS have tongue fasciculations, as well as atrophy (see Fig. 5–4).

The most frequently occurring conditions in which one hypoglossal nerve is damaged are lower brainstem infarctions, penetrating neck wounds, and nasopharyngeal tumors. Guillain-Barré syndrome, myasthenia gravis, and ALS usually injure both hypoglossal and other bulbar cranial nerves.

QUESTIONS and ANSWERS: CHAPTERS 1 to 4

1–7. Match the description with the visual field pattern (a–f):

1. Right homonymous hemianopsia

2. Bilateral superior nasal quadrantanopia

3. Right homonymous superior quadrantanopia

4. Blindness of the right eye

5. Left homonymous superior quadrantanopia

6. Bilateral inferior nasal quadrantanopia

7. Visual field deficit produced by a protuberant nose

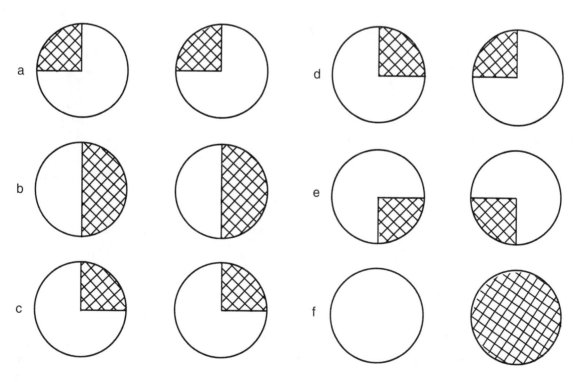

ANSWERS: 1-b, 2-**d**, 3-c, 4-f, 5-a, 6-e, 7-e

8. A 68-year-old man has sudden, painless onset of paresis of the right upper and lower face, inability to abduct the right eye, and paresis of the left arm and leg. Where is the lesion?

a. Cerebrum (cerebral hemispheres)
b. Cerebellum
c. Midbrain
d. Pons
e. Medulla
f. None of the above

> **ANSWER:** d. The damaged structures include the right-sided abducens (VI) and facial (VII) nerves and the corticospinal tract destined to supply the left limbs. The corticospinal tract has a long course during which an injury would produce left hemiparesis; however, cranial nerves VI and VII originate in the pons and have a relatively short course. A small lesion, such as a stroke, in the right side of the pons could damage all these structures. (If the lesion pictured in Fig. 4–10 extended more laterally, it would create these deficits.)

9. An elderly man has left ptosis and a dilated and unreactive left pupil with external deviation of the left eye, right hemiparesis, and right-sided hyperactive DTRs and Babinski sign. He does not have either aphasia or hemianopsia. Where is the lesion?

a. Cerebrum
b. Cerebellum
c. Midbrain
d. Pons
e. Medulla
f. None of the above

> **ANSWER:** c. Because the patient has only a left oculomotor nerve palsy and right hemiparesis, the lesion must be in the left midbrain. He does not have a language or visual field deficit because the lesion is in the brainstem, nowhere near the cerebrum.

10. In which two lobes might a lesion cause a left superior homonymous quadrantanopia?

a. Frontal lobe
b. Parietal lobe
c. Occipital lobe
d. Temporal lobe
e. None of the above

> **ANSWER:** c, d. This visual field loss is usually found with destruction of the right temporal or inferior occipital lobe, which would be caused by a brain tumor or occlusion of the posterior cerebral artery. Alternatively, an optic tract lesion may occasionally be responsible.

11. A 20-year-old woman has right eye "blindness," right hemiparesis, and right hemisensory loss. Pupil and deep tendon reflexes are normal. She does not press down with her left leg while attempting to lift her right leg. Where is the lesion?

a. Cerebrum
b. Cerebellum
c. Midbrain
d. Pons
e. Medulla
f. None of the above

> **ANSWER:** f. The symptoms cannot be explained by a single lesion, cannot be confirmed by objective signs, and lack the usual accompanying symptom of right hemiparesis, aphasia. If she had had a left cerebral lesion, the visual impairment would have been a right homonymous hemianopsia. Moreover, she fails to exert maximum effort with one leg while "trying" to lift the other against resistance (Hoover's sign, see Fig. 3–2). Neurologic disease is probably absent.

12. A 50-year-old woman describes having many years of gait impairment and right-sided decreased hearing. The right corneal reflex is absent. The entire right side of her face is weak. Auditory acuity is diminished on the right. There are left-sided hyperactive DTRs with a Babinski sign, and right-sided difficulty with rapid alternating movements. What structures are involved?

a. Optic nerves
b. Cerebellopontine angle structures
c. Extraocular motor nerves
d. Bulbar cranial nerves
e. None of the above

> **ANSWER:** b. The right-sided corneal reflex loss, facial weakness, and hearing impairment indicate damage to the trigeminal, facial, and acoustic cranial nerves, respectively. These nerves (V, VII, VIII) emerge together from the brainstem at the cerebellopontine angle. The right-sided dysdiadochokinesia reflects right-sided cerebellar damage. The

left-sided DTR abnormalities are caused by compression of the pons. Common cerebellopontine lesions are meningiomas and acoustic neuromas, which are often manifestations of neurofibromatosis (particularly the NF2 variant).

13. A 60-year-old man has interscapular back pain, paraparesis with hyperreflexia, loss of sensation below the umbilicus, and incontinence. Where is the lesion?

a. C7
b. T4
c. T10
d. L1
e. S2
f. None of the above

ANSWER: c. The lesion affects the thoracic spinal cord at the T10 level. The umbilicus is the landmark for T10.

14. After a minor motor vehicle crash, a young man describes having visual loss, paralysis of his legs, and loss of sensation to pin and position below the waist; however, sensation of warm versus cold is intact. He can see only 2 m^2 at every distance. He is unable to raise his legs or walk. He has brisk DTRs, but his plantar responses are flexor. Where is the lesion?

a. C7
b. T4
c. T10
d. L1
e. S2
f. None of the above

ANSWER: f. Many features of the examination indicate that the basis of his symptoms and signs is not neurologic: (1) the constant area (2 m^2) of visual loss at all distances—tunnel vision—is contrary to the optics of vision, in which a greater area of vision is encompassed at greater distances from the eye, (2) the sensory loss to pain (pin) is inconsistent with preservation of temperature sensation because pain and temperature sensory systems are contained in the same pathway, and (3) despite his apparent paraparesis, the normal plantar response indicates that both the UMNs and LMNs are intact. His DTRs are typically brisk because of anxiety.

15. A 50-year-old man with mild dementia has absent reflexes, loss of position and vibration sensation, and ataxia. Which areas are affected?

a. Cerebrum only
b. The entire CNS
c. The entire CNS and PNS
d. The cerebrum and the spinal cord's posterior columns
e. Autonomic nervous system

ANSWER: d. Conditions that cause dementia and dysfunction of the posterior columns of the spinal cord and the cerebellar system are combined system disease (pernicious anemia), tabes dorsalis, some spinocerebellar degenerations, and heavy metal intoxication. The posterior columns seem to be especially vulnerable to environmental toxins and are frequently damaged by hereditary illnesses.

16. A 55-year-old woman, thought to have depression, is then found to have right-sided optic atrophy and left-sided papilledema. Where is the lesion?

a. Frontal lobe
b. Parietal lobe
c. Occipital lobe
d. Temporal lobe
e. None of the above

ANSWER: a. She has the classic Foster-Kennedy syndrome. Probably a right frontal lobe tumor compresses the underlying right optic nerve, causing optic atrophy, and raised intracranial pressure causes papilledema of the left optic nerve.

17. A middle-aged man is distraught because he has developed impotence. He has been in excellent health except for hypertension. He has orthostatic hypotension and lightheadedness, but the neurologic examination is otherwise normal. Which neurologic system is most likely impaired?

a. Cerebrum only
b. The entire CNS
c. The entire CNS and PNS
d. The cerebrum and the spinal cord's posterior columns
e. Autonomic nervous system

ANSWER: e. Impotence in the presence of orthostatic hypotension is likely to be the result of autonomic nervous system dysfunction. In this patient, antihypertensive medications may be responsible.

18. A 60-year-old man with right upper lobe pulmonary carcinoma has the rapid development of lumbar spine pain, weak and areflexic legs, loss of sensation below the knees, and urinary and fecal incontinence. Where is the lesion?

a. Cerebrum
b. Brainstem
c. Spinal cord

d. Peripheral nervous system
e. Neuromuscular junction

ANSWER: d. The lumbar spine pain and absent DTRs suggest that the lesion is in the cauda equina. This structure is composed of lumbosacral nerve roots, which is part of the peripheral nervous system.

19. Subsequently, the man in question 18 develops a flaccid, areflexic paresis of the right arm and a right Horner's syndrome. Where is the lesion?

a. Cerebrum
b. Brainstem
c. Spinal cord

d. Peripheral nervous system
e. Neuromuscular junction
f. None of the above

ANSWER: d. His problem is now a lesion of the right C4–6 nerve roots and the thoracic sympathetic chain. He has a Pancoast tumor. He should have a chest x-ray film or computed tomography (CT).

20. Of the following, which two structures comprise the posterior columns of the spinal cord?

a. Spinothalamic tract
b. Fasciculus cuneatus
c. Fasciculus gracilis

d. Posterior horn cells
e. Lateral spinothalamic tract

ANSWER: b, c

21. Of the structures listed in question 20, which one carries temperature sensation?

ANSWER: e

22. A 40-year-old man has interscapular spine pain, paraparesis with hyperactive DTRs, bilateral Babinski signs, and a complete sensory loss below his nipples. What is the location of the lesion?

a. C7
b. T4
c. T10

d. L1
e. S2
f. None of the above

ANSWER: b. The lesion clearly affects the spinal cord at the T4 level. The nipples are the T4 landmark. Common causes include benign and malignant mass lesions (a herniated thoracic intervertebral disk or an epidural metastatic tumor), infections (abscess or tuberculoma), and inflammations (transverse myelitis or multiple sclerosis). Human immunodeficiency virus (HIV) infection itself does not produce such a discrete lesion; however, complications of acquired immunodeficiency syndrome (AIDS), such as lymphoma, toxoplasmosis, and tuberculosis, might create a mass lesion that would compress the spinal cord. Magnetic resonance imaging (MRI) of the thoracic spine or myelography is routinely performed to rule out mass lesions compressing the spinal cord.

23. Which cranial nerves are covered totally or partly by CNS-generated myelin?

a. Optic and acoustic
b. Facial, acoustic, and trigeminal
c. Bulbar

d. All
e. None

ANSWER: a

24. An elderly, hypertensive man has vertigo, nausea, and vomiting. He has a right-sided Horner's syndrome, loss of the right corneal reflex, and dysarthria because of paresis of the palate. Which way does the palate deviate?

a. Right
b. Left

c. Up
d. Down

ANSWER: b. The patient has a right-sided lateral medullary (Wallenberg's) syndrome. This syndrome includes crossed hypalgesia (right-facial and left-truncal, in this case) and right-sided ataxia. The palate deviates to the left because of right-sided palatal muscle weakness. Because the cerebrum is spared, patients do not have emotional or cognitive impairment or physical signs of cerebral damage, such as visual field cuts or seizures.

25. A 28-year-old physician, in her last trimester of a normal pregnancy, developed pain in her low back. Immediately before delivery, the pain spread down her right anterolateral thigh. That quadriceps muscle was slightly weak and its DTR was reduced. By 2 weeks post partum, after delivery of a healthy 11-pound girl, all signs and symptoms resolved. Which of the following was the most likely diagnosis?

a. A herniated disk with sciatic nerve compression
b. Compression of the lateral femoral cutaneous nerve (meralgia paresthetica)
c. Compression of the femoral nerve or its nerve roots
d. Multiple sclerosis

ANSWER: c. An enlarged uterus can compress the lumbosacral plexus in the pelvis or the femoral nerve as it exits from the inguinal area. Meralgia paresthetica, which results from nerve compression in the inguinal region, is painful but not associated with weakness or DTR loss. Herniated disks occur in pregnancy because of weight gain, hyperlordosis, and laxity of ligaments; however, sciatica usually causes low back pain that radiates to the posterior portion of the leg. The pain and hypoactive DTRs exclude multiple sclerosis.

26. Where is the primary damage in Wilson's disease, Huntington's chorea, and choreiform cerebral palsy?

a. Pyramidal system
b. Extrapyramidal system

c. Entire CNS
d. Cerebellar outflow tracts

ANSWER: b. These diseases, like Parkinson's disease, damage the basal ganglia, which are the foundation of the extrapyramidal motor system. Basal ganglia dysfunction causes tremor, chorea, athetosis, rigidity, and bradykinesia. In contrast, corticospinal tract dysfunction causes spasticity, DTR hyperreflexia, clonus, and Babinski signs.

27. What are the frontal lobe release reflexes? Are they pathologic?

ANSWER: The frontal release reflexes involve the face (snout, suck, and rooting reflex), jaw (jaw jerk), and palm (palmomental and grasp reflexes). Almost all frontal release signs are normally present in infants. In adults, none of the frontal release reflexes reliably indicates the presence of a pathologic condition. However, if several are detected, a congenital cerebral injury, frontal lobe lesion, or cerebral degenerative condition may be present.

28–39. Match the condition with its description (a–l):

28. Anosognosia

29. Aphasia

30. Astereognosis

31. Athetosis

32. Bradykinesia

33. Chorea

34. Dementia

35. Dysdiadochokinesia

36. Gerstmann's syndrome

37. Dysarthria

38. Ataxia

39. Dysmetria

a. Slowness of movement that is usually seen with many basal ganglia diseases and is characteristic of parkinsonism.

b. An involuntary movement disorder characterized by slow writhing, sinuous movement of the arm(s) or leg(s) that is more pronounced in the distal part of the limbs. It usually results from basal ganglia damage from perinatal jaundice, anoxia, or prematurity.

c. Impairment in pronouncing words that may result from lesions in the cerebrum, brainstem, cranial nerves, or even vocal cords.

d. It is a disorder of verbal or written language rather than simply pronunciation. It almost always results from discrete lesions in the dominant cerebral hemisphere's perisylvian language arc. However, occasionally degenerative conditions, including Alzheimer's disease, may cause aspects of it.

e. It is an impairment of memory and judgment, abstract thinking, and other cognitive functions of a degree sufficient to impair social activities or interpersonal relationships.

f. It is a disorder of involuntary movement characterized by intermittent, random jerking of the limbs, face, or trunk. Medications, such as levodopa and typical neuroleptics, and many basal ganglia diseases may cause it.

g. Inability to identify objects by touch. It is a variety of cortical sensory loss that is found with lesions of the contralateral parietal lobe.

h. It consists primarily of irregularity of voluntary movement. It is often a sign of cerebellar injury and associated with intention tremor, hypotonia, and impaired rapid alternating movements.

i. Impairment of rapid alternating movements that is characteristic of cerebellar injury, but may be result of red nucleus damage.

j. Failure to recognize a deficit or disease. The most common example is ignoring a left hemiparesis from a right cerebral infarction. Another example is denial of the sudden onset of blindness (Anton's syndrome) from occipital lobe infarctions.

k. Irregularities on performing rapid alternating movements. The term does not refer to a measure of distance, but to rhythm.

l. Combination of agraphia, finger agnosia, dyscalculia, and inability to distinguish right from left.

ANSWERS: 28-j, 29-d, 30-g, 31-b, 32-a, 33-f, 34-e, 35-i, 36-l, 37-c, 38-h, 39-k

40. Which of the following neurologic diseases are genetically transmitted and, if so, in what manner?

a. Alzheimer's disease
b. ALS
c. Cluster headaches
d. Creutzfeldt-Jakob disease
e. Down syndrome
f. Duchenne muscular dystrophy
g. Adrenoleukodystrophy
h. Tay-Sachs disease
i. Phenylketonuria (PKU)
j. Guillain-Barré syndrome
k. Huntington's disease
l. Migraine without aura (common migraine)
m. Sturge-Weber disease
n. Subacute sclerosing panencephalitis
o. Wilson's disease

ANSWERS:

a. Nongenetic, except autosomal dominant in certain families
b. Nongenetic, except autosomal dominant in 10% of cases
c. Nongenetic
d. Nongenetic, except autosomal dominant in 10% of cases. This illness probably represents an interaction of genetic vulnerability and an atypical virus infection.
e. Nondysjunction (trisomy 21)

f. Sex-linked recessive
g. Sex-linked recessive
h. Autosomal recessive
i. Autosomal recessive
j. Nongenetic (probably infectious)
k. Autosomal dominant
l. Frequently familial, but not entirely genetic
m. Autosomal dominant with variable penetration, but most cases are sporadic
n. Nongenetic (probably infectious)
o. Autosomal recessive

41. Three months after a young man sustained closed head injury, he has insomnia, fatigue, cognitive impairment, and personality changes. He also reports that food is tasteless. What is the most specific origin of his symptoms?

a. Posttraumatic stress disorder
b. Frontal lobe, head, and neck trauma
c. Partial complex seizures
d. Frontal lobe and olfactory nerve trauma

ANSWER: d. He probably has had a contusion of both frontal lobes resulting in a postconcussion syndrome manifested by changes in mentation and personality. The anosmia results from shearing of the thin fibers of the olfactory nerve in their passage through the cribriform plate.

42. A middle-aged woman has increasing blindness in the right eye, where the visual acuity is 20/400 and the optic disc is white. The right pupil does not react either directly or consensually to light. The left pupil reacts directly, although not consensually. All motions of the right eye are impaired. In which area is the lesion?

a. Neuromuscular junction
b. Orbit
c. Retro-orbital structures
d. Cerebrum

ANSWER: c. She evidently has right-sided optic nerve damage. She has right-sided impaired visual acuity, optic atrophy, and loss of direct light reflex in that eye with loss of the indirect (consensual) light reflex in the other. In addition, the complete extraocular muscle paresis indicates oculomotor, trochlear, and abducens nerve damage. Only a lesion located immediately behind the orbit, such as a sphenoid wing meningioma, would be able to damage all these nerves.

43. In which of the following conditions do pupils usually accommodate but not react to light?

a. Psychogenic disturbances
b. Oculomotor nerve injuries
c. Midbrain lesions
d. Argyll-Robertson

ANSWER: d

44. In which of the following conditions is a patient in an agitated, confused state with abnormally large pupils?

a. Heroin overdose
b. Multiple sclerosis
c. Atropine, scopolamine, or sympathomimetic intoxication
d. Hyperventilation

ANSWER: c

45. In what condition is a patient typically comatose with respiratory depression and pinpoint-sized pupils?

a. Heroin overdose
b. Multiple sclerosis
c. Atropine, scopolamine, or sympathomimetic intoxication
d. Hyperventilation

ANSWER: a. Heroin, barbiturate, and other overdoses are the most common cause of the combination of coma and miosis. Infarctions and hemorrhages in the pons also produce the same picture.

46. Match the reflex limb (a–f) with the cranial nerve (1–9) that carries it.

a. Afferent limb of the light reflex
b. Efferent limb of the light reflex
c. Afferent limb of the corneal reflex
d. Efferent limb of the corneal reflex
e. Afferent limb of the accommodation reflex
f. Efferent limb of the accommodation reflex

1. Optic nerve
2. Oculomotor nerve
3. Trochlear nerve
4. Trigeminal nerve
5. Abducens nerve
6. Facial nerve
7. Acoustic nerve
8. Olfactory nerve
9. Hypoglossal nerve

   ANSWERS: a-1, b-2, c-4, d-6, e-1, f-2

47. What is the name of the object that hangs down in the back of the throat?

a. Hard palate
b. Soft palate
c. Vallecula
d. Uvula

   ANSWER: d

48. On looking to the left, a patient has diplopia without nystagmus. Which nerve or region is paretic?

a. Left III or right VI
b. Right III or left VI
c. Left medial longitudinal fasciculus
d. Right medial longitudinal fasciculus

   ANSWER: b

49. Which nerve is responsible when the left eye fails to abduct fully on looking to the left?

a. Left III
b. Right III
c. Left VI
d. Right VI

   ANSWER: c

50. The patient's right eyelid has ptosis, the eye is abducted, and its pupil is dilated. Which nerve or region is injured?

a. Left III
b. Right III
c. Left VI
d. Right VI

   ANSWER: b

51. A 15-year-old girl is lethargic and disoriented, walks with an ataxic gait, and has slurred speech. She also has bilateral, horizontal, and vertical nystagmus. What is the most likely cause of her findings?

a. Multiple sclerosis
b. A cerebellar tumor
c. A psychogenic disturbance
d. None of the above

   ANSWER: d. She may be intoxicated with alcohol, barbiturates, or other drugs. A cerebellar tumor is an unlikely possibility without signs of raised intracranial pressure or corticospinal tract damage. Multiple sclerosis is unlikely because of her lethargy, disorientation, and young age.

52. A young man has suddenly developed vertigo, nausea, vomiting, and left-sided tinnitus. He has nystagmus to the right. What is the lesion?

a. Multiple sclerosis
b. A cerebellar tumor
c. A psychogenic disturbance
d. Labyrinthine dysfunction

ANSWER: d. The unilateral nystagmus, hearing abnormality, nausea, and vomiting are most likely caused by left-sided inner ear disease, such as labyrinthitis, rather than by neurologic dysfunction.

53. A 21-year-old soldier has vertical and horizontal nystagmus, mild spastic paraparesis, and ataxia of finger-to-nose motion bilaterally. Which region of the CNS is not affected?

a. Cerebrum
b. Brainstem
c. Cerebellum
d. Spinal cord

ANSWER: a. This patient has lesions in the brainstem causing nystagmus, in the cerebellum causing ataxia, and in the spinal cord causing paraparesis. The picture of scattered or "disseminated" lesions is typical of but not diagnostic of multiple sclerosis.

54. What is the lowermost (caudal) level of the CNS?

a. Foramen magnum
b. Slightly caudal to the thoracic vertebrae
c. The sacrum
d. None of the above

ANSWER: b. The spinal cord, which is one of the two major components of the CNS, has a caudal extent to the T12–L1 vertebrae.

55. A 35-year-old man, who has been shot in the back, has paresis of the right leg and loss of position and vibration sensation at the right ankle. Pinprick sensation is lost in the left leg. Where is the lesion?

a. Right side of the cervical spinal cord
b. Left side of the cervical spinal cord
c. Right side of the thoracic spinal cord
d. Left side of the thoracic spinal cord
e. Right side of the lumbosacral spinal cord
f. Left side of the lumbosacral spinal cord
g. One or both lumbar plexuses

ANSWER: c. The gunshot wound has caused hemitransection of the right side of the thoracic spinal cord (the Brown-Séquard syndrome, see Fig. 2–16). Occasionally, to alleviate intractable pain, neurosurgeons purposefully sever the lateral spinothalamic tract.

56–58. Match the numbered structures with their description.

a. Diencephalon
b. Midbrain
c. Pons
d. Medulla
e. Spinal cord
f. Anterior horn cells
g. Pyramids
h. Cerebellum
i. Locus ceruleus
j. Lateral ventricles
k. Third ventricle
l. Fourth ventricle
m. Subarachnoid space
n. Cranial nerve three
o. Cranial nerve four
p. Cranial nerve six
q. Aqueduct of Sylvius
r. Periaqueductal gray matter
s. Inferior olivary nucleus
t. Inferior cerebellar peduncle
u. Medial lemniscus
v. Caudate and putamen
w. Globus pallidus and putamen
x. Substantia nigra
y. Thalamus
z. Medial longitudinal fasciculus

56.

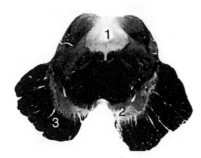

1. What is the name of the entire structure?
2. Which regions of the brain does structure "1" connect?
3. What is the region that surrounds structure "1"?

4. Where do the axons terminate that originate in structure "2"?
5. What is the termination of most of the axons that pass through structure "3"?

ANSWERS:

1. b. This is the midbrain, which is one of four regions of the brainstem (a–d). The midbrain's configuration is characterized by the ventral cleft, unstained semilunar regions, and the upper, central aqueduct.
2. k and l. Structure "1" is the aqueduct of Sylvius, which is the channel for cerebrospinal fluid (CSF) to flow from the third to fourth ventricles.
3. r. Periaqueductal gray matter
4. v. Structure "2" is the substantia nigra. Its neurons form the nigrostriatal tract, which terminates in the striatum (caudate and putamen).
5. f. Structure "3" is the cerebral peduncle, which carries the corticospinal tract. Most of its axons cross in the pyramids and terminate on the contralateral anterior horn cells of the spinal cord.

57.

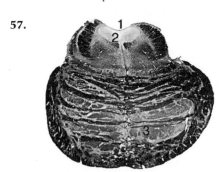

1. What is the name of the entire structure?
2. What is the name of the fluid-filled structure designated structure "1"?
3. Which structure lies dorsal to structure "1"?
4. Which cranial nerve nucleus is located at structure "2"?
5. Which white matter tract that connects the third and sixth cranial nerve nuclei lies near structure "2"?
6. In which two structures do axons passing through structure "3" terminate?

ANSWERS:

1. c. This is the pons. Its configuration is characterized by the bulbous ventral portion, the basis pontis.
2. l. The fourth ventricle lies dorsal to the pons and medulla.
3. h. The cerebellum forms the roof of the fourth ventricle (see Fig. 21–2 and Chapter 20).
4. p. The nuclei of the abducens nerves (cranial nerves VI) are located as a pair of midline dorsal structures in the pons. The nuclei of the other cranial nerves involved in ocular motility, the third and fourth cranial nerves, are similarly located as paired midline dorsal structures, but in the midbrain.
5. z. The MLF, a heavily myelinated tract, connects the sixth and contralateral third cranial nerve nuclei. It is essential for conjugate vision.
6. f and h. Structure "3," the basis pontis, contains the corticospinal tract that is descending and the pontocerebellar fibers that terminate in the cerebellum.

58.

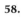
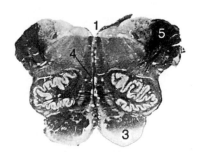

1. What is the name of the entire structure?
2. What is the name of the fluid-filled structure designated structure "1"?
3. Which structure lies dorsal to structure "1"?
4. What is the name of the pair of scalloped nuclei designated structure "2"?
5. Which structure, which transmits proprioception, is shown in structure "4"?
6. What is the common name of structure "5," which is also called the restiform body?

ANSWERS:

1. d. This is the medulla. The unique pair of scalloped nuclei (see below) readily identifies it.
2. l. The fourth ventricle lies dorsal to both the pons and medulla.
3. h. The cerebellum forms the roof of the fourth ventricle.
4. s. They are the inferior olivary nuclei. Although conspicuous and complex, they seem to be involved in only a few neurologic illnesses, such as olivopontocerebellar degeneration and palatal myoclonus.
5. u. Structure "4" is the decussation of the medial lemniscus where ascending proprioception and vibration sensation tracts cross to terminate in the contralateral thalamus.
6. t. The inferior cerebellar peduncle is located in the lateral medulla and contains fibers ascending from the spinal cord to the cerebellum.

59. Match the gait abnormalities (1–6), which are important neurologic signs, with their descriptions (a–f).

1. Apraxic
2. Astasia-abasia
3. Ataxic
4. Festinating
5. Hemiparetic
6. Steppage

a. Short-stepped, narrow-based with a shuffle
b. Impaired alternation of feet
c. Broad-based and lurching
d. Seeming to be extraordinarily unbalanced, but without falling
e. Swinging one leg outward with excessive wear on the inner sole
f. Excessively lifting the knees to raise the feet

ANSWERS: 1-b, 2-d, 3-c, 4-a, 5-e, 6-f

60. Match the neurologic conditions (a–f) with the gait abnormalities (1–6) they induce.

a. Cerebral infarction
b. Cerebellar degeneration
c. Parkinsonism
d. Normal pressure hydrocephalus
e. Hysteria
f. Tabes dorsalis

1. Apraxic
2. Astasia-abasia
3. Ataxic
4. Festinating
5. Hemiparetic
6. Steppage

ANSWERS: a-5, b-3, c-4, d-1, e-2, f-6. Normal pressure hydrocephalus is characterized by dementia, incontinence, and, most strikingly, apraxia of gait. Gait apraxia is characterized by an inability to alternate leg movements and inappropriately attempting to lift the weight-bearing foot. The feet are often immobile because the weight is not shifted to the forward foot, and the patient attempts to lift the same foot twice. The feet seem magnetized to the floor (see Fig. 7–7).

Astasia-abasia is a psychogenic pattern of walking in which the patient seems to alternate between a broad base for stability and a narrow, tightrope-like stance, with contortions of the chest and arms that give the appearance of falling (see Fig. 3–2).

Ataxia of the legs and trunk in cerebellar degeneration force the feet widely apart (in a broad base) to maintain stability. Because coordination is also impaired, the gait has an uneven, unsteady, lurching pattern (see Fig. 2–13).

Festinating gait, also called *marche à petits pas,* a feature of Parkinson's disease, is a shuffling, short-stepped gait with a tendency to accelerate.

Hemiparesis and increased tone (spasticity) from cerebral infarctions force patients to swing (circumduct) a paretic leg from the hip. Circumduction permits hemiparetic patients to walk if they can extend their hip and knee. The weak ankle drags the inner front surface of the foot (see Fig. 2–4).

Patients with tabes dorsalis have impairment of position sense. To prevent their toes from catching, especially when climbing stairs, patients raise their legs excessively.

61. Match the descriptions or characteristics (a–f) with the pictures (1, 2, 3).

a. Cerebral infarction
b. Loss of taste on one side of tongue
c. Idiopathic inflammation

d. Normal
e. Overexposure and drying of eye
f. Loss of the corneal reflex

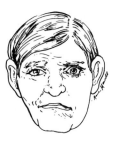 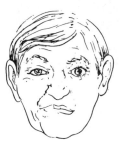 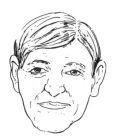

ANSWERS: a-2, b-1, c-1, d-3, e-1, f-1. Patient No. 1, who has weakness of his left upper and lower facial muscles, has Bell's palsy. With facial nerve damage, taste sensation is lost in the ipsilateral anterior two thirds of the tongue. Paresis of the eyelid muscles prevents spontaneous or reflex eyelid closure, which potentially results in corneal dehydration and foreign body irritation. Patient No. 2 has weakness of his left lower facial muscles. This pattern of facial weakness is typical of contralateral cerebral injuries and is usually accompanied by arm and leg weakness (i.e., hemiparesis). Patient No. 3 is normal.

62–67. This patient is looking slightly to her right and attempting to raise both arms. Her left eye deviates across the midline to the right, but her right eye cannot abduct. (The answers are provided after Question 67.)

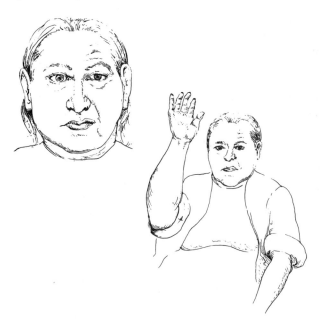

62. Paresis of which extraocular muscle prevents the affected eye from moving laterally?

a. Right superior oblique
b. Right abducens
c. Left abducens

d. Left lateral rectus
e. Right lateral rectus

63. The left face does not seem to be involved by the left hemiparesis. Why might the left side of the face be uninvolved?

a. It is. The left forehead and mouth are contorted.
b. The problem is in the right cerebral hemisphere.
c. The corticospinal tract is injured only after the corticobulbar tract has innervated the facial nerve.
d. The problem is best explained by postulating two lesions.

64. On which side of the body would a Babinski sign most likely be elicited?

a. Right
b. Left
c. Both
d. Neither

65. What is the most likely cause of this disorder?

a. Bell's palsy
b. Hysteria
c. Cerebral infarction
d. Medullary infarction
e. Pontine infarction
f. Midbrain infarction

66. With which conditions is such a lesion associated?

a. Homonymous hemianopsia
b. Diplopia
c. Impaired monocular visual acuity
d. Intellectual impairment
e. Aphasia if the patient were right cerebral dominant
f. Various nondominant hemisphere syndromes

67. Sketch the region of the damaged brain, inserting the damaged structures and the area of damage.

> **ANSWERS:** This patient has weakness of the right eye that prevents it from moving laterally, weakness of the right upper and lower face, and paresis of the left arm. She has injury of the right abducens and facial cranial nerves and the corticospinal tract before it crosses in the medulla. The lesion is located in the base of the pons and caused by an occlusion of a small branch of the basilar artery. 62-e, 63-c, 64-b, 65-e (A right pontine infarction would produce this condition by injuring the right sixth and seventh cranial nerves and corticospinal tract.), 66-b. Diplopia would be present on right lateral gaze.

PONS

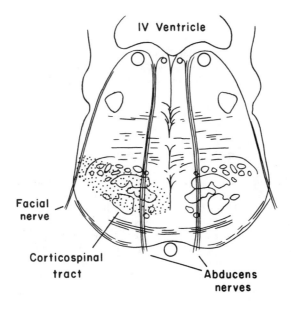

68. Where does the corticospinal tract cross as it descends?

a. Internal capsule
b. Base of the pons

c. Pyramids
d. Anterior horn cells

ANSWER: c. Because each corticospinal tract crosses in the pyramids, it is often called the "pyramidal tract."

69. Which artery supplies Broca's area and the adjacent corticospinal tract?

a. Anterior cerebral
b. Middle cerebral
c. Posterior cerebral

d. Basilar
e. Vertebral

ANSWER: b. The left middle cerebral artery

70. Which group of illnesses are all suggested by the presence of spasticity, clonus, hyperactive deep tendon reflexes, and Babinski signs?

a. Poliomyelitis, cerebrovascular accidents, spinal cord trauma
b. Bell's palsy, cerebrovascular accidents, psychogenic disturbances
c. Spinal cord trauma, cerebrovascular accidents, congenital cerebral injuries
d. Brainstem infarction, cerebellar infarction, spinal cord infarction
e. Parkinson's disease, cerebrovascular accidents, cerebellar infarction

ANSWER: c. The common denominator is UMN injury.

71. Which group of illnesses is suggested by the presence of muscles that are paretic, atrophic, and areflexic?

a. Poliomyelitis, diabetic peripheral neuropathy, traumatic brachial plexus injury
b. Amyotrophic lateral sclerosis, brainstem infarction, psychogenic disturbance
c. Spinal cord trauma, cerebrovascular accidents, congenital cerebral injuries
d. Brainstem infarction, cerebellar infarction, spinal cord infarction
e. Parkinson's disease, cerebrovascular accidents, cerebellar infarction
f. Guillain Barré syndrome, multiple sclerosis, and uremic neuropathy

ANSWER: a. The common denominator is LMN injury.

72. Match the location of the nerve, nucleus, or lesion (a–k) with its brainstem location (1–3):

a. Cranial nerve nucleus III
b. Cranial nerve nucleus IV
c. Cranial nerve nucleus VI
d. Cranial nerve nucleus VII
e. Cranial nerve nucleus IX
f. Cranial nerve nucleus X
g. Cranial nerve nucleus XI
h. Abducens paresis and contralateral hemiparesis
i. Abducens and facial paresis and contralateral hemiparesis
j. Palatal deviation to one side, contralateral Horner's syndrome, and ataxia
k. Miosis, ptosis, anhidrosis

1. Midbrain
2. Pons
3. Medulla

ANSWERS: a-1, b-1, c-2, d-2, e-3, f-3, g-3, h-2, i-2, j-3, k-3

73. During "Spring Break," a college student dove into the shallow end of a swimming pool. He struck his forehead firmly against the bottom. His friends noted that he was unconscious and resuscitated him. On recovery in the hospital several days later, he noticed that he had weakness in both hands. A neurologist finds that the intrinsic muscles of the hands are weak and DTRs in the arms are absent. Also, pain sensation is diminished, but position and vibration sensations are preserved. He has mild, aching neck pain. The legs are strong and have normal sensation, but their DTRs are brisk. Plantar reflexes are equivocal. There is a large, tender ecchymotic area on the forehead. Which of the following is the most likely cause of the hand weakness?

a. Cerebral concussion
b. Intoxication
c. Syringomyelia
d. Herniated intervertebral disk

ANSWER: c. Striking a forehead against the bottom of a swimming pool produces a forceful hyperextension (extreme backward bending) injury to the neck, as well as head trauma. In this case, the spinal cord developed a hematomyelia or syringomyelia (syrinx) probably because of bleeding into the center of the spinal cord. The cervical spinothalamic tracts as they cross the spinal cord are ripped by the hematoma as it expands the central canal of the spinal cord. The corticospinal tracts destined for the legs are compressed. In this type of swimming pool accident, victims should be evaluated for alcohol and drug intoxication and for sequelae of head trauma. Similar situations occur in motor vehicle crashes where the victim's forehead strikes the inside of the windshield and in sports accidents where the athlete's head and neck are snapped backward.

74. A 65-year-old man describes many problems, but his most bothersome is loss of hearing in both ears during the previous 6 to 12 months. This problem began with his being unable to distinguish his dinner partner's conversation in restaurants. It progressed to his being unable to hear telephone conversations. He began to withdraw from social occasions. Audiometry shows bilateral high-tone hearing loss. In addition, he has difficulty recalling names of recent acquaintances, impaired vibratory sense in his toes, and mild bilateral anosmia. However, he does not have dementia. What should the physician do first?

a. Obtain an MRI of the head
b. Do a spinal tap
c. Obtain a serum vitamin B_{12} level
d. Advise him to obtain a hearing aid

ANSWER: d. His symptoms are attributable to "normal changes of old age." The initial manifestation of age-related hearing loss, *presbycusis,* is loss of speech discrimination, especially in crowded situations. It interferes with social and cognitive function. It is severe enough at times to give the false impression of dementia. In presbycusis, audiometry initially shows loss of high tones but eventually loss in all frequencies. Without delay, he should be fitted for a hearing aid.

75. In the examination of a patient, which maneuver reveals most about the function of the patient's motor system?

a. Testing plantar reflexes
b. Manual muscle testing
c. Deep tendon reflex testing
d. Observation of the patient's gait

ANSWER: d. To walk normally a person must have normal corticospinal tracts and LMNs, coordination, proprioception, and balance.

76. Which structure separates the cerebrum from the cerebellum?

a. CSF
b. Foramen magnum
c. Falx
d. Tentorium

ANSWER: d. The tentorium lies above the cerebellum (see Fig. 20–16).

77. Which of the structures in question 76 separate the two cerebral hemispheres?

ANSWER: c. The falx cerebri, which often gives rise to meningiomas, separates the cerebral hemispheres.

78. Which two cranial nerves convey taste sensation from the tongue to the brain?

a. V and VII
b. VII and IX
c. IX and X
d. IX and XI

ANSWER: b. The facial nerve (VII) conveys taste sensation from the anterior two thirds of the tongue and the glossopharyngeal nerve (IX) from the posterior one third.

79. Which will be the pattern of a myelin stain of the cervical spinal cord's ascending tracts several years after a thoracic gunshot wound?

a. The entire cervical spinal cord will be normal.
b. The myelin will be unstained.
c. The fasciculus cuneatus will be black, and the f. gracilis will be unstained.
d. The f. gracilis will be black, and the f. cuneatus will be unstained.

ANSWER: c. Because the f. cuneatus arises from the arms and upper trunk, it will be un-injured and normally absorb stain. Therefore, the ascending tracts, being normal, will be stained black. In contrast, the f. gracilis will be unstained because myelin will be lost distal (downstream) from the lesion. The corticospinal tracts, which are descending, will be normally stained black because they originate proximal to the lesion.

80. A 20-year-old man has become progressively dysarthric during the previous 2 years. He has no mental impairments or cranial nerve abnormalities. His legs have mild weakness and Babinski signs but poorly reactive DTRs. All his limbs are ataxic and his speech is scanning. He has impaired position and vibration sensation in his hands and feet. His feet have a high arch, elevated dorsum, and retracted first metatarsal. His two younger brothers seem to have the same problem. Both his parents, three aunts and uncles, and two older siblings have no neurologic symptoms or physical abnormalities. Which of the following genetic features will probably be found on further evaluation of the patient?

a. Excessive trinucleotide repeats on both alleles of chromosome 9
b. Excessive trinucleotide repeats on only one allele of chromosome 6
c. Two Y chromosomes, giving him an XYY karyotype
d. Two X chromosomes, giving him an XXY karyotype

ANSWER: a. The patient and his two younger brothers have Friedreich's ataxia, which is characterized by posterior column sensory abnormalities, Babinski signs, limb ataxia, scanning speech, and the characteristic foot deformity, "pes cavus." Friedreich's ataxia is an autosomal recessive condition resulting from excessive trinucleotide repeats on chromosome 9. Spinocerebellar ataxia, which has at least six varieties, is an autosomal dominant disorder with predominantly cerebellar dysfunction.

81. A man with diabetic neuropathy is unable to stand erect with feet together and eyes closed. When attempting this maneuver, he tends to topple, but he catches himself before falling. What is the name of this sign (a–d), and to which region of the nervous system (1–5) is it referable in this patient?

a. Hoover's
b. Babinski's
c. Chvostek's
d. Romberg's

1. Cerebrum
2. Cerebellum
3. Spinal cord
4. Labyrinthine system
5. Peripheral nerves

ANSWER: d, 5. He has a Romberg's sign, but it results from PNS rather than CNS disease. Falling over when standing erect and deprived of visual sensory input suggests a loss of joint position sense from the legs. When deprived of vision and joint position sense, people must rely on labyrinthine (vestibular) input, but that input is effective only with rapid or relatively large changes in position. It is activated when people start to fall and prevents their tumbling over.

Romberg's sign was classically attributed to injury of the spinal cord's posterior columns because position sense from the feet would not be conveyed to the brain. It is a classic sign of combined system disease and tabes dorsalis—conditions in which the posterior columns are destroyed. Romberg's sign is now detected most often in people with peripheral neuropathy who have lost position sense, as well as other sensations, in their feet and ankles.

82. In which conditions would Romberg's sign be detectable?

a. Tabes dorsalis
b. Multiple sclerosis
c. Combined system disease
d. Alcoholism

e. Diabetes
f. Uremia
g. Cerebellar disease
h. Blindness

ANSWER: a–f. Impairment of either the peripheral nerves (d–f) or the posterior columns of the spinal cord (a–c) can cause Romberg's sign. However, closing the eyes will not make a person more unstable with either cerebellar disease or blindness.

83. A 25-year-old man who has had diabetes mellitus since childhood develops erectile dysfunction. He has been found previously to have retrograde ejaculation during an evaluation for sterility. Examination of his fundi reveals hemorrhages and exudates. He has absent DTRs at the wrists and ankles, loss of position and vibration sensation at the ankles, and no demonstrable anal or cremasteric reflexes. Which three other conditions are likely to be present?

a. Urinary bladder hypotonicity
b. Bilateral Babinski signs
c. Gastroenteropathy
d. Dementia
e. Anhidrosis

ANSWER: a, c, e. He has a combination of peripheral and autonomic system neuropathy because of diabetes mellitus. A peripheral neuropathy is suggested by the distal sensory and reflex loss and the absent anal and cremasteric reflexes. Autonomic neuropathy is suggested by the retrograde ejaculation. Common manifestations of autonomic neuropathy are erectile dysfunction, urinary bladder hypotonicity, gastroenteropathy, and anhidrosis.

5

Peripheral Nerve Disorders

By relying on clinical findings, physicians can distinguish peripheral nervous system (PNS) from central nervous system (CNS) disorders. In PNS disorders, damage to one, a group, or all peripheral nerves causes readily identifiable patterns of paresis, deep tendon reflex (DTR) loss, and sensory impairments. Some PNS disorders are associated with mental changes, systemic illness, or a fatal outcome.

ANATOMY

The spinal cord's *anterior horn cells* form the motor neurons of the peripheral nerves. These nerves are the final links in the neuron chain that transmit motor commands from the brain through the spinal cord to muscles (Fig. 5–1). Anterior spinal cord "roots" mingle within the brachial or lumbosacral plexuses to form the major peripheral nerves, such as the femoral and radial nerves. Although peripheral nerves are quite long, especially in the legs, they faithfully conduct electrochemical impulses over considerable distances. The impulses are not dissipated because *myelin*, which is a lipid-based sheath made by Schwann cells, surrounds peripheral nerves and acts as insulation.

When stimulated, the nerves release acetylcholine (ACh) in packets from storage vesicles at the neuromuscular junction. The ACh packets traverse the neuromuscular junction and bind onto specific ACh receptors on the muscle end plate. The interaction of ACh and its receptors depolarizes the muscle membrane and initiates a muscle contraction (see Chapter 6). Neuromuscular transmission culminating in muscle depolarization is a deliberate, discrete, and quantitative action. Thus, ACh does not merely ooze out of the presynaptic terminal as loose molecules and drift across the neuromuscular junction.

Sensory information is also transmitted by peripheral nerves, but in reverse direction, from the PNS to the CNS. Impulses from the various types of receptors—pain, temperature, vibration, and position, which are located in the skin, tendons, and joints—flow through peripheral nerves to the spinal cord.

MONONEUROPATHIES

Disorders of single peripheral nerves, *mononeuropathies*, are characterized by flaccid paresis, DTR loss *(areflexia)*, and reduced sensation, particularly pain *(hypalgesia or analgesia*, Table 5–1). However, sometimes mononeuropathies and other peripheral nerve injuries lead paradoxically to spontaneously occurring painful sensations *(painful paresthesias)* or the misperception of neutral stimulation as pain *(dysesthesia)*.

Penetrating and blunt injuries often cause mononeuropathies. Another common nerve injury is compression, especially of those nerves protected only by overlying

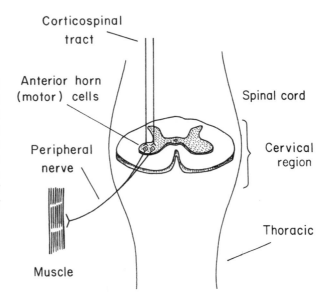

FIGURE 5–1. The corticospinal tracts, as discussed in Chapter 2 and as their name indicates, consist of upper motor neurons (UMNs) that travel from the motor cortex to the spinal cord. They synapse on the spinal cord's *anterior horn cells,* which give rise to the lower motor neurons. These neurons join sensory fibers to form peripheral nerves.

skin and subcutaneous tissue. People most susceptible to compression injuries are diabetics; those rapidly losing weight, which depletes nerves' protective myelin covering; or those found in disjointed positions for long periods possibly because of drug or alcohol abuse. For example, the radial nerve is compressed where it winds around the humerus. People in an alcohol-induced stupor who lean against their upper arm for several hours are apt to develop a *wrist drop* (Fig. 5–2, left). *Foot drop,* the lower extremity counterpart, is caused by an injury to the common peroneal nerve by prolonged leg crossing or a constrictive cast compressing the nerve as it winds around the neck of the fibula.

A variation on the theme of pressure-induced mononeuropathy is the *carpal tunnel syndrome,* which results from entrapment of the median nerve as it travels through the carpel tunnel of the flexor surface of the wrist. The median nerve may be injured by repetitive stresses, such as keyboarding and some kinds of assembly line work, or by fluid retention, especially during pregnancy.

In carpal tunnel syndrome, paresthesias and pain usually shoot from the wrist to the palm, thumb, and adjacent two fingers (Fig. 5–2, right). Symptoms are characteristically worse at night. Typically, pain awakens victims who shake their hands in

TABLE 5–1. *Major Mononeuropathies*

Nerve	Motor Paresis	DTR Lost	Pain or Sensory Loss	Examples
Median	Thumb and wrist flexor (thenar atrophy)	None	Thumb, second and third fingers	Carpal tunnel syndrome
Ulnar	Finger and thumb adduction ("claw hand")	None	Fourth and fifth fingers	
Radial	Wrist and thumb extensors	Brachioradialis*	Dorsum of hand	Wrist drop from overdose
Femoral	Knee extensors	Quadriceps (knee)	Anterior thigh, medial calf	
Sciatic	Ankle dorsiflexors and plantar flexors ("flail ankle")	Achilles (ankle)	Buttock, lateral calf, and most of foot	Sciatica from a herniated disk
Peroneal	Ankle dorsiflexors and evertors	None	Dorsum of foot and lateral calf	Foot drop from lower knee injury

*When the radial nerve is damaged by compression in the spiral groove of the humerus, the triceps DTR is spared.

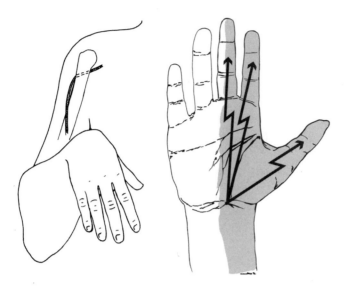

FIGURE 5–2. *Left,* As the radial nerve winds around the humerus, it is vulnerable to compression. Radial nerve damage leads to the readily recognizable *wrist drop* that results from paresis of the extensor muscles of the wrist, finger, and thumb. *Right,* The usual sensory distribution of the median nerve is the medial palmar surface of the lower forearm and palm, thenar eminence (thumb base), thumb, and adjacent two fingers. In carpal tunnel syndrome, with median nerve entrapment, pain typically spreads downward from the wrist in the median nerve distribution. However, the pattern is variable within the hand and fingers, and sometimes the paresthesias spread upward (proximal) from the wrist.

attempting to find relief. The characteristic *Tinel's sign* may be elicited by percussing the wrist, which generates electric sensations that shoot into the palm and fingers. With chronic carpal tunnel syndrome, prolonged median nerve entrapment leads to thenar (thumb) muscle weakness and atrophy.

Mononeuropathies can also result from systemic illnesses, such as diabetes mellitus, vasculitis (e.g., lupus erythematosus, polyarteritis nodosa), and lead intoxication (see below). In most of these conditions, the symptoms are painful and sudden in onset but apt to resolve spontaneously or with specific treatment. Vasculitis and other illnesses can cause stroke-like CNS insults as well as PNS injuries.

MONONEURITIS MULTIPLEX

This complex PNS condition consists of multiple peripheral injuries that are often accompanied by cranial nerve injuries. For example, a patient with injury of the left radial, right sciatic, and right third cranial nerve would have mononeuritis multiplex. It is usually the result of a systemic illness, such as diabetes mellitus, vasculitis, or, in Africa and Asia, leprosy.

POLYNEUROPATHIES (NEUROPATHIES)

The most frequently occurring PNS disorder, *polyneuropathy* or, for short, *neuropathy,* is generalized, symmetric involvement of all peripheral nerves. In certain neuropathies, cranial nerves may also be involved. Many neuropathies first affect the ends of nerves, so that patients' earliest symptoms are in the toes and feet and then in the fingers and hands.

Patients' symptoms can reflect both sensory and motor impairment, but in many neuropathies one or the other impairment may predominate. Patients with "sensory neuropathy" usually have numbness and paresthesias in the distal part of their arms or legs and typically describe "burning" or "numbness" in their fingers and toes (i.e., *stocking-glove hypalgesia*) (Fig. 5–3). Sometimes the paresthesias are so disconcerting that they provoke involuntary leg movements, such as in *restless leg syndrome* (see

Chapter 17). In contrast to their distressing sensory problems, these patients have little or no weakness.

Patients with "motor neuropathy" have distal limb weakness that impairs fine, skilled movements (e.g., buttoning a shirt). In addition, because their ankle and toe muscles are much weaker than their hip muscles, they will have difficulty raising their feet when they walk or climb stairs. Neuropathy usually leads to muscle weakness, atrophy, and flaccidity. It also diminishes wrist and ankle DTRs because of lower motor neuron injury (see Fig. 2–2, C).

Mental Status Usually Unaffected

Most neuropathies are usually unaccompanied by mental status changes and do not give rise to consultations with psychiatrists (Table 5–2). Nevertheless, several of these neuropathies should be particularly important to psychiatrists because they are common, exemplify general neurologic principles, and are occasionally associated with mental status changes that only prepared physicians will appreciate.

Guillain-Barré Syndrome.   Acute inflammatory demyelinating polyradiculoneuropathy (AIDP) or postinfectious demyelinating polyneuropathy, commonly known as Guillain-Barré syndrome, is the quintessential PNS illness. Although often idiopathic, this syndrome typically follows an upper respiratory or gastrointestinal illness. Cases following a week's episode of watery diarrhea are apt to be associated

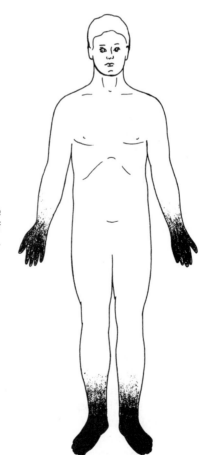

FIGURE 5–3. In polyneuropathy, pain and other sensations are lost symmetrically and most severely in the distal portions of the limbs. The legs are more severely affected than the arms. This disturbance is termed *stocking-glove hypalgesia.*

TABLE 5–2. *Important Causes of Neuropathy*

Endogenous toxins
  Acute intermittent and variegate porphyria*
  Diabetes mellitus
  Uremia*
Nutritional deficiencies
  Combined system disease/pernicious anemia*
  Starvation: dieting, malabsorption, alcoholism*
Medicines
  Antibiotics: Anti-human immunodeficiency virus (HIV) (dideoxyinosine, dideoxycyti-
    dine), tuberculosis (isoniazid), nitrofurantoin
  Antineoplastic agents
  Vitamin B_6 (pyridoxine), in high doses
Industrial or chemical toxins†
  Metals: lead, arsenic, organic and inorganic mercury
  Nitrous oxide (anesthesia)
  Organic solvents: *n*-hexane, toluene,* and others
Infectious/inflammatory conditions
  Infectious: mononucleosis, hepatitis, Lyme disease,* idiopathic (Guillain-Barré), leprosy,
    syphilis,* acquired immunodeficiency syndrome*
  Vasculitis: systemic lupus erythematosus, polyarteritis*
Genetic diseases
  Charcot-Marie-Tooth disease
  Friedreich's ataxia and other spinocerebellar degenerations
  Metachromatic leukodystrophy*

*Associated with mental status abnormalities.
†May be substances of abuse.

with a gastrointestinal *Campylobacter jejuni* infection and be more extensive, severe, and slower to recover. Similarly, Guillain-Barré syndrome is an occasional complication of mononucleosis, Lyme disease, hepatitis, cytomegalovirus (CMV), or human immunodeficiency virus (HIV) infection.

In general, young and middle-aged adults first develop paresthesias and numbness in the fingers and toes and then areflexic, flaccid paresis of their feet and legs. Weakness, which then becomes a much greater problem than numbness, ascends to involve the hands and arms. Many patients develop respiratory distress from involvement of the phrenic and intercostal nerves and must be intubated for respirator assistance. If weakness ascends further, patients develop cranial nerve involvement that leads to dysphagia and other aspects of bulbar palsy (see Chapter 4), facial weakness, and ocular immobility. Nevertheless, possibly because optic and acoustic nerves are protected by myelin generated by the CNS—not the PNS—patients continue to see and hear. Despite total paralysis, they are typically conscious. They are in a *locked-in syndrome* (see Chapter 11). Their cerebrospinal fluid (CSF) exhibits elevated protein concentration but few white cells (i.e., classic "albuminocytologic dissociation") (see Table 20–1).

This illness usually resolves almost completely within 3 weeks to 3 months as the PNS myelin is regenerated. The severity and duration of the paresis can be reduced by plasmapheresis (plasma exchange), which presumably filters a toxic antibody from the serum, or by intravenous administration of human immunoglobulin (IVIG), which "blocks" the antibody.

The significance of the Guillain-Barré syndrome is not only that it is a life-threatening illness but that it epitomizes the distinction between PNS and CNS diseases. Although paraparesis or quadriparesis might be a common feature, brain or spinal cord injuries and neuropathies cause different patterns of muscle weakness, change in reflexes, and sensory distribution (Table 5–3). Also, in Guillain-Barré syndrome, as in most neuropathies other than diabetic neuropathy (see below), bladder, bowel, and sexual function are preserved. These pelvic organs might be spared in neuropathies because the nerves innervating them are the relatively short fibers of the autonomic nervous system. In contrast, patients with spinal cord disease usually have incontinence and impotence at the onset of the injury.

Another distinction is seen between demyelinating diseases of the CNS and PNS. Despite performing a similar insulating function, CNS and PNS myelin differ in chemical composition, antigenicity, and cells of origin. Oligodendrocytes produce CNS myelin, and Schwann cells produce PNS myelin (i.e., oligodendrocytes are to Schwann cells as the CNS is to the PNS). From a clinical viewpoint, although damaged PNS myelin is regenerated and patients with Guillain-Barré syndrome usually recover, damaged CNS myelin is not regenerated and impairment is permanent.

CNS demyelination, as in multiple sclerosis (MS), results in recurring, cumulative deficits referable to several CNS areas, including the optic nerves (see Chapter 15). The partial or even complete recovery that MS patients achieve between episodes results more from the resolution of the inflammatory response rather than the regeneration of myelin. When MS affects large areas of cerebral CNS myelin, it routinely results in dementia and other mental changes.

From another perspective, patients with uncomplicated cases of Guillain-Barré syndrome, despite profound motor impairment, should not develop mental aberrations because it is a disease of the PNS. However, mental changes do develop in patients who have complications, which include cerebral anoxia from respiratory insufficiency, "steroid psychosis" from high-dose steroid treatment (now outdated), hydrocephalus from impaired CSF reabsorption, fluid and electrolyte imbalance, or sleep deprivation. Therefore, psychiatric consultants should look for hypoxia and other serious medical complications in patients with Guillain-Barré syndrome who develop mental aberrations. Also, unless the patient is already on a respirator, they should avoid prescribing sedatives and neuroleptics that might further depress respiration.

Diabetes.   Although rigid treatment of diabetes may forestall or even prevent development of diabetic neuropathy, most patients who have diabetes for more than 10 years lose sensation and DTRs in their feet and ankles. In contrast, strength remains relatively normal. With long-standing diabetic neuropathy, sensation in the fingertips is impaired, preventing blind diabetics from "reading" Braille. In addition

TABLE 5–3. *Differences between CNS and PNS Signs*

	CNS	**PNS**
Motor system	*Upper motor neuron*	*Lower motor neuron*
Paresis	Patterns*	Distal
Tone	Spastic†	Flaccid
Bulk	Normal	Atrophic
Fasciculations	No	Sometimes
Reflexes		
DTRs	Hyperactive	Hypoactive
Plantar	Babinski sign(s)	Absent
Sensory loss	Patterns*	Hands and feet

*Examples: motor and sensory loss of one side or lower half of the body (e.g., hemiparesis or paraparesis) and hemisensory loss.
†May be flaccid initially.

to neuropathy, diabetic patients suffer from suddenly occurring painful mononeuropathies and mononeuritis multiplex. By a different mechanism—damaging blood vessels—diabetes can lead to cerebrovascular disease that may cause multi-infarct (vascular) dementia.

Diabetic neuropathy often causes painful paresthesias. Typically patients feel a burning sensation in their feet, which is especially distressing at night. Various pain-relieving strategies are helpful, but none help the majority of patients. Several tricyclic antidepressants and an antiepileptic drug, gabapentin (see Chapter 10), may reduce the pain and promote sleep. Selective serotonin reuptake inhibitors (SSRIs) rarely help, except perhaps when depression is a major component of the problem. A skin cream containing capsaicin (Zostrix), which depletes the putative neurotransmitter for pain, substance P, is analgesic. If these remedies fail, prescribing narcotics is justifiable (see Chapter 14).

Patients can also have autonomic nervous system damage that includes impaired gastrointestinal mobility, bladder muscle contraction, and sexual function. In fact, erectile dysfunction is sometimes the first or most disturbing symptom of diabetic autonomic neuropathy (see Chapter 16).

Toxic-Metabolic Disorders.   Neuropathies also result from numerous toxins, metabolic derangements, and medications. Uremia is a common cause of neuropathy, and it is almost universal in patients undergoing maintenance hemodialysis. Neuropathy also commonly results from medications used for chemotherapy of neoplasms and HIV treatment (see below), but it has not complicated neuroleptic or antidepressant usage.

Lead poisoning is a neurologic condition that has reached the level of a public health problem because young children with pica (craving for unnatural foods), possibly from hunger, eat lead-pigment paint chips from decaying tenement walls. (Lead paint on interior walls has been illegal for decades in most cities.) These children develop lead poisoning that causes mental retardation and poor school performance. In contrast, because lead has a different deleterious effect on the mature nervous system, adults with lead poisoning develop mononeuropathies, such as a foot drop or wrist drop. Adults usually develop lead poisoning from industrial exposure or drinking homemade alcohol distilled with lead pipes ("moonshine").

Aging-Related Changes.   Although the condition is not yet considered a neuropathy and has not yet received a name, as people age they develop sensory loss from peripheral nerve degeneration. Almost all people who are older than 80 years have lost some joint position and a great deal of vibratory sensation in their feet. This sensory neuropathy, which is accompanied by absent ankle DTRs, prevents them from standing with their feet placed closely together, impairs their gait, and predisposes them to falling.

Mental Status Usually Affected

Although the neuropathies described in the previous section may be painful, incapacitating, or otherwise devastating to the PNS, they generally do not cause mental aberrations. Most people who are old, diabetic, on hemodialysis, or receiving chemotherapy, remain intelligent, thoughtful, and competent. The combination of dementia and neuropathy, reflecting both CNS and PNS damage, is found in only a few disease categories (see Table 5-2). An analogous, useful perspective is the combination of dementia and movement disorders, which indicates cerebral cortex and basal ganglia damage (see Table 18-4).

Nutritional Deficiencies.   Deficiencies of thiamine (vitamin B_1), niacin (nicotinic acid, vitamin B_3), or vitamin B_{12} each produce a neuropathy that is predominantly sensory and accompanied by dementia or other mental status abnormality. Gastrectomy, gastric bypass surgery, and inflammatory bowel disease can lead to malabsorption of these vitamins or their carrier-fats. Starvation can also lead to vitamin deficiency; however, few patients with anorexia nervosa or self-imposed extreme diets develop a neuropathy, possibly because of a selective, possibly secret, intake of food or vitamin pills.

Alcohol-induced neuropathy is virtually synonymous with thiamine deficiency because almost all cases result from alcoholics subsisting on alcohol and carbohydrate foods that are devoid of thiamine. Similarly, starvation or malabsorption causes thiamine deficiency neuropathy. Contrary to popular opinion, alcohol itself may not cause a neuropathy.

Patients with alcohol-induced neuropathy have loss of position sensation and absent DTRs. The disorder is usually asymptomatic until patients walk in the dark when they must rely on position sense generated in the legs and feet. In the well-known *Wernicke-Korsakoff syndrome*, alcohol-induced neuropathy is accompanied by amnesia, dementia, cerebellar degeneration, and, in the acute illness, nystagmus and ocular-motor paresis (see Chapter 7).

Niacin deficiency causes *pellagra*. In this disorder, starved people suffer from dementia, dermatitis, and diarrhea—the "three D's." Although a neuropathy has also often been attributed to pellagra, it may actually be the result of other vitamin deficiencies.

Combined system disease (pernicious anemia) or vitamin B_{12} deficiency causes a neuropathy overshadowed by anemia, dementia, or spinal cord impairment (see Fig. 2–17, *B*). Vitamin B_{12} deficiency usually results from pernicious anemia, malabsorption, a pure vegetarian diet, or even a brief exposure to nitrous oxide (N_2O), the common gaseous dental anesthetic.

The screening test for vitamin B_{12} deficiency is simply to determine the serum vitamin B_{12} level. In equivocal cases, especially where mental or spinal cord abnormalities are not accompanied by anemia, determining the serum homocysteine and methylmalonic acid levels is useful because they will both be elevated in vitamin B_{12} deficiency. Intrinsic factor antibodies, a classic finding, will be detectable in only about 60% of cases. The standard confirmatory test is the Schilling test. Most important, combined system disease is best known as a "correctable cause of dementia" because vitamin B_{12} injections can reverse the cognitive impairment, as well as its physical CNS and PNS manifestations.

Excessive intake of certain vitamins is also deleterious. Several food faddists developed a profound sensory neuropathy from excessive vitamin B_6 (pyridoxine) intake. Although the normal adult daily requirement of this vitamin is only 2 to 4 mg daily, they had been consuming several grams. Similarly, high vitamin A intake may cause pseudotumor cerebri (see Chapter 9) or induce fetal abnormalities (see Chapter 13).

Infectious Diseases.   Several common organisms that generally spare the CNS have a predilection for infecting the peripheral nerves. For example, *herpes zoster* infects a single nerve root or a branch of the trigeminal nerve, usually in people older than 65 years or those with an impaired immune system. It causes an ugly red vesicular eruption ("shingles"), which may be excruciatingly painful long after the infection (see Chapter 14). Leprosy, infection with *Mycobacterium leprae* (Hansen's disease), causes anesthetic, hypopigmented patches of skin, anesthetic fingers and toes, and palpable nerves. The cool portions of the body, such as the nose, ear lobes, and digits, are the most severely affected.

Some systemic infections involve the CNS as well as the PNS. Named for the town in Connecticut where it was discovered, *Lyme disease* has become endemic in New England, eastern Long Island, Wisconsin, Minnesota, and the Pacific Northwest. Caused by a spirochete, *Borrelia burgdorferi*, whose vector is a tick, Lyme disease's peak incidence is June through September, when people walk in wooded areas. Reminiscent of the dreaded spirochete infection, syphilis, Lyme disease has indolent, multisystem manifestations that include malaise, low-grade fever, cardiac arrhythmias, arthritis, and a pathognomonic bull's-eye-shaped rash, *erythema migrans* (moving red rash), surrounding the tick bite.

PNS involvement, its most common neurologic manifestation, induces facial nerve palsy, similar to Bell's palsy, either unilaterally or bilaterally (see Fig. 4–14). It also causes paresthesias, weakness, and, in extreme cases, Guillain-Barré syndrome. When the CNS is involved, patients may have dementia and other mental status abnormalities (see Chapter 7), headache, and chronic fatigue (see Chapter 6) but few physical signs.

In many cases of neurologic involvement, the CSF will have pleocytosis, abnormal protein and glucose concentrations, and Lyme antibodies, which is indicative of meningitis. Serologic tests for Lyme disease are notoriously inaccurate. Also, because a spirochete is the infectious agent, patients may have biologic false-positive tests for syphilis (see Chapter 7).

The most widespread infection of the CNS and PNS is *acquired immunodeficiency syndrome (AIDS)*. In it, HIV or CMV infection, abnormal immune mechanisms, or a necrotizing vasculitis produce a variety of debilitating PNS problems. Neuropathy is the most common AIDS-associated peripheral nerve disorder, but patients sometimes develop mononeuritis multiplex or Guillain-Barré syndrome. Paradoxically, several anti-HIV medications, such as ddI (dideoxyinosine, Videx) and ddC (dideoxycytidine, Hivid), sometimes cause temporary anesthesia and burning paresthesias. AIDS also predisposes to the meningovascular varieties of syphilis (acute meningitis or encephalitis) rather than the chronic varieties (dementia or tabes dorsalis).

Inherited Metabolic Illnesses.   Although numerous genetically determined illnesses cause neuropathy, two are notorious because they also cause psychosis.

Acute intermittent porphyria (AIP), the classic autosomal dominant genetic disorder of porphyrin metabolism, causes dramatic attacks of colicky abdominal pain, psychosis, and quadriparesis. During attacks, the urine turns red because, as the Watson-Schwartz and other tests show, it contains porphyrins. Although attacks may be exacerbated if the patient is given barbiturates, phenothiazines may be given for psychosis. Despite its prominence as an examination question, AIP is rare in the United States.

Metachromatic leukodystrophy (MLD), an autosomal recessive illness, is named for the metachromatic granules that accumulate in the brain, peripheral nerves, and many nonneurologic organs. MLD, like MS (see Chapter 15), causes demyelination of the CNS white matter (*leuko*dystrophy), and, to a lesser extent, of the PNS. It also causes extensive nonneurologic problems.

MLD usually becomes apparent in infants and children, but it often develops in young adults (typically, age 30 years). In them, MLD causes progressively severe personality changes, cognitive impairment, or psychosis. These MLD-induced mental disturbances are usually accompanied by peripheral neuropathy. Physical signs of CNS demyelination—commonly spasticity and ataxia—complicate the clinical picture and eventually overshadow both the mental disturbances and peripheral neuropathy.

In MLD, activity of the enzyme arylsulfatase A is markedly decreased in the urine, leukocytes, serum, and amniotic fluid, leading to abnormalities in the gallbladder, testicles, retinas, and other organs. MLD is diagnosed by showing reduced arylsulfatase A activity in leukocytes and finding metachromatic lipid material in biopsy specimens of peripheral nerves. As in MS, magnetic resonance imaging (MRI) shows lesions in the cerebral and cerebellar myelin (see Chapters 15 and 20). The pathology has been delineated, but no treatment arrests the illness.

Volatile Substance Exposure.   Industrial organic solvents, which are generally lipophilic and volatile at room temperature, enter the body through inhalation, absorption through the skin, or occasionally by ingestion. Workers most liable to be exposed include those in electronic assembly, paint and varnish manufacturing, and metal-part degreasing. However, toxic exposures are related more to poor ventilation or inadequate safety barriers than particular industries. Also, many of these neurologic disorders are self-inflicted during substance abuse.

Industrial solvents, such as ethylene oxide and carbon disulfide, can attack both the PNS and CNS. Besides causing a neuropathy, they can bring about various neuropsychologic symptoms—cognitive impairment, personality changes, inattention, depression, headaches, and fatigue—together termed "solvent-induced encephalopathy." In addition, carbon disulfide, unlike almost all other solvents, can cause psychosis.

Because symptoms of solvent-induced encephalopathy are usually nonspecific, inconsistent between workers, and largely subjective, diagnostic criteria have been controversial. Another diagnostic problem is that common conditions, such as depression and alcohol abuse, can mimic or contribute to solvent-induced encephalopathy. In addition, concentrations to which workers can be safely exposed for long periods have not been established and the neuropsychologic tests are often unreliable.

However, neurologic damage from recreational abuse or, in the extreme, addictive compulsive inhaling of certain volatile substances ("huffing") is unequivocal. In "glue sniffing," a classic example, the intoxicating component is the common hydrocarbon solvent, *n*-hexane. Sensation-seekers and overexposed industrial workers develop neuropathy because *n*-hexane damages PNS myelin.

Likewise, toluene, which is a component of spray paint and glue, damages CNS myelin. Its victims develop cognitive impairment, pyramidal and cerebellar injury, and even optic nerve damage. In chronic abusers, toluene induces dementia that is proportional to cerebral myelin injury. Severe toluene-induced cerebral demyelination can be seen on MRI.

Another potentially hazardous volatile substance is N_2O, which is often abused to produce a few minutes of euphoria. In addition to being administered by dentists for anesthesia, it is readily available as the gas in cartridges used to make whipped cream at home. Inhaling nitrous oxide, even intermittently for several weeks, may induce a profound neuropathy. Brief exposures can cause vitamin B_{12} deficiency, as previously mentioned. Succumbing to N_2O abuse, with its neurologic consequences, is an occupational hazard for dentists.

MOTOR NEURON DISORDERS

Amyotrophic Lateral Sclerosis

Amyotrophic lateral sclerosis (ALS) was known for decades as "Lou Gehrig's disease" because the famous baseball player Lou Gehrig had this dreadful, untreatable illness at the height of his career. Among neurologists, ALS is known as the classic *motor neuron disease* because both upper and lower motor neurons (UMN and LMN) degenerate while other neurologic systems—notably mental faculties—are spared.

The etiology of ALS remains an enigma, but one clue includes the 5% to 10% of patients with an autosomal dominant inheritance pattern. These patients carry an abnormal gene (the Cu, Zn superoxide dismutase [SOD1] gene), located on chromosome 21, that normally assists in detoxifying superoxide free radicals. Clues indicating that ALS is not an autoimmune disease are the absence of inflammatory reaction around degenerating motor neurons and lack of positive serologic test results. The response of patients, albeit modest, to blocking the excitatory neurotransmitter glutamate (see Chapter 21), suggests that glutamate "excitotoxicity" is somehow responsible for the disorder

People develop ALS at a median age of 66 years. The first symptoms are weakness, atrophy, and subcutaneous muscular twitching *(fasciculations)*—a sign of degenerating anterior horn cells—in one arm or leg (Fig. 5–4). Surprisingly, even in these atrophic muscles, physicians can elicit brisk DTRs and Babinski signs—signs of upper motor degeneration—because undamaged LMNs are supplied by damaged UMNs. The weakness, atrophy, and fasciculations spread asymmetrically to other limbs and also to the face, pharynx, and tongue. Eventually, dysarthria and dysphagia (bulbar palsy) develops in most patients. When pseudobulbar palsy superimposes itself on bulbar palsy, patients' speech becomes unintelligible and interrupted by "demonic" laughing and crying (see Chapter 4). Despite the extensive motor impairment, ocular muscle control and bladder and bowel function, as well as cognitive capacity, remain normal.

No treatment cures or even arrests ALS. However, riluzole (Rilutek), seems to slow progression, delaying the time until tracheostomy or death. By inhibiting presynaptic glutamate release and possibly also blocking postsynaptic receptors, riluzole presumably reduces glutamate excitotoxicity and preserves motor neuron function.

The outstanding clinical feature of ALS is that patients tragically remain alert, mentally competent, and completely aware of their plight throughout the course of the illness. As consulting psychiatrists who are drawn into this extremely painful situation will find, patients with ALS have the cognitive capacity to chose their medical care and make other important decisions. In particular, many patients having con-

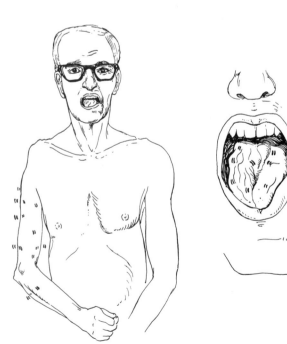

FIGURE 5–4. This elderly gentleman with ALS has typical (right arm) asymmetric limb atrophy, paresis, and fasciculations. His tongue also has fasciculations and atrophy, as indicated by clefts and furrows.

fronted their situation refuse resuscitation measures, mechanical ventilation, and other life-support devices. After lengthy, complicated litigation, several patients have hastened the inevitable process. About 80% of ALS patients receiving standard medical care die, usually from respiratory complications or sepsis, within 5 years from the time of diagnosis.

Several other motor neuron diseases also cause extensive loss of anterior horn cells (LMNs) while, however, sparing UMNs and extraocular muscle movement. For example, hereditary varieties of motor neuron disease in infants (Werdnig-Hoffmann disease) and children (Kugelberg-Welander disease) are characterized by exclusively LMN involvement: flaccid quadriplegia with atrophic, areflexic muscles, and fasciculations. Both are autosomal recessive disorders carried on chromosome 5.

Poliomyelitis

The most frequently occurring motor neuron disease until development of the Salk vaccine, poliomyelitis (polio), is a viral infection of the anterior horn (motor neuron) cells of the spinal cord and lower brainstem (the bulb). Polio patients, who were mostly children, had an acute, febrile illness with ALS-type LMN signs: paresis that was typically asymmetric, muscle fasciculations, and absent DTRs. Patients with bulbar polio had respiratory muscle paralysis that forced them to be placed in the "iron lung." (The iron lung is essentially a large airtight, approximately 3 feet in diameter and 5 feet long, metal tube that extended from the patient's neck, which was covered by airtight rubber, to their feet. A pump would withdraw air from the inside of the iron lung to create negative pressure that forced room air into the patient's lungs.)

In polio, as in ALS, oculomotor, bladder, bowel, and sexual functions are normal (see Chapters 12 and 16). Likewise, polio patients, no matter how devastating their illness, retain normal mental function. For example, Franklin Roosevelt, handicapped by polio-induced paraplegia, served as president of the United States. Unfortunately, some middle-aged individuals who had poliomyelitis in childhood tend to develop further weakness and fasciculations of muscles initially affected or spared. An ALS-like condition, the *post-polio syndrome*, has been postulated to explain this late deterioration, but if this syndrome exists at all, it is rare. In actuality, the deterioration can almost always be reasonably attributed to common nonneurologic conditions, such as lumbar spine degeneration.

Benign Fasciculations

These commonplace, innocuous muscle twitchings are precipitated by excessive physical exertion, psychologic stress, use of tobacco, excessive coffee intake, or exposure to some insecticides. Diagnosis may be difficult because they mimic ALS-induced fasciculations and are sometimes associated with cramps, fatigue, muscle aches, and hyperactive DTRs. In contrast to those induced by ALS, benign fasciculations are unaccompanied by weakness, atrophy, or pathologic reflexes, and they usually last for only several days to weeks, thus calming the fears of medical students and others acquainted with ALS.

A similar benign disorder consists of fasciculations confined to the eyelid muscles (orbicularis oculi) that create an annoying twitching or jerking movement around one eye. However, if the movements are bilateral, forceful enough to close the eyelids, or exceed a duration of 1 second, they may represent a facial dyskinesia, such as blepharospasm, hemifacial spasm, or tardive dyskinesia (see Chapter 18, "Involuntary Movement Disorders").

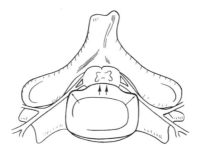

FIGURE 5–5. In cervical spondylosis, bony proliferation damages upper and lower motor neurons. Intervertebral ridges of bone *(double arrows)* compress the cervical spinal cord. At the same time, narrowing of the foramina *(single arrows)* constrict cervical nerve roots.

Orthopedic Disturbances

Cervical spondylosis is the age- and occupation-related degenerative condition, often termed "osteoarthritis," in which bony encroachment leads to narrowing (stenosis) of the vertebral foramina and spinal canal (Fig. 5–5). In this disorder, cervical spine "wear and tear" narrows the nerve and spinal cord passages or tunnels. Stenosis of the neural foramina can "pinch" cervical nerve roots. That stenosis leads to neck pain with arm and hand paresis, atrophy, hypoactive DTRs, and fasciculations—signs of LMN injury. In addition, compression of nerve roots or the spinal cord leads to sensory loss in the hands and often the legs. Spinal canal stenosis, when it occurs, can compress the spinal cord and lead to leg spasticity, hyperreflexia, and Babinski signs—signs of UMN injury.

Similarly, patients with *lumbar spondylosis* have lumbar nerve compression and low back pain. Although they could not have spinal cord compression (because the spinal cord terminates at the first lumbar vertebra [see Fig. 16–1]), patients will have signs of lumbar peripheral nerve damage: leg and feet paresis, atrophy, fasciculations, sensory loss, and paresthesias.

In addition to being common, disabling, and often painful, cervical and lumbar spondylosis, by causing both PNS and CNS signs, mimic ALS. Their distinguishing features are neck or low back pain, sensory loss, and absence of abnormalities in the facial, pharyngeal, and tongue muscles.

Herniated intervertebral disks ("herniated disks") are usually precipitated or caused by trauma, strain, poor posture, or obesity that extrudes the gelatinous intervertebral disk material. Instead of cushioning vertebral bodies like a shock absorber, herniated disk material presses against the adjacent nerve root and neighboring structures. More than 90% of disk herniations occur at either the L4–5 or L5–S1 intervertebral space (Fig. 5–6).

Lumbar herniated disks usually cause low back pain that radiates to the buttocks and down the leg along the compressed nerve. The pain in the buttock and leg pain as well as in the low back is characteristically increased by coughing, sneezing, or elevating the straightened leg because these maneuvers press the herniated disk more strongly against the nerve root (Fig. 5–7). Pain that radiates in the distribution of the sciatic nerve, *sciatica*, is indicative of a lumbar herniated disk and distinguishes it from other causes of low back pain. Large herniations can lead to paresis, incontinence, and, rarely, sexual dysfunction.

Cervical intervertebral disks are also sometimes herniated. "Whiplash" automobile injuries and other trauma are the most common cause. Although any soft tissue injury of the neck causes pain, patients with cervical herniated disks, in addition, have pain that radiates down their arms and loss of an upper extremity DTR.

However, neither cervical nor lumbar disks are usually responsible for the pain, chronic disability, sexual dysfunction, and multitudinous other symptoms blamed on them. In fact, herniated disks may be an innocuous chance finding in many people: MRI studies have revealed a herniated disk in about 20% of asymptomatic indi-

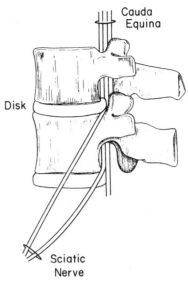

FIGURE 5–6. The cauda equina (horse's tail) consists of the bundle of lumbar and sacral nerve roots in the spinal canal. The nerve roots leave the spinal canal through foramina where they might be compressed by intervertebral disk herniations. Herniated disks usually produce pain in the low back that radiates along the distribution of the sciatic nerve. Common movements that momentarily further herniate the disk, such as coughing, sneezing, or straining at stool, intensify the pain.

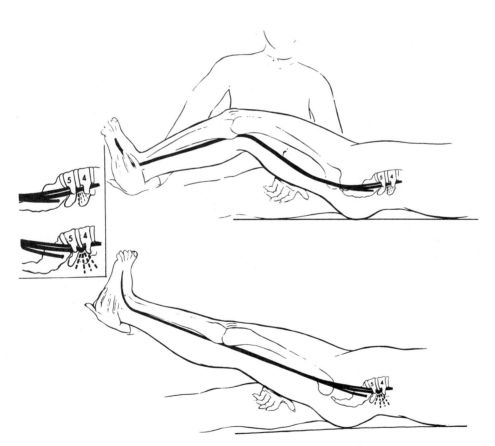

FIGURE 5–7. With herniated disks, the low back pain is intensified and often made to radiate to the buttocks if an examiner raises the patient's *straightened* leg (Lasègue's sign). In this maneuver the nerve root is compressed and irritated because it is drawn taut against the edge of the herniated disk.

viduals younger than 60 years. Even more so, bulging and desiccated disks, which do not compress nerve roots, certainly cannot be held responsible for chronic back pain and sciatica. Alternative potential causes include soft tissue injury, normal largely age-related degenerative changes of the spine, and retroperitoneal abnormalities, such as endometriosis.

As much as in any other neurologic condition, psychologic factors contribute to etiology, disability, and prognosis of low back pain. Work-related low back pain, in particular, is resistant to prevention and treatment. Of all the problem's aspects, disability associated with low back pain is consistently greatest in workers who describe their job as "unsatisfying."

For acute low back pain, nonopioid analgesics, anti-inflammatory drugs, and reduction in physical activity is usually helpful. Opinion varies as to whether the most effective approach is at most a 2-day course of bed rest, continuing routine activities when physically tolerable, or performing certain exercises. Epidural injections of steroids improve pain but do not alter the outcome. Whatever the particular course, conservative treatment helps 90% of cases of acutely herniated disks.

For chronic low back pain, patients may be best approached by accepting it as a chronic illness that the physician might ameliorate but cannot cure (see Chapter 14). The goal of treatment would be improving function rather than abolishing pain. For example, goals, which would be kept modest, could be completing only a 6-hour workday, swimming 10 laps, or playing 9 holes of golf.

Opioids and surgery should be avoided. For chronic pain alone, the Minnesota Multiphasic Personality Inventory (MMPI) and other psychologic screening tests are unreliable in identifying those patients who will have a good surgical outcome.

Antidepressant medications, at doses that are smaller than those used for depression, provide an analgesic effect. Physical therapy is very useful and can become the mainstay of treatment. Finally, physicians and patients should acknowledge, when relevant, that litigation often implicitly promises large amounts of money for *permanent* pain, suffering, and disability. This incentive naturally weighs against accurate reporting, effective treatment, and returning to work.

REFERENCES

Abramowicz M (ed): Treatment of Lyme disease. Med Lett *39:* 47, 1997

Albert SM, Murphy PL, DelBene ML: A prospective study of preferences and actual treatment choices in ALS. Neurology *53:* 278–283, 1999

Aubourg P, Adamsbaum C, Lavallard-Rousseau MC, et al: A two-year trial of oleic and erucic acids ("Lorenzo's oil") as treatment for adrenomyeloneuropathy. N Engl J Med *329:* 745–752, 1993

Broadwell DK, Darcey DJ, Hudnell HK: Work-site clinical and neurobehavioral assessment of solvent-exposed microelectronics workers. Am J Ind Med *27:* 677–698, 1995

Carette S, LeClaire R, Marcoux S, et al: Epidural corticosteroid injections for sciatica due to herniated nucleus pulposus. N Engl J Med *336:* 1634–1640, 1997

Dawson DM: Entrapment neuropathies of the upper extremities. N Engl J Med *329:* 2013–2018, 1993

Filley CM, Heaton RK, Rosenberg NL: White matter dementia in chronic toluene abuse. Neurology *40:* 532–534, 1990

Galer BS: Neuropathic pain of peripheral origin: Advances in pharmacologic treatment. Neurology *45* (12 Suppl 9): S17–25, 1995

Ganzini L, Johnston WS, Hoffman WF: Correlates of suffering in amyotrophic lateral sclerosis. Neurology *52:* 1434–1440, 1999

Green R, Kinsella LJ: Current concepts in the diagnosis of cobalamin deficiency. Neurology *45:* 1435–1440, 1995

Halstead LS: Post-polio syndrome. Sci Am *April:* 42–47, 1998

Hyde TM, Ziegler JC, Weinberger DR: Psychiatric disturbances in metachromatic leukodystrophy. Arch Neurol *49:* 401–406, 1992

Jacobs BC, Rothbarth PH, Van der Meché FGA, et al: The spectrum of antecedent infections in Guillain-Barré syndrome. Neurology *51:* 1110–1115, 1998

Jensen MC, Brant-Zawadzki MN, Obuchowski N, et al: Magnetic resonance imaging of the lumbar spine in people without back pain. N Engl J Med *331*: 69–73, 1994

Low PA, Dotson RM: Symptomatic treatment of painful neuropathy. JAMA *280*: 1863–1864, 1998

Merriam AE, Hegarty AM, Miller A: The mental disabilities of metachromatic leukodystrophy. Neuropsychiatry Neuropsychol Behav Neurol *3*: 217–225, 1990

Miller RG, Rosenberg JA, Gelinas DF, et al: Practice parameter: The care of the patient with amyotrophic lateral sclerosis. Report of the Quality Standards Subcommittee of the American Academy of Neurology. Neurology *52*: 1311–1323, 1999

Murata K, Araki S, Yokoyama K, et al: Autonomic and peripheral nervous system dysfunction in workers exposed to mixed organic solvents. Int Arch Occup Environ Health *63*: 335–340, 1991

Quality Standards Subcommittee of the American Academy of Neurology: Practice advisory on the treatment of amyotrophic lateral sclerosis with riluzole. Neurology *49*: 657–659, 1997

Reinvang I, Borchgrevink HM, Aaserud O, et al: Neuropsychological findings in a non-clinical sample of workers exposed to solvents. J Neurol Neurosurg Psychiatry *57*: 614–616, 1994

Russell RW, Flattau PE, Pope AM (eds): Behavioral measures of neurotoxicity. Washington, DC, National Academy Press, 1990

Schaumburg HH, Berger AB, Thomas PK: Disorders of peripheral nerves (2nd ed). Philadelphia, F.A. Davis, 1992

Therapeutics and Technology Assessment Subcommittee, American Academy of Neurology: Assessment of plasmapheresis. Neurology *47*: 840–843, 1996

Vroomen PCAJ, De Krom MCTFM, Wilmink JT: Lack of effectiveness of bed rest for sciatica. N Engl J Med *340*: 418–423, 1999

White RF, Proctor SP: Solvents and neurotoxicity. Lancet *340*: 1239, 1997

Windeban AJ, Litchy WJ, Daube JR, et al: Lack of progression of neurologic deficit in survivors of paralytic polio: A five-year prospective population-based study. Neurology *46*: 80–84, 1996

Web Sites

Agency for Toxic Substances and Disease Registry: http://atsdr1.atsdr.cdc.gov:8080/cx.html

---

QUESTIONS and ANSWERS: CHAPTER 5

1. After recovering from an overdose, a 21-year-old heroin addict has paresis of his right wrist, thumb, and finger extensor muscles. All DTRs are normal except for a depressed right brachioradialis reflex. Where is the lesion and what is the cause?

ANSWER: The patient has a wrist drop from compression of the radial nerve as it winds around the humerus. This is a common problem for drug addicts and alcoholics who lean against their arm while stuporous. Drug addicts are also liable to develop brain abscesses, AIDS, and cerebrovascular accidents—but these are all diseases of the CNS that cause hyperactive DTRs, a different pattern of weakness, and, usually when the *right* arm is involved, aphasia.

2. An 18-year-old waiter who had 8 days of watery diarrhea has a profound Guillain-Barré syndrome. Which is the most likely cause of her illness?

a. Lyme disease
b. Mononucleosis
c. A viral respiratory tract infection
d. *Campylobacter jejuni*

ANSWER: d. *Campylobacter jejuni* infections, which cause diarrhea, lead to more severe, extensive, and slowly resolving deficits than other antecedents of the Guillain-Barré syndrome.

3. A 24-year-old woman has the sudden onset of low back pain with inability to dorsiflex and evert her right ankle. Raising her straightened right leg produces back pain that radiates down the lateral leg. Sensation is diminished on the dorsum of her right foot. No alteration in DTRs is detectable. What is her problem?

ANSWER: The paresis, pain on straight leg raising (Lasegue's sign), and sensory loss indicate that the low back pain involves nerve root injury rather than merely muscle strain, degenerative spine disease, or retroperitoneal conditions such as endometriosis. She probably has an L4–5 herniated intervertebral disk compressing the L5 nerve root.

4. A 54-year-old man with pulmonary carcinoma has had 2 weeks of midthoracic back pain. He describes the sudden onset of abnormal sensation in his legs and difficulty walking. He has weakness of both legs, which are areflexic, and hypalgesia from the toes to the umbilicus. What process is evolving?

> **ANSWER:** He has acute spinal cord compression from a metastatic tumor with paraparesis, sensory loss below T10, and areflexia from "spinal shock." His problem is not a neuropathy because of the absence of symptoms in the upper extremities, the presence of a sensory level (rather than a stocking-glove sensory loss), and his localized back pain.

5. After recovering consciousness, while still sitting on a toilet, a 27-year-old drug addict is unable to walk. He has paresis of the knee flexor (hamstring) muscles and all ankle and toe muscles. His knee DTRs are normal, but the ankle DTRs and plantar reflexes are absent. Sensation is absent below the knees. Where is (are) the lesion(s) and what is the cause?

> **ANSWER:** He has sustained bilateral sciatic nerve injury, which often happens to drug addicts who take an overdose when sitting on a toilet. This injury, the toilet seat neuropathy, is the lower extremity counterpart of the wrist drop (see Question 1).

6. A 58-year-old carpenter reports weakness of his right arm and hand. He has fasciculations and atrophy of the hand and triceps muscles and no triceps reflex. There is mild sensory loss along the medial surface of his right hand. What process is occurring?

> **ANSWER:** He has symptoms and signs of cervical spondylosis with nerve root compression, which is an occupational hazard among laborers. Cervical spondylosis resembles ALS because of the atrophy and fasciculations, but the sensory loss precludes that diagnosis. In cervical spondylosis, depending on the degree of foraminal compression, DTRs may be either hyperactive or hypoactive. In ALS, despite the loss of anterior horn cells, DTRs are almost always hyperactive.

7. A 30-year-old computer programmer describes a painful tingling in both her palms and all her fingers that often wakes her from sleep. In addition, she frequently drops small objects. She has mild paresis of her thumb (thenar) flexor and opposition muscles. Percussion of the wrist recreates the paresthesias. DTRs are normal. Where is (are) the lesion(s) and what is the cause?

> **ANSWER:** Despite the mild and indefinite symptoms, she has bilateral carpal tunnel syndrome (i.e., median nerve compression at the wrist). She has sensory disturbances, which typically do not strictly conform to the textbook median nerve's distribution and an almost pathognomonic Tinel's sign (percussion of the flexor surface of the wrist creates a tingling sensation in the median nerve distribution). The carpal tunnel syndrome frequently occurs when fluid accumulates in the carpal tunnel (e.g., during pregnancy, before menses, and after trauma to the wrist, including "repetitive stress injuries," such as assembly-line handwork, word processing, knitting, or gardening). Acromegaly or hypothyroidism also leads to tissue or fluid accumulation in the carpal tunnel, but those conditions are rare. The diagnosis in this case, and in most others, is based on the occupation, sensory symptoms, and Tinel's sign. Weakness and atrophy of the thenar muscles develop inconsistently but usually late in the disorder. Nerve conduction velocity studies that demonstrate slowing across the flexor surface of the wrist confirm the diagnosis.

8. A young woman has confusion and hallucinations, flaccid paresis, and abdominal pain. Her urine has turned red. What is the diagnosis and which test would confirm it?

> **ANSWER:** She has acute intermittent porphyria that may be confirmed with a Watson-Schwartz test or determination of total urinary porphyrins. Phenothiazines may be used to treat the psychotic symptoms, but barbiturates are contraindicated.

9. A 31-year-old neurosurgeon has the sudden onset of inability to elevate and evert her right ankle. Her DTR and plantar reflexes are normal, but she has hypalgesia on the lateral aspect of the calf and dorsum of the foot. Where is the lesion and what are possible causes?

> **ANSWER:** She has had the sudden, painless onset of a peroneal nerve injury. It commonly results from nerve compression by crossing the legs, leaning against furniture, or wearing a cast. The nerve is injured at the lateral aspect of the knee where it is cov-

ered only by skin and subcutaneous tissue. When patients lose weight, the nerve is vulnerable to compression because subcutaneous fat is depleted. Sometimes diabetes, Lyme disease, or a vasculitis causes this or other mononeuropathy.

10. Several workers in a chemical factory describe tingling of their fingers and toes and weakness of their feet. Each worker has a stocking-glove hypalgesia and absent ankle DTRs. Which objective finding suggests that they have a neuropathy? What are the common causes of industrial neuropathies?

ANSWER: The loss of ankle DTRs is objective. Although the hypalgesia and other symptoms and signs can be mimicked, areflexia cannot. Heavy metals, organic solvents, *n*-hexane, and other hydrocarbons are industrial toxins that cause neuropathies.

11. A 29-year-old woman, recently found to have hypertension, rapidly develops a paresis of the dorsiflexors and evertors of the right foot, paresis of the extensors of the wrist and thumb of the left hand, and paresis of abduction of the right eye. Where is (are) the lesion(s) and what are the possible causes?

ANSWER: Because several different nerves are abnormal—the right common peroneal, left radial, and right abducens nerve—she has mononeuritis multiplex, which usually results from vasculitis, diabetes, or leprosy.

12. A 17-year-old man, after a (losing) fist fight, states that he has inability to walk or feel anything below his waist. He has complete inability to move his legs, which have normally active DTRs and flexor plantar responses. He has no response to noxious (pinprick) stimulation below his umbilicus, but sensation of position, vibration, and temperature is preserved. Where and what is the lesion?

ANSWER: This is neither a peripheral neuropathy nor a spinal cord lesion. There is no objective evidence of neurologic disease in this man, such as changes in the DTRs or the presence of Babinski signs. Moreover, he is able to feel temperature change but not pinprick, although the same neurologic pathway carries both sensations.

13. A 68-year-old diabetic man has the sudden onset of pain in the anterior right thigh. He has weakness of knee extension, an absent (quadriceps) knee DTR, and hypalgesia of the anterior thigh on the right. Where is the lesion and what is its cause?

ANSWER: The knee weakness and especially the loss of its DTR indicate that the femoral nerve, rather than any CNS injury, has led to his deficits. Diabetes causes infarctions most often of the femoral, sciatic, peroneal, oculomotor, and abducens nerves.

14. A 34-year-old man with chronic low back pain has a sudden exacerbation while raking leaves. He has difficulty walking and pain that radiates from the low back down the left posterior thigh to the lateral ankle. He has paresis of plantar flexion of the left ankle and an absent ankle DTR. He has an area of hypalgesia along the left lateral foot. What has happened to him?

ANSWER: He probably has a herniated L5–S1 intervertebral disk that compresses the S1 root on the left. The radiating pain, paresis, and loss of an ankle DTR characterize an S1 nerve root compression that usually results from a herniated disk. In contrast, compression of the L5 nerve root does not lead to an absent ankle DTR.

15. A 62-year-old man has a gradual onset of weakness of both arms and then the left leg. On examination he is alert and oriented but has dysarthria. His jaw jerk is hyperactive and his gag reflex is absent. The tongue is atrophic and has fasciculations. The muscles of his arms and left leg have atrophy and fasciculations. All DTRs are hyperactive, and Babinski signs are present. Sensation is intact. What disease process is occurring? How extensive is it? What is the chance that one of his parents had this illness?

ANSWER: He obviously has ALS with both bulbar and pseudobulbar palsy and wasting of his limb as well as cranial muscles. The corticobulbar and corticospinal tracts, brainstem nuclei, and spinal anterior horn cells are all involved. Characteristically, he has normal ocular movements and mental faculties. Approximately 10% of ALS cases are familial.

16. A 47-year-old watchmaker has become gradually unable to move his thumbs and fingers. He has sensory loss of the fifth and medial aspect of the fourth fingers but no change in reflexes. Where is (are) the lesion(s) and what is the cause?

ANSWER: He has bilateral "tardy" (slowly developing) ulnar nerve palsy, which is an injury caused by pressure on the ulnar nerves at the elbows. Tardy ulnar palsy is an occupational hazard of old-time watchmakers, draftsmen, and other workers who must continuously lean on their elbows. (See Question 7 for occupations that predispose to median nerve compression [carpal tunnel syndrome].)

17. Which one of the following characteristics renders volatile solvents dangerous to the nervous system?

a. Hydrophilia
b. Lipophilia
c. Ability to block neuromuscular transmission
d. Tendency to generate free radicals

ANSWER: b. Volatile solvents are generally hydrocarbons, relatively odorless, and lipophilic. Several of them, such as *n*-hexane, cause inhalation chemical dependency. Because they are lipophilic, which is why they are a solvent, these substances readily permeate the nervous system. They cause two major problems: neuropathy and encephalopathy, which is manifested by cognitive and personality changes.

18. Which one of the following is an effect of superoxide free radicals?

a. Accelerates aging and death of neurons
b. Alzheimer's disease
c. Diabetes
d. Hypoxia

ANSWER: a. Superoxide free radicals accelerate aging and promote premature death of neurons. They are toxic byproducts of normal metabolism that are usually neutralized by superoxide dismutase. They tend to accumulate in elderly people and those with certain diseases because this system fails. Superoxide free radicals have been implicated in the etiology of Parkinson's disease and familial cases of ALS.

19. A 24-year-old man who distills and drinks moonshine (illegal whisky) suddenly develops an inability to extend his right wrist, thumb, and fingers. He is not aphasic. His DTRs remain intact. What is the problem?

ANSWER: He has sustained a "wrist drop" from a radial nerve injury. During a drunken stupor, he may have compressed his radial nerve as it winds around the humerus. Alternatively, he may have developed a mononeuropathy from the lead pipes in illegal distillation. (In children, lead intoxication usually results from their eating paint chips or other lead-containing substances [pica]. In them, lead ingestion causes mental retardation and seizures.)

20. Pat, a 25-year-old anxious medical student who is in psychotherapy, describes fasciculations in the limb muscle, calf cramps at night, and muscle aches during the day. A classmate found that Pat's strength was normal and that no muscle was atrophic; however, all DTRs were brisk. Pat's father, who had been a house painter, had developed arm muscle weakness and fasciculations before he died of pulmonary failure. Which is the most likely cause of Pat's fasciculations?

a. ALS
b. Psychotropic medications
c. Anxiety and fatigue
d. Cervical spondylosis

ANSWER: c. In view of the lack of atrophy and weakness, the fasciculations are probably benign fasciculations. This commonly occurring disorder in young adults, which strikes fear into the heart of almost every medical student, may be accompanied by aches, cramps, and hyperactive DTRs. Incidentally, Pat is also much too young to have contracted ALS. The father probably had cervical spondylosis, which is an occupational hazard of painters who must daily, for many hours, extend their head and neck. As for Pat's fasciculations, hearing a diagnosis of benign fasciculations epitomizes the medical adage that the three greatest words in the English language are not "I love you" but "It is benign."

21–25. Match the cause with the illness.

21. White lines of the nails (Mees' lines)

22. Lyme disease

23. Nitrous oxide neuropathy

24. *n*-Hexane neuropathy

25. Metachromatic leukodystrophy (MLD)

a. Genetic abnormality
b. Glue sniffing
c. Spirochete infection

d. Dental anesthetic abuse
e. Arsenic poisoning

    ANSWERS: 21-e, 22-c, 23-d, 24-b, 25-a

26–36. Which conditions are associated with fasciculations? (Yes or No)

26. Acute inflammatory demyelinating polyradiculoneuropathy (AIDP)

27. Spinal cord compression

28. ALS

29. Insecticide poisoning

30. Werdnig-Hoffmann

31. Fatigue

32. Porphyria

33. Psychologic stress

34. Cervical spondylosis

35. Post-polio syndrome

36. Poliomyelitis

    ANSWERS: 26-no, 27-no, 28-yes, 29-yes, 30-yes, 31-yes, 32-no, 33-yes, 34-yes, 35-yes, 36-yes

37. Found with his suicide note, a 42-year-old man is brought to the hospital in coma with cyanosis, bradycardia, and miosis; flaccid, areflexic quadriplegia; and pronounced muscle fasciculations. How has he attempted suicide, and how should he be treated?

    ANSWER: Most likely, he has taken a common anticholinesterase-based insecticide that might be reversed with atropine. Most insecticides block neuromuscular transmission and create generalized paralysis, which mimics an acutely developing neuropathy; however, they characteristically also cause fasciculations and increased parasympathetic activity (miosis and bradycardia).

38. Which of the following conditions are associated with sexual dysfunction?

a. Peroneal nerve palsy
b. Carpal tunnel syndrome
c. Diabetes
d. Poliomyelitis

e. MS
f. Post-polio syndrome
g. ALS
h. Myasthenia gravis

    ANSWERS: a-no, b-no, c-yes, d-no, e-yes, f-no, g-no, h-no

39. A 40-year-old man with rapidly advancing Guillain-Barré syndrome has confusion, overwhelming anxiety, and then agitation. Which two of the following statements are correct?

a. He should be treated with a benzodiazepine.
b. He may be developing hypoxia, hypercapnia, or both because of chest and diaphragm muscle paresis.
c. He probably has "ICU psychosis."
d. Guillain-Barré syndrome is generally not associated with CNS complications.

ANSWER: b and d. Guillain-Barré syndrome, also called AIDP, is not directly associated with central nervous system dysfunction. However, respiratory insufficiency, a common complication, might cause anxiety and agitation. Other complications that can induce mental changes are metabolic aberrations, pain, sleep deprivation, or an adverse reaction to a medication; however, these complications are not immediately life threatening. Treatment with a benzodiazepine at this stage is contraindicated because it might completely inhibit respirations. "ICU psychosis," which is a misnomer, implies that psychosis results from the psychologic stress of a life-threatening illness.

40. After admission to the hospital for several months of progressively severe polyneuropathy, a 43-year-old man develops agitation, hallucinations, and disorientation. Of the various causes of neuropathy, which one leads to mental changes after hospitalization?

ANSWER: Alcoholic neuropathy is associated with delirium tremens (DTs) when hospitalized alcoholic patients are deprived of their usual alcohol consumption. They may also develop alcohol withdrawal seizures that precede DTs.

41. Why is "glue sniffing" associated with neuropathy and occasionally with cognitive impairment?

ANSWER: "Glue sniffing," the chronic inhalation of vapors from cements or paint thinners leads to neuropathy because these substances contain *n*-hexane, toluene, and other solvents. Because these chemicals are lipophilic, they damage the lipid-rich myelin coat of peripheral nerves. In addition, dementia accompanied by cerebellar signs may develop if toluene or certain other solvents are inhaled for periods of at least 2 months.

42–45. A 60-year-old man who has had mitral valve stenosis and atrial fibrillation suddenly developed quadriplegia with impaired swallowing, breathing, and speaking. He required tracheostomy and a nasogastric feeding tube during the initial part of his hospitalization. Four weeks after the onset of the illness, although quadriplegic with hyperactive DTRs and Babinski signs, he appears alert, establishes eye contact, and blinks appropriately to questions. His vision is intact.

42. What findings indicate that the problem is caused by CNS injury?

43. Is the lesion within the cerebral cortex or the brainstem?

44. Does the localization make a difference?

45. Which neurologic tests would help distinguish brainstem from extensive cerebral lesions?

ANSWERS: 42-The hyperactive DTRs and Babinski signs indicate that there is CNS rather than PNS damage. 43-A brainstem injury has caused oculomotor paresis, quadriparesis, and apnea. This injury spared his mental, visual, and upper brainstem functions, such as blinking his eyes. He has the well-known "locked-in syndrome" (see Chapter 11) and should not be mistaken for being comatose, demented, or vegetative. 44-If the lesion is confined to the brainstem, as in this case, intellectual function is preserved. With extensive cerebral damage, he would have had irreversible dementia. 45-Although a computed tomographic scan might be performed to detect or exclude a cerebral lesion, only an MRI is sensitive enough to detect a brainstem lesion. An electroencephalogram in this case would be a valuable test because, since the cerebral hemispheres are intact, it would show a relatively normal pattern. Visual-evoked responses will determine the integrity of the entire visual system. Brainstem auditory-evoked responses will determine the integrity of the auditory circuits, which are predominantly brainstem pathways. Positron emission tomography and single-photon emission computed tomography can be very helpful.

46–60. Which conditions are associated with MS, Guillain-Barré syndrome, both, or neither?

a. MS
b. Guillain-Barré syndrome

c. Both
d. Neither

46. Areflexic DTRs

47. Typically follows an upper respiratory tract infection

48. Unilateral visual loss

49. Paresthesias

50. Internuclear ophthalmoplegia

51. Paraparesis

52. Cognitive impairment early in the course of the illness

53. Produced by Lyme disease

54. Quadriparesis

55. Recovery through remyelination

56. Leads to pseudobulbar palsy

57. Leads to bulbar palsy

58. Where emotional lability of pseudobulbar palsy is frequently mistaken for "euphoria"

59. Typically, a monophasic illness that lasts several weeks

60. Sexual dysfunction can be the only or primary persistent deficit

> *ANSWERS:* 46-b, 47-b, 48-a, 49-c, 50-a, 51-c, 52-d, 53-b, 54-c, 55-c, 56-a, 57-b, 58-a, 59-b, 60-a

61. A 16-year-old waiter, who has been subsisting on minimal quantities of food and megavitamin treatments, develops symptoms and signs of a neuropathy. In what way can the neurologic picture be ascribed to an eating disorder?

> *ANSWER:* Teenagers who develop a neuropathy may have any of the usual causes (see Table 5–2), but several might be given special consideration. Mononucleosis, a common condition of young adults, may be complicated by the development of a neuropathy that is akin to Guillain-Barré syndrome. Substance abuse—alcohol, glue, paint thinners, or N_2O—might be responsible, particularly when neuropathy develops concurrently in several teenagers. Even abuse of supposedly nutritious foods, such as pyridoxine (vitamin B_6), should be considered as a potential cause of neuropathy.

62. After gastric partitioning for morbid obesity, a 30-year-old man seems depressed and has signs of a neuropathy. Which conditions might be responsible?

> *ANSWER:* Surgical resection of the stomach or duodenum for either morbid obesity or ulcers may be complicated in the acute period by Wernicke-Korsakoff syndrome (thiamine deficiency) or electrolyte imbalance. After 6 months, when their stores of vitamin B_{12} are depleted, patients may have combined-system disease. Thus, a change in mental status after gastric surgery for obesity may be a manifestation of a potentially fatal metabolic aberration.

63. A 29-year-old lifeguard at Cape Cod had profound malaise for 1 week, an expanding rash, and then bilateral facial weakness (facial diplegia). Blood tests for mononucleosis, Lyme disease, AIDS, and other infective illnesses were negative. What should be the next step?

> *ANSWER:* The patient has a typical history, dermatologic signature (erythema migrans), and neurologic findings for Lyme disease, which is endemic on Cape Cod and other areas of the Northeast coast. Serologic tests are notoriously inaccurate for Lyme disease. Blood tests are frequently negative early in the illness and even throughout its course. Another possibility is that she has Guillain-Barré syndrome that began in a small fraction of cases with involvement of the cranial nerves rather than with the lower spinal nerves. Myasthenia gravis is a possibility, but it is unlikely because of the absence of oculomotor paresis. Sarcoidosis is a rare cause of facial diplegia. The next steps would be to perform a lumbar puncture to test the CSF for Lyme disease and look for the characteristic protein elevation of Guillain-Barré syndrome and to obtain a chest x-ray film and other tests for sarcoidosis. If the diagnosis remains unclear, the best course would be to treat for Lyme disease.

64. In which ways are CNS and PNS myelin similar?

a. They both derive from the same cells.
b. They possess the same antigens.
c. They insulate electrochemical transmissions.
d. They are affected by the same illnesses.

ANSWER: c

65. Which is the correct relationship?

a. Oligodendrocytes are to glia cells as CNS is to PNS
b. Oligodendrocytes are to Schwann cells as PNS is to CNS
c. Oligodendrocytes are to Schwann cells as CNS is to PNS
d. Oligodendrocytes are to neurons as CNS is to PNS

ANSWER: c

66. Which of the following statements is false concerning the neuropathy that affects otherwise normal people older than 75 years?

a. It includes loss of ankle DTRs.
b. It contributes to their tendency to fall.
c. Position sensation is lost more than vibration sensation
d. The peripheral nerves' sensory loss is greater than their motor loss.

ANSWER: c. The normal elderly often develop a subtle neuropathy that causes loss of ankle DTRs and vibration sensation more than position sense. It contributes to their gait impairment and lack of stability. However, strength is relatively preserved.

67–70. Match the illness with the skin lesion.

a. Pellagra   c. Herpes zoster
b. Lyme disease   d. Leprosy

67. Erythema migrans

68. Dermatitis

69. Depigmented anesthetic areas on ears, fingers, and toes

70. Vesicular eruptions in the first division of the trigeminal nerve

ANSWERS: 67-b, 68-a, 69-d, 70-c

71. The wife of a homicidal neurologist enters psychotherapy because of several months of fatigue and painful paresthesias. She also describes numbness in a stocking-glove distribution, darkening of her skin, and the appearance of white lines across her nails (Mees' lines). In addition to a general medical evaluation, which specific test should be performed?

ANSWER: The astute psychiatrist suspected arsenic poisoning and ordered analysis of hair and nail samples.

72. Which is the most common PNS manifestation of AIDS?

a. Guillain Barré syndrome
b. Myopathy
c. Neuropathy
d. Myelopathy

ANSWER: c

73. Regarding low back pain, which one of the following statements is true?

a. If an MRI shows a herniated disk, the patient should have surgery.
b. MMPI results will be a reliable guide to recommending surgery.
c. Work-related low back pain is relatively resistant to treatment.
d. A traditional 7- to 10-day course of bed rest, despite its simplicity, is more effective than a day course.

ANSWER: c. In about 20% of asymptomatic individuals, an MRI will show a herniated disk. Therefore, there is not always a causal relationship. Moreover, surgery will improve patients in the immediate postoperative period, but at 4 years and longer, patients who have surgical and conservative treatment will have a similar status. Work- and litigation-related low back pain is resistant to conservative and surgical treatment. At most, a 2-day course of bed rest is beneficial. In fact, merely continuing with a modified schedule may be the best treatment in most cases of low back pain.

6

Muscle Disorders

The clinical evaluation can distinguish muscle disorders from both central nervous system (CNS) and peripheral nervous system (PNS) disorders (Table 6–1). It can then divide them into disorders of the neuromuscular junction and those of the muscles themselves, *myopathies* (Table 6–2). Surprisingly, considering their physiologic distance from the brain, several disorders are associated with mental retardation, cognitive decline, personality changes, or use of psychotropic medications.

NEUROMUSCULAR JUNCTION DISORDERS

Myasthenia Gravis

Neuromuscular Transmission Impairment. Normally, discrete amounts—packets or *quanta*—of *acetylcholine (ACh)* are released across the neuromuscular junction to trigger a muscle contraction (Fig. 6–1). Afterward, acetylcholinesterase (AChE) enzymes or cholinesterases inactivate the ACh. In myasthenia gravis, the classic neuromuscular junction disorder, *ACh receptor antibodies* block or inactivate ACh receptors (Fig. 6–2). These destructive antibodies are selective in that they attack only *nicotinic*—not muscarinic—ACh receptors and those receptors located predominantly in certain muscle groups, particularly the extraocular and facial muscles. Therefore, ACh can produce only weak, unsustained muscle contractions of certain muscle groups.

Standard medicines for myasthenia are aimed at maintaining normal ACh concentrations at the neuromuscular junction or restoring the quantity or sensitivity of ACh receptors. The most frequently used medications, *anticholinesterases* (anti-AChE medicines) or simply "cholinesterase inhibitors," such as edrophonium (Tensilon) and pyridostigmine (Mestinon), inhibit AChE and thus retard ACh metabolism. By prolonging ACh activity, they restore strength. In the complementary approach, which is similar to treatment of the Guillain-Barré syndrome (see Chapter 5), steroids, plasmapheresis, or infusions of human immunoglobulins deactivate the ACh receptor antibodies. Freed of their toxic antibodies, the ACh receptors' activity is

TABLE 6–1. *Signs of CNS, PNS, and Muscle Disorders*

	CNS	PNS	Muscle
Paresis	Pattern*	Distal	Proximal
Muscle tone	Spastic	Flaccid	Sometimes tender or dystrophic
DTRs†	Hyperactive	Hypoactive	Normal or hypoactive
Babinski signs	Yes	No	No
Sensory loss	Hemisensory	Stocking-glove	None

*Hemiparesis, paraparesis, etc.
†DTRs, Deep tendon reflexes.

TABLE 6–2. *Common Muscle Disorders*

Neuromuscular Junction Disorders
Myasthenia gravis
Botulism
Tetanus
Nerve gas poisoning

Muscle Diseases (Myopathies)
Inherited dystrophies
  Duchenne's muscular dystrophy
  Myotonic dystrophy
Polymyositis
  Polymyositis
  Eosinophilia-myalgia syndrome
  Trichinosis
  AIDS* myopathy
Metabolic
  Steroid myopathy
  Hypokalemic myopathy
  Alcohol myopathy
Mitochondrial myopathies
  Primary mitochondrial myopathies
  Progressive ophthalmoplegia
  MELAS* and MERRF*
Neuroleptic malignant syndrome

*AIDS, Acquired immunodeficiency syndrome; MELAS, mitochondrial encephalomyelopathy, lactic acidosis, and strokelike episodes; MERRF, myoclonic epilepsy and ragged-red fibers.

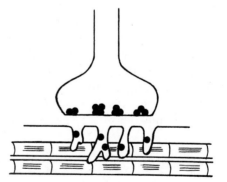

FIGURE 6–1. Peripheral nerve endings contain discrete *packets* or *quanta* of ACh that are released in groups of about 200 in response to nerve impulses. The ACh packets cross the synaptic cleft of the neuromuscular junction to reach numerous, deep, and convoluted ACh receptor binding sites. ACh-receptor interactions open cation channels, which induce an *end-plate potential*. If the potential is large enough, it will trigger an *action potential* along the muscle fiber. Action potentials open calcium storage sites, which produces muscle contractions.

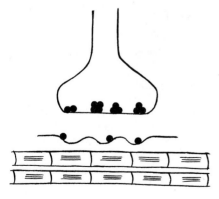

FIGURE 6–2. In myasthenia gravis, antibodies block or inactivate neuromuscular ACh receptors. The remaining receptors are wide and shallow with less effective binding sites. In addition, the synaptic cleft is greater, making neuromuscular transmission less efficient.

ACh receptor antibodies. Freed of their toxic antibodies, the ACh receptors' activity is restored.

Changes in ACh neuromuscular transmission may also be caused by other illnesses or may be purposefully induced by medications. For example, *botulinum toxin*, as both a naturally occurring food poison and a medication, blocks the release of ACh packets from the presynaptic membrane and causes paresis (see below). At the postsynaptic side of the neuromuscular junction, *succinylcholine*, the muscle relaxant often used in conjunction with major surgery or electroconvulsive therapy (ECT), binds to the ACh receptors to relax (weaken) muscles. Like ACh, succinylcholine depolarizes the muscle membrane until AChE deactivates it.

Unlike dopamine and serotonin, ACh is a transmitter at the neuromuscular junction, as well as in the CNS, and its action is terminated predominantly by metabolism instead of by reuptake. Furthermore, in myasthenia gravis, antibodies impair ACh transmission at nicotinic neuromuscular receptors but they do not impair CNS ACh transmission. One reason is that cerebral ACh receptors are muscarinic (see Chapter 21).

This distinction between neuromuscular and CNS ACh activity is reflected in myasthenia gravis by profound weakness strikingly coexisting with normal cognitive capacity. Similarly, most anti-AChE medications for myasthenia gravis have no effect on CNS ACh activity or cognitive capacity because they do not penetrate the blood-brain barrier. One of the few exceptions, physostigmine, penetrates into the CNS, where it increases ACh activity. Physostigmine has been proposed as a treatment for conditions with low CNS ACh levels, such as Alzheimer's disease. In various experiments with Alzheimer's disease, however, physostigmine increased cerebral ACh concentrations, but it produced virtually no clinical benefit (see Chapter 7).

Clinical Features.   Myasthenia gravis is characterized by fluctuating, asymmetric weakness of the extraocular, facial, and bulbar muscles. The muscle weakness may be induced by repeated activity, and thus it is usually worse at the end of the day. Rest temporarily alleviates the weakness. Almost 90% of patients, who are typically either young women or older men, first notice diplopia and ptosis. These symptoms result from extraocular muscle paresis. Because of facial and neck muscle weakness, patients grimace when attempting to smile (Fig. 6–3) and have nasal speech. In moderately advanced cases, the neck, shoulder, and swallowing and respiratory muscles become weak (i.e., bulbar palsy) (see Chapter 4). In severe cases,

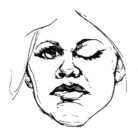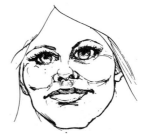

FIGURE 6–3. *Left,* Examination of this young woman after several weeks of intermittent double vision reveals left-sided ptosis and bilateral facial muscle weakness that is especially evident in the loss of the contour of the right nasolabial fold and sagging lower lip. Her weakness is characteristically asymmetric. *Right,* Intravenously administered edrophonium (Tensilon) 10 mg—the Tensilon test—produced a 60-second restoration of eyelid, ocular, and facial strength. This typical brief but dramatic strengthening results from edrophonium transiently inhibiting AChE to increase ACh availability.

patients have respiratory distress, quadriplegia, and an inability to speak (anarthria). Paralysis can be so extensive and severe that patients can become "locked-in" (see Chapter 11).

Absence of certain findings is equally important. Again, in contrast to the physical incapacity, neither the disease nor the medications directly produce mental changes. In addition, although extraocular muscles may be paretic, intraocular muscles are spared. Thus, patients may have complete ptosis and no eyeball movement, but their pupils are normal in size and reactivity to light. Another oddity is that even though patients may be quadriparetic, bladder and bowel sphincter muscle strength will be normal. In myasthenia gravis, unlike other muscle disorders, deep tendon reflexes (DTRs) are normal. Of course, there is no sensory loss.

Patients with myasthenia gravis can experience exacerbations that occur spontaneously in conjunction with intercurrent illnesses or possibly as the result of psychologic stress. In addition, about 20% of pregnant women with myasthenia gravis undergo a flare-up. On the other hand, about 40% of pregnant women with myasthenia gravis experience a remission.

Clinical diagnosis can be confirmed by a positive Tensilon (edrophonium) test (Fig. 6–3), by detecting serum ACh receptor antibodies, or by obtaining certain results on electromyograms (EMGs). About 5% of patients have underlying hyperthyroidism, and 10% have a mediastinal thymoma. If these conditions are detected and treated, myasthenia will be improved.

Differential Diagnosis. Lesions of the oculomotor nerve (cranial nerve III), which result from midbrain infarctions (see Fig. 4–4) or compression by posterior communicating artery aneurysms, can also cause extraocular muscle paresis. These disorders are identifiable by a subtle finding: the pupil will be widely dilated and unreactive to light because of intraocular (pupillary) muscle paresis (see Fig. 4–5). In addition, many other illnesses cause facial or bulbar palsy: amyotrophic lateral sclerosis (ALS), Guillain-Barré syndrome, Lyme disease, Bell's palsy, Lambert-Eaton syndrome, botulism, and brainstem lesions. However, only myasthenia gravis consistently responds to the Tensilon test.

Lambert-Eaton Syndrome and Botulism

The physiologic opposites of myasthenia gravis are Lambert-Eaton syndrome and botulism, where impaired *release* of ACh packets from the presynaptic membrane reduces ACh activity. The ensuing weakness in these conditions shares some clinical features with myasthenia gravis.

Lambert-Eaton syndrome, a *paraneoplastic syndrome* (see Chapter 19), is an autoimmune disorder closely associated with small-cell carcinoma of the lung and rheumatologic illnesses. Unlike the weakness in myasthenia gravis, impairment of ACh transmission in Lambert-Eaton syndrome leads to weakness primarily in the limbs, autonomic nervous system dysfunction, and increasing strength with repetitive exertion.

The infamous, often fatal disorder *botulism* is caused by paralytic toxin elaborated by *Clostridium botulinum* spores. Victims have oculomotor, bulbar, and respiratory paralyses that resemble the Guillain-Barré syndrome, as well as myasthenia gravis. However, the botulism symptoms arise explosively 18 to 36 hours after ingestion of contaminated food and include dilated unreactive pupils. Often several family members simultaneously develop the weakness after systemic and gastrointestinal symptoms, particularly nausea, vomiting, diarrhea, and fever. Botulism poisoning is almost always the result of eating contaminated food.

Neurologists are able to turn botulinum-induced paresis to advantage. They inject pharmaceutically prepared botulinum toxin to alleviate focal dystonias and dyskinesias, such as blepharospasm, spasmodic torticollis, and writer's cramp (see Chapter 18).

Tetanus

In this disorder, *Clostridium tetani* toxin blocks presynaptic release—not of ACh—but of inhibitory neurotransmitters, such as glycine. Uninhibited muscle contractions cause trismus, facial grimacing, an odd but characteristic smile (risus sardonicus), and muscle spasms.

Thus, psychiatrists must not attribute all acutely developing facial or jaw muscle spasmodic contractions to a dystonic reaction from neuroleptics. The differential diagnosis includes tetanus (particularly for drug addicts and others with open wounds), strychnine poisoning, and rabies.

Nerve Gas and Other Wartime Issues

Like many common insecticides that attack neuromuscular junctions and produce fatal, generalized paralysis, *nerve gases* that threatened soldiers from World War I through the Persian Gulf War are poisonous organophosphates that bind and inactivate AChE. The common ones—GA, GB, GD, and VX—affect both the CNS and PNS. Some are gaseous, but others, such as the Tokyo subway poison sarin (GB), are liquid. Malathion (Ovide), the common shampoo for head lice, is actually an irreversible AChE inhibitor. Individuals committing suicide, especially in India, often ingest organophosphate pesticides.

These poisons' anti-AChE activity causes excessive cholinergic stimulation that produces tearing, pulmonary secretions, muscle weakness, fasciculations, and, when the CNS is involved, unconsciousness and convulsions. Pyridostigmine (Mestinon), if taken before exposure to nerve gases, protects ACh by temporarily occupying the vulnerable site on AChE. After exposure, first aid consists of washing exposed skin with dilute bleach (hypochlorite) and injections of atropine to block the excessive cholinergic activity.

Agent Orange, the herbicide sprayed extensively in Southeast Asia during the Vietnam War, allegedly produced peripheral neuropathy, cognitive impairment, psychiatric disturbances, and brain tumors in hundreds of soldiers. Although large scientific reviews found no evidence that it actually caused any of those problems, advocacy groups have prodded Congress into accepting a causal relationship.

A recent counterpart, *Persian Gulf War syndrome*, had similar notoriety. Veterans described varied symptoms, including fatigue, weakness, and myalgias. Again, exhaustive studies have found no consistent, significant clinical sign or laboratory evidence of any neurologic disorder. One briefly popular theory was that in anticipation of a nerve gas attack, soldiers had taken a "neurotoxic" antidote, pyridostigmine; however, numerous myasthenia gravis patients have been taking that common medicine for years without ill effects.

The notion that silicone toxicity from breast implants causes a neuromuscular disorder and other neurologic illness is discussed in the differential diagnosis of multiple sclerosis (see Chapter 15).

Chronic Fatigue Syndrome

Myasthenia and other neurologic disorders are sometimes unconvincingly invoked as an explanation of one of the most puzzling clinical problems: *chronic fatigue syndrome.* Individuals with this condition typically describe a generalized sense of weakness sometimes preceded by flulike symptoms with *myalgias* (painful muscle aches). In addition, many complain of impaired memory and inability to concentrate (i.e., symptoms of cerebral dysfunction).

Unlike myasthenia gravis, chronic fatigue syndrome does not produce weakness in the face or extraocular muscles, nor does it cause asymmetric weakness. In contrast to most neurologic illnesses, symptoms of different individuals vary greatly. In addition, their symptoms are unaccompanied by objective findings. Manual muscle testing typically elicits an inconsistent, weak exertion. Blood tests, EMGs, and magnetic resonance imaging (MRI) reveal no significant abnormalities. Finally, many studies have attributed symptoms, in most cases, to depressive disorders.

Regardless of whether chronic fatigue syndrome is a distinct entity, several neurologic illnesses induce unequivocal fatigue, sometimes as the primary symptom, that may be accompanied by cognitive impairment: Lyme disease, acquired immunodeficiency syndrome (AIDS), mononucleosis, multiple sclerosis, sleep apnea and other sleep disturbances, and eosinophilia-myalgia syndrome. In addition, simple deconditioning from limited physical activity, including weightless space travel and confinement to a hospital bed, frequently causes weakness and loss of muscle bulk.

MUSCLE DISEASE (MYOPATHY)

Although myopathies occasionally involve particular regions of the body, in most patients' shoulder and hip girdle muscles—large, "proximal" muscles—are affected first, most severely, and often exclusively. Patients have difficulty performing tasks depending on these muscles: standing, walking, climbing stairs, combing their hair, and reaching upward. Even when weakness is extensive and severe, there is usually no oculomotor or sphincter paresis, and patients retain the use of their hands and feet. (Hand and feet muscles are "distal" and are affected by neuropathies.)

Acute inflammatory myopathies cause myalgias and tenderness. Eventually, both inflammatory and noninflammatory myopathies lead to muscle weakness and atrophy, also known as *dystrophy*. DTRs are hypoactive roughly in proportion to the weakness. Patients do not have Babinski signs or sensory loss because the corticospinal and sensory tracts are not involved. With most myopathies, serum concentrations of muscle-based enzymes, such as creatine phosphokinase (CPK), are elevated and EMGs are abnormal. Finally, with a few exceptions (see below), myopathies are not associated with mental disorders (see below).

Inherited Dystrophies

Duchenne's Muscular Dystrophy. Well known simply as *muscular dystrophy,* Duchenne's muscular dystrophy is the most frequently occurring myopathy. A sex-linked genetic illness with expression in childhood, it is a chronic, progressively incapacitating, ultimately fatal illness that develops in some boys whose mothers carried the abnormal gene.

Dystrophy, which typically first affects boys' thighs and shoulders, usually becomes evident in early childhood. The first symptom is trouble with standing and walking. In a characteristic finding, *muscle pseudohypertrophy,* affected muscles increase in size because they are infiltrated with fat cells and connective tissue. Yet, paradoxically, these apparently excellently developed muscles are drastically weak (Fig. 6–4, *top*). Instinctively learning *Gower's maneuver* (Fig. 6–4, *bottom*), boys with the illness arise from sitting only by pulling themselves upward or climbing up their own legs.

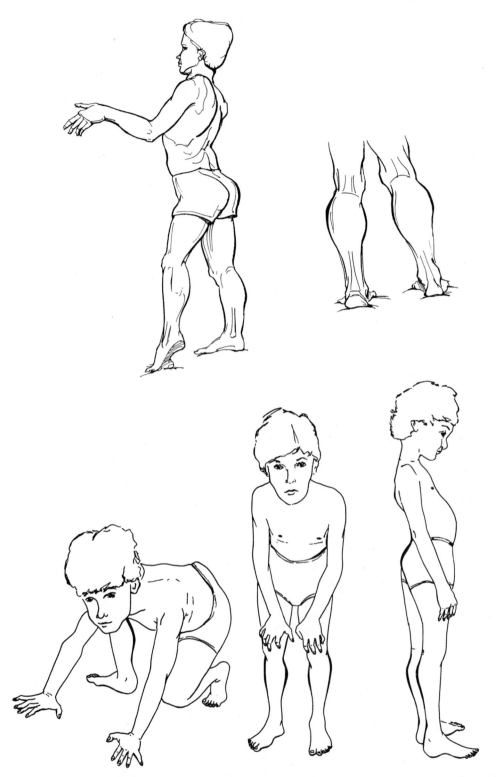

FIGURE 6–4. *Top,* This 10-year-old boy with typical Duchenne's muscular dystrophy has a waddling gait and inability to raise his arms above his head because of weakness of the shoulder and pelvic girdle muscles (i.e., his proximal muscles). His weakened calves are paradoxically enlarged by fat and connective tissue infiltration, not by exercise. This *pseudohypertrophy* of the calf muscles is a signature of the disorder. There is also a typical exaggeration of the normal inward curve of the lumbar spine, *hyperlordosis*. Children with Duchenne's muscular dystrophy are frequently pictured on fund-raising posters. *Bottom, Gower's maneuver,* a classic sign of Duchenne's muscular dystrophy, consists of young boys pushing or pulling themselves to a standing position. They must use their arms and hands because their hip and thigh muscles are weakened early in the disease.

Usually by age 12, when their musculature can no longer support their maturing frame, they become wheelchair-bound and finally develop respiratory insufficiency.

Muscular dystrophy is accompanied by psychomotor retardation and, in one-third to one-half of patients, mental retardation. The children's mental disabilities can overshadow their weakness. Of course, some cognitive, psychologic, social impairment is attributable to isolation, lack of education, and being afflicted with a progressively severe handicap. No cure is available, but investigations include the transplantation of muscle cells (myoblast transfer) and gene therapy.

Genetic Studies and Testing.   The location of the abnormal gene for Duchenne's dystrophy on the X chromosome had long been assumed because only boys developed the illness. Sophisticated techniques have isolated the genetic defect—a deletion in most cases—to the short arm of the X chromosome.

Duchenne's dystrophy causes a pathognomonic absence of a particular muscle-cell membrane protein, *dystrophin*. A relatively benign variant of Duchenne's dystrophy that results from an abnormality in the same gene, *Becker's dystrophy*, causes abnormal dystrophin.

A diagnosis of Duchenne's dystrophy can also be based on a muscle biopsy that shows little or no staining for dystrophin (the *dystrophin test*). Testing blood samples for the DNA deletions on the X chromosome can identify affected fetuses and females who carry the gene (carriers), as well as potential victims.

Myotonic Dystrophy.   The most frequently occurring myopathy of adults is *myotonic dystrophy*. Although also an inherited muscle disorder, it differs in several respects from Duchenne's dystrophy. The median age of appearance of symptoms is 20 to 25 years, and both sexes are equally effected. Also, rather than having proximal muscle weakness and pseudohypertrophy, patients develop facial and distal limb muscle dystrophy. Myotonic dystrophy is named after its unique characteristic, *myotonia*, an involuntary prolonged muscle contraction. Physicians can elicit this phenomenon by asking patients for a strong handshake or by lightly percussing their thenar muscle. Patients are unable to release their grip for several seconds after shaking hands or opening a door. In addition, their tongue and palm muscles have long-lasting ridges if tapped with a reflex hammer.

A further unique feature, caused by hair loss over the temples and facial muscle atrophy, is a sunken and elongated face, ptosis, and a prominent forehead that form a "hatchet face" (Fig. 6–5). Neurologic and nonneurologic manifestations may vary.

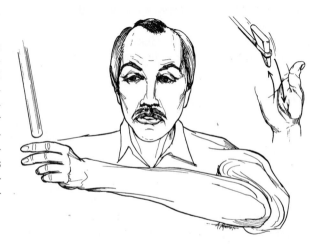

FIGURE 6–5. This 25-year-old man with myotonic dystrophy has the typically elongated, "hatchet" face caused by temporal and facial muscle wasting, frontal baldness, and ptosis. Because of myotonia, when his thenar eminence muscle is struck with a percussion hammer, it undergoes a forceful, sustained contraction that pulls the thumb for 3 to 10 seconds. Myotonia also prevents him from rapidly releasing his grasp.

The latter include cataracts, cardiac conduction system disturbances, and endocrine organ failure, such as testicular atrophy, diabetes, and infertility. Treatment is limited to replacement of endocrine deficiencies and reducing myotonia.

Contrasting somewhat with the mental retardation of Duchenne's dystrophy, patients with myotonic dystrophy tend to have limited intelligence, increased cognitive impairment with age, and changes in personality characterized by lack of initiative and progressive blandness. Their cognitive impairment correlates with an early age for appearance of symptoms but not with severity of dystrophy.

Genetics.   Myotonic dystrophy is an autosomal dominant genetic disorder carried on chromosome 19. A particularly interesting aspect of this disease's genetic basis is that it and several other neurologic illnesses result from excessive repetition of a particular nucleotide base triplet *(trinucleotide repeat)* in the abnormal gene's DNA. In the case of myotonic dystrophy, the trinucleotide base CTG is excessively repeated on chromosome 19.

Other disorders that result from different excessive trinucleotide repeats include those that are inherited in an autosomal recessive pattern (Friedreich's ataxia), autosomal dominant pattern (spinocerebellar atrophies and Huntington's disease), and sex-linked pattern (fragile X syndrome) (see Chapters 2, 13, and 18, and Appendix 3D). Whichever the particular trinucleotide base and pattern of inheritance, these illnesses can be easily and reliably diagnosed in symptomatic and asymptomatic individuals by testing white blood cells' DNA.

The illnesses in this group have several features that stem from the expanded trinucleotide sequences. One feature is that sperm are more likely than eggs to increase their DNA repeats, as if sperm DNA were more genetically unstable than egg DNA. Thus, children who have inherited the abnormal gene from their father rather than from their mother develop the illness at a younger age and eventually in a more severe form. Similarly, fathers are more apt than mothers to pass along a more severe form of the illness.

Another feature, *amplification,* is that the genetic abnormality is unstable and tends to expand further when transmitted. Thus, in successive generations, individuals carrying the abnormal gene show signs of the illness at a progressively younger age *(anticipation)*. For example, the grandfather may not have been diagnosed with myotonic dystrophy until age 38 years. At that age, he already had a son and daughter who both carried the gene. The son may not have shown signs of the illness until he was 26 years old but still had conceived children. The affected daughter's children would not show signs of myotonic dystrophy until they were also 26. The amplification would be demonstrated when the son's children showed signs in their teenage years.

Physicians' finding signs of myotonic dystrophy in progressively younger individuals is due to the actual earlier manifestation of the illness in successive generations. It is not due to heightened vigilance for the condition. An apparent increased incidence resulting from closer scrutiny is an epidemiologic error called *ascertainment bias.*

Polymyositis

Some infectious and inflammatory illnesses affect only the muscles. These illnesses can cause weakness accompanied by myalgias, as in the common "flu," but rarely mental status changes.

Polymyositis is a nonspecific, generalized muscle inflammation or infection characterized by myalgia and weakness. Muscle problems are sometimes overshadowed by systemic symptoms, such as fever and malaise. In many cases, polymyositis is caused by a benign, self-limited systemic viral illness, but it may be a complication of polymyalgia rheumatica, polyarteritis nodosa, and other inflammatory diseases.

When it is accompanied or preceded by a rash on the face and extensor surfaces of the elbows and knees, it is called *dermatomyositis*, which, in adults, is associated with underlying pulmonary or gastrointestinal malignancies.

Trichinosis, a variety of polymyositis, is caused by a *Trichinella* infection of muscles. It stems from eating undercooked pork or game. In the United States, trichinosis is found in hunters, unfortunate diners, and recent immigrants from South and Central America.

The *eosinophilia-myalgia syndrome*, which is more of a toxic than an inflammatory disorder, results from tryptophan or tryptophan-containing products. These substances, which are usually taken by insomniacs and health food devotees, commonly cause several days of severe myalgias and a markedly elevated number and proportion of eosinophils in the blood. Patients often have fatigue, rash, neuropathy, and cardiopulmonary impairments.

More than half the patients with eosinophilia-myalgia syndrome display mild depressive symptoms that are not correlated with physical impairments, eosinophil counts, or concurrent psychiatric disorders. These patients are in danger of being mislabeled as having chronic fatigue syndrome because of their variable symptoms and, except for the eosinophilia, lack of objective findings.

AIDS myopathy, associated with human immunodeficiency virus (HIV), causes myalgia and weakness associated with weight loss and fatigue. In most patients, the myopathy results from an infection with HIV, but in some it seems to have been caused by moderate to large doses of zidovudine (popularly known as AZT). In the AZT group, muscle biopsies often show abnormalities in mitochondria. Withdrawing the medicine leads to partial improvement.

Metabolic Myopathies

Muscle metabolism is usually independent of cerebral metabolism, but some disorders induce combinations of muscle and cerebral impairments. For example, prolonged steroid treatment—for organ transplantation, brain tumors, vasculitis, or asthma—frequently produces proximal muscle weakness and wasting *(steroid myopathy)*. This treatment also causes a round face, acne, and an obese body with spindly limbs ("cushingoid" appearance). In high doses, steroids can cause mood changes, agitation, and irrational behavior—loosely termed "steroid psychosis." These mental changes are most apt to occur in patients with brain tumors, cerebral vasculitis, and other CNS disorders.

Testosterone and other steroids, when taken in conjunction with exercising, can increase muscle size and strength. Athletes and body-builders use this regimen, often surreptitiously, to enhance dramatically their power and appearance. These people also subject themselves to steroid myopathy and steroid psychosis.

An example of the delicate nature of muscle metabolism, notably independent of cerebral metabolism, is that a low serum potassium concentration (hypokalemia) leads to profound weakness, *hypokalemic myopathy*, and cardiac arrhythmias. Hypokalemic myopathy is often an iatrogenic condition that is caused by administration of diuretics without potassium supplements. Also, diuretics, as well as steroids, are sometimes taken surreptitiously. Another cause of hypokalemia is chronic alcoholism. Unlike hypokalemia, which does not alter the mental status, sodium depletion (hyponatremia) causes stupor and seizures.

An interesting variety of hypokalemic myopathy is *hypokalemic periodic paralysis*, in which patients have dramatic episodes, lasting several hours to 2 days, of areflexic quadriparesis associated with hypokalemia. Despite widespread paralysis, they remain alert and fully cognizant, breathing normally and purposefully moving their eyes.

Usually transmitted in an autosomal dominant pattern, hypokalemic periodic paralysis becomes apparent in adolescent boys. The disorder's genetic basis is a defect in the calcium ion channel gene that is cited as an example of a new disease category, "ion channelopathy." An adult-onset variety is associated with hyperthyroidism.

Attacks of periodic hypokalemic paralysis follow exercise, sleep, or large carbohydrate meals. They tend to occur every few weeks but, contrary to the illness' name, timing is irregular. In other words, periodic paralysis attacks do not occur in a "periodic" pattern. Episodes resemble sleep paralysis and cataplexy but are differentiated by a longer duration and a diagnostic electrolyte disturbance. (All these conditions differ from psychogenic episodes by their areflexia.)

Other common metabolic myopathies sometimes have indirectly related mental status changes. For example, alcoholism leads to limb and cardiac muscle wasting (alcohol cardiomyopathy). In *hyperthyroid myopathy,* weakness develops as part of hyperthyroidism. When this disorder occurs, symptoms of hyperthyroidism, such as heat intolerance and hyperactivity, are usually evident. However, particularly with older individuals, in *apathetic hyperthyroidism,* signs of overactivity are remarkably absent. As a general rule, metabolic myopathies resolve when normal metabolism is restored.

Some medications, such as clozapine, may cause an elevation of the serum CPK concentration but rarely a clinically detectable myopathy.

Mitochondrial Myopathies

Whereas chromosomal DNA is derived equally from both parents and is arranged in the familiar strands, mitochondrial DNA (mtDNA) is derived entirely from the mother and is ring-shaped. In mitochondrial disorders, mtDNA is passed to daughter cells in mixtures of normal and abnormal DNA. Thus, mtDNA disorders deviate from standard Mendelian (chromosomal) inheritance patterns.

The CNS, followed by the heart and voluntary muscle, is the body's greatest energy consumer. Mitochondria, using their enzymes for the high-energy cytochrome cycle, lipid metabolism, and especially oxidative phosphorylation, produce about 90% of the body's energy requirement, mostly in the form of adenosine-triphosphate (ATP). In generating energy, mitochondria must constantly remove *free radicals,* which are highly toxic by-products of their own metabolism. Failure to remove them may lead to Parkinson's disease (see Chapter 18) and other illnesses.

The vital energy-producing enzymes of mitochondria are delicate and easily poisoned (e.g., by a minute quantity of cyanide). Cyanide, used for executions in gas chambers, has also been taken by individuals committing suicide, including several hundred cultists in the murder-suicide massacre in Jonestown, Guyana, in 1978.

MtDNA abnormalities can produce tragic *mitochondrial myopathies,* characterized by combinations of impaired muscle metabolism, abnormal lipid storage, and brain damage. In these disorders, muscle mitochondria are unusually numerous, misshapen, or filled with ragged-red fibers.

Although some overlap occurs, we may differentiate first the *primarily mitochondrial myopathies,* which result from deficiencies of lipid storage enzymes and cytochrome oxidase, cause weakness and exercise intolerance, short stature, epilepsy, and episodes of lactic acidosis. Next come *progressive ophthalmoplegia* and related disorders, which cause ptosis and other extraocular muscle palsies along with numerous nonneurologic manifestations: retinitis pigmentosa, short stature, cardiomyopathy, and endocrine abnormalities. The related mitochondrial DNA disorder, Leber's optic atrophy, causes hereditary optic atrophy in young men (see Chapter 12).

A third group of mitochondrial disorders characterized by progressively severe *encephalopathy* usually appears between infancy and 12 years. Their most prominent physical manifestations are seizures, strokes, and other brain injuries. Mental status examinations usually reveal mental retardation or progressive cognitive impairment. In other words, mitochondrial disorders can cause dementia in children. This group has two infamous varieties known best by their acronyms:

- *MELAS: m*itochondrial *e*ncephalomyelopathy, *l*actic *a*cidosis, and *s*trokelike episodes.
- *MERRF: m*yoclonic *e*pilepsy and *r*agged-*r*ed *f*ibers

Neuroleptic Malignant Syndrome (NMS)

This condition, which is not always caused by neuroleptics, consists of intense muscle rigidity, fever, and autonomic dysfunction. Rigidity is so powerful that the muscles crush themselves to the point of *rhabdomyolysis* (muscle necrosis). Crushed muscles release their *myoglobin* (muscle protein) into the blood, producing *myoglobinemia* (muscle protein in the blood). Most myoglobin passes through the kidneys, causing *myoglobinuria* (muscle protein in the urine), but some myoglobin precipitates in the renal tubules. At a high enough concentration, especially if a patient is dehydrated, myoglobin impairs renal clearance and often causes renal failure.

This series of events is evident in several routine laboratory tests. Rhabdomyolysis causes an elevated concentration of CPK. Renal impairment raises the blood urea nitrogen (BUN) and creatinine concentrations. Myoglobin can be detected in the blood and the urine. The EEG remains normal or shows only diffuse slowing, which is a mild and nonspecific abnormality indicative either of a toxic disorder or the use of psychotropic medicines (see Chapter 10).

The autonomic dysfunction produced by NMS causes hyperthermia, tachycardia, and possibly cardiovascular collapse. Body temperatures reaching 107° F cause cerebral cortex damage. Not surprisingly, the mortality rate has been 15% to 20%.

The *Diagnostic and Statistical Manual, Fourth Edition (DSM-IV)* describes muscle rigidity and fever as "essential features" of NMS. Other features include "changes in level of consciousness ranging from confusion to coma," autonomic dysfunction, leukocytosis, and elevated CPK. This description is consistent with the usual uncodified clinical criteria of neurologic and internal medical services in acute care hospitals.

NMS has been found most often in agitated, dehydrated men who have received neuroleptics in large doses over a brief period. Medications regularly implicated are the "typical" neuroleptics that primarily block the D_2 receptor. In addition, NMS has been associated in case reports with nonpsychotropic dopamine-blocking medications, such as metoclopramide (Reglan); "atypical" neuroleptics, such as clozapine; and fluoxetine, lithium, and other psychotropics not known primarily as dopamine-blocking agents. Abruptly withdrawing dopamine precursors, such as L-dopa (Sinemet), which is comparable to initiating dopamine-blocking neuroleptics, has also precipitated NMS.

Although no explanation accounts for all cases, one credible theory is that NMS is an extreme Parkinson-like reaction to sudden dopamine deficiency. Basal ganglia dopamine deficiency produces intense muscular rigidity, and hypothalamus dopamine deficiency impairs body heat dissipation and other autonomic functions. Alternatively, dopamine-blocking psychotropics alter the calcium distribution in muscle cells.

Recommended treatment has included administering L-dopa and the dopamine agonist bromocriptine (Parlodel) in an effort to restore dopamine-like activity. Dantrolene (Dantrium) has also been advocated because it restores intracellular calcium distribution to correct the muscular abnormalities. Several studies have advocated ECT, but the rational has been unclear.

Other Causes of Rhabdomyolysis, Hyperthermia, and Altered Mental States

Serotonin Syndrome.   This disorder, like NMS, is iatrogenic and consists of combinations of muscle rigidity with rhabdomyolysis and autonomic instability. In addition, it produces tremulousness, myoclonus, hyperactive DTRs, and agitated confusion. Serotonin syndrome has generally been attributed to excessive CNS serotonin stimulation from administration of serotonin reuptake inhibitors, serotonin agonists, tricyclic antidepressants, and tryptophan, occasionally alone, but typically along with a monoamine oxidase inhibitor (see Chapter 21). As with NMS, the serotonin syndrome might develop in patients treated with neuroleptics or antidepressants for nonpsychiatric conditions, such as Parkinson's disease, migraines, chronic pain, and neuropathy. Possibly reflecting the disorder's recent description, variable features, and other unresolved aspects, the *DSM-IV* does not offer diagnostic criteria for it.

Unlike NMS, the serotonin syndrome typically causes myoclonus and little or no fever or CPK elevation. Treatments for the serotonin syndrome attempt to support vital functions, decrease the muscle rigidity, and reduce agitation—rather than reverse the excessive CNS serotonin activity. Some authors recommend ECT as a last resort.

Malignant Hyperthermia (MH).   MH, the disorder most often contrasted to NMS, is precipitated by general anesthesia or by the muscle relaxant succinylcholine. Like NMS, MH leads to rhabdomyolysis, hyperthermia, brain damage, and death. It differs not only in etiology but also because a vulnerability to MH is inherited as an autosomal disorder carried on chromosome 19. Its cause is excessive calcium release by a calcium channel. Because MH is an inherited condition, the family history of patients should be reviewed before ECT when succinylcholine is to be administered. Dantrolene may be an effective treatment.

Other causes of hyperthermia, altered mental status, and a muscle abnormality other than rigidity, include meningitis and other infections, hallucinogen ingestion, heat stroke, and delirium tremens (DTs).

LABORATORY TESTS

Nerve Conduction Velocity (NCV) Studies

The NCV can determine the site of nerve damage, confirm a clinical diagnosis of polyneuropathy, and distinguish polyneuropathy from myopathy. NCV is normally 50 to 70 m/s (Fig. 6–6). If a nerve is damaged, NCV is slowed at the point of injury, which can be located by proper placement of the electrodes (e.g., across the carpal tunnel). In a polyneuropathy, NCV of all nerves is slowed, typically to 30 m/s. In a myopathy, in contrast, NCV is normal.

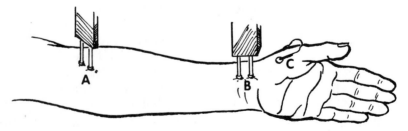

FIGURE 6–6. In determining nerve conduction velocity (NCV), a stimulating electrode that is placed at two points (*A* and *B*) along a nerve excites the appropriate muscle *(C)*. The distance between the electrode and responding muscle is divided by the time interval between nerve stimulation and muscle response to calculate the NCV, which is normally 50 to 70 m/s.

Electromyography

EMGs are performed by inserting fine needles into selected muscles. The examiner observes the consequent electrical discharges on an oscilloscope during complete muscle rest, voluntary contractions, and stimulation of the innervating peripheral nerve. In a myopathy, muscles produce abnormal, *myopathic*, EMG patterns. Several diseases—myasthenia, ALS, and myotonic dystrophy—produce distinctive EMG patterns.

Abnormal EMG patterns may also be found with mononeuropathies and peripheral neuropathy because muscles deteriorate if the nerves that innervate them are damaged. In other words, the EMG can detect denervated muscles. In those cases, it can also determine which peripheral nerve or nerve root is damaged. This test is often used in cases of lumbar or cervical pain when attempting to document nerve damage from herniated disks.

Serum Enzyme Determinations

Lactic dehydrogenase (LDH), aspartate aminotransferase (AST, SGOT), and CPK, enzymes concentrated within muscle cells, escape into the bloodstream when muscles are damaged. Increases in their serum concentration are roughly proportional to the severity of muscle damage and are greatest in NMS. Elevated CPK concentrations are characteristic in Duchenne's dystrophy patients, affected fetuses, and women carriers. Patients with peripheral neuropathy, of course, have normal enzyme concentrations. Therefore, for patients with unexplained, ill-defined weakness, as well as those with myopathy or neuroleptic malignant syndrome, one of the first laboratory tests should be a determination of the serum CPK concentration.

Muscle Biopsy

In expert hands, the microscopic examination of muscle is useful when muscular atrophy might be the result of a neuropathy, ALS, or certain myopathies. Specific muscle disorders that might be diagnosed in this way include Duchenne's muscular dystrophy, polymyositis, trichinosis, collagen-vascular diseases, and the rare glycogen-storage diseases. Electron microscopy is necessary to diagnose the mitochondrial disorders. In many conditions, genetic testing may obviate the need for a muscle biopsy, and it is superior to a biopsy in identifying carriers of the Duchenne's gene. A nerve biopsy is useful in uncovering only a few rare diseases.

Thermography

Although infrared thermography is frequently performed on the head, neck, lower spine, and limbs, it has little or no value. In particular, thermography is unreliable in the evaluation of herniated disks, headache, or cerebrovascular disease.

REFERENCES

Abramowicz M (ed): Treatment of nerve gas poisoning. Med Lett *37*: 43, 1995
Amato AA, McVey A, Cha C, et al: Evaluation of neuromuscular symptoms in veterans of the Persian Gulf War. Neurology *48*: 4–12, 1997
Bertorini TE: Myoglobinuria, malignant hyperthermia, neuroleptic malignant syndrome and serotonin syndrome. Neurol Clin *15*: 649–671, 1997
Goetz CG, Bolla KI, Rogers SM: Neurologic health outcomes and Agent Orange: Institute of Medicine report. Neurology *44*: 801–809, 1994
Gunderson CH, Lehmann CR, Sidell FR, et al: Nerve agents: A review. Neurology *42*: 946–950, 1992

Hyams KC, Wignall FS, Roswell R: War syndromes and their evaluation: From the U.S. Civil War to the Persian Gulf War. Ann Intern Med *125*: 398–405, 1996

Kartsounis LD, Troung DD, Morgan-Hughes JA, et al: The neuropsychological features of mitochondrial myopathies and encephalomyopathies. Arch Neurol *49*: 158–160, 1992

Koo B, Becker LE, Chuang S, et al: Mitochondrial encephalopathy, lactic acidosis, stroke-like episodes (MELAS): Clinical, radiological, pathological, and genetic observations. Ann Neurol *34*: 25–32, 1993

Krilov LR, Fisher M, Friedman SB, et al: Course and outcome of chronic fatigue in children and adolescents. Pediatrics *102*: 360–366, 1998

Krup LB, Masur DM, Kaufman LD: Neurocognitive dysfunction in the eosinophilia-myalgia syndrome. Neurology *43*: 931–936, 1993

LoCurto MJ: The serotonin syndrome. Emerg Med Clin North Am *15*: 665–675, 1997

Rose MR: Mitochondrial myopathies. Arch Neurol *55*: 17–24, 1998

Sachdev P, Mason C, Hadzi-Pavlovic D: Case-control study of neuroleptic malignant syndrome. Am J Psychiatry *154*: 1156–1158, 1997

Shapiro RL, Hatheway C, Swerdlow DL: Botulism in the United States: A clinical and epidemiologic review. Ann Intern Med *129*: 221–228, 1998

Therapeutics and Technology Assessment Subcommittee, American Academy of Neurology: Assessment of plasmapheresis. Neurology *47*: 840–843, 1996

Wallace DC: Mitochondrial DNA in aging and disease. Sci Am 40–47, August, 1997

QUESTIONS and ANSWERS: CHAPTER 6

1–3. A 17-year-old woman intermittently has double vision when gazing to the left for more than one minute. In each eye alone, her visual acuity is normal. Her examination reveals that she has right-sided ptosis and difficulty keeping her right eye adducted. Her pupils are 4 mm, round, and reactive. Her speech is nasal and her neck flexor muscles are weak. There are no paresis or reflex abnormalities of the limbs.

1. Which diseases might explain the ocular abnormalities?

a. Multiple sclerosis
b. Psychogenic weakness
c. Myasthenia gravis
d. Right posterior communicating artery aneurysm

> **ANSWER:** c. This is a classic case of myasthenia gravis with ocular, pharyngeal, and neck flexor paresis but no pupil abnormality. She develops diplopia when one or more ocular muscles fatigue. By way of contrast, this pattern of neck flexor paresis, ocular muscle weakness, and ptosis does not occur in multiple sclerosis (MS). Although internuclear ophthalmoplegia does occur frequently in MS, it causes nystagmus in the abducting eye as well as paresis of the adducting eye (see Chapters 12 and 15). As for psychogenic disturbances, people cannot mimic paresis of one ocular muscle or ptosis. Compression of the third cranial nerve by an aneurysm produces ptosis and paresis of adduction, but it has a painful onset and the pupil becomes large and unreactive to light. Furthermore, the bulbar palsy could not be explained by an aneurysm.

2. Which three tests are helpful in confirming the diagnosis?

a. ACh receptor antibodies
b. Nerve conduction velocities (NCV)
c. Electromyograms (EMG)
d. Tensilon test
e. Muscle enzymes: CPK, LDH, AST
f. CSF analysis

> **ANSWER:** a, c, d. More than 80% of myasthenia patients have demonstrable serum antibodies to ACh receptor, but their concentration does not correlate with the severity of the illness. The EMG will show a pattern of a rapid decrease in motor response to repetitive nerve stimulation in myasthenia. The Tensilon test is almost always positive.

3. Which two conditions often underlie the illness?

a. Hypothyroidism
b. Hyperthyroidism
c. Bell's palsy
d. Thymoma

> **ANSWER:** b, d. Correction of coexistent hyperthyroidism or thymoma will improve or eliminate myasthenia.

4–5. An 18-year-old dancer develops progressive weakness of her toes and ankles. On examination, she has loss of the ankle reflexes, unresponsive plantar reflexes, and decreased sensation in the toes and feet.

4. Which two diseases are likely causes of her symptoms and signs?

a. Myasthenia gravis
b. Toxic polyneuropathy
c. Polymyositis
d. Guillain-Barré syndrome
e. Thoracic spinal cord tumor
f. Psychogenic mechanisms

ANSWER: b, d. She has distal lower extremity paresis, areflexia, and hypalgesia, which are signs of a polyneuropathy. Common causes are alcohol, chemicals, and inflammation, for example, Guillain-Barré syndrome (acute inflammatory demyelinating polyradiculoneuropathy [AIDP]). Myasthenia rarely affects the legs alone and does not cause a sensory loss. Likewise, the sensory loss and pattern of distal paresis preclude a diagnosis of muscle disease. A spinal cord tumor is unlikely because her ankle reflexes are unreactive, Babinski signs are not present, and she has no "sensory level" or urinary incontinence.

5. Which single test would be most likely to be helpful in making a diagnosis?

a. EEG
b. NCV
c. EMG
d. Tensilon test
e. Muscle enzymes: CPK, LDH, AST
f. Positron emission tomography (PET)

ANSWER: b. NCV will probably confirm the presence of a peripheral neuropathy, but it will not suggest a particular cause.

6–11. A 5-year-old boy begins to have difficulty standing upright. He has to push himself up on his legs in order to stand. He cannot run. A cousin of the same age has a similar problem. The patient seems to be unusually muscular and has a normal examination aside from paresis of his upper leg muscles and decreased quadriceps (knee) reflexes.

6. Which single disease is he likely to have?

a. Porphyria
b. Peripheral neuropathy
c. Spinal cord tumor
d. Duchenne's muscular dystrophy
e. A psychogenic disorder
f. Myotonic dystrophy

ANSWER: d. The boy and his cousin probably have Duchenne's muscular dystrophy because he has the typical findings: Gower's sign (pushing against one's own legs to stand), pseudohypertrophy, and areflexia of weak muscles.

7. Which three tests will help diagnose the case?

a. Muscle dystrophin test
b. NCV
c. EMG
d. Tensilon test
e. Muscle enzymes
f. CSF analysis

ANSWER: a, c, e. In a definitive finding of Duchenne's muscular dystrophy, muscle dystrophin will be absent on examination of a muscle biopsy. In its variant, Becker's dystrophy, dystrophin will be abnormal. In addition, in Duchenne's muscular dystrophy, EMGs will show abnormal (myopathic potential) patterns and the CPK will be markedly elevated. Genetic analysis of blood samples will show deletions in the X chromosome.

8. What is the sex of the cousin?

a. Male
b. Female
c. Either

ANSWER: a. Duchenne's muscular dystrophy is a sex-linked trait. Becker's dystrophy, which is probably carried on an allele of the Duchenne's gene, is then also a sex-linked trait. In contrast, myotonic dystrophy is an autosomal dominant trait that is inherited through the chromosomes in a classic Mendelian pattern of transmission. Progressive external ophthalmoplegia is probably inherited through mitochondrial DNA (mtDNA), which is derived entirely from the mother: this is non-Mendelian inheritance.

9. Who is the carrier of this condition?

a. Father

b. Mother

c. Either

d. Both

ANSWER: b

10. If a sister of the patient is a carrier and the father of all her children does not have the illness, what percent of her female children (girls) will be carriers of Duchenne's dystrophy?

a. 0%

b. 25%

c. 50%

d. 75%

e. 100%

ANSWER: c

11. If a sister of the patient is a carrier and the father of all her children does not have the illness, what percent of her children will develop Duchenne's dystrophy?

a. 0%

b. 25%

c. 50%

d. 75%

e. 100%

ANSWER: b. One half of the boys and one half of the girls will inherit the abnormal X chromosome. The boys who inherit it will develop the disease, but the girls who inherit it will only be carriers. Therefore, 25% of the children (one half of the boys) will have the disease.

12–15. A 68-year-old man has aches and tenderness of the shoulder muscles. He is unable to lift his arms above his head. There is a blotchy red rash about his head, neck, and upper torso.

12. Which two diseases should be considered?

a. Steroid myopathy

b. Dermatomyositis

c. Polyneuropathy

d. Periodic paralysis

e. Myasthenia

f. Trichinosis

ANSWER: b, f. The muscle pain, tenderness, and paresis suggest an inflammatory myopathy, such as dermatomyositis and trichinosis. In contrast, steroid myopathy and most other metabolic myopathies are painless.

13. Which two tests are most likely to confirm the diagnosis?

a. EEG

b. NCV

c. EMG

d. Tensilon test

e. Muscle enzymes

f. Skin and muscle biopsy

g. Nerve biopsy

ANSWER: e, f. There will be a marked elevation in the CPK serum concentration. A biopsy will permit the diagnosis of dermatomyositis, vasculitis, and trichinosis.

14. Which conditions are associated with dermatomyositis in the adult?

a. Dementia

b. Pulmonary malignancies

c. Diabetes mellitus

d. Gastrointestinal malignancies

e. Delirium

f. Polyarteritis nodosa

ANSWER: b, d, f

15. Which of the above conditions are associated with polymyositis in the child?

ANSWER: None. In children, polymyositis is associated only with viral illnesses.

16–24. Which medications are associated with myopathy or neuropathy?

16. Prednisone

17. Chlorpromazine

18. Nitrofurantoin

19. Isoniazid (INH)

20. Hydrochlorothiazide

21. Amitriptyline

22. Thyroid extract

23. Lithium carbonate

24. Vitamin B_6

a. Neuropathy   c. Neither
b. Myopathy   d. Both

ANSWERS: 16-b, 17-c, 18-a, 19-a, 20-b (via hypokalemia), 21-c, 22-b (hyperthyroid myopathy), 23-c, 24-a

25–27. A 50-year-old man has developed low thoracic back pain and difficulty walking. He has mild weakness in both legs, a distended bladder, diminished sensation to pinprick below the umbilicus, and equivocal plantar and DTRs. He has tenderness of the midthoracic spine.

25. Which single condition do his symptoms most clearly indicate?

a. Polymyositis   c. Idiopathic polyneuropathy
b. Herniated lumbar intervertebral disk   d. Thoracic spinal cord compression

ANSWER: d. The patient has spinal cord compression at T10. The reflexes are equivocal because in acute spinal cord compression reflexes are diminished in a phenomenon called "spinal shock." The level is indicated by the sensory changes at the umbilicus. Metastatic tumors are the most frequent cause of spinal cord compression, but herniated intervertebral thoracic disks, multiple sclerosis, tuberculous abscesses, and trauma are sometimes responsible. In contrast, polymyositis affects the arms as well as the legs and does not involve the bladder muscles, produce loss of sensation, or cause spine pain or tenderness.

26. If the routine history, physical examination, and laboratory tests, including a chest x-ray, were normal, which of the following tests should be performed next?

a. CT of the spine   d. Tensilon test
b. X-rays of the lumbosacral spine   e. MRI of the spine
c. NCV   f. PET of the spine

ANSWER: e. MRI is usually the first test, but sometimes CT-myelograms are performed.

27. The diagnostic test confirms the clinical impression. If the condition does not receive prompt, effective treatment, which complications might ensue?

a. Sacral decubitus ulcers   c. Permanent paraplegia
b. Urinary incontinence   d. Hydronephrosis and urosepsis

ANSWER: a, b, c, d

28. Which of the following are potential complications of excessive or prolonged use of steroids?

a. Obesity, especially of the face and trunk
b. Steroid myopathy
c. Compression fractures of the lumbar spine
d. Opportunistic lung and CNS infections
e Gastrointestinal bleeding
f. Opportunistic mouth and vaginal infections

ANSWER: All

29. A 31-year-old woman who has systemic lupus erythematosus (SLE) has been treated for 10 months with prednisone (40 mg daily). She has developed agitation, combative behavior, hallucinations, confusion, and a temperature of 100.5° F. The routine history, general physical examination, neurologic examination, and laboratory tests do not reveal the cause.

Which of the following tests or procedures should be attempted and in which order should they be performed?

a. Stop the steroids
b. Begin haloperidol or another major tranquilizer
c. Do a CT scan of the head
d. Perform a lumbar puncture
e. Raise the steroid dosage

> **ANSWER:** b, e, c, d. The real problem is determining whether the patient suffers from too much or too little steroids (i.e., steroid psychosis versus lupus cerebritis). Another consideration is whether the steroid treatment has been complicated by an opportunistic CNS infection, such as tuberculous or cryptococcal meningitis. While diagnostic tests are being undertaken, psychosis must be controlled with major tranquilizers. The question of stopping or raising steroids is best answered by raising them because lupus cerebritis is more common than steroid psychosis, and prednisone at only 40 mg daily is unlikely to have caused steroid psychosis. Moreover, because the patient is under physical and psychiatric stress, she might develop adrenal crisis if her long-standing steroid medication were abruptly stopped.
>
> A CT or MRI scan should be performed to exclude an intracranial mass lesion, such as an abscess or a subdural hematoma. If no mass lesion is detected, a lumbar puncture should be performed to examine the CSF for evidence of infection and other abnormalities.

30. A 75-year-old woman is hospitalized for congestive heart failure, placed on a low-salt diet, and given a potent diuretic. Although her congestive heart failure resolves, she develops somnolence, disorientation, and generalized weakness. Which of the following is the most likely cause of her mental status change?

a. Hypokalemia
b. A cerebrovascular infarction
c. A subdural hematoma
d. Cerebral hypoxia from congestive heart failure
e. Dehydration, hyponatremia, and hypokalemia

> **ANSWER:** e. Administration of potent diuretics to patients on low-salt diets eventually leads to hypokalemia, hyponatremia, and dehydration. Diuretics are particularly apt to cause obtundation and confusion in the elderly. Hypokalemia alone, however, does not cause mental abnormalities.

31. Which two myopathies are associated with mental impairment?

a. Polymyositis
b. Duchenne's muscular dystrophy
c. Carpal tunnel syndrome
d. Myotonic dystrophy
e. Periodic paralysis
f. Trichinosis

> **ANSWER:** b, d. Duchenne's muscular dystrophy and myotonic dystrophy are associated with congenital intellectual impairments. Moreover, myotonic dystrophy is associated with cognitive impairment and personality changes.

32–37. Match the illness with its probable or usual cause:

32. MERRF

33. Myotonic dystrophy

34. Hypokalemic myopathy

35. Cytochrome oxidase deficiency

36. Progressive ophthalmoplegia

37. Periodic paralysis

a. Autosomal inheritance
b. Sex-linked inheritance
c. mtDNA abnormality
d. Viral illness
e. Underlying malignancy
f. ACh receptor antibodies
g. Medications

> **ANSWERS:** 32-c, 33-a, 34-g, 35-c, 36-c, 37-a

38. Which of the following illnesses is not transmitted by excessive trinucleotide repeats?

a. Huntington's disease
b. Myotonic dystrophy
c. Duchenne's muscular dystrophy

d. Spinocerebellar atrophy (type 1)
e. Friedreich's ataxia
f. Fragile X

ANSWER: c

39. Which pattern of inheritance precludes transmission by excessive trinucleotide repeats?

a. Autosomal dominant
b. Autosomal recessive

c. Sex-linked
d. None of the above

ANSWER: d. Illnesses transmitted by excessive trinucleotide repeats include autosomal dominant (Huntington's disease and most spinocerebellar atrophies), autosomal recessive (Friedreich's ataxia), and sex-linked (myotonic dystrophy) disorders.

40. What is the role of edrophonium in the Tensilon test?

a. Edrophonium inhibits cholinesterase to prolong ACh activity.
b. Edrophonium inhibits cholinesterase to shorten ACh activity.
c. Edrophonium inhibits choline acetyltransferase to prolong ACh activity.
d. Edrophonium inhibits choline acetyltransferase to shorten ACh activity.

ANSWER: a. Edrophonium, which is the generic name for Tensilon, prolongs ACh activity by inhibiting its destructive enzyme, cholinesterase (AChE). Choline acetyltransferase (CAT) is the enzyme that catalyzes the synthesis of ACh.

41. Which type of acetylcholine receptor is damaged in myasthenia gravis?

a. Muscarinic
b. Nicotinic
c. Both
d. Neither, the problem is in the presynaptic neuron

ANSWER: b. The number of nicotinic receptors is reduced, and those remaining are rendered less effective.

42. Which two of the following conditions might explain an illness becoming apparent at an earlier age in successive generations?

a. Ascertainment bias
b. Age-related vulnerability

c. Mitochondria DNA inheritance
d. Anticipation

ANSWER: a, d. Ascertainment bias is earlier detection from heightened vigilance for a condition that does not change its age of onset. Anticipation is an actual earlier development of an illness, usually because of expansion of an abnormal DNA segment in successive generations.

43. In which three of the following conditions is plasmapheresis therapeutic?

a. Schizophrenia
b. Barbiturate overdose
c. Manic depressive illness

d. Guillain-Barré illness
e. Myasthenia gravis

ANSWER: b, d, e

44. Poisoning with which substance causes mental retardation in young children but mononeuropathy in adults?

a. Copper
b. Silicone

c. Lead
d. Narcotics

ANSWER: c. Children may develop lead poisoning from eating lead-based paint chips. These children will have cognitive slowing and subsequent school difficulties. Adults may develop lead-induced mononeuropathies, such as a wrist drop, from moonshine or industrial exposure.

45. Which type of ACh receptors predominate in the cerebral cortex?

a. Nicotinic
b. Muscarinic
c. Both
d. Neither

ANSWER: b. Muscarinic receptors predominate in the cerebral cortex. They are depleted in Alzheimer's disease. Antibodies directed against nicotinic receptors, which predominate in neuromuscular junctions, characterize myasthenia gravis.

46. Which one of the following is not a characteristic of the Lambert-Eaton syndrome?

a. Because Lambert-Eaton syndrome is typically found in conjunction with small cell lung carcinoma and other forms of cancer, it is considered a paraneoplastic syndrome.
b. The syndrome is associated with rheumatologic diseases.
c. It results, like myasthenia, from deactivation of ACh at the postsynaptic neuromuscular junction ACh receptor.
d. The weakness in Lambert-Eaton syndrome primarily involves the limbs. The disorder also causes autonomic nervous system dysfunction.

ANSWER: c. Although it mimics myasthenia, Lambert-Eaton syndrome differs in the pattern of weakness, involvement of the autonomic nervous system, and basic abnormality being the impaired ACh release from the presynaptic neuron at the neuromuscular junction.

47. Which neurotransmitter system do common nerve gases poison?

a. Glycine
b. GABA
c. Serotonin
d. Acetylcholine

ANSWER: d. Nerve gases are typically organophosphorous agents that inactivate acetylcholinesterase (AChE) to produce excessive ACh activity. Tetanus blocks the release of the inhibitory neurotransmitter, glycine. Botulinum toxin blocks the release of acetylcholine.

48. Called to a subway station because of a terrorist attack, a physician is confronted with dozens of passengers in a state of panic who all have abdominal cramps, dyspnea, miosis, weakness, and fasciculations. Many passengers are unconscious and several are having seizures. Which medication should she administer?

a. Large doses of a minor tranquilizer
b. Small doses of a major tranquilizer
c. Atropine
d. Naloxone

ANSWER: c. The passengers have been exposed to a terrorist nerve gas poison that has produced PNS dysfunction from excessive ACh activity. In some passengers, the nerve gas has penetrated into the CNS to cause loss of consciousness and seizures. The antidote to excessive ACh activity is atropine. It penetrates the blood-brain barrier and thus is able to restore CNS as well as PNS ACh activity.

49. A 52-year-old woman with a history of several episodes of psychosis is brought to the emergency room with agitated confusion, muscle rigidity, and a temperature of 105° F. Her white blood count is 18,000. Although she has marked muscle rigidity and tremulousness, her neck is supple. Her family said that her medications had been changed, but they could provide no other useful information. A head CT and lumbar puncture revealed no abnormalities. Her urine was dark brown. Of the following tests, which one should be performed next?

a. Urine analysis
b. An MRI of the brain
c. An EEG
d. An HIV test

ANSWER: a. The key to the case is the nature of the urinary pigment. Is it myoglobin or hemoglobin? Are there signs of inflammatory renal damage? The serum chemistry profile might reveal an elevated CPK, long-standing renal insufficiency, or other abnormality. In addition to the standard analysis, the urine should be tested for metabolites of cocaine, PCP, and other intoxicants. The other tests are too time-consuming or nonspecific to be helpful for this desperately ill woman. Although meningitis is unlikely in view of the supple neck and normal CSF, many clinicians would administer antibiotics while further evaluation is undertaken. Similarly, whatever the cause, her temperature should be lowered to avoid brain damage.

50. Concerning the preceding question, which two conditions might cause myoglobinuria?

a. Neuroleptic malignant syndrome
b. Porphyria
c. Serotonin syndrome
d. Glomerular nephritis
e. Malaria

ANSWER: a, c. All these conditions (a–e) can be associated with psychosis and dark urine, but several pigments may darken urine. Neuroleptic malignant syndrome (NMS) and the serotonin syndrome cause myoglobinuria, although the degree is greater in NMS. Acute intermittent porphyria produces porphyrins in the urine. Glomerular nephritis and falciparum malaria produce hemoglobinuria.

51–56. Match the myopathy with the phenomenon:

51. Unilateral ptosis

52. Facial rash

53. Waddling gait

54. Inability to release a fist

55. Pseudohypertrophy of calf muscles

56. Premature balding and cataracts

a. Myasthenia gravis
b. Duchenne's dystrophy
c. Myotonic dystrophy
d. Polymyositis

ANSWERS: 51-a, 52-d, 53-b, 54-c, 55-b, 56- c

57. Myasthenia gravis is a disorder in which antibodies damage the postsynaptic neuromuscular ACh receptor. Which of the following therapies would not be helpful?

a. Giving steroids to reduce the abnormal immunologic reaction
b. Performing plasmapheresis to extract ACh antibodies from the bloodstream
c. Giving medications that enhance cholinesterase (AChE)
d. Giving medications that impair cholinesterase (AChE)
e. Giving medications that cross the blood-brain barrier
f. Performing a thymectomy whether or not a thymoma is detected

ANSWER: c, e.
a. Giving steroids in large doses is a powerful, effective treatment.
b. Plasmapheresis can be effective even when all other modalities have failed.
c. No. They would reduce the concentration of ACh at the neuromuscular junction.
d. By reducing the effectiveness of cholinesterase, the concentration of ACh would increase. Muscle strength would increase as more ACh stimulated ACh receptors.
e. No. Being a disorder of the neuromuscular junction, myasthenia gravis does not involve the brain. The anticholinesterases in common use, such as Mestinon (pyridostigmine), do not cross the blood-brain barrier and do not precipitate mental abnormalities.
f. Removal of thymomas or even persistent but otherwise normal thymus tissue improves myasthenia gravis patients.

58. A 50-year-old man has developed impotence. As a child, he had poliomyelitis that caused scoliosis and atrophy of his right leg and left arm. DTRs are absent in the affected limbs. What role do the polio-induced physical deficits play in his symptom?

ANSWER: The polio-induced muscle weakness and atrophy are typically confined to the voluntary muscles of the trunk and limbs. Polio victims have no sensory loss, autonomic dysfunction, or sexual impairment. Although polio survivors sometimes develop a "postpolio" ALS-like syndrome in middle age, it does not cause sensory, autonomic, or sexual dysfunction. This patient's impotence must have an explanation other than polio.

59. A corporation's chief executive officer develops ALS. His left arm begins to weaken. Then a multinational conglomerate that claims the executive is losing his mental capabilities initiates a hostile takeover bid. Can this contention be supported by the facts known about ALS?

a. Yes
b. No

> ***ANSWER:*** b. Because ALS is strictly a motor neuron disease, no intellectual deterioration can be attributed to it. Although this illness can cause dysarthria and apparent loss of emotional control because of pseudobulbar palsy, ALS does not cause cognitive impairment.

60. A psychiatrist has been called to evaluate a 30-year-old woman for agitation and bizarre behavior. She had been admitted to an intensive care unit for exacerbation of myasthenia gravis and treated with high-dose anticholinesterase medications (e.g., pyridostigmine [Mestinon] and neostigmine). When no substantial improvement occurred, she was given plasmapheresis. Nevertheless, the next day she became confused and agitated. Which is the most likely cause of her mental status change?

a. Anticholinesterase medications
b. Plasmapheresis
c. Cerebral hypoxia
d. Alzheimer-like dementia from CNS depletion of ACh

> ***ANSWER:*** c. Behavioral thought disturbances are a relatively common neurologic problem in severe, poorly controlled myasthenia gravis, Guillain-Barré syndrome, and other neuromuscular diseases, even though the CNS is not directly involved. Mental status changes that occur in myasthenia gravis are not attributable to the illness, anticholinesterase medications, or plasmapheresis. However, generalized weakness, extreme fatigue, or respiratory distress could cause cerebral hypoxia; high-dose steroids could produce psychotic behavior; or being confined to an intensive care unit may create a psychologically stressful situation that, superimposed on medical illnesses and sleep deprivation, might precipitate "ICU psychosis."

61. Match the process with its terminology:

a. Breakdown of muscle cells
b. Determination of abnormal gene location
c. Arising from lying or sitting position by pushing against one's own thighs

1. Restriction fragment length polymorphism (RFLP)
2. Rhabdomyolysis
3. Gower's maneuver

> ***ANSWER:*** a-2, b-1, c-3

62. Which one of the following is *not* common to neuroleptic malignant syndrome and malignant hyperthermia?

a. Fever
b. Muscle rigidity
c. Brain damage
d. Elevated CPK
e. Tachycardia
f. Familial tendency

> ***ANSWER:*** f. Malignant hyperthermia, but not neuroleptic malignant syndrome, has a genetic basis. A vulnerability to the disorder is carried on chromosome 19.

63. Which of the following is a neurotransmitter at the neuromuscular junction as well as CNS?

a. Dopamine
b. Serotonin
c. GABA
d. Acetylcholine

> ***ANSWER:*** d

64. Which of the following is deactivated more by metabolism than reuptake?

a. Dopamine
b. Serotonin
c. GABA
d. Acetylcholine

> ***ANSWER:*** d

65. In myasthenia gravis, against which site are antibodies directed?

a. Muscarinic ACh receptors
b. All acetylcholine (ACh) receptors
c. Nerve endings
d. Nicotinic ACh receptors

ANSWER: d

66. Which of the following treatments is not associated with the development of neuroleptic malignant syndrome (NMS)?

a. Metoclopramide
b. L-dopa
c. Haloperidol
d. Risperidone

ANSWER: b. The NMS is generally attributable to sudden deprivation of dopamine effect. Almost all cases are caused by dopamine-blocking antipsychotic medications. Similarly, nonpsychiatric dopamine-blocking agents, such as metoclopramide, can produce NMS. Another cause of dopamine deprivation and the NMS, although by a different mechanism, is sudden withdrawal of dopamine precursor therapy, such as suddenly stopping L-dopa treatment in Parkinson's disease patients.

67. Which are characteristics of myotonic dystrophy but not of Duchenne's dystrophy?

a. Dystrophy
b. Cataracts
c. Baldness
d. Myotonia
e. Infertility
f. Autosomal inheritance
g. Dementia
h. Distal muscle weakness
i. Pseudohypertrophy

ANSWER: b–f, h

68. Which conditions are associated with episodic quadriparesis in teenage boys?

a. Low potassium
b. REM activity
c. Hypnopompic hallucinations
d. Hypnagogic hallucinations
e. Hyponatremia
f. 3 Hz spike-and-wave EEG discharges

ANSWER: a–d. Hypokalemic periodic paralysis and narcolepsy-cataplexy syndrome cause episodic quadriparesis. Hypokalemia causes episodes lasting many hours to days rather than a few minutes. Hyponatremia, when severe, causes stupor and seizures but not quadriparesis. Three-Hz spike-and-wave EEG discharges are associated with absence or petit mal seizures, which do not cause episodic quadriparesis.

69. Which statement concerning mitochondria is not true?

a. They produce energy mostly in the form of adenosine triphosphate (ATP).
b. Their DNA is inherited exclusively from the mother.
c. Their DNA is in a circular pattern.
d. They generate and must remove toxic free radicals.
e. Compared to the massive energy consumption of the heart and voluntary muscles, the brain's consumption is low.

ANSWER: e. The brain has the body's greatest energy consumption. The heart and voluntary muscles have the next greatest energy consumption.

70. On which two of the following can a firm diagnosis of Duchenne's dystrophy be based?

a. Elevated serum CPK
b. Deletion in the DNA of the short arm of the X chromosome
c. Deletion in the DNA of the short arm of the Y chromosome
d. Deletion in mtDNA
e. Absent dystrophin in a muscle biopsy
f. Abnormal dystrophin in a muscle biopsy

ANSWER: b, e. The CPK will be elevated in patients with a variety of muscle disorders as well as both carriers and patients with Duchenne's dystrophy. The diagnosis of Duchenne's dystrophy can be based on an absence of dystrophin in a muscle biopsy.

71. Which four of the following statements are true regarding dystrophin?

a. Dystrophin is located in the muscle surface membrane.
b. Dystrophin is absent in Duchenne's dystrophy.
c. Dystrophin is absent in myotonic dystrophy.
d. Dystrophin absence in voluntary muscle is a marker of Duchenne's dystrophy.
e. Dystrophin is present but abnormal in Becker's dystrophy, which results from the same gene as Duchenne's dystrophy.
f. Dystrophin is present but abnormal in myotonic dystrophy, which results from the same gene as Duchenne's dystrophy.

ANSWER: a, b, d, e

72. In regard to the genetics of myotonic dystrophy, which are three consequences of its particularly unstable gene?

a. Males are more likely than females to inherit the illness.
b. Mitochondrial DNA might be affected.
c. In successive generations the disease becomes apparent at an earlier age (i.e, genetic anticipation).
d. In successive generations, the disease is more severe.
e. When the illness is transmitted by the father rather than the mother, its symptoms are worse.

ANSWER: c, d, e. The excessive trinucleotide repeats' instability leads to the illness becoming apparent at an earlier age with more severe symptoms (i.e., anticipation) in successive generations. In addition, as in other conditions that result from excessive trinucleotide repeats, when the illness is inherited from the father, its symptoms are more severe because the DNA in sperm is less stable than the DNA in eggs.

73. Which statement concerning mitochondrial abnormalities is not true?

a. Abnormalities affect the brain, muscles, and retinae in various combinations.
b. Abnormalities can produce combinations of myopathy, lactic acidosis, and epilepsy.
c. Mitochondrial myopathies are characterized by ragged-red fibers.
d. Mitochondrial encephalopathies can cause mental retardation or dementia.
e. The dementia induced by mitochondrial encephalopathies is characterized by certain neuropsychologic deficits.

ANSWER: e. Although the dementia may be superimposed on mental retardation, it is often severe and accompanied by numerous physical deficits but nonspecific in its characteristics.

74. Which of the following may be the result of body-builders taking steroids?

a. Muscle atrophy
b. Muscle development
c. Mood change
d. Euphoria
e. Depression
f. Acne
g. Compression fractures in the spine
h. Oral and vaginal infections

ANSWER: a–h. If taken in excess, steroids produce myopathy, mental changes, infections, and a Cushing's disease appearance.

75–79. Match the muscle disorder and its cause:

75. Steroid abuse

76. HIV infection

77. Tryptophan-containing products

78. Alcohol

79. *Trichinella*

a. Trichinosis
b. Eosinophilia-myalgia syndrome
c. AIDS-associated myopathy
d. Body building
e. Cardiac myopathy

ANSWERS: 75-d, 76-c, 77-b, 78-e, 79-a

80. The serotonin syndrome shares several features with the neuroleptic malignant syndrome (NMS). Which one distinguishes the serotonin syndrome?

a. Results from treatment of nonpsychiatric illnesses
b. Fever and autonomic nervous system dysfunction
c. Muscle rigidity and myoglobinuria
d. Myoclonus
e. Response to dopaminergic medications
f. Response to serotonin

ANSWER: d. Myoclonus is characteristic of the serotonin syndrome but is not found in the NMS. Both conditions may result from medications used in nonpsychiatric diseases. Both produce fever, autonomic nervous system dysfunction, muscle disorders, and psychosis. The NMS may respond to restoration of dopamine activity, but neither responds to serotonin stimulation.

81. Which of the following statements regarding mitochondria is false?

a. They satisfy the entire body's energy requirement.
b. Oxidative phosphorylation produces most of their energy stores.
c. Oxidative phosphorylation leads to adenosine triphosphate (ATP).
d. Most mitochondrial myopathies impair production of ATP.

ANSWER: a. Mitochondria produce about 90% of the body's energy requirement.

Major Neurologic Symptoms

The second half of this book focuses on symptoms that are common, illustrate neurologic principles, or indicate serious illnesses. Many are likely to be encountered by psychiatrists because they produce neuropsychologic changes or are so common that they are invariably encountered in any medical practice. In addition, several are included specifically because, possibly contrary to expectations, they are *not* associated with any neuropsychologic changes.

Each chapter discusses the symptoms' essential neuropsychologic aspects, physical neurologic features, appropriate laboratory tests, differential diagnosis, and underlying neuroanatomy. All this material is important. Psychiatrists familiar with it will be better able to perform evaluations that are reliable, informative, effective, and helpful.

These discussions intentionally do not present an encyclopedic review. Textbooks offering complete descriptions are listed in Notes About the References (in the Preface).

Questions and answers at the end of chapters recapitulate the material. Those at the end of the book compare information presented in several chapters. In keeping with the current problem-based method of teaching medicine, this approach allows readers to induce the general neurologic principles from individual cases.

Self-help groups for each illness are listed in Appendix 1. Costs of the diagnostic tests, which can be considerable, are listed in Appendix 2. Genetics—chromosomal and mitochondrial—of inherited illnesses are tabulated in Appendix 3. Physicians are reminded about warnings, reservations, and precautions in the section Physician-Readers, Please Note (in the Preface).

Dementia

7

Dementia is not an illness itself but a clinical condition or syndrome of a decline in cognitive function that interferes with day-to-day activities. The neurologic and psychiatric communities both have similar functional or descriptive diagnostic criteria. As stated in the *Diagnostic and Statistical Manual of Mental Disorders-IV (DSM-IV)*, the diagnosis of dementia requires deficits in memory plus at least one of the following cognitive deficits: aphasia, apraxia, agnosia, or impaired executive functioning (see Chapter 8). It also requires that the cognitive decline interfere with social or occupational function. The dementia due to various illnesses, such as Alzheimer's disease or Huntington's disease, is defined by the same criteria, but an addendum stipulates the course of the illness and identification of any underlying neurologic, medical, or psychiatric disorder. These criteria differentiate dementia from normal aging, related disorders, and toxic-metabolic encephalopathies.

DISORDERS RELATED TO DEMENTIA

Mental Retardation

In contrast to dementia, mental retardation consists of *stable* cognitive impairment that has been present since infancy or childhood. Especially when profound, mental retardation is often accompanied by other signs of cerebral injury, such as seizures and cerebral palsy (see Chapter 13). In cases of genetic anomalies, which constitute a small subgroup, mental retardation may be accompanied by distinctive abnormalities in behavior and the appearance of the face, skin, skeleton, and other nonneurologic organs.

The *DSM-IV* diagnostic criteria for mental retardation are a general intelligence quotient (IQ) of approximately 70 or less; impairment of several adaptive functions, such as social skills and personal care; and onset before 18 years of age. (In contrast, neurologists generally extend the age of onset to 5 years.) Whatever the definition, mentally retarded children may, in later life, develop dementia. For example, individuals who have been mentally retarded as a result of Down's syndrome (trisomy 21) characteristically develop dementia in their fourth or fifth decades (see below).

Amnesia

Memory loss with otherwise preserved intellectual function constitutes *amnesia*. People with amnesia typically can no longer recall events that have recently occurred and cannot remember newly presented information. The *DSM-IV* list of criteria for amnesia requires, in addition, that amnesia impairs social or occupational functioning and excludes episodes that have occurred exclusively during delirium. The *DSM-IV* recognizes an "amnestic disorder" due to various medical conditions and a "substance-induced" amnesia from drugs or medications.

Amnesia is related to dementia, but these clinical conditions are different. The rule is that *memory loss alone is not equivalent to dementia*. Many individuals with amnesia retain sufficient cognitive function so as not to be classified as having dementia. On the other hand, virtually all patients with dementia have memory loss sufficient to be classified as having amnesia.

Neurologists usually attribute amnesia to temporary or permanent dysfunction of the *hippocampus* and other portions of the limbic system, which are based in the temporal and frontal lobes (see Fig. 16–5). Dementia is usually the result of extensive cerebral cortical dysfunction (see below).

Depending on whether limbic system dysfunction is temporary or permanent, amnesia may be transient or chronic. The *DSM-IV* defines amnesia lasting 1 month or less as transient and that lasting longer as chronic. For neurologists, in contrast, *transient amnesia* is an important, relatively common disturbance consisting of a suddenly occurring period of amnesia lasting several minutes to several hours that has developed in previously healthy individuals. Besides having several possible medical and neurologic causes (Table 7–1) transient amnesia might also be mistaken for a psychogenic disorder (see below).

An obvious, well-known cause of amnesia lasting several days to several weeks is electroconvulsive therapy (ECT). Although effective for treating mood disorders, ECT almost invariably produces a transient amnesia, especially for memories acquired shortly before and after treatment. The amnesia is more pronounced with high electrical dosage and with bilateral rather than unilateral, nondominant hemisphere treatment.

Despite the nonequivalence rule, most cases of chronic amnesia are, in fact, found in conjunction with dementia, other neuropsychologic abnormalities, and physical signs. Posttraumatic amnesia, for example, which is due primarily to contusion of the frontal and temporal lobes' anterior surfaces after they are thrown against the inner surfaces of the frontal and middle fossae, is associated with behavioral disturbances, headache, epilepsy, hemiparesis, ataxia, and pseudobulbar palsy (see Chapter 22). Similarly, Wernicke-Korsakoff's syndrome, in addition to the distinctive amnesia, includes ataxia and signs of a peripheral neuropathy (see below).

An important cause of amnesia lasting for many months, if not permanently, is *herpes simplex* encephalitis, which is the most common, sporadically occurring (nonepidemic) viral encephalitis. (HIV encephalitis is, of course, epidemic.) *Herpes simplex* enters the undersurface of the brain through the nasopharynx and invades the frontal and temporal lobes. Destruction of these regions can be so severe that amnesia, which is inevitable, may be accompanied by other manifestations of temporal lobe damage, such as the Klüver-Bucy syndrome (see Chapters 12 and 16), personality changes, and partial complex seizures.

Nevertheless, not all amnesia is a manifestation of neurologic disease. A certain degree of memory impairment is a common, benign condition beginning in people older than 50 years (see section below titled Normal Aging).

Another example of nonneurologic amnesia is psychogenic amnesia, which may occur in people who are depressed, distraught, inattentive, or subject to a somatization disorder. In addition, *DSM-IV* describes "dissociative amnesia," a condition in

TABLE 7–1. *Commonly Cited Causes of Transient Amnesia*

Alcohol abuse	Medications
Wernicke-Korsakoff syndrome	Partial complex seizures
Alcoholic blackouts	Transient global amnesia
Head trauma (e.g., concussion)	

which individuals have one or more episodes of amnesia concerning personal information, such as their name and address. In this disorder, traumatic or stressful information, such as the circumstances of a family member's death, is especially vulnerable. In a closely related condition, "dissociative fugue," victims, who are also amnestic for personal information, may travel away from home and sometimes assume new identities.

Psychogenic amnesia differs from neurologic (organic) amnesia in that loss of memory is predominantly of personal information or emotionally laden events. In addition, psychologic amnesia typically produces inconsistent results on formal memory testing. Amytal infusions may temporarily reverse amnesia in certain psychogenic disorders. In neurologic amnesia, recently learned facts are usually the first to be lost. Also, Amytal, other sedatives, and medications with anticholinergic side effects will exacerbate neurologic memory impairment.

Neuropsychologic Conditions

Confabulation is a neuropsychologic condition, frequently precipitated by amnesia, in which patients offer implausible explanations in a sincere, forthcoming, typically jovial manner. They are not being deceitful but are merely concealing memory impairment. Confabulation is a well-known aspect of Wernicke-Korsakoff's syndrome, Anton's syndrome (see cortical blindness, Chapter 12), and anosognosia (see Chapter 8). Because these conditions are referable to entirely different regions of the brain, confabulation lacks a consistent anatomic correlation.

Aphasia, especially the nonfluent variety, *anosognosia, apraxia,* and other neuropsychologic conditions occur within the spectrum of impairments associated with dementia (see Chapter 8). These disorders may be so severe that they incapacitate cognitive functioning or communication. In addition, their presence indicates that a dementia originates in cortical rather than subcortical dysfunction (see below). However, each of these neuropsychologic conditions is a discrete impairment that alone does not meet the criteria for dementia. Physicians must use skillful testing, which may require nonverbal components, to identify these disorders and detect cases where they coexist with dementia.

NORMAL AGING

The aging process subjects people to a variety of naturally occurring neurologic, psychologic, and physical impairments beginning in some at about age 45 and in most by age 65 (when individuals may arbitrarily be considered "old"). These impairments are usually normal variants, but some may be the prelude to Alzheimer's disease.

Many cognitive functions are vulnerable to age. However, some seem to be more fragile than others. Also, those that decline do so at different rates and uneven trajectories.

The most common, normal, age-related change is a mild, relatively specific memory impairment termed *benign senescence, forgetfulness of old age,* or *age-associated memory impairment.* This variety of amnesia is characterized by forgetfulness for people's names and other isolated facts. It also impairs ability to recall lists of words, especially after a delay. This memory impairment probably reflects slowed retrieval of specific information and, although troublesome, is not incapacitating.

Individuals with benign senescence, unlike those with dementia, continue to function, and their cognitive capacities other than memory are preserved. Nevertheless, some individuals with this condition progress to dementia (see below).

Another age-related change is shortened attention span. Duration and strength of attention is tested by asking a subject to circle a particular letter of many presented in sequence. Other changes are slower learning, which leads to slower or imperfect acquisition of new information, and decreased ability to perform complex tasks.

On the other hand, several cognitive processes normally resist aging. For example, older people have little or no loss of vocabulary, language ability, reading comprehension, or general information. In addition, as determined by the *Wechsler Adult Intelligence Scale-Revised (WAIS-R)*, older individuals' general intelligence declines only slightly. Social deportment and political and religious beliefs continue—stable in the face of a changing society. The elderly remain almost as well-spoken, well-read, and knowledgeable as ever, although possibly becoming set in their ways.

Another normal, age-related change is that sleep is fragmented, sleep and awakening times are phase-advanced (earlier than usual), and there is less stage 4 NREM sleep (see Chapter 17). Older people usually lose muscle mass and develop atrophy of the small muscles of their hands and feet. These changes reduce strength in their limbs. The elderly lose deep tendon reflex (DTR) activity in their ankles and perception of vibration in their legs. They also have impaired postural reflexes and loss of balance. Most cannot stand on one foot with their eyes closed, which is a standard, simple test.

These motor and sensory losses, especially when combined with age-related skeletal changes, lead to a common walking pattern of older people called senile gait. This gait pattern, which is largely compensatory and nonspecific, is characterized by increased flexion of the trunk and limbs, diminished arm swing, and shorter steps. Many instinctively compensate by using a cane.

Their gait impairment might lead to falls, which can be incapacitating and potentially fatal. Other major risk factors for falling are cognitive impairment, use of sedatives, and a previous fall. (Antidepressants, like many other medications, have been implicated as a risk factor. Among them, selective serotonin reuptake inhibitors [SSRIs] carry the same risk as tricyclic antidepressants.)

Age-related deterioration of sensory organs impairs hearing and vision. Older individuals typically have small, less reactive pupils, and some retinal degeneration. They require greater light, more contrast, and sharper focusing to be able to read, drive, and perform other activities. Their hearing tends to be poorer, especially for speech discrimination. Their sense of taste and smell is also impaired.

Vision and hearing must be tested in elderly patients because loss of these special senses can mimic dementia or accentuate psychologic and physical disabilities. Extreme sensory deprivation can cause depression, sleep impairment, and perceptual disturbances, including hallucinations.

In the elderly, the electroencephalogram (EEG) typically shows slowing of the normal background alpha activity (from 8–12 Hz to about 7–8 Hz). Computed tomography (CT) and magnetic resonance imaging (MRI) may be normal, but often these studies reveal decreased volume of the frontal and parietal lobes, atrophy of the cerebral cortex, expansion of the sylvian fissure, and concomitant increased volume of the lateral and third ventricles (see Figs. 20–2, 20–3, and 20–16). In addition, MRIs reveal white matter hyperintensities. Although often striking, none of these abnormalities indicate early Alzheimer's disease.

With advancing age, brain weight decreases to about 85% of normal. Age-associated histologic changes include loss of large cortical neurons and the presence of lipofuscin granules, granulovacuolar degeneration, senile plaques that contain amyloid, and a limited number of neurofibrillary tangles. These changes affect the frontal and temporal lobes more than the parietal lobe.

DEMENTIA

Causes and Classifications

Seemingly innumerable illnesses can cause dementia, making traditional classification by etiology only slightly more enlightening than an alphabetical list. Although quality and depth of the intellectual deficits are interesting, such information is not distinctive enough for a diagnosis. The following classifications based on salient clinical features, although overlapping, are practical and easy to learn:

- *Prevalence:* The most common causes of dementia are Alzheimer's disease; its variants, such as Lewy body disease; and multiple cerebral infarctions (multi-infarct or vascular dementia, see Chapter 11).

- *Patient's age at the onset of dementia:* At age 65 years or older, dementia is most often caused by Alzheimer's disease, its variants, or multiple infarctions; between 21 and 65 years, by acquired immunodeficiency disease (AIDS), drug and alcohol abuse, head trauma, multiple sclerosis, and other demyelinating diseases; for adolescents see Table 7–2; and for younger children see Chapter 13.

- *Accompanying physical manifestations:* Dementia can be associated with gait apraxia (see below), myoclonus (see below), peripheral neuropathy (see Table 5–2), chorea and other involuntary movement disorders (see Table 18–4), and lateralized signs in brain tumors and head trauma.

- *Genetics:* Dementia is transmitted in an autosomal dominant pattern in all patients with Huntington's disease and in some families with Alzheimer's disease, Creutzfeldt-Jakob's disease, and frontotemporal dementia (see below); and in an autosomal recessive pattern in Wilson's disease.

- *Reversibility:* The most common reversible causes of dementia are medications, depression, hypothyroidism, and other metabolic abnormalities. Dementia due to many conditions, including subdural hematomas and normal pressure hydrocephalus, is theoretically reversible, but substantial, sustained improvement is unusual. Overall, reversible dementias are rightfully sought, but the results are discouraging. Using current, relatively strict criteria, only about 8% of dementia cases are partially reversible and even fewer—less than 3%—are fully reversible. Also, most reversible cases consist of only mild cognitive impairment of less than 2 years duration.

- *Cortical and subcortical dementias:* In this somewhat dubious distinction, cortical dementias are accompanied by other neuropsychologic signs of cortical injury, typically aphasia, agnosia, and apraxia. Because the brain's deeper areas are relatively untouched, patients remain alert, attentive, and ambulatory. The prime

TABLE 7–2. *Common Causes of Dementia in Adolescents*

Metabolic abnormalities
   Wilson's disease
   Drug and alcohol abuse, including overdose
Degenerative illnesses
   Huntington's disease
   Metachromatic leukodystrophy
   Other rare, usually genetically transmitted, illnesses
Head trauma, including abuse
Infections
   Subacute sclerosing panencephalitis (SSPE)
   AIDS dementia

example is Alzheimer's disease. In contrast, subcortical dementias are supposedly typified by less severe intellectual and memory dysfunction but prominent apathy, affective changes, slowed mental processing, and gait abnormalities. Examples include Huntington's disease, Parkinson's disease, normal pressure hydrocephalus, vascular dementia, multiple sclerosis, and AIDS encephalopathy.

The cortical-subcortical classification persists, but it has been slipping into disuse for several reasons. The presence or absence of aphasia, agnosia, and apraxia does not reliably predict the category of dementia. In addition, because the *DSM-IV* requires these neuropsychologic deficits for the diagnosis of dementia, whatever the etiology, it would classify virtually all patients with dementia as being cortical. Moreover, this system cannot account for the prominent exceptions inherent in several illnesses, including subcortical pathology in Alzheimer's disease, motor problems in diffuse Lewy body disease, and cortical abnormalities in Huntington's disease.

This chapter discusses Alzheimer's disease and other commonly occurring or otherwise important neurologic illnesses that cause dementia. In addition, under separate headings, it includes discussions of the closely related topics of pseudodementia and toxic-metabolic encephalopathy. Subsequent chapters discuss other dementia-producing illnesses, which are usually identified by the physical signs, such as vascular dementia (see Chapter 11); several childhood illnesses (see Chapter 13); Huntington's, Parkinson's, and Wilson's diseases (see Chapter 18); brain tumors (see Chapter 19); and head trauma (see Chapter 22).

Mental Status Testing

Screening Tests.   Screening tests, which can be administered in 5 to 10 minutes, are useful in detecting and estimating severity of cognitive deficits. In addition to being specific and sensitive for the diagnosis of dementia, they are predictive of dementia.

However, several caveats must be noted. Screening tests tend to overestimate cognitive impairment in people who are older, poorly educated (8 years or less of school), or members of ethnic minorities. Dementia produced by Alzheimer's disease cannot be distinguished from that produced by multiple infarctions or other dementia-producing illnesses. Moreover, in some circumstances, such as evaluating a highly educated person, screening tests may not distinguish age-related memory impairment from dementia. Also, the tests do not distinguish depression-induced memory impairment. (In their favor, gender has no significant effect, a Spanish edition of some tests is available, and corrections may be applied for age and education.)

The *Blessed Mental Status Test*, one of the first tests corroborated by autopsy material, remains in use in some clinical settings and investigational studies despite being somewhat outdated and restricted in its survey of cognitive functions (Fig. 7–1). In this test, increased cognitive impairment correlates with greater neuritic plaque concentration (see below).

The *Mini-Mental State Examination (MMSE)* also correlates cognitive impairment with histologic changes (Fig. 7–2). Its results closely parallel Blessed test results. The MMSE is so widely used that it is considered the standard. However, critics describing the test as "too easy" assert that it permits mild dementia to escape detection.

These screening tests may also have a predictive value. For example, when well-educated individuals' scores are borderline normal, as many as 10% to 25% may develop dementia in the next 2 years. In addition, these tests can cast doubt on a diagnosis of Alzheimer's disease as the cause of dementia under certain circumstances: (1) If scores on successive tests remain stable for 2 years, the diagnosis of Alzheimer's disease should be reconsidered because this illness almost always causes a progressive decline. (2) If successive scores decline precipitously, illnesses that cause a

Patient Initials [F | M | L]

| (1) Observation Date | | (2) Patient Study Number |
| Month / Day / Year | | |

Score each item 0 if correct, 1 if wrong.   Starting Time _____

☐ Name _____

Correct Name, if wrong _____

☐ Age _____ (D.O.B. _____)

☐ When born? _____ (Month, Year)

☐ Where born? _____ Say: Some questions will be easy, some will be hard.

☐ Name of this place _____

☐ What street is it on? _____

☐ How long are you here? _____ (How long today?)

☐ Name of this city? _____

☐ Today's date? _____ (Within a day)

☐ Month _____

☐ Year _____

☐ Day of Week _____

☐ Part of Day _____

☐ Time? (best guess) _____ (Time: (Within 1 hour)

☐ Season _____

Something to remember (Score: immediate repetition-0; phrase by phrase-1; word by word-2; no repetition-3)

☐ ____ John   ____ Brown   ____ 42   ____ Market St.   ____ Chicago   Repetition Score _____

☐ Mother's first name _____ (Any sensible response)

☐ How much schooling did you have? _____

☐ Name of one specific school _____

☐ What kind of work have you done? _____

☐ Who is the president now? _____

☐ Who was the last president? _____

☐ Date of WW I (1914-18) _____ ☐ Date of WW II (1939-45) _____

Next 3 items: For uncorrected errors, score 2; for corrected errors, score 1.

☐ Months of the year, backwards. Start with December . . . .

   D   N   O   S   A   Jl   Jn   M   Ap   Mch   F   Ja

☐ Count 1–20

☐ Count 20–1 (20 19 18 17 16 15 14 13 12 11 10 9 8 7 6 5 4 3 2 1)

☐ Recall name & address __ J __ B __ 42 __ M __ C (Cue with "John Brown" only. Score up to 5 errors.)

TOTAL BLESSED [   ]   Finishing Time _____

FIGURE 7–1. Blessed Mental Status Test. Each incorrect answer adds one point to the dementia score. Scores for normal middle-aged adults are 3 points or fewer. Studies have shown that older individuals with these scores have little probability of developing dementia. People with scores of 5 to 7 have approximately a 10% to 25% chance of developing dementia within 2 years. The scores for people with dementia are 8 points or more. When they die, their brains have increased numbers of neuritic plaques. The critical questions are those requiring the repetition of the John Brown phrase, which requires recall of five items, and saying the months backward. Note that the dates of World Wars I and II are those of Britain's participation, and thus, with time and increasing cultural differences, the test will become less valid. (Reprinted from Blessed G, Tomlinson BE, Roth M: The association between quantitative measures of dementia and senile change in the cerebral gray matter of elderly subjects. Br J Psychiatry *114:* 797–811, 1968. With permission of Dr. Blessed and *The British Journal of Psychiatry.*)

Maximum Score	Patient's Score	Ask the patient, "Please . . . (tell me) . . ."
		Orientation
5	_____	What is the day, date, month, year, and season?
5	_____	Where are we: city, county, state; floor of hospital/clinic?
		Registration
3	_____	Repeat the names of 3 common objects that I say.
		Attention and Calculation
5	_____	Either subtract serial 7's from 100 or spell backward the word "World."
		Recall
3	_____	Repeat the 3 names learned in "registration."
		Language
2	_____	Name a pencil and a watch.
1	_____	Repeat "No and's, if's, or but's."
3	_____	Follow this 3-step request: "Take a paper in your right hand, fold it in half, and put it on the floor."
1	_____	Read and follow this request: "Close your eyes."
1	_____	Write any sentence.
1	_____	Copy this figure:
30	_____	**Patient's total score**

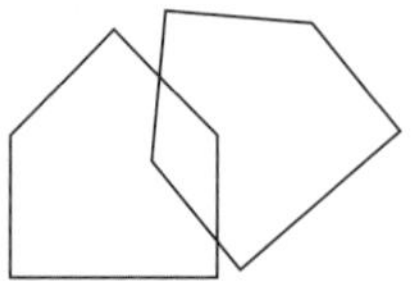

FIGURE 7–2. Mini-Mental State Examination (MMSE). In this test, which has become the standard, points are assigned for correct answers. Scores of 20 points or fewer indicate dementia, delirium, schizophrenia, or affective disorders alone or in combination. These low scores are not found in normal elderly people or in those with neuroses or personality disorders. Note that the MMSE includes, unlike the Blessed, some assessment of visual-spatial relationships and language function. (Adapted from Folstein MF, Folstein SE, McHugh PR: "Mini-Mental state": A practical method for grading the cognitive state of patients for the clinician. J Psychiatr Res *12:* 189–198, 1975. ©1975, 1998 MiniMental LLC.)

rapidly advancing dementia, such as a glioblastoma or Creutzfeldt-Jakob disease, are more likely than Alzheimer's disease.

Further Testing.   Besides yielding borderline results, screening tests for dementia are sometimes simply inadequate. At times, individuals suspected of having dementia should undergo a battery of neuropsychologic tests. This further testing, which usually requires at least 2 to 3 hours, assesses the major realms of cognitive function, such as language (which should be tested first to assure the validity of the entire test), memory, calculations, judgment, perception, and construction. Neuropsychologic tests, while not required to render a diagnosis of dementia and not part of a standard evaluation, are indicated in the following situations:

- For highly intelligent, well-educated, or highly functional individuals with symptoms of dementia whose screening tests fail to show a cognitive impairment. (The *Graduate Record Examination [GRE]* might be administered to them. The results should be compared to prior tests, which are often available.)

- For individuals whose ability to execute critical occupational or personal decisions (legal competency) must be assured.

- For individuals with confounding problems, such as mental retardation, minimal education, deafness, or aphasia.

- In distinguishing dementia from depression, other psychiatric disturbances, and malingering.

- In distinguishing Alzheimer's disease from frontal lobe dementia.

- In distinguishing between cortical and subcortical dementia.

Numerous neuropsychologic tests are administered in various combinations. One of the most widely used tests is the WAIS-R. In early dementia, as measured by this test, performance scales are lower than verbal scales and intelligence is decreased from estimated premorbid levels.

A format complementing traditional neuropsychologic tests evaluates the *functional status* of patients measuring patients' performance of daily activities that require judgment, memory, and attentiveness. Several activities, ranked in degree of difficulty, reflect functional status (Fig. 7–3). Other tests, such as the *Clinical Dementia Rating (CDR)*, provide a view of the impact of cognitive impairment on daily activities.

Laboratory Evaluation

When no particular cause of dementia is suggested by the clinical evaluation, neurologists generally request a series of laboratory tests (Table 7–3). Although these tests are expensive and unlikely to disclose a correctable cause of dementia, they are cost-effective compared to the huge annual charge for nursing home care (see Appendix 2).

CT is reliable in detecting most structural abnormalities, including brain tumors, subdural hematomas, and normal pressure hydrocephalus. An MRI is superior because it is better able to diagnose multiple infarctions, demyelinating diseases, and small lesions. However, neither CT nor MRI can diagnose Alzheimer's disease because cerebral atrophy, which is virtually the only abnormality evident on CT or MRI, is also present in people with normal age-related changes, Down's syndrome, alcoholic dementia, AIDS dementia, some varieties of schizophrenia, and numerous other conditions.

The EEG is not indicated for routine evaluation of dementia because in Alzheimer's disease and most other causes it shows only nonspecific abnormalities that are often indistinguishable from normal age-related changes. On the other hand, an EEG is indicated for patients showing unusual clinical features, such as seizures or myoclonus; a rapid decline in cognitive function; or stupor. In particular, it is indicated in suspected cases of Creutzfeldt-Jakob disease or subacute sclerosing panencephalitis (SSPE) (see below), where patients have myoclonus and the EEG shows relatively specific periodic complexes or burst-suppression patterns (see Fig. 10–6).

FUNCTIONAL CAPACITY ASSESSMENT

Fulfills professional/occupational responsibilities
Maintains financial records: checkbook, credit accounts, etc.
Continues hobbies
Shops, keeps house, cooks
Travels independently to work, friends, or relatives

FIGURE 7–3. The Functional Capacity Assessment is not a quantitative assessment but a survey. The physician should determine whether the patient performs or at least tolerates these common activities. If an activity cannot be performed, the physician should determine if the reason is impaired intellectual ability, emotional disturbance, social isolation, or physical incapacity, including impaired special senses.

TABLE 7–3. *Screening Laboratory Tests for Dementia*

Routine tests
  Chest x-ray
  Complete blood count
  Chemistry profile of electrolytes, glucose, liver function, renal function
  Urine analysis
Specific blood tests
  Thyroid function (e.g., T_4)
  Syphilis test*
  B_{12} level[†]
  Human immunodeficiency virus (HIV) antibodies[‡]
  Lyme titers[‡]
Neurologic tests
  Electroencephalogram (EEG)[‡]
  Computed tomography (CT)[§]

*In testing for neurosyphilis, either the FTA-ABS or MHA-TP test is preferred to the VDRL or RPR (see text).
[†]Serum folate level determinations are indicated only if patients have anemia or nutritional impairments.
[‡]For individuals in risk groups (see text).
[§]The MRI is not standard because the CT is usually sufficient.

The EEG can also contribute to a diagnosis of pseudodementia, where a patient's poor performance on mental status tests contrasts with the EEG's normal or only mildly slowed background activity. It might also help in diagnosing a metabolic encephalopathy.

A lumbar puncture (LP) is not a routine test because it cannot add direct support to the diagnosis of Alzheimer's disease or vascular dementia. However, it should be performed to inspect the cerebrospinal fluid (CSF) when patients with dementia have signs of certain infections, such as neurosyphilis, meningitis, SSPE, Creutzfeldt-Jakob's disease, or sometimes AIDS.

Many tests should be reserved for particular indications. For instance, if adolescents or young adults develop dementia, evaluation might include blood tests for AIDS; serum ceruloplasmin determination and slit-lamp examination for Wilson's disease; urine toxicology screens for drug abuse; and, rarely, urine analysis for metachromatic granules and arylsulfatase-A activity for metachromatic leukodystrophy (see Chapter 5). Likewise, systemic lupus erythematosus (SLE) preparations, serum Lyme disease titer determinations, and other tests for systemic illness should be requested judiciously.

ALZHEIMER'S DISEASE

Because a "definite" diagnosis of Alzheimer's disease requires histologic examination of brain tissue, this criterion is rarely met in clinical practice. Instead, a probable diagnosis, which is accepted for clinical purposes and is consistent with psychiatric criteria, is offered if (1) adults have the insidious onset of a progressively worsening dementia and (2) clinical and laboratory evaluations (Table 7–3) have excluded other neurologic and systemic illnesses that could account for the dementia. These criteria yield an antemortem diagnostic accuracy of almost 90%.

Clinical Features

Cognitive Decline.   Alzheimer's disease typically causes a progressive loss of cognitive function but its rate of progression can differ among individuals. Also, in many patients the decline is uneven, with about 10% experiencing several years of plateau.

In the early stage, patients may remain conversant, sociable, able to perform routine work-related tasks, and physically intact. Nevertheless, they suffer from memory impairment for facts, words, and ideas; a tendency to lose their bearings at night and in new surroundings; and slowness in coping with new situations. Without further evaluation, these impairments are liable to be misinterpreted as depression or normal age-related changes. However, mental status testing will disclose impaired judgment or other cognitive function.

As Alzheimer's disease progresses, it causes a disabling memory loss, unequivocal impairment in other cognitive functions, and psychopathology. Language impairment, which is common, includes a decrease in spontaneous verbal output, an inability to find words *(anomia)*, and the use of incorrect words *(paraphasic errors)*—elements of aphasia (see Chapter 8). When patients try to circumvent forgotten words or phrases, they may lapse into loquaciousness. However, patients' verbal output eventually declines until they become mute.

Several Alzheimer's disease symptoms stem from deterioration in visual-spatial abilities (see Chapter 8). This impairment causes patients to lose their way in familiar surroundings or while following well-known routes. It also causes *constructional apraxia*, which is the inability to translate an idea or mental picture into a physical object, organize visual information, or integrate visual and motor functions. Constructional apraxia is usually revealed by tests requiring patients to draw or manipulate small objects, such as matchsticks, to produce figures or recreate models. Evidence of constructional apraxia includes simplification, impaired perspective, perseverations, and sloppiness. The copy-a-design section in the MMSE tests for constructional apraxia, but the Blessed test does not, which is a shortcoming.

Although aphasia and constructional apraxia are each frequent and prominent manifestations of Alzheimer's disease, they have at least one drawback as diagnostic criteria. Aphasia is much more closely associated with cerebral infarctions and other lesions in the dominant hemisphere. Similarly, constructional apraxia is often a manifestation of similar lesions in the nondominant parietal lobe or other regions of the brain. Therefore, both these symptoms are frequently hallmarks of vascular dementia. Nevertheless, Alzheimer's disease's characteristic impairments in language and construction, which are cortical functions, have allowed it to be considered the quintessential cortical dementia.

Other Mental Aberrations.   Alzheimer's disease patients commonly develop psychopathology. The *Neuropsychiatric Inventory (NPI)* has shown that the majority of them have apathy, agitation, or both. In addition, the disease may induce dysphoria and abnormal behavior. These symptoms have neurologic implications beyond their close association with dementia.

Delusions occur in about 20% to 35% of patients. Dementia-induced delusions are relatively simple but often incorporate paranoid ideation. Hallucinations, which occur only about half as frequently as delusions, are usually visual but sometimes auditory or even olfactory. Whatever their form, hallucinations are ominous because they are associated with delusions, behavioral disturbances, a rapid decline of cognitive function, severely abnormal EEGs, and a poor prognosis.

There are several warning signs about hallucinations that develop in Alzheimer's disease patients. Although "sundowning" has probably been overestimated, hallucinations may be triggered by a sudden, unexpected change in the environment. Also, they are often precipitated by a superimposed toxic-metabolic condition, such as pneumonia, rather than progression of the dementia. Moreover, development of visual hallucinations may indicate that a patient actually has Lewy body disease (see below), in which hallucinations are a commonplace characteristic.

A particularly troublesome behavioral manifestation of Alzheimer's disease is *wandering*. A sign of moderately advanced dementia, wandering probably originates in a combination of memory impairment, visual-spatial difficulties, delusions, and hallucinations; possibly akathisia or other medication side effect; or mundane activities, such as looking for food or seeking old friends. Wandering is dangerous to the patient and disruptive to caregivers.

Alzheimer's patients lose the normal, circadian sleep-wake pattern to a greater degree than unaffected elderly people (see Chapter 17). Their sleep becomes fragmented throughout the day and night. Breakdown in sleep parallels severity of dementia.

Disturbingly, Alzheimer's patients who drive tend to be involved in motor vehicle accidents. Their accident rate is greater than comparably aged individuals, and it increases with the duration of their illness. (Yet, 16- to 24-year-old men have an even higher rate of motor vehicle accidents than Alzheimer's patients!) Several states require that physicians report patients with medical impairments that would interfere with safe driving, presumably including Alzheimer's disease, to the motor vehicle bureau.

Physical Signs.   Patients with Alzheimer's disease characteristically have few physical abnormalities until the end stage of the illness. For example, until then, they are ambulatory. The common sight of a patient walking aimlessly through a neighborhood characterizes the disparity between intellectual and motor deficits. Physicians can typically elicit only frontal release signs (Fig. 7–4), increased jaw jerk reflex (see Fig. 4–12), and Babinski signs. Unlike patients with vascular dementia, those with Alzheimer's disease do not have lateralized signs, such as hemiparesis or homonymous hemianopsia.

When patients reach the end stage, their physical as well as cognitive deficits become profound. They then become mute, fail to respond to verbal requests, take to bed, and assume a decorticate (fetal) posture. They frequently slip into a persistent vegetative state (see Chapter 11).

Tests

Testing for Alzheimer's disease is a misnomer because no test possesses the requisite diagnostic sensitivity and specificity. Tests performed when it is suspected serve rather to exclude other causes.

The first EEG change in Alzheimer's disease, slowing of background activity, is not universal and is difficult to distinguish from expected age-related slowing. In advanced disease, the EEG usually shows slow, disorganized background activity, which is also nonspecific.

The CT shows nonspecific cerebral atrophy. Serial studies typically show a rapidly progressive, yet still nonspecific atrophy.

The MRI similarly shows a sequential, progressive atrophy: first the hippocampus, then the temporal and parietal lobes, and eventually frontal lobes. As can be seen with both the CT and MRI, cerebral atrophy produces widening of the third ventricle. The gyri thin to ribbonlike structures and the sulci widen and deepen. Although

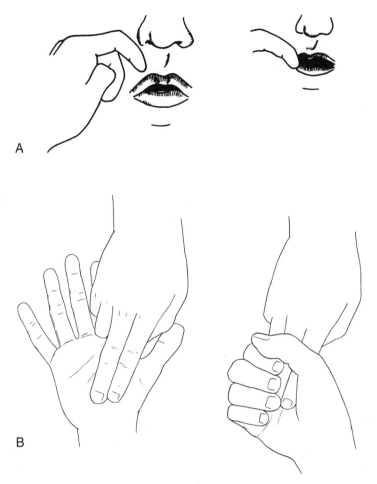

FIGURE 7–4. The frontal lobe release reflexes that are found frequently in elderly individuals with severe dementia are the snout and grasp reflexes. **A,** The snout reflex is elicited by tapping the patient's upper lip with a finger or a percussion hammer. This reflex causes the patient's lips to purse and the mouth to pout. **B,** The grasp reflex is elicited by stroking the patient's palm crosswise or the fingers lengthwise. The reflex causes the patient to grasp the examiner's fingers and fail to let go despite requests.

obvious, the cerebral atrophy is not specific for Alzheimer's disease. Even in established cases, it has no predictive value.

In about one-half of Alzheimer's patients, positron emission tomography (PET) shows areas of decreased cerebral oxygen and glucose metabolism in the parietal and temporal cortical association cortex bilaterally. These areas of hypometabolism are vague at first, but as the disease progresses they become more distinct and spread to the frontal lobe cortex. Nevertheless, PET remains unsuitable for routine use mostly because of poor sensitivity and specificity (see Chapter 20).

Single photon emission computed tomography (SPECT) is a less expensive and less cumbersome version of PET. It, too, produces nonspecific results and is an unsatisfactory test for Alzheimer's disease.

Cerebral cortex biopsies for diagnostic purposes are virtually never indicated—mostly because routine evaluation is about 90% reliable. In addition, histologic findings of Alzheimer's disease differ only quantitatively rather than qualitatively from age-related changes. As a rare last resort, cerebral cortex biopsies can provide a diagnosis of Creutzfeldt-Jakob disease or, mostly by excluding other illnesses, might help establish cases of familial Alzheimer's disease.

Various other less invasive tests—psychologic, serologic, and radiographic—are constantly proposed to diagnose Alzheimer's disease. However, they lack the specificity or sensitivity to surpass the current reliability of about 90%.*

Pathology

Compared with age-matched controls, brains of Alzheimer's disease patients are more atrophic. Moreover, Alzheimer's disease atrophy characteristically preferentially affects the cerebral cortex association areas, such as the parietal-temporal junction, and the limbic system, especially the hippocampus. In contrast, the cortex governing primary motor, sensory, or visual functions is relatively spared. Consequently, the atrophy causes the lateral and particularly the third ventricles to be dilated.

Although found in normal aging and other conditions, plaques and tangles remains the most conspicuous histologic feature of Alzheimer's disease. Alzheimer's disease plaques and tangles are dense and, like the atrophy, found mostly in the cortex association areas and limbic system, especially the hippocampus.

These gross and histologic changes in the limbic system and association areas correlate with Alzheimer's disease's characteristic impairment of memory and more complex cognitive function. Similarly, the relative sparing of the motor and visual areas correlates with the lack of paresis and blindness.

Neurofibrillary tangles are composed of paired helical filaments within neurons (i.e., they are "intraneuronal"). The filaments contain abnormally phosphorylated tau protein. In Alzheimer's disease, neurofibrillary tangles are concentrated in the hippocampus and, most important, parallel the dementia's duration and severity. Although they are closely associated with Alzheimer's disease, neurofibrillary tangles are also found in dementia pugilistica, SSPE, and other neurologic illnesses, where they affect different populations of neurons.

Neuritic plaques, a form of *senile plaques,* are round extracellular aggregates composed of an amyloid core surrounded by abnormal axons and dendrites *(neurites).* While plaques generally show a poor correlation with dementia, neuritic plaques can be correlated with dementia, although less closely then neurofibrillary tangles.

In Alzheimer's disease, enzymes encoded on chromosome 21 cleave *amyloid precursor protein (APP)* to deposit *β-amyloid* in senile plaques. This amyloid differs from the amyloid deposited in viscera as the result of various systemic illnesses, such as multiple myeloma and amyloidosis. Alzheimer's disease β-amyloid accumulates early and uniformly and may be required for development of the characteristic pathology. In fact, conversion of APP to β-amyloid seems to be an essential step in producing Alzheimer's disease. Nevertheless, despite its being an almost invariable finding in Alzheimer's disease, β-amyloid concentration does not correlate with severity of dementia.

Loss of neurons in the frontal and temporal lobes and particularly in the *nucleus basalis of Meynert* (also known as the *substantia innominata*)—a group of large neurons located near the septal region beneath the globus pallidus—is characteristic of Alzheimer's disease. Of all histologic features, loss of these neurons' synapses correlates most closely with dementia.

---

*Sensitivity $= \dfrac{\text{true-positives}}{\text{(true-positives + false-negatives)}}$

Specificity $= \dfrac{\text{true-negatives}}{\text{(true-negatives + false-positives)}}$

Biochemical Abnormalities.   Under normal circumstances, neurons in the basal nucleus of Meynert (the substantia innominata) synthesize *acetylcholine (ACh)*. Using the enzyme *choline acetyltransferase (ChAT)*, they convert acetylcoenzyme-A (acetyl-CoA) and choline to ACh:

$$\text{Acetyl-CoA} + \text{Choline} \xrightarrow{\text{ChAT}} \text{ACh}$$

The axons of these neurons project upward to virtually the entire cerebral cortex and the limbic system to provide cholinergic (i.e., acetylcholine [ACh]) innervation. These regions have abundant ACh receptors that are almost entirely *muscarinic* rather than nicotinic. (Nicotinic ACh receptors are found predominantly in the spinal cord and the neuromuscular junction.)

Alzheimer's disease is characterized—virtually identified—by a loss of the neurons in the basal nucleus of Meynert. This loss causes a marked reduction in cerebral cortex ACh concentrations, ChAT activity, and overall cerebral cholinergic activity. (Despite the loss of the presynaptic neurons, cortical postsynaptic muscarinic elements remain intact.) ACh activity is depressed especially in the limbic system and association areas. The ACh and ChAT loss correlates roughly with the degree of dementia.

Other established or putative neurotransmitters also depleted in Alzheimer's disease include somatostatin, substance P, norepinephrine, vasopressin, and several other polypeptides. However, compared to ACh loss, their concentrations are not decreased profoundly or consistently and do not correlate with dementia.

The "cholinergic hypothesis," drawn from these biochemical observations, postulates that dementia in Alzheimer's disease results from reduced cholinergic activity. It is supported by finding that even in normal individuals, blocking cerebral muscarinic ACh receptors causes profound memory impairments. In particular, scopolamine, which has central anticholinergic activity, induces a several-minute episode of Alzheimer-like cognitive impairment that can be reversed with physostigmine (Fig. 7–5).

Although the ChAT deficiency in Alzheimer's disease is striking, it is not unique. Pronounced ChAT deficiencies are also found in the cortex of brains in Down's syndrome and Parkinson's disease dementia (but not Huntington's disease).

Risk Factors and Potential Etiologies

Many risk factors (statistically significant associations)—but not causes (etiologies)—have been established for Alzheimer's disease. The greatest risk factors are advanced age, Down's syndrome, having a twin or a first-degree relative with Alzheimer's disease, and *apolipoprotein E (Apo-E)* 3/4 or 4/4 (see below). Associations have been asserted between Alzheimer's disease and head trauma, myocardial infarction, episodic depression, personality disorder, hypertension, hyperthyroidism, and exposure to aluminum, but these are weak.

The risk attributed to apolipoprotein E (Apo-E) is the most complex. Apo-E is a cholesterol-carrying protein produced in the liver and brain that circulates in the plasma. It binds to β-amyloid and becomes incorporated into neuritic plaques. The gene for Apo-E is encoded on chromosome 19 in three alleles: Apo-E2, Apo-E3, and Apo-E4. Inheriting one of three alleles (E2, E3, E4) from each parent gives everyone one of six possible allele pairs (e.g., E2-E2, E2-E4, E3-E4, etc.). Approximately 10% to 20% of the population has the pair E3-E4 or E4-E4, which is most closely associated with Alzheimer's disease.

Having two alleles (being homozygous) for E4—and to a lesser degree having one allele (being heterozygous) for E4—is associated with an unequivocally increased risk of developing Alzheimer's disease. Risk is accentuated by other factors, such as

Choline + Acetyl-CoA $\xrightarrow{\text{ChAT}}$ ACh $\longrightarrow$ Receptors:
Central
Neuromuscular
Autonomic

ACh $\longrightarrow$ | Scopolamine
Atropine | Receptors

ACh
↓ Cholinesterase
↓ Anticholinesterases:
Edrophonium (Tensilon)
Pyridostigmine (Mestinon)
Physostigmine
Tacrine (Cognex)
Donepezil (Aricept)
Insecticides

FIGURE 7–5. *Top,* The enzyme choline acetyltransferase (ChAT) catalyzes the synthesis of choline and acetyl-coenzyme-A (acetyl-CoA) to form acetylcholine (ACh) in central, peripheral, and autonomic nervous system neurons. When released from its presynaptic neurons, ACh interacts with postsynaptic ACh receptors. *Middle,* However, ACh may be blocked from interacting with the receptors by various substances. For example, scopolamine, which readily crosses the blood-brain barrier, blocks ACh-receptor interaction in the CNS. Atropine blocks ACh receptors but predominantly those in the autonomic nervous system. Unless large quantities are administered, atropine does not cross the blood-brain barrier. *Bottom,* ACh is metabolized by cholinesterase. Thus, its action is terminated under normal conditions by enzyme degradation rather than, as with dopamine and serotonin, being terminated by reuptake. However, if cholinesterase is inhibited or blocked, ACh will be preserved. Various substances—anticholinesterases or cholinesterase inhibitors—block the enzyme and preserve ACh concentrations. For example, edrophonium (Tensilon) and pyridostigmine (Mestinon) are anticholinesterase medications used to treat myasthenia gravis by preserving neuromuscular junction ACh (see Fig. 6–2). Anticholinesterases are also widely used in insecticides that cause paralysis by creating excessive ACh activity at neuromuscular junctions. Physostigmine, a powerful anticholinesterase medication that can cross the blood-brain barrier, is administered to correct ACh deficits in Alzheimer's disease and purported in tardive dyskinesia (see Chapter 18). It might also be administered to counteract excessive anticholinergic activity in tricyclic antidepressant overdose or the effects of scopolamine or atropine.

being older than 80 years, having Down's syndrome, or having had repeated head injury. Overall, having one E4 allele triples the risk of developing Alzheimer's disease by 80 years and having two E4 alleles raises the risk to 90%. An E4 allele is found in more than 50% of Alzheimer's disease patients. Moreover, Alzheimer's disease patients who are Apo-E4 homozygous, compared to those who are not, tend to develop Alzheimer's disease at an earlier age, experience a more rapid decline, and, have greater amyloid content and lower acetylcholine activity.

On the other hand, having one or even two E4 alleles is neither necessary nor sufficient for development of Alzheimer's disease. The association of Apo-E4 with Alzheimer's disease, while very close, is not close enough to be etiologic. Apo-E determinations lack the specificity and sensitivity required for a reliable diagnostic test. Current recommendations are as follows: (1) In individuals who have developed dementia, Apo-E determinations should not be performed to diagnose Alzheimer's disease. (2) In asymptomatic individuals, these determinations should not be performed as a predictive test for Alzheimer's disease.

In contrast, several factors are associated with decreased incidence or postponed onset of the disease. Although its level cannot be determined as yet, formal education seems to offer a measurable degree of protection against dementia in general and Alzheimer's disease in particular. Other protective factors seem to be use of nonsteroidal anti-inflammatory drugs (NSAIDs) and, in postmenopausal women, estrogen replacement therapy (ERT). These medicines' apparent protective value may be converted to preemptive treatment. Surprisingly, smoking is associated with a reduced incidence of Alzheimer's disease, even adjusted for premature death.

Other Genetic Considerations. Family history of Alzheimer's disease is a clear risk factor. Although most cases occur sporadically, about 20% of patients' offspring, 10% of second-degree relatives, and 5% of age-matched controls will develop it.

In some families, the disease is clearly genetically induced. *Familial Alzheimer's disease,* for example, follows an autosomal dominant pattern. This variety theoretically gives offspring a 50% incidence during the course of a 90-year life span. However, the observed incidence is lower probably because susceptible individuals succumb to other conditions before the onset of dementia.

Most familial Alzheimer's disease patients have the cognitive and histologic changes typical of nonfamilial Alzheimer's disease but tend to display an early age of onset and other clinical anomalies. They characteristically develop dementia between ages 40 and 60 years, significantly younger than in sporadic cases. Also, they often run a rapid or fulminant course and develop myoclonus or seizures.

Mutations on at least four chromosomes—1, 14, 19, and 21—have individually been suspected of transmitting or rendering people susceptible to familial Alzheimer's disease. All are associated with β-amyloid deposition in plaques and increased neurofibrillary tangles.

Most familial Alzheimer's disease cases are linked to a mutation on chromosome 14, which contains the *presenilin I gene.* The Apo-E data and other information implicate chromosome 19. A chromosome 21 mutation, despite rare association with Alzheimer's disease, has been implicated because the gene for APP (see above), which is closely associated with amyloid deposition in plaques, is situated on chromosome 21. Also, almost all trisomy 21 (Down's syndrome) individuals develop the clinical and pathologic manifestations of Alzheimer's disease by age 40 (see below). A mutation on chromosome 1, present in several European families (Volga Germans) with familial Alzheimer's disease, contains the *presenilin II gene,* which is similar to the presenilin I gene on chromosome 14.

Although genetic factors are undoubtedly important in Alzheimer's disease pathogenesis, they account for less than 20% of cases. As noted, cases of familial Alzheimer's disease tend to have idiosyncratic features. Even monozygotic twins develop symptoms at greatly different times.

Treatment

Dementia. In light of the plausibility of the cholinergic hypothesis and the finding that postsynaptic muscarinic cholinergic receptors remain relatively intact, several treatments have attempted to restore ACh activity. Researchers have administered ACh precursors, such as choline and lecithin (phosphatidyl choline), and ACh agonists, such as arecoline, oxotremorine, acetyl-L-carnitine, and bethanechol. Whether administered by intraventricular or traditional routes, these substances produced no benefit.

A complementary strategy increased ACh concentration by reducing its metabolism by cholinesterases. Centrally acting anticholinesterases, such as physostigmine, tetrahydroacridine (tacrine [Cognex]), and donepezil (Aricept) increase cerebral ACh concentrations. Moreover, tacrine and donepezil, which are long-acting, orally administered anticholinesterases, produce modest, temporary improvements on performance-based tests, "global evaluations," and measurements of quality of life. They retard cognitive decline and preserve functional capacity, at best, for about 12 months in mild to moderately severe Alzheimer's disease.

Similar therapeutic trials were based on replenishing other deficient presynaptic neurotransmitters, such as somatostatin, vasopressin, and other polypeptides. Despite promise, all were unsuccessful.

Although reduced cerebral blood flow is a result, not a cause, of Alzheimer's disease, attempts have been made to restore normal blood flow with cyclospasmol and Hydergine. A minimal improvement that followed Hydergine, which is an ergot alkaloid, is attributable to its antidepressant properties.

Alternative approaches aimed at preventing cerebral cortical damage are in clinical trials. For example, selegiline (see Chapter 18, deprenyl) and alpha-tocopherol (vitamin E) administration, antioxidants that presumably protect neurons, theoretically will retard any cognitive decline. In view of the reduced incidence of Alzheimer's disease in postmenopausal women who have taken ERT and individuals who have taken NSAIDs, these agents are being evaluated.

Other Symptoms.   Because depression may complicate dementia or even cause cognitive impairment (as in pseudodementia), trials of antidepressants have been justifiably freely given. In view of Alzheimer's disease patients' ACh deficiency, physicians should favor psychotropics with minimal anticholinergic activity. Tricyclic antidepressants provide little benefit in depression, and, predictably, they often cause confusion and orthostatic hypotension in Alzheimer's disease patients. SSRIs may alleviate depression as much or more than tricyclic antidepressants. Although they may cause insomnia and sexual impairment, they produce few cognitive side effects.

Neuroleptics, anxiolytics, or antiepileptic drugs are often administered for agitation, delusions, and aggressive behavior. With an absence of definitive studies comparing one to another medication, only a few general rules can be applied. In consultation with the patient's caregivers, target one symptom. Begin with small doses of a single medication but proceed to effective doses. Do not confuse medication side effects, especially sedation, with disease progression. Periodically reassess need for psychotropics because, as disease progresses, symptoms change or even disappear.

Psychotropic medications provide little benefit for wandering and most other dangerous or disruptive behavior. Alternatives, such as constructing large indoor and outdoor "safe zones," might satisfy the patient and caregivers.

Sleep disturbances, such as hallucinations and REM behavioral disorder (see Chapter 17), deprive the patient of restorative, restful nighttime sleep and lead to daytime sleep. Because patients' sleep disruptions extend to the entire household, they often represent the most burdensome problem for caregivers. When mild and in their early stages, sleep disturbances may be reduced by providing daytime exercise, exposure to sunlight, and restricted naps. Otherwise, for everybody's benefit, these symptoms usually require preemptive early evening administration of sedatives or tranquilizers.

With the various medications and nonpharmacologic interventions providing only palliative care for the progressively severe cognitive and behavioral manifestations of Alzheimer's disease, physicians must, at some time, concede that care at home is not in the patient's or family's best interest. Disruptive behavior—not cognitive decline—is the most compelling reason for families to place these patients in nursing homes. The other reasons are incontinence and nighttime disruptions. Physicians can help families by keeping their expectations realistic, preserving their financial and emotional resources, securing help from social service agencies, and preventing a hopeless situation from dominating family life.

RELATED DISORDERS

Down's Syndrome

Almost all individuals with Down's syndrome, which is almost always the result of chromosome 21 trisomy, develop an Alzheimer-like dementia superimposed on their mental retardation if they live to 40 years (see Chapter 13). Moreover, their brains show Alzheimer's-like changes: atrophy, cholinergic depletion, amyloid plaques, neurofibrillary tangles, and loss of neurons in the nucleus basalis. Likewise, CT, MRI, and PET changes show Alzheimer's-like changes. Even relatives of Down's syndrome individuals have an increased incidence of Alzheimer's disease. These striking similarities between Down's syndrome and Alzheimer's disease were an early suggestion that in certain families Alzheimer's disease resulted from an abnormality on chromosome 21. (Of course, other chromosomes—1, 14, and 19—have also been implicated [see earlier discussion].)

Lewy Body Disease

Also typically causing dementia in individuals older than 65 years is *Lewy body disease* (*diffuse Lewy body disease* or *dementia with Lewy bodies* [the awkward but official title]). Possibly accounting for up to 30% of cases diagnosed as Alzheimer's disease, Lewy body disease may be merely a variant of Alzheimer's disease rather than a distinct illness. It has been described so recently that it is not specifically included in *DSM-IV*.

Unlike Alzheimer's disease, Lewy body disease has relatively rapid development of dementia accompanied by mild extrapyramidal (Parkinson-like) features, such as masked face, bradykinesia, resting tremor, and gait impairment so pronounced that it leads to falls (see Chapter 18). In addition to their extrapyramidal symptoms failing to respond to L-dopa (see Chapter 18), patients are unusually sensitive to dopamine-blocking neuroleptics. If given even small amounts, they develop akinesia and severe rigidity. Another characteristic is that Lewy body dementia is complicated by depression, delusions, and visual hallucinations (see Chapter 12).

Its definitive diagnosis requires an abundant presence and unusual location of Lewy bodies, which are intracytoplasmic inclusions in neurons previously found virtually only in the substantia nigra in Parkinson's disease. In Lewy body disease, Lewy bodies are distributed diffusely throughout the cerebral cortex, are readily detectable, and are confirmed by an *antiubiquitin* antibody stain. Concentration of Lewy bodies in the cerebral cortex correlates with dementia.

OTHER DEMENTIAS

Frontal Lobe Disorders

Injuries. The frontal lobes are one of the main sources of personality, emotions, and executive decisions, as well as the seat of inhibitory systems that suppress certain behaviors. Patients with frontal lobe damage show personality and behavioral changes that are much more stereotyped than those seen in Alzheimer's disease. Although dementia is not necessarily among these changes, understanding them provides a helpful context for discussion of frontotemporal dementia (see below). The basic principle is that, whether or not patients with frontal lobe damage have cognitive impairment, frontal lobe symptoms themselves do not equal dementia.

Lacking spontaneity, patients with frontal lobe damage tend to be reticent. They have impoverished, slowed thoughts and emotions. They are indifferent or unresponsive to their surroundings, ongoing events, and underlying illness. Mental rigidity prevents them, on neuropsychologic testing, from making transitions, changing sets, and adopting alternate strategies.

Movements tend to be reduced or absent (akinetic). When patients initiate movements, they are slow (bradykinetic) and tend to be repeated (perseverated). With extensive frontal lobe damage, patients lack communication and voluntary movement. Patients with such deficits are described as having *abulia* or, in the extreme, *akinetic mutism.*

For patients with mild to moderate frontal lobe injury, walking becomes awkward and uncertain (ataxic or apraxic). Viscous thinking and movement, *psychomotor retardation,* is often accompanied by other signs of frontal lobe injury: pseudobulbar palsy, nonfluent aphasia, and frontal release signs. Also, because of the olfactory nerves' location on the frontal lobes' undersurface, patients with frontal lobe injuries often have anosmia (see Chapter 4).

Impaired inhibitory systems tend to promote flighty and inappropriate comments and thoughts, bladder or bowel incontinence, and unrestrained expression of sexual urges. Because patients cannot inhibit a natural tendency to attend to new stimuli, they are easily distracted from their tasks. They may be so incapable of disregarding new or changing stimuli that they are "stimulus bound." Possibly, because they are uninhibited, patients with frontal lobe injury characteristically display a superficial, odd jocularity with uncontrollable, facetious laughter *(witzelsucht)* that includes elements of pseudobulbar palsy. On a more somber note, on what is a different aspect of uninhibited behavior, neurologic evaluations of murderers have revealed that the majority have frontal lobe dysfunction.

Patients with frontal lobe damage typically retain memory, simple calculation ability, and visual-spatial perception because these cognitive domains are based in the parietal and temporal lobes. Indeed, IQ tests of patients with frontal lobe dysfunction often yield normal results.

Discrete lesions, such as a gunshot wound, glioblastoma multiforme, metastatic tumor, multiple sclerosis plaques, or infarction of both anterior cerebral arteries, commonly cause frontal lobe dysfunction. The now abandoned, infamous *frontal lobotomy,* a group of neurosurgical procedures in which surgeons resected patients' frontal lobe cortex, severed its underlying large white matter tracts, or injected it with sclerosing agents, produced a variety of frontal lobe deficits (see Fig. 20–14). Patients had less agitation but usually at the expense of developing apathy, restricted spontaneous verbal output, indifference to social conventions, and impaired abstract reasoning. Nevertheless, they usually retained their intelligence.

Frontotemporal dementia, a degenerative illness, causes a variety of frontal lobe dysfunction. In contrast, Alzheimer's disease and vascular dementia are not usually responsible for the constellation of frontal lobe symptoms because they produce a different cognitive impairment but not the behavioral changes.

Frontotemporal Dementia.   This degenerative condition encompasses Pick's disease and related illnesses. Its primary clinical feature is a progressively severe dementia that, in addition to memory loss, is accompanied by impaired executive functions and changes in personality and behavior. These noncognitive symptoms, which commonly include aggression or apathy, disinhibition, obsessive or compulsive symptoms, "hyperorality," and other aspects of the Klüver-Bucy syndrome (see Chapters 12 and 16), all reflect frontal and temporal lobe damage. At least in the early stages, its features do not include either constructional apraxia or visual-spatial impairments.

This disease's gross pathologic appearance, so distinctive as to provide its name, closely correlates with the clinical features. The frontal and anterior temporal lobes are atrophic. In contrast, the parietal and occipital lobes, which are unaffected, are relatively prominent. Plaques and tangles are not particularly common. Those cases with neurons containing argentophilic (silver-staining) inclusions *(Pick bodies)*, which are a minority, are designated Pick's disease. In other words, Pick's disease is now considered a histologic variant of frontotemporal dementia rather than a distinct illness.

Frontotemporal dementia, which may account for about 15% of cases of dementia, usually develops in individuals younger than 65 years. It tends to occur in multiple family members and has been linked to chromosome 17. The *DSM-IV* retains the designation dementia due to Pick's disease for this disorder.

CT and MRI changes, which are predictable in view of the gross pathology, consist of frontal and temporal lobe atrophy with normal-sized parietal lobes (see Fig. 20–10, *A*). By contrast, CT and MRI changes in Alzheimer's disease primarily affect the parietal and temporal lobes. Despite an overall poor sensitivity and specificity, PET and SPECT often show hypometabolism in the frontal lobes in cases of unequivocal frontotemporal dementia.

Vascular Dementia

After Alzheimer's and perhaps diffuse Lewy body disease, multiple cerebral infarctions are the most common cause of dementia (see Chapter 11). In *DSM-IV*, multi-infarct dementia seems to be virtually interchangeable with vascular dementia (see Chapter 11). Also, the *DSM-IV* criteria for dementia are the same in vascular dementia, dementia of the Alzheimer's type, and dementia in general.

In vascular dementia, patients sustain multiple cerebrovascular accidents (CVAs) that characteristically produce dementia accompanied by focal or lateralized physical signs, such as hemiparesis, visual field cuts, and ataxia. In addition, pseudobulbar palsy and aphasia are often superimposed on the dementia and alter its expression. Although vascular dementia often evolves as a *stepwise* intellectual deterioration, that pattern is no longer a clinical criterion.

The neuropsychologic picture of vascular dementia, unlike that of most other varieties, is often obscured by aphasia, other specific neuropsychologic deficits, and critical physical impairments, particularly dysarthria. In addition, frequently associated illnesses, such as renal and cardiac disease, and the medications used to treat them can exacerbate the neurologic deficits and produce additional problems.

Wernicke-Korsakoff Syndrome

Chronic, excessive alcohol consumption is complicated by cognitive impairment and other signs of central nervous system (CNS) and peripheral nervous system (PNS) damage. Although any particular neurologic complication may predominate, most are considered elements of the *Wernicke-Korsakoff syndrome*.

Cognitive impairment is proportional to the lifetime consumption of alcohol and develops in about 50% of all chronic alcoholics. It begins with a *global confusional state*, in which patients are apathetic, slow, and oblivious to their difficulties. Contrary to traditional descriptions, confabulation is usually absent or inconspicuous.

The distinctive feature of Wernicke-Korsakoff syndrome is amnesia that includes impaired memory for previously known facts *(retrograde amnesia)* coupled with an inability to remember new ones *(anterograde amnesia)*. Although disabling, amnesia does not constitute dementia. As the syndrome progresses, the amnesia interferes with various memory-based cognitive functions, especially learning. Eventually an Alzheimer-like dementia evolves.

In acute stages, patients may have ataxia and ocular motility abnormalities that include conjugate gaze paresis, abducens nerve paresis, and nystagmus (see Chapters 4 and 12); however, only a minority have all these findings. With chronic alcoholism, patients develop a peripheral neuropathy (see Chapter 5) and cerebellar atrophy. The cerebellar atrophy particularly affects the vermis (see Chapter 2), which leads to the distinctive gait ataxia (see Fig. 2–13).

CTs and MRIs may be normal or show only cerebral atrophy. The EEG is usually normal. The mamillary bodies and structures surrounding the third ventricle and the aqueduct of Sylvius (see *periaqueductal gray matter*, Fig. 18–2) develop petechial hemorrhages. Because these structures support the limbic system, the anatomic basis of the memory circuit, injury to them produces the amnesia (see Fig. 16–5).

Wernicke-Korsakoff syndrome is not restricted to alcoholics. Virtually identical clinical and pathologic changes develop in nonalcoholics who have undergone starvation, dialysis, or chemotherapy.

Therefore, Wernicke-Korsakoff syndrome is not merely the result of alcohol toxicity. In fact, it probably results primarily from a profound nutritional deficiency of thiamine (vitamin B_1), an essential co-enzyme in carbohydrate metabolism. This theory is confirmed by thiamine administration preventing or even partially reversing the condition. Established practice is that thiamine should be administered parenterally as soon as possible in equivocal as well as clear-cut cases. Despite timely treatment, only 25% of patients recover from dementia, and pathologic changes are irreversible.

The *DSM-IV*, accepting the predominance of amnesia and the thiamine deficiency theory, gives the terms "amnestic disorder due to thiamine deficiency" or "alcohol-induced (persisting) amnestic disorder" to Wernicke-Korsakoff syndrome without addressing the ocular and other physical neurologic abnormalities. When alcoholism leads to dementia, the *DSM-IV* term "alcohol-induced persisting dementia" is applicable.

Other Causes of Dementia in Alcoholics.   Alcoholics frequently sustain head trauma that causes contusions and subdural hematomas leading to dementia and other neurologic problems. Likewise, they are prone to motor vehicle accidents because of impaired judgment, slowed physical responses, and a tendency to fall asleep while driving. Those with Laënnec's cirrhosis develop hepatic encephalopathy, especially after gastrointestinal bleeding. The encephalopathy, which may be low-grade or subtle, might continually or intermittently cause cognitive or personality changes.

Rarely, but interestingly, alcoholics can develop degeneration of the corpus callosum that causes a *split brain syndrome* (see Marchiafava-Bignami syndrome, Chapter 8). Alcoholics are also susceptible to seizures from either excessive alcohol or alcohol withdrawal. In either case, because the seizures result from metabolic aberrations, they are more likely to be generalized, tonic-clonic seizures rather than partial complex seizures (see Chapter 10). Finally, infants of severely alcoholic mothers are often born with *fetal alcohol syndrome*, which includes facial anomalies, a low birth weight, microcephaly, and tremors. This disorder can lead to mental retardation, and the others to dementia.

Medication-Induced Dementia

Cognitive impairment from medications is one of the few truly correctable varieties of dementia. Agents designed to act on the CNS—narcotics, anticonvulsants, antiparkinson agents, steroids, and, of course, psychotropics—routinely produce various mental abnormalities. Others, such as cimetidine, do so infrequently and unpredictably. Even medicines instilled into the eye may be absorbed into the sys-

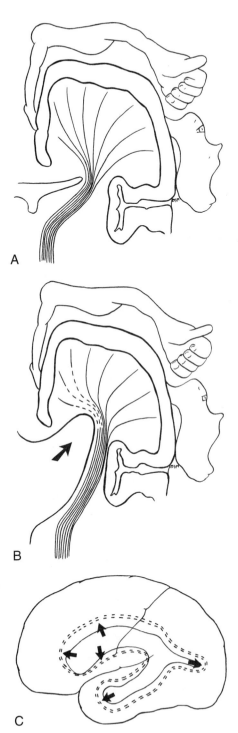

FIGURE 7–6. A and B, Ventricular expansion, as in normal pressure hydrocephalus, results in compression of brain parenchyma and stretching of the myelinated tracts of the internal capsule (see Fig. 18–1). Gait impairment (apraxia) and urinary incontinence are prominent NPH symptoms because the tracts that govern the legs and the voluntary muscles of the bladder are the most stretched. **C,** Also, because the CSF exerts force equally in all directions, pressure on the frontal lobes leads to dementia and psychomotor retardation.

temic circulation and cause mental changes. Over-the-counter medications, which have become numerous, potent, and widely advertised, may produce mental aberrations individually or through interaction.

Normal Pressure Hydrocephalus

Normal pressure hydrocephalus (NPH) is commonly cited both as (1) a cause of dementia clinicians can identify by its physical manifestations and (2) reversible. However, actual patients correctly identified and then successfully treated are few, clinical and laboratory diagnoses are unreliable, and treatment is hazardous and inconsistently effective.

NPH is a clinical syndrome that consists of dementia, urinary incontinence, and *gait apraxia*. It often follows attacks of meningitis or subarachnoid hemorrhage, but most often results from an unknown injury. Apparently, these insults clog the arachnoid villi overlying the brain to impair reabsorption of CSF, thus producing hydrocephalus (Fig. 7–6).

NPH dementia is distinctively characterized as much by psychomotor retardation as cognitive impairment. Consequently, it is accompanied or overshadowed by its physical features. Gait apraxia is usually the first and most prominent symptom of NPH (Fig. 7–7). Similarly, it is the first symptom to improve with treatment. Urinary

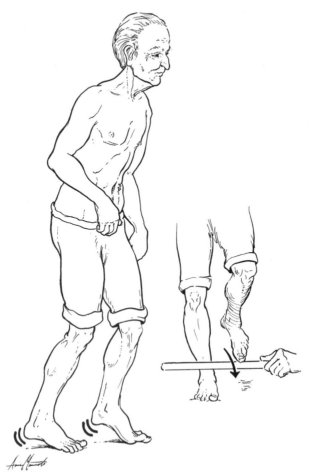

FIGURE 7–7. Gait apraxia, the cardinal manifestation of NPH, can be seen in several aspects of gait testing. Patients with gait apraxia fail to alternate their leg movements and do not shift their weight to the forward foot. They tend to pick up the same leg twice in a row or elevate the weight-bearing foot. When their weight remains on the foot that they attempt to raise, that foot appears to be stuck or "magnetized" to the floor.

Gait apraxia is most pronounced when patients start to walk or begin a turn. However, because their stepping reflex is relatively preserved, they can sometimes step over a stick or other obstacle.

incontinence initially consists of urgency and frequency but, in severe cases, total incontinence.

Urinary incontinence and gait abnormality present at the onset of dementia distinguish NPH from Alzheimer's disease. The gait abnormality and psychomotor retardation also make NPH the quintessential subcortical dementia.

In NPH, CTs and MRIs show ventricular dilation, particularly of the temporal horns (see Figs. 20–4 and 20–15). There is minimal or no cerebral atrophy and sometimes signs of CSF reabsorption across ventricular surfaces. However, identification of NPH by CTs and MRIs is unreliable because this pattern is nonspecific and it resembles cerebral atrophy with resultant hydrocephalus, *hydrocephalus ex vacuo* (see Fig. 20–3). Isotopic cisternography, a technique that outlines the ventricles as well as the cisterns and provides a profile of CSF absorption is also not reliable enough for therapeutic decisions. The CSF pressure and its protein and glucose concentrations are normal. The EEG is also not helpful for a diagnosis.

Common tests are simply to withdraw 30 ml of CSF by a lumbar puncture (LP) or to perform a series of three LPs. Each maneuver would presumably transiently reduce hydrocephalus. Following CSF removal, improvement in the patient's gait—not necessarily the dementia—would indicate NPH and predict benefits from permanent CSF drainage.

NPH can be relieved, at least theoretically, by placement of a shunt into a lateral ventricle to drain CSF into the chest or abdominal cavity, where it can be absorbed. However, a clinically beneficial response to shunt installation is as low as 50% of cases where a cause of NPH, such as a subarachnoid hemorrhage, is established, and only 15% of idiopathic cases. Moreover, despite the apparent simplicity of shunting, neurosurgical complications, which can be devastating, occur in 13% to 28% of patients.

INFECTIONS

Neurosyphilis

Caused by persistent *Treponema pallidum* infection, neurosyphilis had been largely of historic interest until the late 1980s, when it began to be diagnosed in many AIDS patients. Secondary syphilis causes *acute syphilitic meningitis.* Only a small fraction of patients eventually develop tertiary complications, such as meningovascular syphilis or dementia.

If dementia does develop, it initially causes only mild, nonspecific personality changes and amnesia that, over years, evolve into dementia. Delusions of grandeur, despite their notoriety, occur rarely. The dementia may be accompanied by a variety of physical abnormalities that include dysarthria, tremors, Argyll-Robertson pupils (see Chapter 12), tabes dorsalis, and optic atrophy.

In AIDS patients who contract syphilis, compared to others who contract syphilis, neurosyphilis is more likely to develop and follow a more aggressive course. AIDS impairs syphilis patients' ability to suppress the illness at its secondary stage or its emergence from a latent stage. AIDS patients with syphilis require intravenous (IV) rather than intramuscular penicillin. Although complete clinical recovery is rare, vigorous penicillin treatment may improve cognitive impairment and reverse CSF abnormalities.

Diagnosis of neurosyphilis in AIDS patients is difficult in part because they cannot mobilize the immunologic responses that produce positive serologies. Also, CTs in neurosyphilis typically reveal cerebral atrophy but rarely the diagnostic gummas.

Standard serologies for syphilis are the *Venereal Disease Research Laboratory (VDRL)* and the newer *rapid plasma reagin (RPR)* blood tests. However, both are insufficiently sensitive and specific. Only about 85% of neurosyphilis patients have a positive test result. False-negative findings may result from the naturally occurring resolution of serologic abnormalities; prior, sometimes inadequate, treatment; or immunologic incapacity from AIDS. False-positive results, also common, have been attributed to old age, addiction, and autoimmune diseases (the "3 As").

Refinements of the standard tests are the treponemal or confirmatory serologic tests, the *fluorescent treponemal antibody absorption (FTA-ABS)* and the *treponemal microhemagglutination assay (MHA-TP)*. Both more sensitive and more specific, they are positive in more than 95% of neurosyphilis cases. Moreover, false-positive FTA-ABS and MHA-TP tests are exceedingly rare, except in cases of other spirochete infections. In fact, when evaluating a patient for dementia that might result from neurosyphilis, rather than first ordering a VDRL or RPR test, the physician might simply order a FTA-ABS or MHA-TP.

CSF testing should be done when individuals who develop dementia have either clinical evidence of syphilis, test positive on the FTA-ABS or MHA-TP, or have AIDS. The VDRL is the only currently available CSF test. In about 60% of neurosyphilis cases, the CSF has an elevated protein concentration (45 to 100 mg/dl) and a lymphocytic pleocytosis (5 to 200 cells/ml).

A potentially confusing point is that the CSF in AIDS patients *without* syphilis often has an elevated protein concentration and a lymphocytic pleocytosis that might lead to a false-positive diagnosis of syphilis. Moreover, when AIDS patients develop neurosyphilis, the CSF, as well as routine serologic tests, may for various reasons be false-negative.

One guideline is that a positive CSF VDRL test provides an unequivocal diagnosis of neurosyphilis. On the other hand, the CSF VDRL test is false-negative in as many as 40% of cases. Neurosyphilis can nevertheless usually be diagnosed by the clinical situation and the CSF profile. Another guideline is that penicillin remains the best treatment for neurosyphilis. Physicians should administer it even in equivocal situations or if a penicillin-allergic patient must undergo desensitization.

Subacute Sclerosing Panencephalitis (SSPE)

SSPE is a rare infectious illness that develops predominantly in children. Its earliest manifestations are poor schoolwork, behavioral disturbances, restlessness, and personality changes. As the illness progresses, they develop dementia and characteristic *myoclonus* (see Chapter 18). When SSPE develops in adults, which is extraordinarily rare, patients' mean age is 25 years and the clinical manifestations, in addition to myoclonus, are visual impairment and various motor deficits (spastic hemiparesis, bradykinesia, and rigidity).

A clinical diagnosis of SSPE may be confirmed by finding an elevated CSF measles antibody titer and, during the initial illness, periodic complexes or burst-suppression patterns on the EEG (see Fig. 10–6). Although antiviral medications may arrest its course, SSPE is usually fatal in 1 to 2 years.

Several observations point to a defective measles (rubeola) virus as the cause: about 50% of patients contracted measles before 2 years of age, the CSF measles antibody titer is very high in SSPE patients, and almost no children who have been vaccinated against measles have developed SSPE.

Creutzfeldt-Jakob and Related Diseases

In most cases, Creutzfeldt-Jakob disease, like SSPE, causes a triad of dementia, myoclonus, and the distinctive periodic EEG complexes (see Fig. 10–6). Creutzfeldt-

Jakob disease also mimics Alzheimer's disease because cardinal manifestations are progressively severe dementia and victims' average age at onset is 60 to 64 years. However, unlike Alzheimer's disease, it often causes pyramidal, extrapyramidal, or cerebellar impairment, as well as the myoclonus; follows a characteristically rapid fatal course of about 6 months; and is transmissible.

Creutzfeldt-Jakob disease is the primary example of a *transmissible spongiform encephalopathy* induced by a *prion infection* (see below). Its infectious nature has long been established by inoculating laboratory animals with brain tissue from human patients, confirming *interspecies transmission.* Similarly, it has been accidentally transferred between humans (*intra*species transmission) by corneal transplantation, intracerebral EEG electrodes, and neurosurgery specimens. In a famous iatrogenic tragedy, a group of children contracted it from treatment with growth hormone extracted from human cadaver pituitary glands.

Although most cases of Creutzfeldt-Jakob disease are sporadic, approximately 15% are familial. Those and at least one variant, *Gerstmann-Sträussler* disease, follow an autosomal dominant pattern and have an earlier age of onset. They have been attributed to the infected "host" (patient) having a genetic susceptibility, probably owing to a mutation on the PrP gene (see below) on chromosome 20.

Prions and Spongiform Encephalopathies.   Recent, Nobel Prize–winning work has shown that Creutzfeldt-Jakob disease and its variants are caused by a novel group of pathogens, *prions* (proteinaceous infective agents), composed totally or almost totally of protein and lacking DNA and RNA. Unlike conventional agents, prions resist treatments that hydrolyze nucleic acids, as well as routine sterilization, heat, and formaldehyde; however, they are readily susceptible to procedures that denature proteins.

Prion protein, PrP, an amyloid protein encoded on chromosome 20, is the major or sole constituent of prions. Normally, PrP exists in a *PrP^c* isoform, which is soluble and easily digested by proteases. In a pathologic state, it is transformed to the *PrP^{Sc}* isoform, which is insoluble in most detergents and markedly resistant to proteases. It condenses in neurons and causes their death. While not conventionally reproducing, PrP continuously reconfigures soluble PrP^c to insoluble aggregates of PrP^{Sc}.

As prion-induced changes accumulate, the cerebral cortex takes on the distinctive microscopic, vacuolar (spongelike) appearance of *spongiform encephalopathy.* Western blot studies and special histologic stains of specimens reveal the abnormal protein. Surprisingly, histologic specimens lack the inflammatory cells normally seen in infections. Cerebral biopsies might be diagnostic, but because of the dangers in obtaining and processing them and with no effective treatment, they are performed only to resolve diagnostic dilemmas or when alternative diagnoses are treatable.

The CSF in almost 90% of Creutzfeldt-Jakob disease cases contains traces of prion proteins, which can be detected by a routine LP. These markers are sufficiently specific to confirm the diagnosis and make a biopsy unnecessary.

Other Spongiform Encephalopathies.   Several spongiform encephalopathies affecting humans or animals are defined by histology rather than cause (prions). As when 10 years elapsed before infected pituitary extract–induced Creutzfeldt-Jakob, spongiform encephalopathies appear after an incubation period of many years. Manifestations are virtually confined to the CNS and consist primarily of mental deterioration accompanied by myoclonus and ataxia. Their course is relentlessly progressive and ultimately fatal. Because brain tissue can carry infection, the encephalopathies are transmissible.

Interspecies transmission of prion infections rarely occurs naturally. When they do, incubation time is long. In contrast, intraspecies transfer is relatively easy and incubation time is short.

Several spongiform encephalopathies have remained restricted to animals. One example, *scrapie,* causes sheep and goats to scrape against walls to denude themselves. (PrP^{Sc} is named after the scrapie prion.) In *transmissible mink encephalopathy,* affected mink develop more vicious, antisocial behavior than normal and then progressive deterioration of motor function.

Some spongiform encephalopathies are restricted to humans, although possibly only those with a genetic susceptibility. *Fatal familial insomnia* is a recently described sleep disorder that clearly depends on a genetic vulnerability (see Chapter 17). *Kuru,* characterized by dementia, tremulousness, dysarthria, and ataxia, developed in members of the Fore tribe of New Guinea. Until the entire practice was stopped, people preparing for cannibalism rituals evidently had infected themselves with brain tissue through open cuts. The incubation was 4 years to 30 years, but once symptoms were apparent, death ensued in about 1 year.

Bovine spongiform encephalopathy (BSE), commonly known as "mad cow disease," is the notorious veterinarian spongiform encephalopathy that has struck small numbers of various animals, as well as cows. (The human counterpart has another name and is discussed later.) BSE more closely mimics kuru than Creutzfeldt-Jakob disease.

In most cases, after an incubation period of 4 to 5 years, BSE causes normally docile cows to become belligerent, apprehensive, and difficult to handle. They develop tremulousness, then ataxia, before collapsing. Although its origin remains a mystery, the subsequent intraspecies transmission probably resulted from slaughterhouses' incorporating scraps of infected CNS organs, such as spinal cords, into animal feed (offal). The miniepidemic in British cows has been eradicated by their wholesale slaughter.

The alarm over BSE arose when several British citizens succumbed to *new variant Creutzfeldt-Jakob disease* (the human counterpart of BSE). In this possible interspecies transfer or human extension of BSE, victims developed a striking syndrome of behavioral disturbances, thought disorders, painful peripheral sensory disturbances, and ataxia progressing to death. New variant differs from common Creutzfeldt-Jakob disease in that its victims are younger (average age 29 years) and include teenagers; the course is longer (average 1 year); sensory disturbances are prominent; and EEGs fail to show characteristic changes.

Lyme Disease

Neurologic involvement in acute Lyme disease *(neuroborreliosis)* causes facial palsy, headache, peripheral neuropathy, and meningitis (see Chapter 5). In chronic form, presumably because of encephalitis, Lyme disease produces combinations of cognitive problems with prominent memory difficulties; irritability, depressed mood, and lability; sleep disturbances; and chronic fatigue (see Chapter 6). Although symptoms can mimic multiple sclerosis or other neurologic illness, differential diagnosis in practice is Lyme disease versus depression.

Currently available serum and CSF tests for Lyme disease remain insufficient for confirming or refuting a clinical diagnosis. Also, these tests' results do not correlate with memory impairment. Confusing matters further, because the infectious agent, *Borrelia burgdorferi,* is a spirochete as in syphilis, serum FTA-ABS and VDRL tests may be positive. With active CNS infection, the CSF will almost always have pleocytosis, elevated protein concentration, reduced glucose concentration, and Lyme antibodies. The EEG, CT, and MRI are helpful only in excluding other possibilities.

Lyme disease can be considered a correctable cause of dementia because treatment with several weeks of IV antibiotics is effective. (On the other hand, many patients with symptoms or test results consistent with Lyme disease do not respond to treatment because either they did not actually have Lyme disease, had graver problems, or had no medical illness.)

AIDS Dementia

The principal target of *human immunodeficiency virus (HIV)* infection is helper lymphocytes with CD4 receptors *(CD4 cells)*. In HIV infection, the concentration of CD4 cells declines below the normal count of $\geq 1,400/\text{mm}^3$. Patients who have CD4 counts lower than $400/\text{mm}^3$ are subject to opportunistic infections and neoplasms.

The second target of HIV infection is the CNS. Depending on which portion is primarily infected, patients can develop HIV encephalitis, myelitis, or meningitis. Similarly, all CNS tissue, especially the CSF, is infectious.

AIDS dementia, which is also called the *HIV-1-associated dementia, AIDS dementia complex, HIV dementia*, or, according to the *DSM IV, dementia due to HIV disease*, is the most frequent neurologic complication of AIDS. It affects 20% of all AIDS patients, including 30% to 60% of those in late stage illness. Reflecting its tendency to be a manifestation of late stage illness, AIDS dementia is associated with anemia and weight loss, CD4 counts below $200/\text{mm}^3$, and opportunistic infections. AIDS dementia is also disproportionately prevalent in older patients and those who acquired AIDS by intravenous drug abuse. Besides being debilitating, it shortens survival.

Cognitive impairment is rarely an early complication of asymptomatic HIV infection. Dementia occurs in only 0.4% of otherwise asymptomatic HIV-positive individuals but in 3% of those when AIDS is first diagnosed and in 7% during the following year.

AIDS dementia is caused by direct HIV infection of the brain, that is, *HIV encephalitis*. The cells most heavily infected are the macrophages and microglia; however, unlike other viral infections of the brain, neurons are not infected. The concentration of HIV, the *viral load*, in the brain and CSF is greater in AIDS patients with dementia. Also, severity of dementia may be proportional to CSF viral load but not to the systemic (blood) viral load. In some patients, cytomegalovirus (CMV) or toxoplasmic encephalitis may be contributory or responsible for cognitive impairment.

Manifestations. AIDS dementia causes a rapid decline, over weeks to a few months, in concentration and memory, accompanied by psychomotor retardation, apathy, and withdrawal from social interactions. Language function, at least initially, is preserved, and patients remain articulate.

Early AIDS dementia mimics depression because patients tend to have blunted affect, social withdrawal, and vegetative symptoms, such as anorexia and sleeplessness. Although their suicide rate is 17 to 36 times greater than in a healthy population, a proportion of that high suicide rate is attributable, as with other illness causing dementia, particularly Huntington's disease, to dementia-induced impetuousness and impaired judgment. The misleading nature of the apparent overlap is captured by the adage, "If an AIDS patient seems to have depression, he probably has dementia."

Motor impairment of AIDS dementia includes slow limb movements, clumsy and slow gait, ocular motility abnormalities, and awkward finger movements. Neurologic examination usually discloses frontal release signs, ataxia, and, in the legs, increased tone, clonus, and hyperactive reflexes.

Gait difficulties and slow movements have been so consistent that AIDS dementia is classified, by those who value the distinction, as subcortical. Motor impairment, especially accompanying rapid progression of dementia, distinguishes AIDS dementia from most other dementias and from psychiatric disturbances.

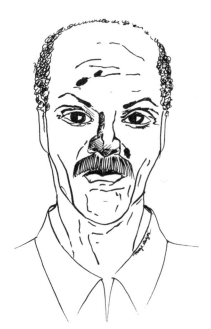

FIGURE 7–8. Kaposi's sarcoma lesions, which appear as small, slightly raised, dry, and purple or red-brown patches, indicate but do not prove AIDS. They are most often found in homosexual male AIDS patients.

Within a year of the onset of HIV dementia, 80% of survivors lose virtually all cognitive function. They often decline into a persistent vegetative state, in which they are akinetic, severely demented, incontinent, paraplegic, and mute (see Chapter 11). Seizures, myoclonus, and parkinsonism may complicate their course (see Chapter 18). In addition, they are beset with systemic or constitutional symptoms, such as weight loss and fever. Although the purple plaques of Kaposi's sarcoma (Fig. 7–8) are characteristic of AIDS, they are not a marker for dementia.

Zidovudine (AZT [Retrovir]), an antiviral medication that acts by inhibiting reverse transcriptase, may slow or possibly reverse AIDS dementia. However, potential side effects include mental aberrations, bone marrow suppression, neuropathy, and myopathy (see Chapters 5 and 6), and its use is costly. The protease inhibitors also improve cognitive function in patients with AIDS dementia. Stimulants, such as dextroamphetamine and methylphenidate, may alleviate psychomotor retardation, social withdrawal, and fatigue. Depression may respond to tricyclic antidepressants or serotonin reuptake inhibitors. After testing excludes a mass lesion, ECT may be appropriate.

Testing.   The standard HIV screening test is an enzyme-linked immunosorbent assay (ELISA); however, results may remain negative for 6 months after HIV infection is contracted, and some results are false-positive. Patients suspected of AIDS dementia must have a positive ELISA test confirmed by the Western blot, polymerase chain reaction (PCR), or other highly specific test. They should also have a CD4 count determination.

Both CTs and MRIs reveal cerebral atrophy with enlarged ventricles, basal ganglia abnormalities, and any coexistent opportunistic infections or neoplasms. MRIs can also show nonspecific scattered white matter abnormalities in uncomplicated AIDS dementia and large white matter plaques (see discussion of progressive multifocal leukoencephalopathy below).

In AIDS dementia, the CSF typically shows a mild lymphocytic pleocytosis and normal or slightly elevated protein concentration. When opportunistic infections are present, the CSF shows abnormalities that are much more pronounced. With *Crypto-*

coccus infections, for example, the CSF often contains antigens. Thus, in contrast to evaluation of Alzheimer's disease patients, an LP is usually indicated in evaluating AIDS patients who develop dementia.

Depending on the circumstances, tests might also be conducted for illnesses other than AIDS that are associated with drug abuse or unsafe sex, such as hepatitis, subacute bacterial endocarditis, and syphilis.

At autopsy, the brain is atrophic and pale. Microscopic examination shows perivascular infiltrates, gliosis of the cerebral cortex, demyelination, microglial nodules, and multinucleated giant cells. HIV can be isolated from the brains and CSF of virtually all AIDS patients with dementia and from many without it. Overall, clinical changes may be more pronounced than histologic abnormalities.

AIDS-Induced Cerebral Lesions.   Infectious or neoplastic AIDS-induced cerebral lesions, like other cerebral lesions, cause headache, focal seizures, lateralized signs, and increased intracranial pressure. Moreover, they can exacerbate AIDS dementia. The symptom of headache is particularly important in AIDS patients. In them, headaches are liable to be misdiagnosed as a manifestation of depression or "tension," but they are actually ominous. About 85% of AIDS patients who have a newly developing headache actually harbor serious underlying pathology, including *Cryptococcus* meningitis and cerebral toxoplasmosis (see below).

After HIV, the protozoan *Toxoplasma gondii* causes the most common AIDS-related CNS infections, *cerebral toxoplasmosis*. This organism typically produces multiple ring-shaped enhancing lesions that are readily visualized by a CT (see Figs. 20–7 and 20–18). Because toxoplasmosis is so common in AIDS, the CT is virtually diagnostic, and antibiotics are highly effective, neurologists usually prescribe a therapeutic antibiotic trial and reserve a cerebral biopsy for patients who do not respond.

Other opportunistic organisms that cause cerebral lesions are fungi, such as *Candida* and *Aspergillus*, and viruses, such as CMV and polyoma virus. A DNA papovavirus, *JC virus*, causes *progressive multifocal leukoencephalopathy (PML)*. As its name suggests, PML produces multiple widespread, but sometimes confluent, lesions in the white *(leuko)* matter—actually myelin—of the brain and spinal cord. Patients develop hemiparesis, spasticity, blindness, and ataxia. Although neurologic findings and MRI appearance of PML mimic multiple sclerosis (see Chapter 15), which is another demyelinating illness of young adults, the different clinical situations and HIV testing should eliminate confusion. PML is one of the conditions where the MRI is clearly superior to CT in detecting the abnormality. The diagnosis can be confirmed by detecting JC virus in the CSF by PCR testing.

Syphilis and tuberculosis, which both develop in AIDS patients, produce virulent illnesses. Syphilis usually causes acute syphilitic meningitis or meningovascular involvement but, because AIDS patients usually do not live long enough, rarely neurosyphilis.

The most common cerebral neoplasm complicating AIDS is *primary cerebral lymphoma*. Although this tumor's clinical and CT features mimic toxoplasmosis, it occurs much less frequently and usually presents as a solitary lesion. Compared to common systemic lymphomas, primary cerebral lymphomas are poorly responsive to radiotherapy, steroids, and other treatment. Lymphomas may also develop in the spinal canal and compress the spinal cord. Less frequently, gliomas, metastatic Kaposi's sarcoma, and other malignancies are associated with AIDS.

Other AIDS-Related Conditions.   The spinal cord is also subject to HIV infection, as well as lymphomas. Spinal cord infection *(myelitis)* with HIV, *vacuolar myelopathy*, produces paraparesis and the Romberg and other signs of spinal cord injury. Damage is located predominantly in the posterior columns (the fasciculus gracilis and f. cuneatus, see Fig. 2–14). Although this pattern resembles combined system disease (see Fig. 2–17, *B*), vitamin B_{12} treatment does not help HIV myelitis.

A virus related to HIV, the *human T cell lymphotrophic virus type 1 (HTLV-1)*, is also transmitted sexually and by blood transfusion. Similarly, HTLV-1 infects the spinal cord and causes paraparesis. Because this form of myelitis is endemic in the Caribbean region and Africa, it has been known as tropical spastic paraparesis.

AIDS patients with or without dementia may develop *meningitis* from HIV infection, TB, syphilis, or cryptococcosis. In addition to causing headache, fever, and malaise, meningitis in AIDS patients brings on delirium or mental aberrations that can mimic or exacerbate dementia. Cryptococcus meningitis, the most common variety of AIDS-related meningitis, often represents its first clinical manifestation.

The PNS is also frequently involved. HIV or CMV infections lead to polyneuropathy, a Guillain-Barré syndrome, mononeuropathies, and myopathies (see Chapters 5 and 6). Many of these AIDS-related PNS conditions, unlike their usual presentation, are extraordinarily painful. Some are iatrogenic. For example, several AIDS medications, such as AZT, can produce neuropathies or myopathies.

PSEUDODEMENTIA

In this condition a psychiatric disturbance mimics or produces cognitive impairment. Although most cases are associated with depression, some have been associated with factitious disorders, anxiety, or schizophrenia. Unlike Alzheimer's disease patients, those with depression-induced pseudodementia typically have experienced previous episodes of depression. In addition, their apparent cognitive impairment is accompanied by affective and vegetative disturbances. Moreover, their impairment fluctuates in severity and extent but usually does not include disorientation.

Also unlike Alzheimer's patients, pseudodementia patients—when encouraged and given additional time—will perform normally on mental status examinations. Their WAIS tests usually show comparably abnormal performance and verbal scales. (However, if psychomotor retardation is present, performance scales may be much lower.)

A potential pitfall for physicians is failure to recognize pseudodementia because of prominent—but inconsequential—age-related neurologic changes, such as benign forgetfulness, mild EEG slowing, and CTs or MRIs showing cerebral atrophy. A further complication is that pseudodementia patients who have responded to antidepressant treatment eventually develop dementia at a rate as much as six times greater than their age-adjusted counterparts, that is, pseudodementia is often a prelude to Alzheimer's disease.

TOXIC-METABOLIC ENCEPHALOPATHY

Characteristics

The term *toxic-metabolic encephalopathy* is commonly applied by neurologists to a fluctuating state of consciousness, confusion, and other mental disturbances without lateralized signs. It is typically induced by an exogenous or endogenous *chemical* imbalance. When the etiology can be determined, neurologists specify the condition, such as uremic or hepatic encephalopathy. They usually call similar disturbances caused by infectious agents encephalitis and those without an identifiable cause an acute confusional state.

In the *DSM-IV,* the criteria for *delirium* are a disturbance of the level of consciousness (usually reduced awareness and attention span) and either change in cognition (such as disorientation) or development of perceptual deficits. These symptoms, which fluctuate, must have developed over hours to days. Delirium must be attributable to a physiologic disturbance. Although the labels—delirium and toxic-metabolic encephalopathy—refer to almost identical states, this text will use the latter term because it conforms to most neurologists' practice.

Toxic-metabolic encephalopathy can be distinguished from dementia primarily by sudden onset, rapid deterioration, and subsequent almost hourly fluctuations in level of consciousness. "Nonmental" distinguishing characteristics include autonomic system hyperactivity, routine laboratory abnormalities, and pronounced EEG changes.

Patients' consciousness usually fluctuates between lethargy and stupor over several hours to several days—a relatively brief period. Even when alert, patients are inattentive and disoriented. Unless comatose, they are apt to misinterpret stimuli and develop delusions and hallucinations. Sometimes patients maintain an abnormally heightened awareness in which they appear hypervigilant. (This altered level of consciousness should be included in the *DSM-IV* definition of delirium.)

Young children, individuals older than 65 years, and those with pre-existing dementia are particularly susceptible. Whether or not dementia pre-exists, manifestations of toxic-metabolic encephalopathy, whatever its cause, are similar.

Despite successful treatment of the underlying medical problem, improvement in a patient's neurologic condition can lag or occasionally deteriorate (Fig. 7–9). The

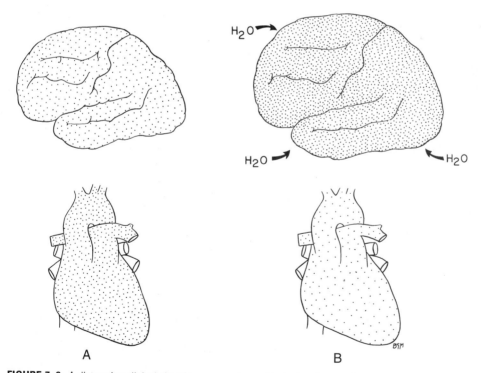

FIGURE 7–9. A distressing clinical situation occurs when patients deteriorate—become confused, lethargic, and agitated—after apparent correction of certain metabolic abnormalities. **A,** As portrayed in the sketches on the left *(A),* in cases of uremia or hyperglycemia, the brain and blood contain an approximately equal concentration of solute *(dots).* **B,** Overly vigorous dialysis or insulin administration clears solute more rapidly from the blood than the brain, leaving the solute concentration in the brain much greater than in the blood. The concentration gradient causes free water to move into the brain, which produces cerebral edema.

encephalopathy can also persist at a low-grade level and mimic dementia. Such chronic encephalopathy can result from renal, hepatic, or pulmonary insufficiency.

Lack of lateralized signs in toxic-metabolic encephalopathy stands in contrast to the prominent mental disturbances. Patients frequently have physical agitation, autonomic imbalance, tremors, tremulousness, and generalized seizures, but these signs are not specific enough to indicate a specific etiology.

Some findings are specific enough to be helpful in making an astute, bedside diagnosis. In Wernicke-Korsakoff syndrome, an encephalopathy often progressing to dementia, patients have oculomotor palsies, nystagmus, ataxia, and polyneuropathy (see Chapters 5 and 12); those with hepatic or uremic encephalopathy have *asterixis* (Fig. 7–10); and some with uremia, penicillin intoxication, meperidine (Demerol) overdose, and other metabolic encephalopathies have myoclonus (see Chapter 18). Narcotic and barbiturate intoxication causes miosis (contracted pupils), and amphetamines, atropine, and other sympathomimetic drugs dilate pupils.

In almost all cases of toxic-metabolic encephalopathy, EEGs show pronounced slowing and other nonspecific abnormalities beginning at the onset of mental aberrations and continuing throughout the course of the illness. In hepatic and uremic encephalopathy, the EEG may have characteristic triphasic waves (see Chapter 10). CTs and MRIs are normal unless they show a co-existing structural lesion, such as a subdural hematoma. The CSF in meningitis, encephalitis, subarachnoid hemorrhage, and severe hepatic encephalopathy is abnormal; however, in most toxic-metabolic encephalopathies it is normal.

Causes

Only a few among myriad causes of toxic-metabolic encephalopathy account for most cases in acute care hospitals (Table 7–4). Most can be diagnosed by reading the chart and examining the patient. Many are iatrogenic. Some are self-induced. Especially in older patients, some may be the first manifestation of a potentially fatal illness.

Medications are outstanding offenders. In practice, they are probably one of the most frequently occurring causes of toxic-metabolic encephalopathy, as well as dementia. Even small doses in previously unexposed patients, interference by another drug with hepatic metabolism, administration by ocular or topical routes, or even medication withdrawal can be responsible. Medications intended to correct CNS disorders—anticholinergic, antiepileptic, antiparkinson, hypnotic, narcotic, and psychopharmacologic—are the ones most likely to produce an encephalopathy. Antihypertensives represent another dangerous group because, through orthostatic

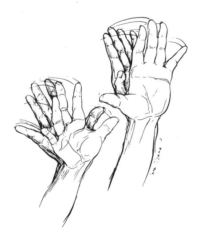

FIGURE 7–10. Asterixis, a sign of a toxic-metabolic encephalopathy, is elicited by having patients extend their arms and hands, as though they were stopping traffic. Their hands intermittently quickly move downward and slowly return, as though waving good-bye.

TABLE 7–4. *Commonly Cited Frequent Causes of Toxic-Metabolic Encephalopathy*

Narcotics and alcohol
Medications
Major surgery
Hepatic or uremic encephalopathy
Fluid or electrolyte imbalance, especially dehydration
Pneumonia or other nonneurologic infection

hypotension and other adverse mechanisms, they can produce mental status changes that mimic depression, as well as dementia.

Hepatic Encephalopathy

A particularly interesting and relatively common variety of toxic-metabolic encephalopathy is *hepatic encephalopathy*. Often, as the liver fails, mental function and consciousness steadily decline into coma. Mild confusion with either lethargy or, less frequently, agitation may precede overtly abnormal liver function tests. The characteristic asterixis and EEG changes develop (see above).

Hepatic encephalopathy has been traditionally attributed to an elevated concentration of ammonia (NH_3). This theory is consistent with the common situation of patients with cirrhosis developing hepatic encephalopathy following gastrointestinal bleeding or meals with a high protein content. In this situation, because of cirrhosis-induced portal hypertension, NH_3 released by protein in food or blood is shunted into the systemic circulation. Being small and nonionic (uncharged), NH_3 is easily able to penetrate the blood-brain barrier. Treatment has been directed at converting ammonia (NH_3) to ammonium (NH_4^+), which is ionic and unable to penetrate the blood-brain barrier.

Alternative explanations include the following: production of false neurotransmitters, production of substances that bind to benzodiazepine—gamma amino butyric acid (GABA) receptors and increase GABA activity, and disturbances in cellular energy generating systems. Clinicians sometimes reduce hepatic encephalopathy when they give flumazenil, a benzodiazepine antagonist that interferes with benzodiazepine-GABA receptors.

REFERENCES

Age-Related Changes and Dementia

Applegate WB, Blass JP, Williams TF: Instruments for the functional assessment of older patients. N Engl J Med *322:* 1207–1214, 1990

Cummings JL, Mega M, Gray K, et al: The Neuropsychiatric Inventory: Comprehensive assessment of psychopathology in dementia. Neurology *44:* 2308–2314, 1994

Grigoletto F, Zappala G, Anderson DW, et al: Norms for the Mini-Mental State Examination in a healthy population. Neurology *53:* 315–320, 1999

Hulette CM, Earl NL, Crain BJ: Evaluation of cerebral biopsies for the diagnosis of dementia. Arch Neurol *48:* 28–31, 1992

Kramer JH, Duffy JM: Aphasia, apraxia, and agnosia in the diagnosis of dementia. Dementia *7:* 23–26, 1996

Marson DC, Chatterjee A, Ingram KK, et al: Toward a neurologic model of competency: Cognitive predictors of capacity to consent in Alzheimer's disease using three different legal standards. Neurology *46:* 666–672, 1996

Masdeu JC, Sudarsky L, Wolfson L: Gait Disorders of Aging. Hagerstown, MD, Lippincott-Raven, 1997

Mega M, Cummings JL, Fiorello T, et al: The spectrum of behavioral changes in Alzheimer's disease. Neurology *46:* 130–135, 1996

Morris JC: The Clinical Dementia Rating (CDR): Current version and scoring rules. Neurology *43:* 2412–2414, 1993

Mungas D, Marshall SC, Weldon M, et al: Age and education correction of Mini-Mental State Examination for English- and Spanish-speaking elderly. Neurology *46:* 700–706, 1996

Quality Standards Subcommittee of the American Academy of Neurology: Practice parameter for diagnosis and evaluation of dementia. Neurology *44:* 2203–2206, 1994

Tinetti M, Baker DI, McAvay ASG, et al: A multifactorial intervention to reduce the risk of falling among elderly people living in the community. N Engl J Med *331:* 821–827, 1994

Weytingh MD, Bossuyt PM, van Crevel H: Reversible dementia: More than 10% or less than 1%? A quantitative review. J Neurol *242:* 466–471, 1995

Alzheimer's Disease

Arriagada PV, Growdon JH, Hedley-Whyte ET, et al: Neurofibrillary tangles but not senile plaques parallel duration and severity of Alzheimer's disease. Neurology *42:* 631–639, 1992

Blessed G, Tomlinson BE, Roth M: The association between quantitative measures of dementia and of senile change in the cerebral gray matter of elderly subjects. Br J Psychiatry *114:* 797–811, 1968

Brugge KL, Nichols SL, Salmon DP, et al: Cognitive impairment in adults with Down's syndrome: Similarities to early cognitive changes in Alzheimer's disease. Neurology *44:* 232–238, 1994

Cobb JL, Wolf PA, Au R, et al: The effect of education on the incidence of dementia and Alzheimer's disease in the Framingham Study. Neurology *45:* 1707–1712, 1995

Craft S, Teri L, Edland SD, et al: Accelerated decline in apolipoprotein E-e4 homozygotes with Alzheimer's disease. Neurology *51:* 149–153, 1998

Drachman DA, Swearer JM: Driving and Alzheimer's disease: The risk of crashes. Neurology *43:* 2448–2456, 1993

Farlow MR, Evans RM: Pharmacologic treatment of cognition in Alzheimer's dementia. Neurology *51*(Suppl 1): S36–S44, 1998

Folstein MR, Folstein SE, McHugh PR: "Mini-Mental State:" A practical method for grading the cognitive state of patients for the clinician. J Psychiatr Res *12:* 189–198, 1975

Gomez-Isla T, West HL, Rebeck GW, et al: Clinical and pathological correlates of apolipoprotein E e4 in Alzheimer's disease. Ann Neurol *39:* 62–70, 1996

Lerner AJ, Koss E, Patterson MB: Concomitants of visual hallucinations in Alzheimer's disease. Neurology *44:* 523–527, 1994

Lopez OL, Becker JT, Brenner RP, et al: Alzheimer's disease with delusions and hallucinations: Neuropsychological and electroencephalographic correlates. Neurology *41:* 906–912, 1991

Mayeux R, Sano M: Treatment of Alzheimer's disease. N Engl J Med *341:* 1670–1679, 1999

Schapiro MB, Ball MJ, Grady CL, et al: Dementia in Down's syndrome. Neurology *38:* 938–942, 1988

AIDS Dementia Complex

Brew BJ, Pemberton L, Cunningham P, et al: Levels of human immunodeficiency virus type 1 RNA in cerebrospinal fluid correlate with AIDS dementia stage. J Infect Dis *175:* 963–966, 1997

Demos DL, John RS, Parker ES, et al: Cognitive function in asymptomatic HIV infection. Arch Neurol *54:* 179–185, 1997

Franzblau A, Letz R, Hershman D, et al: Quantitative neurologic and neurobehavioral testing of persons infected with human immunodeficiency virus type I. Arch Neurol *48:* 263–268, 1991

Holtom PD, Larsen RA, Leal ME, et al: Prevalence of neurosyphilis in human immunodeficiency virus-infected patients with latent syphilis. Am J Med *93:* 9–12, 1992

Lipton SA, Gendelman HE: Dementia associated with the acquired immunodeficiency syndrome. New Engl J Med *332:* 934–940, 1995

Marra CM: Syphilis and human immunodeficiency virus infection. Sem Neurol *12:* 43–50, 1992

McArthur JC, Selnes OA, Glass JD: HIV dementia. Incidence and risk factors. Res Publ Assoc Res Nerv Ment Dis *72:* 251–272, 1994

Other Causes of Dementia

Belman AL, Iyer M, Coyle PK, et al: Neurologic manifestations in children with North American Lyme disease. Neurology *43:* 2609–2614, 1993

Berger JR, David NJ: Creutzfeldt-Jakob disease in a physician: A review of the disorders in health care workers. Neurology *43:* 205–206, 1993

Black DW: Pathologic laughter: A review of the literature. J Nerv Ment Dis *170:* 67–71, 1982

Blake PY, Pincus JH, Buckner C: Neurologic abnormalities in murderers. Neurology *45:* 1641–1647, 1995

Halperin JJ: Neuroborreliosis: Central nervous system involvement. Semin Neurol *17:* 19–24, 1997

Haywood AM: Transmissible spongiform encephalopathies. N Engl J Med *337:* 1821–1828, 1997

Johnson RT, Gibbs CJ: Creutzfeldt-Jakob disease and related transmissible spongiform encephalopathies. N Engl J Med *339:* 1994–2004, 1998

Kaplan RF, Meadows ME, Vincent LC, et al: Memory impairment and depression in patients with Lyme encephalopathy: Comparison with fibromyalgia and nonpsychotically depressed patients. Neurology *42:* 1263–1267, 1992

Kertesz A, Munoz D: Pick's disease, frontotemporal dementia, and Pick complex. Arch Neurol *55:* 302–304, 1998

Klatka LA, Louis ED, Schiffer RD: Psychiatric features in diffuse Lewy body disease. Neurology *47:* 1148–1152, 1996

Kucharski A: History of frontal lobotomy in the United States, 1935–1955. Neurosurgery *14:* 762–772, 1984

Lindqvist G, Anderson H, Bilting M, et al: Normal pressure hydrocephalus: Psychiatric findings before and after shunt operation classified in a new diagnostic system for organic psychiatry. Acta Psychiatr Scand *373*(Suppl): 18–32, 1993

Nicolas JM, Estruch R, Salamero M, et al: Brain impairment in well-nourished chronic alcoholics is related to ethanol intake. Ann Neurol *41:* 590–598, 1997

Ott A, Stolk RP, Harskamp VFV, Pols HAP, et al: Diabetes mellitus and the risk of dementia. Neurology *53:* 1937–1942, 1999

Prusiner SB, Hsiao KK: Human prion diseases. Ann Neurol *35:* 385–395, 1994

Singer C, Lang AE, Suchowersky O: Adult-onset subacute sclerosing panencephalitis. Mov Disord *12:* 342–353, 1997

Tan E, Namer IJ, Ciger A, et al: The prognosis of subacute sclerosing panencephalitis in adults: Report of 8 cases and review of the literature. Clin Neurol Neurosurg *93:* 205–209, 1991

Vanneste J, Augustijn P, Dirven C, et al: Shunting normal pressure hydrocephalus: Do the benefits outweigh the risks? A multicenter study and literature review. Neurology *42:* 54–59, 1992

Victor M, Adams RD, Collins GH: The Wernicke-Korsakoff Syndrome and Related Neurologic Disorders Due to Alcoholism and Malnutrition, 2nd ed. Philadelphia, F.A. Davis, 1989

Toxic-Metabolic Encephalopathy

Abramowicz M (ed): Some drugs that cause psychiatric symptoms. Med Lett *40:* 21–24, 1998

Lipowski ZJ: Delirium: Acute Confusional States. New York, Oxford University Press, 1990

Riordan SM, Williams R: Treatment of hepatic encephalopathy. N Engl J Med *337:* 473–479, 1997

Strub RL, Black FW: The Mental Status Examination in Neurology, 3rd ed. Philadelphia, F.A. Davis, 1993

Trzepacz PT, Mulsant BH, Dew MA, et al: Is delirium different when it occurs in dementia? J Neuropsychia Clin Neurosci *10:* 199–204, 1998

QUESTIONS and ANSWERS: CHAPTER 7

1. What are these illnesses' features in addition to dementia or delirium?

1. CNS lupus
2. Normal pressure hydrocephalus
3. Diffuse Lewy body disease
4. Wilson's disease
5. Huntington's disease
6. Bromism
7. Arsenic poisoning
8. Porphyria
9. Wernicke's encephalopathy
10. Myxedema
11. Tuberous sclerosis
12. Hepatic encephalopathy
13. Subacute sclerosing encephalitis (SSPE)
14. Creutzfeldt-Jakob disease

a. Akinesia, tremor, and postural reflex abnormalities
b. Acne-like skin rash, headache, and lethargy
c. Amnesia with nystagmus, ocular paresis, and ataxia
d. Tremor, rigidity, ataxia, and Kayser-Fleischer rings
e. Nonspecific mental dullness and peripheral neuropathy
f. Adenoma of face and seizures, usually beginning in childhood
g. Seizures, strokes, and psychosis (the three Ss)
h. Chorea but, in young adults, rigidity
i. Recurrent episodes of delirium, seizures, peripheral neuropathy, and abdominal pain with dark red urine
j. Slow mentation, depression, occasionally excited confusion (madness), and "hung-up" deep tendon reflexes (DTRs)
k. Lethargy and asterixis
l. Incontinence and gait apraxia
m. Myoclonus with pyramidal or extrapyramidal findings in individuals older than 65 years
n. Myoclonus, usually in rural boys

ANSWERS: 1-g, 2-l, 3-a, 4-d, 5-h, 6-b, 7-e, 8-i (acute intermittent porphyria only), 9-c, 10-j, 11-f, 12-k, 13-n, 14-m

2. Which tests (a–l) are used to diagnose the illness (1–16) ?

1. Gerstmann-Sträussler disease
2. Combined system disease or subacute combined degeneration
3. Porphyria
4. Arsenic poisoning
5. Lead poisoning
6. Tabes dorsalis
7. SSPE
8. Water intoxication
9. Bromism
10. Subarachnoid hemorrhage
11. Subdural hematomas
12. Creutzfeldt-Jakob disease
13. Wilson's disease
14. Sphenoid wing meningioma
15. Hepatic encephalopathy
16. Cryptococcus meningitis

a. CSF analysis
b. Serum electrolyte determination
c. Serum T_4 level determination
d. CT or MRI
e. Serum heavy metal testing
f. Serum B_{12} level determination
g. Brain biopsy
h. Watson-Schwartz test or urine porphyrin levels
i. Slit-lamp examination
j. Serum ceruloplasmin level
k. EEG
l. Fingernail analysis

ANSWERS: 1-g and k (spongiform changes on brain biopsy), 2-f, 3-h, 4-e and l, 5-e, 6-a, 7-a and k (CSF measles antibody and EEG periodic complexes), 8-b, 9-b (an anion gap), 10-a and d (bloody or xanthochromic CSF or a CT or MRI showing blood), 11-d, 12-g and k (spongiform changes on brain biopsy and EEG periodic complexes), 13-i and j, 14-d, 15-k (EEG triphasic waves. Liver function tests may be helpful, but blood ammonia concentrations are inconsistent), 16-a (CSF cryptococcus antigen is the most specific and occasionally the only positive test).

3. In a 70-year-old man who has normal cognitive and physical function, which sensation is most likely to be lost?

a. Joint position
b. Vibration
c. Pain
d. Temperature

ANSWER: b. Vibration sensation is normally lost to a greater degree than the other sensations; however, loss of position sense is more obvious and, because it leads to gait impairment, more troublesome. Pain and temperature sensations are relatively well preserved.

4. The diagnosis of normal pressure hydrocephalus (NPH) has received much attention in the literature because installation of a ventricular-peritoneal shunt may correct the dementia.

(a) Which conditions predispose a patient to NPH?

1. AIDS dementia
2. Meningitis
3. Subarachnoid hemorrhage
4. Hypothyroidism
5. Unknown causes in the majority of cases

(b) What approximate percentage of patients thought to have NPH benefit from placement of a shunt?

1. 0%
2. 25%
3. 50%
4. 100%

ANSWERS: (a) 2, 3, 5; (b) 2

5. True or False: A cerebral cortex biopsy indicated in the routine diagnosis of Alzheimer's disease.

ANSWER: False. Routine histologic examination cannot be diagnostic because there is no histologic marker for Alzheimer's disease. Even the characteristic plaques and tangles are found in normal aged brains.

6. With which feature is Alzheimer's disease dementia most closely associated?

a. Large ventricles
b. Increased concentration of plaques
c. Increased concentration of tangles
d. Degree of synapse loss

ANSWER: d. Loss of synapses is most closely correlated with dementia, but neurofibrillary tangles are also associated with dementia.

7. A 75-year-old man who had played professional football stated that over the past 3 to 5 years he has become generally weaker and has lost muscle bulk, particularly in his hands. He has also lost his ability to ride his bicycle. Nevertheless, he is still able to play golf, walk a mile, and perform his activities of daily living. A routine medical evaluation reveals no particular abnormality. Which is the most likely explanation for his symptoms?

a. He is describing normal, age-related muscle and coordination changes.
b. He has developed traumatic complications from professional football.
c. The problem is not trauma itself but that CNS trauma has led to an ALS-like condition.
d. A neuropathy that was undetected on the medical evaluation.

ANSWER: a. He has normal age-related changes: loss of muscle bulk that is most obvious in the intrinsic hand muscles, generalized decrease in strength, and mild incoordination. Certain occupations and sports lead to cervical spondylosis, which causes weakness and atrophy of hand muscles and gait impairment. ALS has not been associated with such injuries.

8. What is the pattern of inheritance (a–d) of the following illnesses (1–4)?

1. Wilson's disease
2. Huntington's disease
3. Familial Creutzfeldt-Jakob
4. Familial Alzheimer's disease

a. Sex-linked recessive
b. Autosomal recessive
c. Autosomal dominant
d. None of the above

ANSWERS: 1-b, 2-c, 3-c, 4-c

9. Which feature is *not* common to the dementia of Alzheimer's disease and Down's syndrome?

a. An abnormality referable to chromosome 21
b. Low concentrations of cerebral choline acetyltransferase
c. Presence of cerebral plaques and tangles
d. Low concentrations of cerebral acetylcholine
e. Abnormalities in the nucleus basalis of Meynert
f. Patients having had parents with the same disorder

ANSWER: f. Alzheimer's disease is often found in families. Some varieties are clearly inherited as an autosomal dominant illness. In contrast, Down's syndrome, although genetically based, is virtually never inherited from an affected parent.

10. Which of the following are normal, age-related changes?

a. 8-Hz EEG background
b. Forgetfulness of names and isolated facts
c. MRI hyperintense spots in the cerebrum
d. Slower learning
e. Loss of vocabulary
f. Impaired judgment
g. Hypoactive or absent deep tendon reflexes in the legs
h. Impaired vibration sensation and balance
i. Dilated ventricles
j. Plaques and tangles
k. Gummas in the cerebrum
l. Brain weight of 66% of normal
m. Delayed sleep and awakening times
n. More slow-wave sleep

ANSWER: a, b, c, d, g, h, i, j

11. Which of the following diseases routinely cause dementia that develops in individual's sixth decade in a familial pattern?

a. SSPE
b. Wilson's disease
c. Familial Alzheimer's
d. Parkinson's disease

e. Frontotemporal dementia
f. Gerstmann-Sträussler disease
g. Huntington's disease

ANSWER: c, e, f. SSPE and Wilson's disease cause dementia in children and teenagers. In addition, SSPE is not a familial illness. Parkinson's disease causes dementia, but only 10% of cases follow a familial pattern. Also, its onset is later, and the dementia develops only after the illness has been present for at least 5 years. Although familial, Huntington's disease becomes symptomatic, on the average, in the fourth decade. Frontotemporal dementia, which includes the condition formerly known as Pick's disease, generally develops in the sixth and seventh decades and has a genetic basis (chromosome 17). In addition, alcoholism causes dementia that occurs in families.

12. Match the histologic finding in Alzheimer's disease with its description.

1. Paired helical filaments
2. Cluster of degenerating nerve terminals with an amyloid core
3. Group of neurons beneath the globus pallidus

a. Neurofibrillary tangles
b. Neuritic plaque
c. Substantia innominata or nucleus basalis of Meynert

ANSWERS: 1-a, 2-b, 3-c

13. Which is the most common form of dementia accompanied by a peripheral neuropathy?

a. Alcohol-related neurologic changes
b. Alzheimer's disease

c. Vascular dementia
d. Traumatic brain injury

ANSWER: a. Wernicke-Korsakoff syndrome

14. Which is the most common EEG finding in patients with early Alzheimer's disease?

a. Theta and delta activity
b. Periodic complexes
c. High-voltage fast activity
d. Normal or slight slowing of the background activity
e. K complexes
f. Rapid eye movement (REM) activity

ANSWER: d

15. In which five conditions is cerebral atrophy found on MRIs or CTs?

a. Alzheimer's disease
b. Down's syndrome
c. Normal aging
d. Normal pressure hydrocephalus
e. Encephalitis

f. Pseudotumor cerebri
g. AIDS dementia
h. Cerebral toxoplasmosis
i. Wernicke-Korsakoff syndrome

ANSWER: a, b, c, g, i

16. With which condition is cerebral atrophy, as detected by CT or MRI, most closely associated?

a. Alzheimer's disease
b. Intellectual impairment
c. Old age

ANSWER: c

17. What are the two implications in Alzheimer's disease of positron emission tomography (PET) demonstrating decreased cerebral glucose metabolism and decreased oxygen consumption but normal oxygen extraction?

a. Alzheimer's disease results from cellular hypoxia.
b. Oxygen consumption is low because cerebral requirements are low.
c. When cerebral metabolism is lowered, oxygen consumption is secondarily lowered.
d. Giving oxygen to Alzheimer's disease patients will reverse the dementia.

ANSWER: b, c

18. From which area of the brain do the majority of cerebral cortex cholinergic fibers originate?

a. Hippocampus
b. Basal ganglia
c. Frontal lobe
d. Nucleus basalis of Meynert

ANSWER: d

19–22. What is the affect of the following substances on acetylcholine (ACh) activity?

19. Tacrine

20. Scopolamine

21. Organic phosphate insecticides

22. Physostigmine

a. Increases ACh activity
b. Decreases ACh activity
c. Does not change ACh activity

ANSWERS: 19-a, Tetrahydroacridine (tacrine [Cognex]) is a centrally acting anticholinesterase with a long half-life. Like the other anticholinesterases, it increases ACh activity by interfering with the enzyme cholinesterase, which metabolizes ACh. 20-b, Scopolamine is a centrally acting anticholinergic medication that is similar to atropine. In normal doses, neither cross the blood-brain barrier; however, in high doses, both can cause a toxic psychosis. 21-a, Organic phosphate insecticides are generally anticholinesterases that paralyze the neuromuscular junction with an overabundance of ACh. 22-a, Physostigmine is an anticholinesterase that is centrally acting but has a brief half-life.

23. Which features of vascular dementia are absent in Alzheimer's disease?

a. Prominent physical impairments, e.g., hemiparesis, spasticity, dysarthria
b. History of hypertension and cerebrovascular infarctions
c. Helpfulness of EEG in diagnosis
d. A CT or MRI showing multiple lucencies or frank strokes
e. Improvement in symptoms with antihypertensive treatment
f. Multiple abnormal areas on PET scans

ANSWER: a, b, d, f

24. Which are frequent features of Wernicke-Korsakoff syndrome?

a. A CT or MRI that is normal or shows atrophy
b. Optic nerve dysfunction
c. Hemorrhage into portions of the limbic system
d. Response to thiamine
e. A global confusional state followed by dementia with predominant amnesia

ANSWER: a, c (The mamillary bodies are part of the limbic system.), d, e

25. Which one of the following histologic features of Alzheimer's disease is an intraneuronal abnormality?

a. Neurofibrillary tangles
b. Neuritic plaques
c. Senile plaques
d. β-amyloid deposits

ANSWER: a. Neurofibrillary tangles are composed of intraneuronal paired helical filaments, which are largely composed of abnormally phosphorylated tau proteins. The lesions are extraneuronal. None is diagnostic of Alzheimer's disease.

26. A test for Alzheimer's disease purportedly has a high sensitivity but a low specificity. In a revision of the test, what would be the effect of reducing the proportion of false-positive results?

a. The sensitivity would increase.
b. The specificity would increase.
c. Both the sensitivity and specificity would increase.
d. Neither the sensitivity nor specificity would increase.

ANSWER: b. Specificity would increase because it is calculated by dividing the true-negatives by the sum of true-negatives and false-positives. In simple terms, with fewer false-positives the results would be more specific because a positive result is more likely to be reliable. With Alzheimer's disease, diagnoses based on the neurologic examination and routine testing are approximately 90% accurate. Any new test would have to have a high sensitivity and a high specificity to give additional value to current diagnostic criteria.

27. Of the following, which is the most specific blood test for syphilis?

a. VDRL
b. Microhemagglutination assay (MHA-TP)
c. Wassermann
d. Colloidal gold curve
e. RPR

ANSWER: b. The MHA-TP and FTA-ABS are specific for spirochetes. These tests may also be positive in other spirochete infections, which includes Lyme disease. The Wassermann and colloidal gold curve tests are outdated tests for syphilis. The VDRL and RPR tests are reagin tests that are nonspecific and have a relatively high false-positive rate.

28. Which are early characteristics of frontotemporal dementia that distinguish it from Alzheimer's disease dementia?

a. Relatively preserved directional ability
b. Familial tendency
c. Preserved parietal lobe despite otherwise generalized cerebral atrophy
d. Loss of inhibition (disinhibition)
e. Transmissibility to monkeys
f. Aphasias
g. Personality changes, especially the Klüver-Bucy syndrome
h. Hemiparesis and pseudobulbar palsy

ANSWER: a, c, d, f, g. In frontotemporal dementia, which has subsumed Pick's disease, patients typically present with prominent personality and behavioral disturbances, and language abnormalities. Nevertheless, because the parietal lobes are spared, patients have preserved visuospatial function and do not get lost. Frontotemporal dementia and Alzheimer's disease dementia, at least early in their course, are not associated with physical deficits. Both may be familial: many cases of frontotemporal dementia have a genetic basis (chromosome 17). In Alzheimer's disease, the genetic factors are inconsistent and present only in a minority of cases. Neither illness, unlike Creutzfeldt-Jakob, is transmissible.

29. Which one of the following conditions is not a complication of professional boxing?

a. Dementia pugilistica
b. Intracranial hemorrhage
c. Parkinsonism
d. Slowed reaction times
e. Progression of dementia after retirement
f. Peripheral neuropathy

ANSWER: f

30. During an experiment to reproduce Alzheimer-like cognitive deficits, a subject is administered excessive scopolamine. Of the following, which would be the best antidote?

a. Atropine
b. Edrophonium
c. Neostigmine
d. Physostigmine

ANSWER: d. Scopolamine and atropine block muscarinic acetylcholine receptors. This action reduces cerebral cholinergic activity that, in some respects, mimics the cognitive changes of Alzheimer's disease. It is a *forme fruste* of CNS anticholinergic poisoning that can be reversed with cholinergic-enhancing medications that cross the blood-brain barrier. Edrophonium, neostigmine, and physostigmine inhibit cholinesterase and thus enhance cholinergic activity; however, only physostigmine readily crosses the blood-brain barrier. As general rules, scopolamine and atropine (1) are anticholinergic and (2) counterbalance the cholinesterase inhibitor physostigmine.

31. Which movement disorders are associated with cognitive impairment?

a. Choreoathetosis
b. Parkinson's disease
c. Dystonia musculorum deformans (torsion dystonia)
d. Tourette's syndrome
e. Essential tremor
f. Rigid form of Huntington's disease
g. Wilson's disease
h. Spasmodic torticollis

ANSWER: a (associated with mental retardation in many but not all cases), b (in the middle to late stages), f, g

32. A 65-year-old man was brought to the emergency room by his wife who said that he suddenly became "confused" during sexual intercourse. On examination, he was fully alert and attentive but distraught. He was unable to recall recent or prior events, the date, or any of three objects after a 3-minute delay. His language was normal. At least grossly, his judgment was intact. The symptoms resolved after 2 hours. Which one of the following conditions is this episode most likely to represent?

a. Hysteria
b. Dementia
c. Nondominant hemisphere ischemia
d. Transient global amnesia
e. Transient ischemic attack (TIA)

ANSWER: d. The patient had a 2-hour episode of memory impairment with preservation of consciousness, perception, and judgment. Amnesia is usually caused by temporal lobe dysfunction from ischemia, infarction, epilepsy, hemorrhage, or metabolic imbalance. In this case, the problem is *transient global amnesia (TGA)*. TGA is attributable to ischemia of the posterior cerebral arteries, which supply the temporal lobe; however, some neurologists believe that it is a variety of seizure. It is most common in individuals older than 65 years, and it may be precipitated by sexual intercourse, physical stress, or strong emotions. Other neurologic causes of transient amnesia are partial complex seizures, Wernicke-Korsakoff syndrome, and use of certain medications, such as scopolamine.

33–35. Match the following conditions, which produce confabulation, with the location of the underlying brain damage:

33. Wernicke-Korsakoff syndrome

34. Anton's syndrome

35. Nondominant hemisphere syndrome

a. Right parietal lobe
b. Periventricular gray matter, mamillary bodies
c. Occipital lobes, bilaterally
d. Dominant parietal lobe

ANSWERS: 33-b, 34-c, 35-a

36. Which of the following traits is characteristic of normal 65-year-old individuals?

a. Shorter attention span
b. Slower acquisition of new information
c. Decreased ability to perform new tasks
d. Significant loss of vocabulary
e. Impairment in language ability
f. Decreased general information
g. All of the above

ANSWER: a, b, c. Despite a relatively short attention span and slower acquisition of new information and motor skills, normal older individuals have preserved vocabulary, language function, and reading comprehension.

37. Which one of the following statements is false concerning the results of the WAIS-R testing in patients older than 65 years?

a. As patients become older, WAIS-R results decline.
b. In Alzheimer's disease patients, WAIS-R performance scales are lower then verbal scores.
c. In Alzheimer's disease patients, WAIS-R verbal scales are lower then performance scores.
d. Education has to be considered when evaluating WAIS-R results.

ANSWER: c. Verbal scales remain higher than performance scales in Alzheimer's disease patients. This pattern is similar to normal aging, in which vocabulary, language skills, and general information are preserved relative to memory, attention span, and ability to acquire new skills and information.

38. Match the histologic finding (a–g) with the disease (1–6):

a. Argentophilic intraneuronal inclusions
b. Prions
c. Lewy bodies
d. Neurofibrillary tangles
e. Spongiform encephalopathy
f. Kayser-Fleischer rings
g. Antiubiquitin staining

1. Creutzfeldt-Jakob disease
2. Wilson's disease
3. Frontotemporal dementia
4. Diffuse Lewy body
5. Parkinson's disease
6. Alzheimer's disease

ANSWERS: a-3 (in cases of Pick's disease), b-1, c-4 and 5, d-6, e-1, f-2, g-4

39. Which is the skin malignancy characteristically associated with AIDS?

a. Lymphoma
b. Herpes simplex
c. Kaposi's sarcoma
d. Chancre
e. Herpes zoster

ANSWER: c

40. Which of the following descriptions may be applied to patients in the end-stages of Alzheimer's disease?

a. Locked-in syndrome
b. Persistent vegetative state
c. Electrocerebral silence
d. Slow wave sleep

ANSWER: b. The persistent vegetative state results from extensive cerebral cortex damage. The locked-in syndrome usually results from a massive but incomplete lower brainstem injury. Electrocerebral silence (the absence of EEG activity) characterizes brain death, barbiturate overdose, or deep anesthesia. Slow wave sleep is normal stage 3 and 4 NREM sleep.

41. What is the cause of AIDS-dementia complex?

a. HIV encephalitis
b. Toxoplasmosis
c. Cerebral lymphoma
d. Unknown

ANSWER: a, occasionally b

42. What is the most common cause of multiple, discrete cerebral lesions in AIDS patients?

a. Lymphoma
b. Kaposi's sarcoma
c. Cryptococcus
d. Toxoplasmosis
e. Tuberculosis

ANSWER: d. Toxoplasmosis causes multiple ring-enhancing mass lesions, but the other conditions also form cerebral mass lesions.

43. Which is the most frequently occurring, nonepidemic form of encephalitis?

a. HIV encephalitis
b. *Herpes simplex* encephalitis
c. *Herpes zoster* encephalitis
d. Meningococcal encephalitis

ANSWER: b. *Herpes simplex* is the most common nonepidemic form of encephalitis. It typically invades the temporal lobes and causes partial complex seizures, amnesia, and the Klüver-Bucy syndrome. HIV and meningococcus are epidemic infections. Meningococcus causes meningitis much more often then encephalitis. *Herpes zoster* rarely invades the brain or spinal cord.

44. Which are commonly encountered features of Alzheimer's disease?

a. Lewy bodies
b. Neurofibrillary tangles
c. Amyloid plaques
d. Prions
e. Loss of synapses

ANSWER: b, c, e. Lewy bodies are found in Parkinson's disease and diffuse Lewy body disease. Prions are found in Creutzfeldt-Jakob disease.

45. Which two of the following illnesses that cause dementia are associated with suicide?

a. Alzheimer's disease
b. AIDS
c. Huntington's disease
d. Creutzfeldt-Jakob disease

ANSWER: b, c

46. Amnesia in Alzheimer's disease may be most closely associated with deficiency of which of the following substances?

a. Dopamine
b. Scopolamine
c. Somatostatin
d. Acetylcholine
e. Serotonin

ANSWER: d

47. Which group of drivers has the highest rate of motor vehicle accidents (MVAs)?

a. Healthy individual older than 65 years
b. Alzheimer's disease patients older than 65 years
c. Teenage drivers
d. Men younger than 25 years

ANSWER: d. Individuals older than 65 years have a higher rate of MVAs than the average driver does. Those with Alzheimer's disease have a greater rate than the same-aged drivers, and their rate increases with the duration of their illness. Factors that explain the increased MVA rate include poor judgment, impaired eye-hand-foot coordination, slowed reaction time, and diminished vision and hearing. Teenagers have a high rate, with young adult men having an even higher rate. In addition to often lacking judgment and experience, their use of alcohol probably is a major factor in their increased rate.

48. Of the following, which is the greatest reason that Alzheimer's patients are placed in nursing homes?

a. Dementia
b. Incontinence
c. Hallucinations
d. Sundowning
e. Disruptive behavior

ANSWER: e. Disruptive behaviors—agitation, the interruption of the family's sleep, dangerous activities, and wandering—are the most likely precipitants of placing Alzheimer's patients in a nursing home.

49. Which two of the following statements regarding diffuse Lewy body disease are true?

a. It is possibly 15% as common as Alzheimer's disease.
b. The key feature of the histology is the concentration of Lewy bodies in the substantia nigra.
c. By the time patients are 40 years old, they have all the clinical and neuropathologic features of Alzheimer's disease.
d. Lewy bodies are eosinophilic intracytoplasmic inclusions.

ANSWER: a, d. The defining neuropathologic feature of diffuse Lewy body disease is Lewy bodies dispersed throughout the cerebral cortex. In Parkinson's disease, in contrast, Lewy bodies are confined to the substantia nigra.

50. In the search for the cause of familial Alzheimer's disease, to which chromosome does evidence from studies of amyloid and Down's syndrome point?

a. 14
b. 19
c. 21
d. All of the above

ANSWER: c. Chromosomes 1, 14, 19, and 21 have all been implicated in familial Alzheimer's disease. However, amyloid precursor protein (APP) and trisomy 21 (Down's syndrome) are referable to chromosome 21.

51. Which of the following are significantly reduced in Alzheimer's disease?

a. Glycine
b. Ceruloplasmin
c. Dopamine
d. Nicotine

e. Acetylcholine
f. Vasopressin
g. Norepinephrine
h. Somatostatin

ANSWER: e, f, g, h

52. Regarding the association between apolipoprotein-E (Apo-E) and Alzheimer's disease, which one of the following statements is false?

a. Because people inherit one of three alleles (E2, E3, E4) from each parent, everyone has two alleles (one pair) (e.g., E2-E3, E2-E4, E2-E2).
b. Apolipoprotein binds to β-amyloid and is found in neuritic plaques.
c. Its gene is encoded on chromosome 21.
d. Approximately 10% to 20% of the population has the pair E3-E4 or E4-E4, which are most closely associated with Alzheimer's disease.

ANSWER: c. The gene is encoded on chromosome 19. Down's syndrome, which is also closely associated with Alzheimer's disease, is due to trisomy 21.

53. Through which structure is CSF normally absorbed?

a. Cerebral ventricles
b. The brain parenchyma

c. Choroid plexus
d. Arachnoid villi

ANSWER: d. CSF is produced or secreted through the choroid plexus, which is located mostly in the lateral ventricles. CSF circulates through all the ventricles and then over and around the brain and spinal cord. It is reabsorbed through the arachnoid villi. Blocked arachnoid villi lead to communicating hydrocephalus.

54. Which two of the following are common causes of communicating hydrocephalus?

a. Aqueductal stenosis
b. Chronic meningitis

c. Subarachnoid hemorrhage
d. Glioblastomas

ANSWER: b, c. Aqueductal stenosis, which narrows the aqueduct of Sylvius, causes obstructive hydrocephalus.

55. Which statements are true regarding the gait of the normal elderly?

a. It is characterized by a short stride.
b. Gait impairment frequently causes falls.
c. Orthopedic changes are as important as most neurologic illness.
d. It is characterized by apraxia.

ANSWER: a, b, c

56. Of the following risk factors for falls in the elderly, which is most common?

a. Use of sedatives
b. Transient ischemic attacks

c. Neuropathy
d. Normal pressure hydrocephalus

ANSWER: a. Other risk factors for falls in the elderly are cognitive impairment, musculoskeletal changes, and a history of a fall.

57. Which features are typically present in Creutzfeldt-Jakob disease but not in Alzheimer's disease?

a. Spongiform cerebral cortex
b. Ability to transfer illness to primates by inoculation
c. Myoclonus
d. Dementia
e. Burst suppression pattern or periodic EEG changes
f. Families with an autosomal dominant pattern of illness

g. Survival less than one year
h. Pyramidal or cerebellar signs
i. Association with trisomy 21
j. Association with head trauma
k. PrP^{Sc}
l. Inflammatory cells, indicative of infection, in brain biopsies

ANSWER: a, b, c, e, g, h, k

58. Which statement is *false* regarding the infective agent in spongiform encephalopathies?

a. It is largely, if not totally, composed of protein.
b. It is resistant to formalin fixation and conventional sterilization techniques.
c. Interspecies transfer is possible but associated with a long incubation time.
d. Similar agents cause fatal familial insomnia, bovine spongiform encephalopathy, Gerstmann-Sträussler disease, and SSPE.

ANSWER: d. Prions cause spongiform encephalopathies: fatal familial insomnia, bovine spongiform encephalopathy, and Creutzfeldt-Jakob and its familial variant, Gerstmann-Sträussler disease; however, SSPE is probably caused by a virus.

59. What is the incidence of AIDS dementia in HIV-positive individuals who are otherwise asymptomatic?

a. Less than 1%
b. About 7%
c. About 25%
d. More than 50%

ANSWER: a. Virtually no one who is HIV positive, but otherwise asymptomatic, has cognitive impairment. AIDS dementia is rarely the first or only manifestation of HIV infection.

60. Which one of the following statements is true concerning the usefulness of positron emission tomography (PET) in the diagnosis of Alzheimer's disease?

a. It often shows hypometabolism in the posterior parietal temporal regions.
b. The results are highly sensitive.
c. The results are highly specific.
d. Its results cannot be replicated by single positron emission tomography (SPECT).

ANSWER: a. Both PET and SPECT show hypometabolism in the posterior parietal temporal regions, which are the areas that show the greatest atrophy, even in normal aging.

61. Which of the following are risk factors for AIDS dementia in HIV-positive individuals?

a. Anemia
b. Weight loss
c. Late stages of AIDS
d. Older age at onset of AIDS

ANSWER: a, b, c, d

62. Which one of the following disturbances is most common in dementia?

a. Hallucinations
b. Delusions
c. Apathy
d. Aberrant motor behavior

ANSWER: c. Apathy, the most common disturbance, and the others are each associated with delirium and in a variety of illnesses that cause dementia. Visual hallucinations, for example, are closely associated with Lewy body disease and Parkinson's disease dementia but relatively infrequently with Alzheimer's disease.

63. After being given a medication, a 66-year-old man develops the following side effects: forgetfulness, dry mouth, blurred vision, and urinary retention. Which is the most likely type of medication that he has been taking?

a. Anticholinergic
b. β-blocker
c. Cholinesterase inhibitor
d. Dopamine agonist

ANSWER: a. He has developed classic anticholinergic side effects. These mental and physical changes are most apt to develop in people older than 65 years and those in the early stages of dementia.

64. According to the cortical-subcortical classification of dementia, which of the following illnesses would lead to cortical dementia (c) or subcortical dementia (sc)?

a. Frontotemporal dementia
b. Parkinson's disease
c. Huntington's disease
d. Normal pressure hydrocephalus
e. Alzheimer's disease
f. AIDS dementia

> **ANSWER:** Frontotemporal dementia (including Pick's disease)—c; Parkinson's disease—sc; Huntington's disease—sc; Normal pressure hydrocephalus—sc; Alzheimer's disease—c; AIDS dementia—sc

65. Which three of the following statements are true concerning hepatic encephalopathy?

a. Ammonia (NH_3) crosses the blood-brain barrier more easily the ammonium (NH_4^+).
b. Certain substances bind to benzodiazepine-GABA and increase GABA activity.
c. Ammonia (NH_3) is the primary cause of hepatic encephalopathy, and concentrations of NH_3 directly correlate with its severity.
d. Benzodiazepine receptor antagonists, such as flumazenil, can briefly reverse some of the mental changes of hepatic encephalopathy.

> **ANSWER:** a, b, d

66. A variety of tests are administered to a 30-year-old prisoner of normal intelligence who is being evaluated for violence. In one, the tester deals him four playing cards: 3 of clubs, 7 of clubs, 9 of clubs, and 7 of hearts. The tester asks the patient to point to the one that does not belong. He picks the 7 of hearts after explaining that it is the only red card. The tester deals another four cards: the 5 of clubs, 5 of spades, 5 of hearts, and 6 of clubs. Without an explanation, the patient picks the 5 of hearts. Which disorder does his choice indicate?

a. Frontal lobe dysfunction
b. Visual-spatial impairment
c. Dementia
d. Occipital cortex impairment

> **ANSWER:** a. In this element of the Wisconsin Card Sorting Test, the prisoner cannot change from sorting by color to sorting by number. His inability to "switch sets" is indicative of frontal lobe dysfunction.

67. A 76-year-old right-handed man who had developed confusion was asked to draw a clock. What problem does his drawing most likely represent?

a. Alzheimer's disease
b. Normal aging
c. A dominant frontal lobe infarction
d. A nondominant frontal lobe infarction
e. A dominant parietal lobe infarction
f. A nondominant parietal lobe infarction

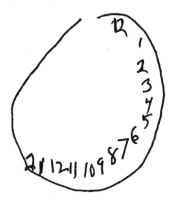

> **ANSWER:** f. The drawing shows a neglect of the left field and constructional apraxia. The clock is an incomplete, poorly drawn circle with uneven spacing between the digits and the circle. There is also perseveration of the digits. Constructional apraxia can be a manifestation of dementia, mental retardation, and both frontal and parietal lobe injuries, on either side; however, it is most closely associated with nondominant parietal lobe lesions. In addition to the constructional apraxia, the left-sided neglect clearly is referable to a nondominant parietal lobe lesion.

68. Which *DSM-IV* criteria distinguish Alzheimer's disease dementia from vascular dementia?

a. Alzheimer's, but not vascular, dementia must include memory impairment.

b. Alzheimer's, but not vascular, dementia must include at least one of the following: aphasia, apraxia, agnosia, or disturbance in executive functioning.

c. Alzheimer's, but not vascular, dementia must impair social or occupational functioning.

d. Alzheimer's, but not vascular, need not be accompanied by focal neurologic symptoms and signs.

e. None of the above.

ANSWER: e. Both Alzheimer's and vascular dementia must include memory impairment and at least one of the following: aphasia, apraxia, agnosia, or disturbance in executive functioning. In addition, both must impair social or occupational functioning. Vascular dementia, but not Alzheimer's disease dementia, must be accompanied by focal neurologic symptoms and signs.

69. Which of the following statements concerning the Mini-Mental State Examination (MMSE) is false?

a. It is sensitive.

b. It closely correlates with the Blessed Mental Status Test.

c. It reliably distinguishes Alzheimer's dementia from vascular dementia, that is, it is specific.

d. Unlike the Blessed, it includes an assessment of visual-spatial relationships and language function.

e. Low scores can reflect metabolic aberrations, thought disorders, or mood disorders, as well as dementia.

ANSWER: c. Although the MMSE will identify most cases of dementia, it cannot determine the cause. Although the MMSE is relatively specific in the diagnosis of dementia, it is nonspecific in terms of dementia's etiology. Moreover, some false-positive results occur.

70. Which of the following is least likely to reduce an individual's score on the Mini-Mental State Examination?

a. Gender

b. Less than an 8th grade education

c. Being an ethnic minority

d. Being over 75 years of age

ANSWER: a. Little education, being a member of a minority group, and advancing age all reduce the score. The individual's gender has least relevance to the score. Correction factors can reduce the effects of age and limited education. Spanish versions of the test are available.

71. A 45-year-old man with AIDS and a CD4 count of 50 cells/mm^3 describes developing a generalized, dull headache and inability to concentrate. The neurologic examination shows no focal findings or indication of increased intracranial pressure. A CT with contrast shows no intracranial pathology. Which of the following would be the best diagnostic test?

a. A lumbar puncture

b. Determining serum toxoplasmosis titers

c. A therapeutic trial of an antidepressant

d. A therapeutic trial of a serotonin agonist

ANSWER: a. About 85% of AIDS patients with headaches have serious intracranial pathology rather than a tension-type headache, migraine, or depression. Almost one-half of them will have *Cryptococcus* meningitis or cerebral toxoplasmosis. In this case, the normal neurologic examination and head CT virtually eliminated toxoplasmosis.

72. A 45-year-old man is brought to the emergency room by his family who state that during the past day he has been confused and behaving strangely. The patient, they state, has not experienced any unusual event, stress, or trauma. A neurologist found no physical abnormalities and extensive testing, including toxicology, EEG, MRI, and LP, showed no abnormality. The patient cannot state his name, birthday, or address. He cannot recall any personal events of the previous six months or any current political events. His affect is appropriate and language function is normal. Although the etiology cannot be stated with certainty, which of the following is the most likely diagnosis?

a. Transient global amnesia
b. Dissociative amnesia
c. Wernicke-Korsakoff syndrome
d. Frontal lobe dysfunction

ANSWER: b. Personal identification—name, birthday, address, and telephone number—is deeply embedded information that is actually "overlearned." Only an extensive, devastating brain injury, such as advanced Alzheimer's disease, would dislodge this information. (It would also impair his affect and language function and produce some physical deficits.) This patient's amnesia does not have an organic basis. However the information at hand is insufficient to make a firm diagnosis of dissociative amnesia, which was formerly known as psychogenic amnesia, or distinguish it from dissociative identity disorder, somatization disorders, or malingering.

73. Which of the following is usually not considered a domain of cognitive function?

a. Language
b. Mood
c. Praxis
d. Visual-spatial conceptualization

ANSWER: b. The traditional domains of cognitive function are memory, calculations, and judgment. Other domains are visual-spatial conceptualization, performing skill, and learned motor actions (praxis). Mood, affect, and emotions, although they originate in cerebral function, are not domains of cognitive function.

74. Some Alzheimer's disease treatments, which are based on the cholinergic hypothesis, attempt to replete ACh concentrations. Which receptors would hopefully benefit from the increased ACh activity?

a. Postsynaptic muscarinic cholinergic receptors
b. Presynaptic muscarinic cholinergic receptors
c. Postsynaptic nicotinic cholinergic receptors
d. Presynaptic nicotinic cholinergic receptors

ANSWER: a. Alzheimer's disease is characterized by a major presynaptic ACh deficiency. Postsynaptic muscarinic cholinergic receptors remain intact. ACh replacement is aimed at these receptors. Nicotinic receptors are virtually confined to the spinal cord and neuromuscular junction. They have little or no role in Alzheimer's disease.

75. A 77-year-old man was asked, as part of an evaluation for dementia, to copy a sequence of four sets of three squares followed by a circle. Almost immediately after beginning the task, he began to tell the physician a joke that was sexually explicit and not very funny. After briefly returning to the task, he was distracted by some defect in the paper and then some noise outside the room. Finally, he excused himself to go the men's room but only after he had let some urine escape and wet his pants. Upon returning, he recounted a similar joke and said he just could not concentrate because of all the distractions. He scored 22 on the Mini-Mental State Examination and had no lateralized neurologic findings. Which area of the brain does this man's behavior reflect?

a. The cortical association areas, as in Alzheimer's disease
b. The parietal lobes, as in hemi-inattention disorders
c. The frontal lobes, as in frontal lobe dysfunction
d. The limbic system, as in the Klüver-Bucy syndrome

ANSWER: c. This man has easy distractibility, marked disinhibition, inappropriate jocularity, and a suggestion of urinary incontinence, in the absence of dementia. The distractibility is a manifestation of inability to suppress attentiveness to new stimuli, which is another form of disinhibition. Alternatively, it is an adult form of attention deficit disorder. In either case, when unable to inhibit shifting attention to new stimuli, patients are "stimulus bound." All these phenomena reflect frontal lobe damage. They are complementary to the patient's difficulties in Question 66. Some elements of frontal lobe damage are similar to limbic system damage largely because the limbic system is partly based in the frontal lobes. Moreover, as is probably the case with this man, frontotemporal dementia causes all these symptoms.

Alzheimer's disease particularly strikes the cerebral cortical association areas; however, while causing dementia, it produces behavioral abnormalities that are less predictable than frontal lobe damage. Damage to the nondominant parietal lobe typically causes a hemi-inattention disorder. Damage to the limbic system typically causes the Klüver-Bucy syndrome.

76. Which one of the following statements concerning pseudodementia is true?

a. The disorder can be diagnosed by neuropsychologic testing.
b. Following successful treatment of pseudodementia, patients subsequently develop true dementia at about three to six times the rate of age-matched controls.
c. If psychomotor retardation is present, verbal scales may be much lower than performance scales.
d. The diagnosis is excluded by a cerebral atrophy on a CT and mild EEG slowing.

> *ANSWER:* b. A markedly increased rate of Alzheimer's disease and other forms of dementia has been found in patients who seemed to have been successfully treated for pseudodementia. Because the nature, extent, and severity of the neuropsychologic deficits are so variable, there is no set of diagnostic criteria for pseudodementia. If psychomotor retardation is present, performance scales may be much lower than verbal scores. Cerebral atrophy on a CT or MRI and mild EEG slowing are age-related changes that are often found in individuals with pseudodementia. They do not exclude a diagnosis of pseudodementia.

77. A 19-year-old exchange student from Britain began to have deterioration in her personality, cognitive impairment, painful burning sensations in her feet, and myoclonic jerks. There was no family history or neurologic or psychiatric illness. The following tests were performed and the results were normal: CT, MRI, CSF, B_{12}, T_4, VDRL and RPR, measles antibodies in serum and CSF, serum ceruloplasmin, urine for metachromatic granules, heavy metal screening, toxicology, porphyrin screening, HIV, Lyme titer, and chromosome studies for excessive trinucleotide repeats. The EEG, lacking distinctive features, was nonspecifically abnormal. After exhaustive noninvasive testing, a cerebral biopsy was performed. It showed microscopic vacuoles. She died after a 1-year course. Which is the most likely etiology of her neurologic illness?

a. A retrovirus
b. A prion
c. Drug or alcohol abuse
d. A psychiatric illness

> *ANSWER:* b. The clinical presentation of progressive, fatal mental deterioration with burning paresthesias and myoclonus is consistent with only several illnesses, but the biopsy showing spongiform changes (microscopic vacuoles) indicates that her diagnosis is the *new variant Creutzfeldt-Jakob disease.* Unlike classic Creutzfeldt-Jakob disease, this prion illness, which probably represents an interspecies transmission of bovine spongiform encephalopathy (BSE), occurs in teenagers and young adults, has a sensory component, and lacks the characteristic EEG changes (periodic complexes).

78. An 80-year-old retired janitor who has developed mild forgetfulness scores 19 on the Mini-Mental Status Examination. The physical portion of the neurologic examination discloses no abnormalities. The standard blood tests and head CT are unremarkable; however, the apolipoprotein E (Apo-E) test shows one E4 allele. Which statement is the most valid in this case?

a. The diagnosis of Alzheimer's disease must be based on both alleles.
b. A single Apo-E4 determination, with dementia, is diagnostic of Alzheimer's disease.
c. Little or no education and Apo-E4 alleles are associated with Alzheimer's disease.
d. Determining Apo-E4 alleles never have a role in cases of Alzheimer's disease.

> *ANSWER:* c. Being uneducated and having one or both Apo-E4 alleles are risk factors for Alzheimer's disease; however, neither causes the disease. Most important, having one or both Apo-E4 alleles is not a diagnostic test for Alzheimer's disease. Apo-E determinations have a role in investigating cases of familial, early onset Alzheimer's disease.

79. What do the following conditions have in common? Toluene abuse, multiple sclerosis (MS), progressive multifocal leukoencephalopathy (PML), metachromatic leukodystrophy, and adrenoleukodystrophy?

a. All are commonly associated with seizures.
b. All are infectious illnesses.
c. All are leukoencephalopathies.
d. All cause dementia early in their course.

ANSWER: c. All these conditions primarily injure CNS white matter. At least early in their course, seizures and dementia are infrequent. PML is an opportunistic infection. MS is only suspected of being infectious. Metachromatic leukodystrophy and adrenoleuko-dystrophy are inherited illnesses.

80. In Alzheimer's disease, which region of the brain contains the greatest concentration of β-amyloid plaques?

a. Frontal lobe

b. Parietal lobe

c. Hippocampus

d. Nucleus basalis

e. Caudate nuclei

ANSWER: c. The greatest concentration of β-amyloid plaques and neurofibrillary tangles is in the hippocampus. Other sites of high concentrations are the cerebral cortex association areas.

81. Which chromosome carries the gene that encodes apolipoprotein E (Apo-E)?

a. 4

b. 19

c. 21

d. X

e. Y

ANSWER: b

8

Aphasia and Related Disorders

Neurologists have studied anatomic and physiologic correlations of language, language impairment *(aphasia)*, and related disorders to deduce how the normal brain functions and advance linguistics studies. Clinically, they test for language-related disorders, which can be dramatic, to help localize and diagnose neurologic disease.

Although the *Diagnostic and Statistical Manual of Mental Disorders-IV (DSM-IV)* includes Developmental Language Impairment, it omits a definition of the frequently occurring adult-onset aphasia. Like Dementia, defined in *DSM-IV*, aphasia is an important neuropsychologic disturbance that can disrupt cognition, halt certain functions, and produce mental aberrations. Language disturbances are also important in many psychiatric conditions. Patients with an aphasia or related disturbance, whatever the underlying cause, often must undergo psychiatric assessment.

LANGUAGE AND DOMINANCE

The *dominant hemisphere* governs language function and integrates it with intellect, emotion, and tactile, auditory, and visual sensation. The dominant hemisphere thus provides the primary avenue for expression of thoughts, emotions, and most cognitive activity. Dominant hemisphere damage often results in aphasia. More important, virtually all cases of aphasia are attributable to dominant hemisphere damage.

Language includes not only speaking, listening, reading, writing, but also sign language and languages based on written symbols, such as Chinese. All are processed in the dominant hemisphere's *perisylvian language arc* (see below) and roughly equally impaired by dominant hemisphere lesions. Deficits in reading, for example, are almost always paralleled by comparable deficits in writing. (The primary exception is alexia without agraphia [see below].)

In contrast, the dominant hemisphere does not necessarily govern languages learned as adults, including "second languages," or use of obscenities, which is usually an expression of strong emotions. The nondominant hemisphere probably bestows the mixture of inflection and rhythm comprising the "tone of voice" or affective component of speech *(prosody)*. In addition, although musically gifted people process music, as language, in their dominant hemisphere, most others rely on the nondominant hemisphere for their modest ability to carry a tune.

Cerebral hemisphere dominance for language is accompanied by control of fine, rapid hand movements (handedness) and, to a lesser degree, reception of vision and hearing. For example, right-handed people, who have left cerebral hemisphere dominance, not only rely on their right hand for writing and throwing a ball but also use their right foot for kicking, right eye when peering through a telescope, and right ear for listening to words spoken simultaneously in both ears *(dichotic listening)*.

Anatomically, the dominant hemisphere is distinctive in being virtually the only exception to the general left-right symmetry of the brain. The dominant temporal lobe's superior surface—the *planum temporale*—has a greater cortical area than its nondominant counterpart because of more gyri and deeper sulci (see Fig. 20–13). However, this normal asymmetry is lacking or even reversed in many individuals with dyslexia, autism, and chronic schizophrenia—conditions with prominent language abnormalities.

Handedness

About 90% of all people are right-handed, which means that they are left hemisphere dominant. In addition, most left-handed people are left hemisphere dominant.

Left-handed people may have naturally occurring right hemisphere dominance, or their right hemisphere may have become dominant from congenital injury to their left hemisphere (see Chapter 13). Left-handedness is overrepresented among children with an overt impairment, such as mental retardation, epilepsy, and certain major psychiatric disorders, including autism. Moreover, it is overrepresented among children with more subtle abnormalities, such as dyslexia, other learning disabilities, stuttering, and general clumsiness.

Left-handed people are also disproportionately represented among musicians, artists, mathematicians, and athletes. Left-handed athletes tend to be more successful than right-handed ones in sports involving direct confrontation, such as baseball, tennis, fencing, and boxing, because they benefit from certain tactical advantages, such as a left-handed batter being closer to first base. However, they have no greater success in sports without direct confrontation, such as swimming, running, and pole vaulting.

In comparison to right-handed people, left-handed ones become aphasic if either cerebral hemisphere is injured. In addition, if they develop aphasia, its variety does not closely relate to the specific injury site (see below). Prognosis in these people is relatively good.

A few individuals are either mixed dominant or ambidextrous. Seemingly endowed with language, music, and motor skill function in both hemispheres, they excel in certain sports and performing on musical instruments.

Although the left hemisphere is dominant in almost all people (and the rest of this chapter assumes it always is), sometimes dominance must be established with certainty. For example, when the temporal lobe must be partially resected because of intractable partial complex epilepsy (see Chapter 10), only a limited resection of the dominant temporal lobe would be permissible without creating aphasia. Cerebral dominance can be established with the *Wada test*, in which sodium amobarbital is injected directly into each carotid artery. When the dominant hemisphere is perfused, the patient becomes temporarily aphasic. A potential safer alternative is functional magnetic resonance imaging (fMRI), in which subjects essentially undergo language evaluation during an MRI.

APHASIA

The Perisylvian Language Arc

Impulses conveying speech, music, and simple sounds travel from the ears along the acoustic (eighth cranial) nerves into the brainstem. Crossed and uncrossed brainstem tracts bring the impulses to the primary auditory cortex, *Heschl's gyri*, in each temporal lobe (see Fig. 4–15). Most music and some other sounds remain in the nondominant hemisphere. Language impulses are transmitted to *Wernicke's* area,

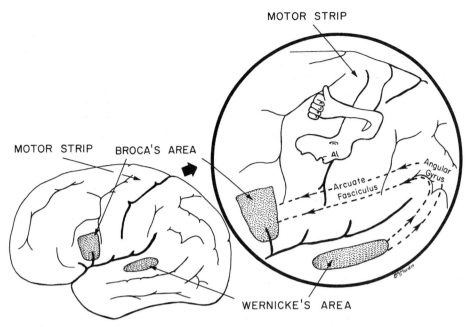

FIGURE 8–1. The left cerebral hemisphere contains *Wernicke's area* in the temporal lobe and *Broca's area* in the frontal lobe, where it sits between Heschl's gyrus (see Fig. 4–15) and the cerebral cortex motor area for the right hand, face, and language. The *arcuate fasciculus,* the "language superhighway," connects Wernicke's and Broca's areas. It curves rearward from the temporal lobe to the parietal lobe. It then passes through the angular gyrus and forward to the frontal lobe. These structures surrounding the sylvian fissure, which comprise the *perisylvian language arc,* form the central processing unit of the language system.

which is in the dominant temporal lobe. They circle in the *arcuate fasciculus,* posteriorly through the temporal and parietal lobes, and then anteriorly to *Broca's area,* which is immediately anterior to the frontal lobe's motor centers for the right arm, face, larynx, and pharynx (Fig. 8–1). Broca's area receives processed, integrated language and governs the articulation of speech. The horseshoe-shaped cerebral cortex surrounding the sylvian fissure, the *perisylvian language arc,* contains Wernicke's area, the arcuate fasciculus, and Broca's area. Language lives in the perisylvian language arc. This region of the cerebral cortex perceives language, integrates it with other cerebral activities, and articulates its expression.

Using the perisylvian language arc model, normal and abnormal language patterns have been established. For example, when normal people repeat aloud what they hear, impulses go to Wernicke's area, pass around the arcuate fasciculus, and arrive in Broca's area for speech production (Fig. 8–2, *A*). Also, when people read aloud, impulses are initially received by the visual cortex in both the left and right occipital lobes (see Fig. 4–1). Those impulses from the left visual field are received by the right occipital cortex and must travel through the posterior corpus callosum to reach the left (dominant) cerebral hemisphere. There, the combined impulses from both the left and right visual cortex travel through the arcuate fasciculus to Broca's area for articulation (Fig. 8–2, *B*).

Patients cannot repeat phrases if they have lesions almost anywhere in the perisylvian arc (see below, Conduction Aphasia). Conversely, when the arc is isolated from the surrounding cerebral cortex, patients can repeat phrases, but they cannot initiate conversation (see below, Isolation or Transcortical Aphasia).

Several frequently occurring injuries simultaneously strike portions of the perisylvian arc and important neighboring structures to create readily recognizable neuro-

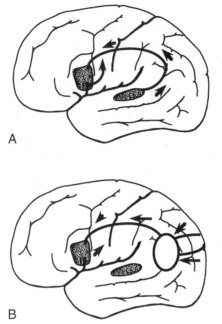

FIGURE 8–2. **A,** When people *repeat aloud,* language is received in Wernicke's area and transmitted through the parietal lobe by the arcuate fasciculus to Broca's area. This area innervates the adjacent cerebral cortex for the tongue, lips, larynx, and pharynx. **B,** When people *read aloud,* visual impulses are received by the left and right occipital visual cortex regions. Both regions send impulses to a left parietal lobe's association region (the oval), which converts text to language. Impulses from the left visual field, which are initially received in the right cortex, must first pass through the posterior corpus callosum to reach the language centers (see Fig. 8–4).

logic deficits that include one or another variety of aphasia. The most common situation, fully predictable from the neuroanatomy, is a left middle cerebral artery stroke that damages Broca's area and the adjacent motor cortex. This lesion produces dysarthria and right hemiparesis, as well as aphasia. Because lesions have a certain depth, they often interrupt the underlying geniculo-calcarine (visual) pathway. Thus, aphasia is often accompanied by a right homonymous hemianopsia.

Clinical Evaluation

Before diagnosing aphasia, the clinician must keep in mind normal language variations. Normal people may struggle and stammer when confronted with a novel experience, such as a neurologic examination. People have their own style and rhythm. Some may be reticent, uneducated, intimidated, or hostile. Some, before speaking, consider each word and formulate every phrase as though carefully considering which item to chose from a menu, but others just impulsively blurt out the first thing on their mind.

In diagnosing aphasia, the clinician can use various classifications. A favorite distinguishes *receptive (sensory)* from *expressive (motor)* aphasia based on relative impairment of verbal reception versus expression. However, a major drawback is that most aphasic patients have mixed impairment

The most clinically useful classification, *nonfluent-fluent,* is based on the patient's verbal output (Table 8–1). Fluent and nonfluent aphasias are usually evident during conversation, history taking, or mental status examination.

A standard series of simple verbal tests identify and further classify these aphasias. This entire test sequence can be repeated with written requests and responses; however, with almost only one exception (described below), written deficits generally parallel verbal ones. The standard aphasia tests evaluate *three basic language functions: comprehension, naming,* and *repetition* (Table 8–2).

- Comprehension is tested by asking the patient to follow simple requests, such as picking up one hand.

TABLE 8–1. *Salient Features of Major Aphasias*

Feature	Nonfluent	Fluent
Previous descriptions	Expressive	Receptive
	Motor	Sensory
	Broca's	Wernicke's
Spontaneous speech	Nonverbal	Verbal
Content	Paucity of words, mostly nouns and verbs	Complete sentences with normal syntax
Articulation	Dysarthric, slow, stuttering	Good
Errors	Telegraphic speech	Paraphasic errors, nonspecific phrases, circumlocutions
Response on testing		
Comprehension	Preserved	Impaired
Repetition	Impaired	Impaired
Naming	Impaired	Impaired
Associated deficits	Right hemiparesis (arm, face > leg)	Hemianopsia, hemisensory loss
Localization of lesion	Frontal lobe	Temporal or parietal lobe Occasionally diffuse

- Naming is tested by asking the patient to say his or her own name and that of common objects, such as a pen or key.

- Repetition is tested by asking the patient to recite several short phrases, such as, "The boy went to the store."

Nonfluent Aphasia

Characteristics.   Paucity of speech characterizes nonfluent aphasia. Patients are nonverbal. Whatever speech is produced consists almost exclusively of single words and short phrases, with preferential use of basic words, particularly as nouns and verbs. Modifiers—adjectives, adverbs, and conjunctions—are missing. Many utterances are only stock phrases or sound bites, such as, "Get out of here."

Nonfluent speech is also slow. Its rate is typically less than 50 words per minute, which is much slower than normal (100 to 150 words per minute). Another hallmark is that the flow of speech is so interrupted by excessive pauses that its pattern is

TABLE 8–2. *Clinical Evaluation for Aphasia*

Spontaneous speech: fluent versus nonfluent
Verbalization tests
  Comprehension
    Ability to follow simple requests: "Please, pick up your hand."
    Ability to follow complex requests: "Please, show me your left ring finger, and stick out your tongue."
  Naming
    Common objects: tie, keys, pen
    Uncommon objects: watchband, belt buckle
  Repetition
    Simple phrases: "The boy went to the store."
    Complex phrases: "No and's, if's, or but's."
Reading and writing (repeat above tests)

termed "telegraphic." For example, in response to a question about food, a patient might stammer "fork . . . steak . . . eat . . . no."

Patients with nonfluent aphasia may be unable to say either their own name or the names of common objects. They cannot repeat simple phrases. At the same time, they have relatively normal comprehension that can be illustrated by their ability to follow verbal requests, such as "Close your eyes" or "Raise your left hand." Nonfluent aphasia was originally designated "expressive" because of this combination of speech impairment and preserved comprehension.

Localization and Etiology.   Lesions responsible for nonfluent aphasia are located in or near Broca's area (Fig. 8–3, *A*). Their etiology is usually a middle cerebral artery stroke or other discrete structural lesion; however, their location, not their nature, produces the aphasia. Whatever their etiology, these lesions tend to be so extensive that they damage neighboring structures, such as the motor cortex and the posterior sensory cortex. Moreover, because they are usually spherical or conical, they damage underlying white matter tracts, including the visual pathway. Diffuse cerebral injuries, such as metabolic disturbances or Alzheimer's disease, are practically never responsible for nonfluent aphasia.

Associated Deficits.   Because the responsible lesion usually damages the motor cortex and other adjacent and underlying regions, nonfluent aphasia is characteristically associated with a right hemiparesis, with particular weakness of the arm and lower face, and with poor articulation (dysarthria). Deep lesions typically induce a right homonymous hemianopsia (visual field cut) and hemisensory loss. One of the

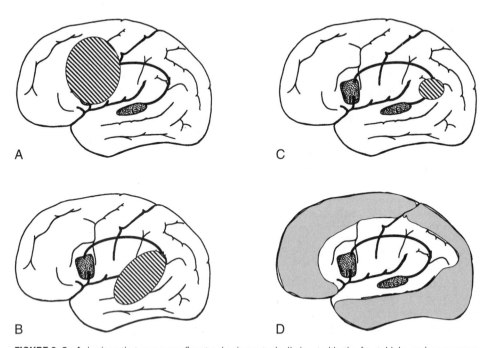

FIGURE 8–3. **A,** Lesions that cause *nonfluent aphasia* are typically located in the frontal lobe and encompass Broca's area and the adjacent cortex motor strip. **B,** Those causing *fluent aphasia* are in the temporoparietal region, may even be a diffuse injury, such as Alzheimer's disease, and encompass Wernicke's areas and the posterior regions. They usually spare the motor strip. **C,** Those causing *conduction aphasia*, which are relatively small, interrupt the arcuate fasciculus in the parietal or posterior temporal lobe. **D,** Those causing isolation aphasia are circumferential injuries of the watershed region that spare the perisylvian language arc.

most common syndromes in neurology is an occlusion of the left middle cerebral artery that produces the combination of nonfluent aphasia and right-sided hemiparesis with the arm much more involved than the leg, visual field cut, and hemisensory impairment. The usual localization and frequently occurring motor problems of this variety of aphasia have given rise to the terms "Broca's" and "motor" aphasia.

Lesions causing nonfluent aphasia often simultaneously produce *buccofacial apraxia,* also called "oral apraxia." This apraxia, like others, is not paresis but the inability to execute normal voluntary movements. When buccofacial apraxia occurs in conjunction with nonfluent aphasia, it impedes facial, lip, and tongue movements, and thus causes poor articulation. Lesions affecting Broca's area proper cause *aphemia* (mutism). Those affecting both frontal lobes cause a paucity or absence of speech, as part of an overall lack of voluntary movement, emotion, and responsiveness *(abulia).*

To demonstrate buccofacial apraxia, the examiner must ask the patient to say "La . . . Pa . . . La . . . Pa . . . La . . . Pa," protrude the tongue in different directions, and pretend to blow out a match and suck through a straw. Those affected will be unable to comply, although they can use the same muscles reflexively or when provided with cues. For example, patients who cannot speak might sing, and those who cannot pretend to suck through a straw might be able to use an actual straw to drink.

Nonfluent aphasia is also characteristically associated with depression. A psychologic explanation is that patients with aphasia, which is usually accompanied by marked physical impairment, have suffered a major loss of bodily function and naturally feel sad, hopeless, and frustrated. A neurologic explanation is that the aphasia-producing lesions are generally located in the frontal lobe, where they also produce apathy and abulia (see Frontal Lobe Disorders, Chapter 7). Alternatively, signs of depression in aphasic patients, particularly those who have had several strokes, may actually be manifestations of dementia or pseudobulbar palsy. In fact, although nonfluent aphasia, dementia, pseudobulbar palsy, and depression may mimic each other, all four are manifestations of frontal lobe injury and may, in various combinations, occur together.

When strokes or trauma cause aphasia, patients recover to a greater or lesser extent because ischemic areas of the brain recover and surviving neurons form new connections. Little or no documentation supports usefulness of speech therapy or medication.

Global Aphasia. An extreme form of nonfluent aphasia is *global aphasia,* in which complete dominant hemisphere damage abolishes language function. Aside from uttering some unintelligible sounds and following an occasional gestured request, patients with global aphasia are mute. Moreover, they tend to be withdrawn, uncommunicative in other ways, and emotionally unresponsive. Comparably severe physical deficits include right hemiplegia, right homonymous hemianopsia, and conjugate deviation of the eyes toward the left. Frequent causes are dominant hemisphere internal carotid or middle cerebral artery occlusions, cerebral hemorrhages, and penetrating injuries.

Fluent Aphasia

Paraphasias and Other Characteristics. Fluent aphasia is characterized by the inability to comprehend language and incessant use of *paraphasic errors* or *paraphasias,* which are incorrect or even nonsensical words. Paraphasias are included within relatively complete, well-articulated, grammatically correct sentences that are spoken at a normal rate. They can render conversation unintelligible.

Paraphasias include word substitution, such as "clock" for "watch" (a related paraphasia); "glove" for "knife" (an unrelated paraphasia); or "that" for any object (a generic substitution). Words may be altered, such as "breat" for "bread" (a literal paraphasia). Most striking are strings of nonsensical coinages (*neologisms*), such as "I want to fin gunt in the fark," and use of words that rhyme (*clang associations*).

Patients may speak in *circumlocutions* to compensate for their word-finding difficulty. They may also tend toward *tangential diversions,* as though once having chosen the wrong word, they pursue the idea triggered by their error.

Nevertheless, since nondominant hemisphere functions are spared, nonverbal expressions are preserved (see above). Patients' prosody or tone of voice is true to their emotions. In addition, whether words are adequate or not, emotions are revealed by facial gestures, body movements, and the "second language" of cursing. Most patients are still able to produce a melody even though they may be unable to repeat the lyrics. For example, patients can hum a tune, such as "Jingle Bells," but if they attempt to sing, their lyrics are strewn with paraphasias.

Associated Deficits.   Unlike nonfluent aphasia, fluent aphasia is not associated with significant hemiparesis because the responsible lesion is distant from the cerebral cortex motor strip. Only right-sided hyperactive deep tendon reflexes (DTRs) and a Babinski sign may be elicited. However, a right-sided sensory impairment and visual field cut may be present because of interrupted sensory and visual cerebral pathways.

Strikingly, patients are strangely unaware of their paraphasias, unable to edit them, and oblivious to their listener's consternation. Concomitantly, they may develop anxiety, agitation, or paranoia. Clinicians not seeing any hemiparesis and unable to capture the patient's attention for detailed testing often do not appreciate the neurologic basis of the abnormal language, thought, or behavior. For many psychiatric consultations, the sudden onset of fluent aphasia often turns out to be the explanation for an "acute psychosis," marked change in behavior, or management problem in a patient on a medical service.

Localization and Etiology.   Usually, discrete structural lesions, such as small strokes, in the temporoparietal region are the cause of fluent aphasia (Fig. 8–3, *B*). Although they do not necessarily damage Wernicke's area, the arcuate fasciculus, or the sensory cortex, fluent aphasia is often termed "Wernicke's" or "sensory" aphasia. Unlike nonfluent aphasia, it is sometimes caused by diffuse cerebral injury, including Alzheimer's disease.

Varieties of Fluent Aphasia

Differences in the varieties of fluent aphasia tend to be subtle, making their diagnosis turn on fine points. Moreover, clinical-pathologic correlations are subject to great individual variations in anatomy, language production, and cognitive capacity.

Anomia.   A common variety, *anomic aphasia* or *anomia*, is simply inability to name objects. Often produced by a small stroke, it can be a symptom of Alzheimer's disease. At times, this variety of aphasia, rather than memory loss, may be responsible for Alzheimer's disease patients' inability to recall the names of places, objects, and people.

Sparing of the Perisylvian Arc.   Another variety, *transcortical* or *isolation aphasia*, results from isolation of the perisylvian arc because the surrounding cerebral cortex is damaged. Often the entire cortex, except for the arc, is devastated, and patients have dementia. Precisely because the language system remains intact, patients with isolation aphasia can characteristically repeat whatever they hear. In contrast, they cannot participate in a conversation, follow requests, or name objects because the language system cannot communicate with the rest of the cerebral cortex. Depending on the injury, patients may have a right hemiparesis or a tendency toward decorticate posturing (see Fig. 11–5). The salient feature of isolation aphasia is remarkable disparity between seeming muteness and ability to repeat long, complex sentences readily, involuntarily, and apparently compulsively. This parrotlike echoing of others' words is called *echolalia*. A cursory examination could understandably confuse such speech with irrational jargon.

The origin of isolation aphasia lies in the precarious blood supply of the cerebral cortex. While the perisylvian arc cerebral cortex is well-perfused by major branches of large cerebral arteries, the surrounding cortex is a large border zone between the middle, anterior, and posterior cerebral arteries (the *watershed area*) tenuously perfused by thin, fragile vessels. Isolation aphasia is usually caused by a *watershed infarction*, which occurs when the cortex receives insufficient cerebral blood flow (Fig. 8–3, *D*). Thus, isolation aphasia is usually the result of a cardiac or respiratory arrest, other hypotensive or hypoxic episodes, or showers of small emboli. It is also found among several neurologic deficits caused by suicide attempts with carbon monoxide, which has a predilection for damaging the globus pallidus, cerebellum, and hippocampus, as well as the cerebral cortex. Occasionally, Alzheimer's disease causes isolation aphasia.

If desired, one can further divide transcortical aphasia. Transcortical *sensory* aphasia is essentially a fluent aphasia characterized by preservation of repetition. Transcortical *motor* aphasia, essentially a nonfluent aphasia, is also characterized, despite paucity of verbal output, by preservation of repetition.

Interruption of the Perisylvian Arc.   If damage to Broca's area, Wernicke's area, or the surrounding cerebral cortex produce varieties of aphasia, the clinician could predict that arcuate fasciculus damage would lead to another variety. In *conduction aphasia*, a small, discrete arcuate fasciculus lesion, usually in the parietal or posterior temporal lobe (Fig. 8–3, *C*), interrupts or *disconnects* Wernicke's and Broca's areas. (It therefore may be seen as one of the *disconnection syndromes* [see below].) Patients are fluent and have good comprehension but cannot repeat phrases or short sentences. In contrast to those with isolation aphasia, they are particularly maladept at repeating strings of syllables.

The most frequent cause of conduction aphasia is a small, embolic stroke in the posterior temporal branch of the left middle cerebral artery. Lesions are so small that they cause little or no physical deficits. At most, patients have right lower facial weakness.

MENTAL ABNORMALITIES WITH LANGUAGE IMPAIRMENT

Dementia

Although aphasia by itself is not equivalent to dementia, it can be a part of dementia or it can mimic dementia. For example, when aphasia impairs common communications, such as saying the date and place, repeating a series of numbers, and following requests, it mimics dementia. At times, aphasia can be so severe that patients appear to be incoherent. Whatever its extent, aphasia also clouds thinking and memory simply because people think in words.

However, unlike dementia, aphasia usually begins suddenly. Nonfluent aphasia, the more common variety, is usually readily recognizable because it is accompanied by dysarthria and obvious lateralized signs: right-sided hemiparesis and visual field cut. Fluent aphasia, although less common, is readily identifiable by characteristic paraphasias.

Likewise, dementia may mimic aphasia. Patients with dementia in its early stages may have anomias while being fully verbal, articulate, and able to perform reasonably well on standard language function tests. Those with severe dementia have a paucity of speech and a limited vocabulary (i.e., are nonverbal).

Occasionally patients have both aphasia and dementia. This combination occurs with multiple infarctions or a stroke superimposed on Alzheimer's disease. These situations are notoriously difficult to clarify because aphasia invalidates many tests of intellectual function.

Distinguishing aphasia from dementia and recognizing when they coexist are more than academic exercises. A diagnosis of aphasia almost always suggests that a patient has had a discrete dominant cerebral hemisphere injury. Since a stroke or other structural lesion would be the most likely cause, the appropriate evaluation would include a computed tomography (CT) or magnetic resonance imaging (MRI). In contrast, a diagnosis of dementia suggests that the most likely cause would be Alzheimer's disease or another diffuse process, and the evaluation might include various blood tests as well as a CT or MRI.

Schizophrenia

Distinguishing fluent aphasia from *schizophrenic speech* can, theoretically at least, be even more troublesome. Circumlocutions, tangential diversions, and neologisms are common to both. As the thought disorder of schizophrenia becomes more pronounced, its language abnormalities increase in frequency and similarity to aphasia. Even in previously healthy people, sudden onset of aphasia can be so frightening and confusing that they become agitated and irrational.

However, many differences can be discerned. Schizophrenic speech usually develops gradually in patients who are relatively young (in their third decade) and have had long-standing illness. Their neologisms and other paraphasias are relatively infrequent and inconspicuous. Unlike most fluent aphasia patients, they can repeat polysyllabic words and complex phrases, such as "Methodist Episcopal Church."

Aphasia usually appears suddenly in the seventh or eighth decade. Except for some with fluent aphasia, patients are aware that they cannot communicate. They often request help in this regard and, possibly because of self-monitoring, keep their responses short and pointed. Any right-sided hemiparesis aids diagnosis.

Other Disorders

Within the category *Pervasive Developmental Disorders*, DSM-IV places *Autistic Disorder*, *Rett's Disorder*, *Childhood Disintegrative Disorder*, and *Asperger's Disorder*. Language abnormalities are a prominent and early symptom of autistic disorder, which neurologists continue to refer to as autism. Rett syndrome (see Chapter 13) and childhood disintegrative disorder are characterized by similar language abnormalities, but they appear only after several years of normal development. In contrast, Asperger's disorder remains relatively free of language abnormalities.

Autistic children begin to speak later than normal and ultimately have impairments in all of its aspects: articulation (phonology), prosody, grammar, reception and especially expression, conversation, and facial and bodily communication. In addition, their speaking is laced with abnormalities, particularly nonsensical repetitions (stereotypies), idiosyncrasies, and echolalia.

Mutism and apparent language abnormalities can also be manifestations of more benign psychologic disturbances (see Chapter 3). In them, language impairment is usually inconsistent and amenable to suggestion. Also, psychogenic language impairment is often complicated by stuttering. For example, a patient with psychogenic aphasia might stutter and be at a loss for words but communicate normally in writing. Sometimes an amobarbital interview might be appropriate.

A much more frequently occurring, psychogenic aphasia-like condition is the sudden, unexpected difficulty in remembering someone's name ("blocking"). The classic example remains the Freudian slip. (Freud himself was an expert on aphasia and its neurologic basis.) Depending on one's viewpoint, everyday word substitutions may be termed either paraphasias or insights into the unconscious. For example, when a physician's former secretary is being evaluated for a neurologic disorder and says that she has been Dr. So-and-So's "medical cemetery," a clinician could interpret the comment as her feelings about the competence of the doctor, an indication of the patient's own fears of death, or a paraphasia that is indicative of a dominant hemisphere lesion.

DISORDERS RELATED TO APHASIA

Alexia and Agraphia

Alexia, inability to read, and *agraphia*, inability to write, are almost always found together as part of aphasia. In an important exception, *alexia without agraphia*, patients who have little or no impairment in comprehending speech or expressing themselves by writing cannot read. For example, although they are unable to read, even their own writing, they can transcribe dictation and write their thoughts. Alexia without agraphia, which should really be called "alexia with graphia," results from a destructive lesion encompassing the dominant (left) occipital lobe and adjacent posterior corpus callosum (Figs. 8–4 and 20–10, *B*). Aside from a right homonymous hemianopsia, patients have no physical deficits.

Gerstmann's Syndrome

Agraphia may also occur in *Gerstmann's syndrome*. In this condition, which has been attributed to lesions in the *angular gyrus* of the dominant parietal lobe (Fig. 8–1), agraphia is accompanied by three other abnormalities: *acalculia* (impairment of arithmetic skills), *finger agnosia* (inability to identify fingers), and *left/right confusion*.

The status of Gerstmann's syndrome as a distinct clinical entity has been questioned because patients rarely display all four components, and those patients with

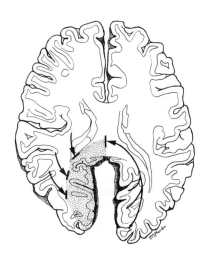

FIGURE 8–4. *Alexia without agraphia* is caused by lesions that damage the left occipital lobe and the posterior corpus callosum. Patients are unable to see anything in their right visual field because of the left occipital cortex damage. Left visual images still reach the right cortex, but they cannot be transmitted to the left cerebral language centers because the critical posterior corpus callosum is damaged. Thus, patients cannot comprehend written material presented to either visual field. In contrast, they can still write full sentences from memory, imagination, or dictation because these forms of information still reach the language centers. (See Fig. 20–10*B* for the corresponding CT.)

many components usually also have aphasia or dementia. Nevertheless, the constellation of Gerstmann's signs, even if they do not constitute a syndrome, is useful because they may be sought in adults with strokes. Also, in evaluating children for learning disabilities, those with dyscalculia frequently also have poor handwriting (agraphia) and left/right confusion accompanied by physical signs of dominant hemisphere injury, such as right-sided hyperactive DTRs and a Babinski sign (see Chapter 13).

Apraxia

Roughly the motor system's equivalent of nonfluent aphasia, *apraxia* is inability to execute learned actions despite normal strength, sensation, coordination, and, more important, comprehension. It is attributable to disruption of motor areas and their disconnection from each other and from language centers.

Although apraxia can be readily differentiated from simple paresis, it is often inseparably associated with aphasia or dementia. An integral aspect of cortical dementia, apraxia is often a symptom of Alzheimer's disease (see Chapter 7). In fact, moderate to severe dementia, whatever the cause, probably can cause apraxia.

In demonstrating apraxia, the examiner generally first tests the patient's buccofacial (lips, face, tongue) and limb movements in making gestures or "symbolic acts" (Table 8–3). Next, the examiner asks the patient to perform actions that are imagined on pretend objects and then actual ones. After seeing the examiner perform an action, patients can copy it. Similarly, when given an object, patients with apraxia can often perform the action because of the cue. Overall, inability to use a common tool, such as a comb or spoon, is the most reliable demonstration of apraxia. Further testing, depending on circumstances, includes performing a series of steps, copying figures, arranging matchsticks, walking, or dressing.

Patients are typically unaware that they have apraxia since they usually do not spontaneously attempt the various tests, such as saluting unseen officers or using an imaginary screwdriver. Moreover, an unsophisticated evaluation might naturally attribute motor impairments to paresis or incoordination.

Despite its complexity, several clinically useful apraxias have been described. *Ideomotor apraxia*, the most frequently occurring, is basically impaired conversion of an idea into an action. It can be pictured as disconnection of cognitive or language regions from motor regions (Fig. 8–5). The underlying lesion is usually a left-sided frontal or parietal lobe infarction. Ideomotor apraxia is thus associated with aphasia, particularly nonfluent aphasia,

One of its two varieties, *buccofacial apraxia*, was discussed as a feature of nonfluent aphasia. In *limb apraxia*, patients are not able to execute simple requests involving their arms or legs. They cannot salute or move their hands in certain abstract patterns. They cannot pretend to brush their teeth, turn a key, comb their hair, or kick a ball.

TABLE 8–3. *Testing for Ideomotor Apraxia*

	Action		
	Gesture*	**Imagined**	**Real**
Buccofacial	Kiss the air	Pretend to blow out a match	Blow out a match
	Repeat "Pa"	Pretend to suck on a straw	Drink water through a straw
Limb	Salute	Pretend to use a comb	Comb the hair
	Stop traffic	Pretend to write	Write with a pencil or pen

*Symbolic acts.

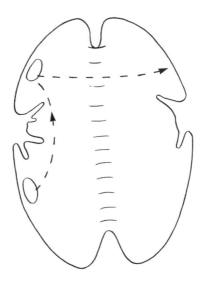

FIGURE 8–5. In a schematic transaxial view, requests for *normal movements* are received by Wernicke's area in the dominant (left) posterior temporal lobe. They are transmitted anteriorly to the motor regions and, through the anterior corpus callosum, to the contralateral motor strip. Interruptions of the path within the left cerebral hemisphere result in ideomotor apraxia of both arms, causing bilateral limb apraxia. Lesions in the anterior corpus callosum interrupt only those impulses destined to control the left arm and leg, which causes unilateral left arm and leg ideomotor apraxia.

When asked to pretend to *use* an object, these patients characteristically use their hands as though they *were* the actual objects. For example, they will brush their teeth with their forefingers instead of pretending to hold a toothbrush. Both varieties are associated with aphasia.

In *ideational apraxia*, patients cannot perform a sequence of steps requiring a simple plan and continual monitoring. For example, they cannot pretend to fold a letter, place it into an envelope, address the envelope, and then affix a stamp. In contrast to ideomotor apraxia, associated with left-sided cerebral lesions and nonfluent aphasia, ideational apraxia usually reflects either frontal lobe injuries or diffuse cerebral disease and is almost inseparable from dementia. In particular, ideational apraxia is often a manifestation of Alzheimer's disease and multiple strokes because the dementia impairs planning and execution.

Several other apraxias are not referable to the dominant hemisphere or diffuse lesions and are covered in more detail elsewhere. *Construction apraxia* is a manifestation of nondominant parietal lobe lesions (see below and Fig. 2–8). *Dressing apraxia*, usually manifested by an inability to clothe the left-sided limbs, is typically a manifestation of nondominant hemisphere lesions (see below). A different but better known condition is *gait apraxia*, which is a hallmark of normal pressure hydrocephalus (see Fig. 7–7).

NONDOMINANT HEMISPHERE SYMPTOMS

Hemi-Inattention

Nondominant hemisphere injury disturbances require considerable clinical acumen to detect because they tend to be short-lived, subtle, and dependent on the patient's premorbid intelligence, personality, and defense mechanisms. Because they occur individually or in various combinations, there is no single nondominant hemisphere syndrome. Neither a syndrome nor the primary disturbances are defined in *DSM-IV.*

Hemi-inattention (hemispatial neglect) is the most prominent manifestation of nondominant hemisphere injury. It usually originates in a stroke of the nondominant parietal lobe cortex and its underlying thalamus and reticular activating system, which are responsible for sensory perception, arousal, and attention.

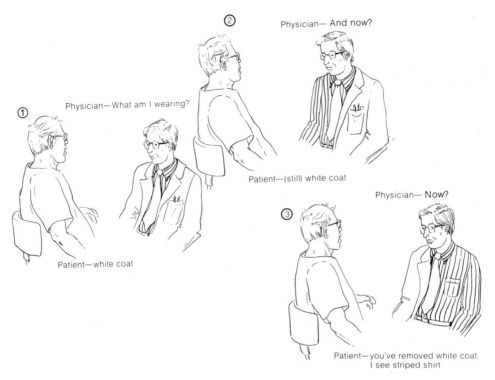

FIGURE 8–6. In a classic demonstration of left *hemi-inattention*, the patient, neglecting left-sided stimulation, perceives only what the examiner is wearing in his right visual field. Even if the patient's problem were simply a left homonymous hemianopsia, he still would have explored and discovered, with his intact right visual field, that the examiner was half-dressed.

Patients with hemi-inattention ignore visual, tactile, and other sensory stimuli that originate from their left side. They disregard, fail to perceive, or misinterpret objects in their left visual field (Fig. 8–6). In contrast to patients with an homonymous hemianopsia, who usually develop some awareness and make compensatory movements to keep objects in the preserved visual field, those with hemi-inattention seem oblivious to their situation and make no normal exploratory eye or limb movements.

Also, when both sides of their body are touched, patients with hemi-inattention neglect the left-sided stimulation *(extinction on double simultaneous stimulation [DSS])* and report that only their right side was touched. Sometimes patients even fail to shave the left side of their face and leave their left side undressed. Their failure to dress completely indicates *dressing apraxia* (inability to dress). In addition to simply leaving their left limbs out of clothing, patients with dressing apraxia put both hands into one sleeve, misalign buttons on a shirt, and become befuddled when presented with their clothing turned inside-out.

An extreme form of hemi-inattention is the *alien hand syndrome.* In this disorder, which typically follows a nondominant hemisphere stroke, a patient's left hand retains some rudimentary motor and sensory functions, but the patient cannot appreciate them. Without the patient's awareness, the limb moves semipurposefully, makes its own explorations, and performs simple tasks, such as scratching and moving bedclothes. In a unique, often quoted example, a patient reported that her hand was attempting to choke her.

The alien hand syndrome rests on the patient having at least two misperceptions: (1) the patient does not possess the hand and (2) the hand's movements are independent or governed by another person (the alien). Most patients feel divorced from the hand or, at least, express a tenuous attachment to it. Several cases have been attributed to corpus callosum injury, suggesting that the alien hand syndrome is another disconnection syndrome.

Anosognosia, inability to accept a physical deficit (usually a left hemiparesis), is an aspect of hemi-inattention. Patients typically cannot identify the affected part of their body (*somatotopagnosia* or *autotopagnosia*). They occasionally claim the examiner's hand and deny ownership of their paretic hand. Sometimes they attribute the weakened hand to a third person.

Patients with anosognosia often refuse to accept physical therapy and other hospital routines, and can become belligerent. They often also have depression. From the other perspective, patients with left hemiparesis, especially those with behavioral problems, should be evaluated for anosognosia and its frequent companion, depression.

Denial and confabulation are not restricted to nondominant hemisphere injury. Both are prominent signs in suddenly occurring cortical blindness (see Anton's syndrome, Chapter 12), and confabulation is found in Wernicke-Korsakoff syndrome (see Chapter 7).

Another manifestation of nondominant hemisphere injury is *constructional apraxia*, a *visual-spatial* perceptual impairment. Patients are unable to organize visual information or integrate it with fine motor skills. For example, they cannot copy simple figures or arrange matchsticks in patterns (Fig. 8–7). Constructional apraxia, however, cannot always be ascribed to a nondominant lesion. It can also be found in patients with diffuse cerebral dysfunction or only left hemisphere injury.

Aprosody

Inability to appreciate or endow speech with emotional or affective qualities is *aprosody*. Nondominant hemisphere lesions, which cause it, interfere with patients' ability to discern emotions from others' tone of voice. For example, a patient with aprosody would be unable to appreciate the contrasting feelings in the question "Are

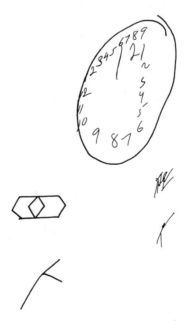

FIGURE 8–7. When asked to draw a clock, a patient with *constructional apraxia* drew an incomplete circle, repeated (perseverated) the numerals, and placed them asymmetrically. When attempting to copy the top left figure, the patient repeated several lines, failing to draw any figure. The patient also misplaced and rotated the position of the bottom left figure (see also Fig. 2–8).

you going home?" asked first by a jealous hospital roommate and then by a gleeful spouse. Unable to express emotionally charged sentences, patients speak without inflection or style. They are unable to sing a song, although they can repeat the lyrics, because they cannot convey its melody.

Aprosody tends to be accompanied by the loss of nonverbal communication, popularly called "body language" and technically *paralinguistic components* of speech, such as facial expression and limb gesture. These physical aspects of communication are similar to prosody. They lend conviction, emphasis, and affect to spoken words. Indeed, gestures seem independent and sometimes more credible than speech. Well-known examples are children crossing their fingers when promising, adults who wink while telling a joke, and people who smile while relating sad events.

To assess prosody, the examiner recreates a short version of the aphasia examination. During spontaneous speech, the examiner notes the patient's variations in volume, pitch, and emphasis. The patient is requested to ask a question such as "May I have the ball?" in the manner of a friend and then a stern schoolteacher using appropriate vocal and facial expressions. The examiner then asks a similar question, impersonating the same characters while the patient tries to identify them. An alternative test is to ask the patient to describe pictures of people displaying extreme emotions.

Extending the concept that the nondominant hemisphere confers affect on language, several authors have suggested it is responsible for perception and expression of emotion and complex nonverbal processes. The dominant hemisphere, they suggest, is responsible for verbal, sequential, analytic cognitive processes and reflection.

DISCONNECTION SYNDROMES

Virtually all mental processes require communication pathways between several areas located within one cerebral hemisphere and often between both hemispheres. The arcuate fasciculus, for example, provides intrahemispheric communication between Wernicke's and Broca's areas. In general, interhemispheric communication is provided by other myelin-coated axonal (white matter) bundles, often called *commissures*, of which the most conspicuous is the *corpus callosum*. Other intercerebral connections are the massa intermedia and the anterior, posterior, and hippocampal commissures.

Injuries that damage these communication pathways but spare the actual neurologic centers cause *disconnection syndromes*. Each is uncommon, but permits examination of the particular neurologic function. Several disconnection syndromes were predicted before actually being demonstrated, much as certain subatomic particles were predicted and then "discovered." Disconnection syndromes that have already been discussed are (1) alexia without agraphia, (2) conduction aphasia, and (3) ideomotor apraxia with its varieties, buccofacial and limb apraxia. In addition, although the medial longitudinal fasciculus (MLF) syndrome or intranuclear ophthalmoplegia (INO) (see Chapters 4, 12, and 15) is strictly a brainstem disorder, it shares many disconnection syndrome characteristics.

Several disconnection syndromes, such as alexia without agraphia and some of the apraxias, result from corpus callosum damage. Another example is the *anterior cerebral artery syndrome*, in which a stroke of the anterior cerebral arteries leads to an infarction of both frontal lobes and the anterior corpus callosum. The infarction obstructs information passing between the left hemisphere language centers and the right hemisphere motor centers. Although the patient's left arm and leg will have normal spontaneous movement, these limbs will not respond to an examiner's verbal or written requests, that is, the patient will have unilateral (left-sided) limb apraxia (Fig. 8–5).

In several corpus callosum disorders, disconnection signs may be present, but they are subtle and variable. The corpus callosum occasionally fails to develop in utero *(congenital absence)*, and sometimes it is damaged by excessive consumption of red wine *(Marchiafava-Bignami syndrome)*.

Split Brain

The most important disconnection syndrome, which also involves the corpus callosum, is the *split brain syndrome*. This disorder usually results from a longitudinal surgical division of the corpus callosum (commissurotomy) for control of intractable epilepsy (see Chapter 10). After a commissurotomy, each cerebral hemisphere is virtually isolated. Examiners may present certain information to only one hemisphere. For example, pictures, writing, and other visual information shown within one visual field will present information to only the contralateral hemisphere (Fig. 8–8). Likewise, tactile information can be presented to only one hemisphere by having a blindfolded patient touch objects with the contralateral hand. However, auditory information cannot be presented exclusively—only predominantly—to one hemisphere. (Because pathways are duplicated in the brainstem [see Fig. 4–15], sounds detected in one ear are ultimately received to some extent by both hemispheres.)

In testing a split brain patients' left cerebral hemisphere function, the examiner writes questions in patients' right visual field and places objects in their right hand. Patients respond correctly by speaking and writing with their right hand. To written requests for right arm and leg movements, patients respond correctly; however, left limbs are unable to follow the same requests because information cannot flow from the left hemisphere to the right hemisphere, that is, the patient has left limb apraxia (Figs. 8–5 and 8–8).

In testing right hemisphere function, visual information is shown in patients' left visual field. Because impulses cannot travel to the language centers, patients cannot read, respond to written requests, or name objects. Similarly, as if they had aphasia, patients cannot name objects placed in their left hand. However, they are able to use their left hand to copy figures and—more striking—discriminate patterns, recognize faces, and perceive emotions.

The interruption of the corpus callosum prevents the right hemisphere from sharing with the entire brain, particularly the left hemisphere's language centers. As could be anticipated, the information, experience, and emotion that the right hemisphere acquires do not reach patients' consciousness, at least to the level of verbal expression. For example, if an object is placed in a blindfolded patient's left hand, the patient cannot name or describe it, and the right hand cannot choose an identical object. Similarly, if one hand learns to follow a maze, the other hand will have to be taught separately.

Not only can each hemisphere separately detect visual and tactile sensations, but each might also perceive emotions separately. For example, if a humorous picture were shown to the right visual field, a patient might laugh and be able to relate the picture's humorous content; however, if the same picture were shown to the patient's left visual field, it might provoke an amused sensation that the patient could not verbalize or even fully comprehend. If a sad picture were shown to the left visual field

Requests Shown In
Left Visual Field

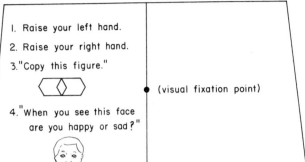

1. Raise your left hand.

2. Raise your right hand.

3. "Copy this figure."

4. "When you see this face are you happy or sad?"

● (visual fixation point)

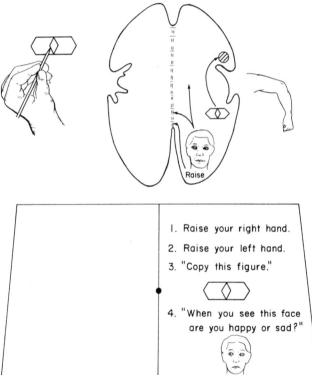

Raise

1. Raise your right hand.

2. Raise your left hand.

3. "Copy this figure."

4. "When you see this face are you happy or sad?"

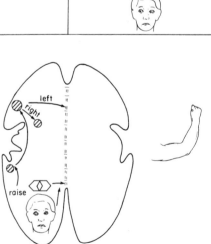

left
right
raise

FIGURE 8–8. After a *commissurotomy,* patients typically have the *split brain syndrome.* Each hemisphere can be tested individually by showing requests, objects, and pictures in the contralateral visual field. *Upper,* Objects and written requests shown in the left visual field are perceived by the right visual field. Since connections to the ipsilateral motor area are intact, the *left* hand can copy figures. However, since the right hemisphere is unable to transmit information through the corpus callosum to the dominant left cerebral hemisphere, which governs language function, patients cannot read the requests or describe the objects. Although patients cannot speak of the feelings evoked by emotionally laden pictures shown in their left visual field, they have sympathetic, nonverbal responses. *Lower,* Written requests and objects shown in the right visual field are perceived by the left hemisphere. Patients can read those written requests, copy those objects with the right hand, and comply with the requests; however, because the language areas cannot send information through the corpus callosum, the left hand cannot comply. When patients describe emotions portrayed in a picture, their language lacks affect, derived from the nondominant hemisphere.

but the humorous one to the right, the patient's amused response would be distorted because of the conflict.

Split brain studies have suggested that normal people have, in their two hemispheres, mental systems that are parallel, nonverbal, and capable of simultaneous reasoning. Although the systems usually complement each other, they have the potential to conflict.

REFERENCES

Absher JR, Benson DF: Disconnection syndromes: An overview of Geschwind's contributions. Neurology *43:* 862–867, 1993

Alexander MP, Baker E, Naeser MA, et al: Neuropsychological and neuroanatomical dimensions of ideomotor apraxia. Brain *115:* 87–107, 1992

Basso A, Scarpa MT: Traumatic aphasia in children and adults: A comparison of clinical features and evolution. Cortex *26:* 501–514, 1990

Basso A, Farabola M, Grassi MP, et al: Aphasia in left-handers. Comparison of aphasia profiles and language recovery in non-right-handed and matched right-handed patients. Brain Lang *38:* 233–252, 1990

Benson DF, Ardila A: Aphasia: A Clinical Perspective. New York. Oxford University Press, 1996

Benton AL: Gerstmann's syndrome. Arch Neurol *49:* 445–447, 1992

Brust JCM: Music and the brain. Brain *103:* 367–392, 1980

Critchley M, Henson RA (eds): Music and the Brain: Studies in the Neurology of Music. London, William Heinemann Medical Books Ltd, 1977

Faber R, Abrams R, Taylor MA, et al: Comparison of schizophrenic patients with formal thought disorder and neurologically impaired patients with aphasia. Am J Psychiatry *140:* 1348–1351, 1983

Feinberg TE, Schindler RJ, Flanagan NG, et al: Two alien hand syndromes. Neurology *42:* 19–24, 1992

Gazzaniga MS: The split brain revisited. Sci Am 51–55, July 1998

Hemenway D: Bimanual dexterity in baseball players. N Engl J Med *309:* 1587, 1983

Klein SK, Masur D, Farber K, et al: Fluent aphasia in children: Definition and natural history. J Child Neurol *7:* 50–59, 1992

Levine DN, Calvanio R, Rinn WE: The pathogenesis of anosognosia for hemiplegia. Neurology *41:* 1770–1781, 1991

Loonen MCB, Dongen HR: Acquired childhood aphasia: Outcome 1 year after onset. Arch Neurol *47:* 1324–1328, 1990

McGuire PK, Shah GMS, Murray RM: Increased blood flow in Broca's area during auditory hallucinations in schizophrenia. Lancet *342:* 703–706, 1993

Motley MT: Slips of the tongue. Sci Am *253:* 116–125, 1985

Portal JM, Romano PE: Patterns of eye-hand dominance in baseball players. N Engl J Med *319:* 655, 1988

Rapin I: Autism. N Engl J Med *337:* 97–104, 1997

Shenton ME, Kikinis R, Jolesz FA, et al: Abnormalities of the left temporal lobe and thought disorder in schizophrenia. N Engl J Med *327:* 604–612, 1992

Starkstein SE, Berthier ML, Fedoroff P, et al: Anosognosia and major depression in two patients with cerebrovascular lesions. Neurology *40:* 1380–1382, 1990

Starkstein SE, Fedoroff JP, Price TR, et al: Neuropsychological and neuroradiologic correlates of emotional prosody comprehension. Neurology *44:* 515–522, 1994

Therapeutics and Technology Subcommittee of the American Academy of Neurology: Melodic intonation therapy. Neurology *44:* 566–568, 1994

Tupper DE, Cicerone KD (eds): The Neuropsychology of Everyday Life. Norwell, MA, Kluwer Academic Publishers, 1991

QUESTIONS and ANSWERS: CHAPTER 8

1–5. Formulate the following cases:

Case 1
A 68-year-old man suddenly develops right hemiparesis. He only utters "Oh, Oh!" when stimulated. He makes no response to questions or requests. His right lower face is paretic, and his right arm and leg are flaccid and immobile. He is inattentive to objects in his right visual field.

Case 2

A 70-year-old man, since suffering a CVA the previous year, can only say "weak, arm," "go away," and "give . . . supper me." His speech is slurred. He can raise his left arm, protrude his tongue, and close his eyes. He can name several objects, but he cannot repeat phrases. His right arm is paretic, but he can walk.

Case 3

Over a period of 6 weeks, a previously healthy 64-year-old woman has developed headaches, progressively severe difficulty in finding words, and apparent confusion. She speaks continuously and incoherently: "Go to the warb," "I can't hear," "My heat hurts." She is unable to follow commands, name objects, or repeat phrases. On examination, there is pronation of the outstretched right arm, a right Babinski sign, and papilledema. Visual fields cannot be tested.

Case 4

A 34-year-old man with mitral stenosis has the sudden onset of aphasia after a transient left-sided headache. Although articulate and able to follow requests and repeat phrases, he has difficulty in naming objects. For example, when a pen, pin, and penny are held up in succession, which is a frequently used test, he substitutes the name of one for the other and repeats the name of the preceding object; however, he can point to the "money," "sharp object," and "writing instrument" when these objects are placed in front of him. No abnormal physical signs are present.

Case 5

A 54-year-old man, over several months, has developed difficulty in thinking and the inability to remember the word he desires. Although his voice quivers, he is fully conversant and articulate. He is able to write the correct responses to questions; however, he has slow and poor penmanship. He is able to name six objects, follow double requests, and repeat complex phrases. On further testing, he has difficulty recalling six digits, three objects after 3 minutes, and both recent and past events. Judgment seems intact. The remainder of the neurologic examination is normal.

ANSWERS:

Case 1. He has complete loss of language function, *global aphasia,* accompanied by right hemiplegia and homonymous hemianopsia. The cause is probably an occlusion of the left internal carotid artery creating an infarction of the entire left hemisphere. However, the lesion's particular etiology is much less important than its location in determining the presence and variety of aphasia.

Case 2. Because he can manage only a few phrases or words in a telegraphic pattern, this man has nonfluent aphasia. Only about one-third of cases of aphasia can be neatly characterized; this man has a "textbook case." As with other textbook cases, his nonfluent aphasia is accompanied by right hemiparesis, in which the arm is more paretic than the leg. Nonfluent aphasia is usually caused by an occlusion of the left middle cerebral artery. An underlying infarction would encompass Broca's area and the adjacent cortical motor region but spare the cortical fibers for the leg, which are supplied by the anterior cerebral artery. However, as mentioned in the preceding case, trauma, tumors, and other injuries in this location would produce the same aphasia.

Case 3. The patient has fluent aphasia characterized by a normal quantity of speech interspersed with paraphasic errors but only subtle right-sided corticospinal tract abnormalities. She probably has a lesion in the left parietal or posterior temporal lobe. The headaches and papilledema, given her age and the course of the illness, suggest that it is a mass lesion, such as a glioblastoma multiforme, rather than a CVA.

Case 4. He has anomic aphasia, which is a variety of fluent aphasia in which language impairment is restricted to the improper identification of objects (i.e., a naming impairment). Its origin may be Alzheimer's disease but, in view of the history of mitral stenosis and headache, the origin was probably a small embolic CVA (see Chapter 11).

Case 5. The patient does not have aphasia. His difficulty with memory could be either an early dementia or psychogenic inattention. Further evaluations might include neuropsychologic studies and evaluation for dementia.

6–10. Match the lesions that are pictured schematically with those expected in cases 1–5.

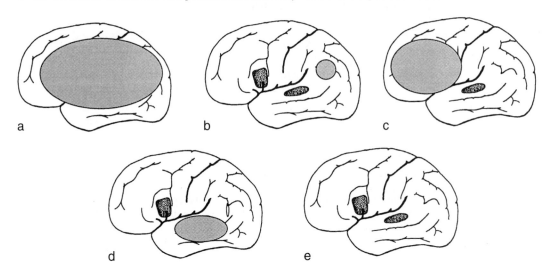

a   b   c

d   e

ANSWERS: Case 1, drawing a; *Case 2*, drawing c; *Case 3*, drawing d; *Case 4*, drawing b or d; *Case 5*, drawing e

11–26. Match the lesion with the expected associated finding(s).

11. Paresis of one recurrent laryngeal nerve

12. Pseudobulbar palsy

13. Bulbar palsy

14. Dominant hemisphere temporal lobe lesion

15. Lateral medullary syndrome

16. Laryngitis

17. Dominant hemisphere angular gyrus lesion

18. Dominant hemisphere parietal lobe lesion

19. Nondominant hemisphere parietal lobe lesion

20. Bilateral frontal lobe tumor

21. Bilateral anterior cerebral artery infarction

22. Streptomycin toxicity

23. Alcohol intoxication

24. Periaqueductal hemorrhagic necrosis (Wernicke's encephalopathy)

25. Phenytoin (Dilantin) toxicity

26. Infarction of left posterior cerebral artery

a. Dysarthria, including hoarseness
b. Dysphagia
c. Dementia
d. Dyscalculia
e. Fluent aphasia
f. Constructional apraxia
g. Dyslexia
h. Deafness
i. Mutism
j. Left-right disorientation

k. Finger agnosia
l. Hyperactive reflexes
m. Sixth cranial nerve palsy
n. Alexia
o. Ataxia
p. Dressing apraxia
q. Anosognosia
r. Hemi-inattention
s. Left limb apraxia

ANSWERS: 11-a; 12-a, b, l; 13-a, b; 14-e; 15-a, b, o; 16-a; 17-d, j, k (Gerstmann's syndrome); 18-d, e, g, j, k; 19-f, p, q, r; 20-c, possibly also a, b, and i; 21-s and possibly c and i; 22-h, o; 23-a, d, o; 24-c, m, o; 25-o; 26-n

27. A 34-year-old man was revived after attempting suicide by sitting in a garaged car with the motor running. During the next week he only sat in bed and looked out of the window. He displayed no emotion and did not respond to requests. Although he was otherwise virtually mute, he seemed to repeat in intricate detail whatever he was asked and occasionally whatever was said on television. His deep tendon reflexes were brisk, and he had bilateral palmomental reflexes. His plantar reflexes were equivocal.

The examiner was uncertain whether the patient had depression, dementia, or other neuropsychologic abnormality. Please discuss the case and suggest further evaluation.

> **ANSWER:** The patient was probably exposed to excessive carbon monoxide. As in cases of cardiac arrest and strangulation where patients survive, any form of cerebral anoxia creates cerebral cortex damage. When patients permanently lose all intellectual and voluntary motor function, they are said to be in the *persistent vegetative state* (see Chapter 11).
>
> In this case, the cerebral damage was incomplete. It probably isolated the perisylvian language arc of the cerebral cortex comprising Wernicke's area, the arcuate fasciculus, and Broca's area. Isolation of this crucial region from the rest of the cerebral cortex causes *transcortical* or *isolation aphasia* that permits repetition of words and phrases, no matter how complex, but because language information cannot connect with the rest of the brain's language system, patients cannot name objects or follow requests. Because a large portion of the cerebral cortex is damaged, patients usually also have dementia, paresis, and frontal release signs.
>
> In cases where cerebral cortex damage is superimposed on depressive illness or other psychologic aberrations, the clinical picture is unpredictable. In these patients, detailed testing of language function must be part of the mental status examination.

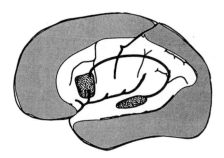

Fig. (above): In isolation aphasia, which is usually induced by hypoperfusion-induced hypoxia, the most vulnerable portions of the cerebral cortex are damaged, sparing the perisylvian language arc. Language processes may continue within this region, but they receive no input from other regions of the cerebral cortex.

28. A left-handed 64-year-old male schoolteacher sustained a cerebral thrombosis of the right middle cerebral artery. What might be predicted regarding language function?

a. He will certainly develop aphasia.
b. He will have left hemiparesis if he has aphasia.
c. If he develops aphasia, his prognosis is relatively good.
d. If he has aphasia, he will have a homonymous hemianopsia.

> **ANSWER:** c. Left-handed individuals who have normal intelligence are often still predominantly left-hemisphere dominant or they have mixed cerebral dominance. Moreover, language centers in the right hemisphere are not arranged consistently with respect to those on the left or to the motor and visual tracts within the hemisphere. If left-handed individuals suffer an infarction of the right cerebral hemisphere, they do not necessarily develop aphasia or the usual associated deficits. In fact, they may develop aphasia if they have an infarction in the left cerebral hemisphere. Left-handed individuals, compared to right-handed individuals, have a better prognosis for the resolution of aphasia.

29. If the patient in the previous question were discovered to have a resectable tumor in the right temporal lobe, how could language function of the right cerebral hemisphere be established before surgery?

a. An MRI could be performed.
b. A CT could show differences in the *planum temporale*.
c. Barbiturates infused into the carotid artery of the dominant hemisphere would cause aphasia.
d. A PET study would indicate cerebral dominance for language.

ANSWER: c. Infusion of barbiturates directly into the dominant carotid artery produces aphasia (the *Wada test*). This test can determine if a cerebral hemisphere is dominant before removal of cerebral neoplasms or an epilepsy scar focus. PET scans are difficult to perform because they require short-lived cyclotron-generated substrates. The scan shows relatively poor resolution of metabolic function. Although the *planum temporale* (the superior surface of the temporal lobe cortex) has a greater area in the dominant than nondominant temporal lobe, the difference is not always present. Even when present, the difference cannot be reliably visualized with a CT or MRI. Functional MRI (fMRI), which is noninvasive, may replace the Wada test in locating the language regions.

30. In which conditions are confabulations *not* found?

a. Anton's syndrome
b. Gerstmann's syndrome
c. Anosognosia
d. Wernicke-Korsakoff syndrome

ANSWER: b. Gerstmann's syndrome is a controversial entity that consists of the combination of right and left confusion, dyslexia, dyscalculia, and finger agnosia. It is usually attributed to lesions in the angular gyrus of the parietal lobe of the dominant hemisphere. In denial of blindness (Anton's syndrome), blind patients typically confabulate or fantasize about the appearance of objects presented to them. It occurs most often in elderly people who undergo ophthalmologic surgical procedures and cannot temporarily see out of either eye. Failure to acknowledge a left hemiparesis or similar deficit (anosognosia) is often accompanied by confabulation, denial, and other defense mechanisms. Although confabulations are described in the Wernicke-Korsakoff's syndrome, they are an uncommon symptom. When they do occur, the patients usually also have marked memory impairment.

31. Match the speech abnormality (dysarthria) (a–d) with the illness (1–4).

a. Hypophonia
b. Scanning speech
c. Nasal speech
d. Strained and strangled speech
1. Myasthenia gravis
2. Parkinsonism
3. Multiple sclerosis
4. Spasmodic dysphonia

ANSWERS: a-2, b-3, c-1, d-4

32. Which conditions *usually* cause aphasia?

a. Chronic subdural hematomas
b. Myasthenia gravis
c. Multiple sclerosis
d. Parkinsonism
e. None of the above

ANSWER: e. Subdural hematomas are located in the extra-axial space. Although chronic subdural hematomas typically cause headaches and dementia, they usually do not cause aphasia or other localized neurologic symptoms. Myasthenia gravis is a disorder of the neuromuscular junction and therefore does not cause dementia, aphasia, or other signs of a CNS dysfunction. Multiple sclerosis (MS) affects the cerebral white matter to a large extent only late in its course. Although MS may then cause dementia, it rarely causes aphasia. Parkinsonism may cause dysarthria (hypophonia and tremor) and, late in the illness, dementia; however, it rarely causes aphasia.

33. A 45-year-old airplane pilot reported that when she awoke earlier in the morning, for approximately 5 minutes she had "expressive aphasia," by which she meant that she was unable to speak or gesture, but she understood most of the news on the radio. During that time, she had no other symptoms. Which of the following conditions are reasonable explanations for her episode?

a. Seizure
b. TIA
c. Migraine
d. Sleep disorder

ANSWER: All. She might have had a partial seizure originating in the left frontal lobe. During a postictal period, she might have had aphasia and a right hemiparesis that prevented her from gesturing. A TIA in the distribution of the left carotid artery might also have caused aphasia with or without right hemiparesis. Hemiplegic migraines, which can cause speech impairment, can occasionally affect adults. An episode of "sleep paralysis," such as hypnopompic cataplexy, may cause brief quadriparesis and mutism. The etiologies of transient aphasia and transient hemiparesis are similar (see Hemiplegic Migraines, Chapter 9, and Carotid Artery TIAs, Chapter 11).

34. A 70-year-old man suddenly developed inability to read. Although he can write his name and most sentences that are dictated to him, he cannot read aloud or copy written material. His speech is fluent and contains no paraphasic errors. He can see objects only in his left visual field. What is this man's difficulty, and where is the responsible lesion(s)?

ANSWER: He clearly has alexia, as demonstrated by his inability to read, and also a right homonymous hemianopsia. He does not have agraphia because he can transcribe dictation and write words from memory. Nor does he have aphasia. Thus, he has the syndrome of alexia without agraphia. This syndrome is caused by a lesion in the left occipital lobe and posterior corpus callosum. The left occipital lesion would explain the failure of visual information to pass from the intact right visual cortex through the corpus callosum to the left (dominant) hemisphere for integration (see Fig. 8–4). Since memory and auditory circuits, as well as the corticospinal system, are intact, he can write words that he hears or remembers. Such lesions are usually caused by infarctions of the left posterior cerebral artery or by infiltrating brain tumors, such as a glioblastoma multiforme.

35. A 68-year-old man had a car accident because he drifted into oncoming traffic. He has a left homonymous hemianopsia and a mild left hemiparesis, which he fails to recognize. Which neuropsychologic problem describes his denying his left arm weakness?

a. Anosognosia   c. Anton's syndrome
b. Aphasia   d. Alexia

ANSWER: a. After having the accident because a left homonymous hemianopsia prevented him from seeing oncoming traffic, he fails to recognize his deficits, which is anosognosia. This perceptual distortion is a characteristic manifestation of a parietal lobe lesion.

36. Which one of the following statements concerning Heschl's gyrus is false?

a. Heschl's gyrus is bilateral and located adjacent to the planum temporale.
b. In almost all individuals, the left-sided Heschl's gyrus, like the left-sided planum temporale, has greater surface area than its right-sided counterpart.
c. Each Heschl's gyrus reflects auditory stimulation predominantly from the contralateral ear.
d. Heschl's gyrus appears to sort auditory stimuli for direction, pitch, loudness, and other acoustic properties rather than words for their linguistic properties.

ANSWER: b. The dominant hemisphere planum temporale, which is integral to language function, has greater surface area than its counterpart. Each hemisphere's Heschl's gyrus, which processes the auditory qualities of sound, is symmetric (see Figs. 4–15 and 8–1).

37. Patients with nondominant hemisphere lesions are reported to have loss of the normal inflections of speech and diminished associated facial and limb gestures. What are the technical terms used to describe these findings?

ANSWER: Aprosody and loss of paralinguistic components of speech

38. A man who has undergone a commissurotomy for intractable seizures is shown a written request to raise both arms. What will be his response when the request is shown in his left visual field? In the right visual field?

ANSWER: When the request is shown in his left visual field, he will not raise either arm because the written information does not reach the left hemisphere language centers. When the request is shown in his right visual field, the information reaches the language centers and he will raise his right hand; however, the command to move his left hand may not reach the right hemisphere's motor center (Fig. 8–8).

39–44. With which conditions are the various forms of apraxia (a–h) associated?

39. Gait

40. Constructional

41. Ideational

42. Limb

43. Buccofacial

44. Ideomotor

a. Aphasia
b. Hemi-inattention
c. Dementia
d. Dysarthria

e. Incontinence
f. Left homonymous hemianopsia
g. Right homonymous hemianopsia
h. Aprosody

ANSWERS: 39-c, e; 40-b, f, h; 41-c; 42-a, g; 43-a, d, g; 44-a, g

45. How does aphasia in left-handed people differ from aphasia in right-handed people?

a. Aphasia can result from lesions in either hemisphere.
b. The variety of aphasia is less clearly related to the site of cerebral injury.
c. The prognosis is better.
d. The etiologies are different.

ANSWER: a, b, c

46. Which of the following are disconnection syndromes?

a. Internuclear ophthalmoplegia
b. Conduction aphasia
c. Split brain syndrome

d. Isolation aphasia
e. Alexia without agraphia
f. Global aphasia

ANSWER: a, b, c, e. Disconnection syndromes usually refer to disorders in which connections between primary neuropsychologic centers are severed. Although not generally considered a disconnection syndrome, internuclear ophthalmoplegia has the same features: Centers or nuclei are normal, but interconnecting fasciculi are damaged. In contrast, isolation aphasia results from extensive cerebral cortex injury that preserves the language arc, and its elements remain connected. Global aphasia results from extensive destruction of the entire language arc.

47. Which artery supplies most of the perisylvian language arc?

a. Anterior cerebral artery
b. Middle cerebral artery

c. Posterior cerebral artery
d. Vertebrobasilar artery system

ANSWER: b

48. What is the term applied to the area of the cerebral cortex between branches of the major cerebral arteries?

a. Watershed area
b. Limbic system

c. Cornea
d. Arcuate fasciculus

ANSWER: a. "Watershed" originally referred to a geographic region or divide drained by a river or stream. To neurologists, the term refers to areas of the cerebral cortex that are perfused by the terminal branches of arteries. During hypotension or anoxia, the already tenuous blood supply falls to the insufficient level.

49. Which is/are true regarding sign language?

a. Sign language, like spoken language, is based in the dominant hemisphere.
b. Middle cerebral artery occlusions in deaf people typically causes aphasia in sign language.
c. Sign language relies on visual rather than auditory input.
d. American Sign Language (ASL) is the proper name for the common, gesture-based sign language.
e. All of the above.

ANSWER: e

50. In nonfluent aphasia, why is the arm typically more paretic than the leg?

a. The motor cortex for the arm is supplied by the middle cerebral artery, which is usually occluded. The motor cortex for the leg is supplied by the anterior cerebral artery, which is usually spared.
b. The arm has a larger cortical representation.
c. The infarct occurs in the internal capsule.
d. The motor cortex for the arm is supplied by the anterior cerebral artery, which is usually occluded. The motor cortex for the leg is supplied by the middle cerebral artery, which is usually spared.

ANSWER: a

51. After a right parietal infarction, patients may develop an alien hand syndrome. Which two of the following characteristics describe this phenomenon?

a. Persistent pain in an amputated hand
b. The misperception that a paralyzed hand is normal
c. Attraction to another person's hand
d. A perception that the paralyzed hand is not the patient's
e. A perception that the paralyzed hand acts independently or under another person's control

ANSWER: d, e. The perception of one's hand seems to be particularly vulnerable.

52. Which variety of apraxia is most closely associated with normal pressure hydrocephalus?

a. Ideational
b. Dressing
c. Ideomotor
d. Buccofacial
e. Oral
f. Gait

ANSWER: f. Gait apraxia, incontinence, and dementia are the primary manifestations of normal pressure hydrocephalus. Gait apraxia is usually the first and most prominent symptom. It is also the first symptom to resolve following successful treatment.

53. In which disorders is echolalia a symptom?

a. Autism
b. Isolation aphasia
c. Dementia
d. Tourette's syndrome
e. All of the above

ANSWER: e. Echolalia, an involuntary repetition of visitors' or examiners' words, is a manifestation of diverse neurologic conditions.

54. Which two disconnection syndromes stem from corpus callosum damage?

a. Alexia without agraphia
b. Internuclear ophthalmoplegia (INO)
c. Conduction aphasia
d. Split brain syndrome

ANSWER: a, d. All the conditions are disconnection syndromes. Conduction aphasia results from an intrahemispheric disconnection, and INO results from a disconnection in the brainstem's medial longitudinal fasciculus.

55. Which conclusion has stemmed from studies of patients who have undergone a commissurotomy?

a. The corpus callosum is vital to the auditory system.
b. Patients with the split brain have gross, readily identifiable physical and cognitive abnormalities.
c. Emotions generated in the right hemisphere are not as readily described as those generated in the left hemisphere.
d. Emotions generated in the left hemisphere are not as readily described as those in the right hemisphere.

ANSWER: c

56. A 60-year-old man who has undergone a commissurotomy has his hands placed in a closed box containing many objects. A set of keys is placed in his left hand. By voice and gesture, he is asked to identify them. Which would be his most accurate response?

a. He would say, "A set of keys."
b. With his right hand, he would write, "A set of keys."
c. Although unable to say, "A set of keys," he would be able to pick another set of keys from the various objects.
d. He would be unable to comply with the request under any circumstance.

> **ANSWER:** c. The commissurotomy isolates the language center from his right hemisphere, but he is still capable of comprehending the request, especially if it is gestured.

57. A 74-year-old woman is seen in psychiatric consultation because of her complaints of intruders in her nursing home room despite several checks having found no evidence of any intruders. She had been placed in the nursing home following partial recovery from a left parietal stroke. Its residual deficits were a mild left hemiparesis and hemisensory impairment but no dementia.

The psychiatrist found that she has a tenuous relationship to her hand, which moves freely and explores the adjacent clothing, without her knowledge. She does not deny that she had a stroke but denies that the hand is hers. "I am not moving it. Who is?" she finally asked. Which is the most likely explanation for her perception?

a. Delusions or hallucinations associated with a nondominant hemisphere infarction
b. The alien hand syndrome
c. Anosognosia
d. Dementia

> **ANSWER:** b. She has the alien hand syndrome because of a nondominant stroke. She proposes the only plausible explanation: The independently moving hand, which she does not fully feel or control, belongs to someone else, such as an intruder.

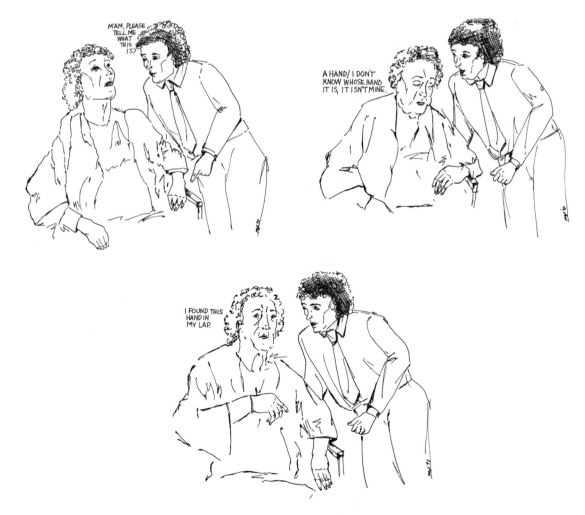

9

Headaches

More than 90% of Americans have at least one headache each year. Most are beset with *tension type, migraine,* or *cluster headaches.* Such attacks *(Chronic Recurring Headaches*)* may be severely painful and incapacitating but are not life-threatening. These headaches are diagnosed not by physical or laboratory tests, which are characteristically normal, but by their distinctive symptoms.

Acutely occurring or steadily progressive headaches, in contrast, often signal life-threatening disease. Included among them are *temporal arteritis, intracranial mass lesions, pseudotumor cerebri, meningitis,* and *subarachnoid hemorrhage (Headaches Secondary to Organic Disease).* With less specific symptoms, their diagnosis rests on abnormal physical findings or laboratory test results. (*Postconcussion* headaches, which could be considered in this group, are discussed in Chapter 22, Head Trauma.)

CHRONIC RECURRING HEADACHE

Tension-Type Headache

These are the almost universal headaches, characterized by intermittent, frontal, cervical, or generalized dull pain. They plague women more than men and affect multiple family members. Symptoms are almost exclusively pain with little or no photophobia, hyperacusis, or phonophobia (sensitivity to noise); autonomic disturbances, such as nausea, but never vomiting; or prostration. Patients with tension-type headaches complain, but they usually go about their business.

These headaches have traditionally been attributed to contraction of the scalp, neck, and face muscles (Fig. 9–1) and emotional "tension." Physical factors, such as fatigue, cervical spondylosis, bright light, loud noise, and, at some level, emotional factors were said to produce or precipitate them.

Nevertheless, because some scientific studies have demonstrated that these headaches are due to neither muscle contractions nor psychologic tension, the designation "muscle contraction" or "tension" headache probably represents a misnomer. At the very least, the term "tension-type" headache is more appropriate. In fact, some current concepts place these headaches at the opposite end from migraine on a headache spectrum, where both result from a common, underlying, but unknown, physiologic disorder.

Treatment. Neurologists generally assure patients that their headaches do not represent a brain tumor or other potentially fatal illness, which are frequently un-

---

*The classification, within parentheses in the introduction, is taken from the International Headache Society (see references). Although accepted in academic neurologic circles, the terminology is often descriptive, arbitrary, and, in some areas, controversial. In particular, the term "Headaches Secondary to Organic Disease" implies that migraines and other headaches are not the result of physiologic disease.

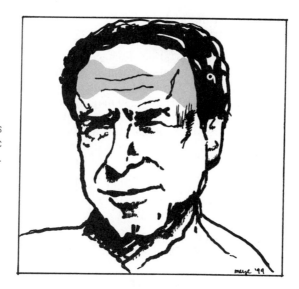

FIGURE 9–1. Tension-type headaches produce a bandlike, squeezing, symmetric pressure at the neck, temples, or forehead.

spoken fears. On prescribing medications (Table 9–1), they commonly also refer patients to formal or informal counseling about emotional factors, general health, diet, and exercise.

For headaches that occur less than twice a week, neurologists usually prescribe "abortive therapy"—medicine taken only at onset. Most often, they prescribe simple analgesics, such as aspirin, aspirin-caffeine compounds, acetaminophen, or, especially for menses-related headaches, nonsteroidal anti-inflammatory drugs (NSAIDs). These medicines should be kept in the car, at work, and in pocketbooks to be taken at the first inkling of a headache to prevent its full development. However, physicians should be mindful that daily use of such readily accessible analgesics may lead to daily, rebound or withdrawal headaches (see below).

Preventive (prophylactic) therapy—medicine taken daily—is recommended if severe headaches occur more frequently than once weekly, abortive therapy is ineffective, or medication consumption is excessive. Neurologists usually avoid prescribing benzodiazepines, except for limited periods. Instead, they often recommend NSAIDs or, even if patients have no history of depression, antidepressants in small nighttime doses.

Biofeedback, relaxation, physical therapy, and stress reduction may be helpful. Insight-oriented psychotherapy and psychoanalysis directed toward headaches do not reduce the headaches but might provide insight, reduce anxiety, treat depression, and offer other benefits.

Migraines

The characteristic feature distinguishing migraines from other chronic recurrent headaches is that sensory, psychologic, and autonomic symptoms accompany the headaches and may actually precede, overshadow, or even replace them. Two major migraine varieties—defined primarily by presence or absence of an *aura*—and several variations can be discerned by their different symptoms (Table 9–2). Although migraine symptoms are complex and variable, they are usually constant for the individual patient.

Classic Migraine (Migraine with Aura)

In the *classic variety* of migraine, which affects only about 15% of migraine patients, a headache is preceded by an aura that can be almost any symptom of brain

TABLE 9–1. *Headache Medications* *

Analgesics

Aspirin	Aspirin (one 5-g tablet = 325 mg)
Bufferin	Aspirin (325 mg), aluminum glycinate, magnesium carbonate
Esgic	Butalbital, acetaminophen, caffeine (40 mg)
Excedrin	Aspirin (250 mg), acetaminophen, caffeine (65 mg)
Fioricet	Butalbital, acetaminophen, caffeine (40 mg)
Fiorinal	Butalbital, caffeine (40 mg), aspirin (325 mg)
Midrin	Isometheptene, dichloralphenazone, acetaminophen

β-Blockers[†]
Propranolol[‡]

Calcium Channel Blockers[†]

Calan	Verapamil[‡]

Antiepileptic Drugs

Depakote	Divalproex

Anti-Inflammatory Agents[†]
Nonsteroidal Anti-Inflammatory Drugs (NSAIDs)
Ibuprofen[‡]
Naproxen[‡]

Steroids
Prednisone
Dexamethasone

Serotonin-Active Medications

Ergots

Cafergot	Ergotamine, caffeine (100 mg)
DHE	Dihydroergotamine
Sansert[†]	Methysergide
Wigraine	Ergotamine, caffeine (100 mg)

"Triptans"[‡]

Naratriptan	Amerge
Rizatriptan	Maxalt
Sumatriptan	Imitrex
Zomig	Zolmitriptan

Tricyclic Antidepressants
Amitriptyline[†]

Miscellaneous
Lithium[†]

*Consult package insert for indications, dosage, contraindications, precautions, and side effects. Several are widely prescribed for headaches without FDA indication.

[†]Prophylactic therapy of migraines. The other medications are generally used as abortive treatment. However, the NSAIDs, including aspirin, may be used as either prophylactic or abortive treatment.

[‡]Example(s).

dysfunction. The subsequent headache is similar to migraines without an aura (see below).

Auras usually evolve gradually over 4 to 10 minutes, persist for less than 1 hour, and evaporate before the headache's onset, although they often linger through and beyond the headache. Typically visual phenomena, they can consist of any particular transient alteration in sensory and language function; sensory distortions, misperceptions, and complex hallucinations; or overwhelming, unprovoked personality changes (Table 9–3).

TABLE 9–2. *Diagnostic Criteria for Migraines With and Without Aura**

Migraines Without Aura: At least five headaches that have the following:
1. Duration of 4 to 72 hours, if untreated
2. Have at least two of the following symptoms:
   a. Unilateral location
   b. Pulsating pain
   c. Moderate or severe pain, which disrupts daily activities
   d. Aggravation of the headache by routine physical activities
3. The headache is accompanied by at least one of the following symptoms:
   a. Nausea or vomiting
   b. Photophobia or phonophobia
4. There is no alternative cause of the headache

Migraines With Aura: At least two headaches that have the following:
1. At least three of the following symptoms:
   a. At least one aura referable to cortex or brainstem dysfunction
   b. At least one aura evolves over more than 4 minutes
   c. The aura lasts less than 1 hour
   d. A headache begins before, during, or within 1 hour of the aura
2. There is no alternative cause of the headache

*Adapted from Olesen J (ed): Classification and diagnostic criteria for headache disorders, cranial neuralgias and facial pain. Cephalalgia 8 (Suppl 7): 13–96, 1988

When auras are not followed by a headache, which often happens, they may consist of recurrent, free-standing hallucinations. In either instance, auras are important because they are a distinctive neurologic symptom, can mimic other neurologic disorders (transient ischemic attacks [TIAs], drug ingestion, and partial complex or occipital seizures), and are an "organic cause" of altered perception, mood, and behavior.

The most common migraine auras, which are visual hallucinations (see Chapter 12), can consist of a graying of a region of the visual field *(scotoma)* (Fig. 9–2, A), flashing zigzag lines *(scintillating fortification scotomata)* (Fig. 9–2, B), crescents of brilliant colors (Fig. 9–2, C), tubular vision, or distortion of objects *(metamorphopsia)*. Patients each have a consistently appearing individual, particular aura: they do not switch between scintillating scotoma and metamorphopsia in successive migraines. Olfactory hallucinations can represent a migraine aura; however, they are more likely a manifestation of a partial complex seizure. In children, recurrent colicky or "cyclic abdominal pain" with nausea and vomiting can constitute auras.

TABLE 9–3. *Varieties of Migraine Aura*

Sensory phenomena
  Special senses
    Visual, olfactory, auditory, gustatory
  Paresthesias, especially lips and hand
Motor deficits
  Hemiparesis, hemiplegia
  Ophthalmoplegia
Neuropsychologic changes
  Aphasia
  Perceptual impairment, especially for size, shapes, and time
Emotional and behavioral
  Anxiety, depression, irritability, (rarely) hyperactivity

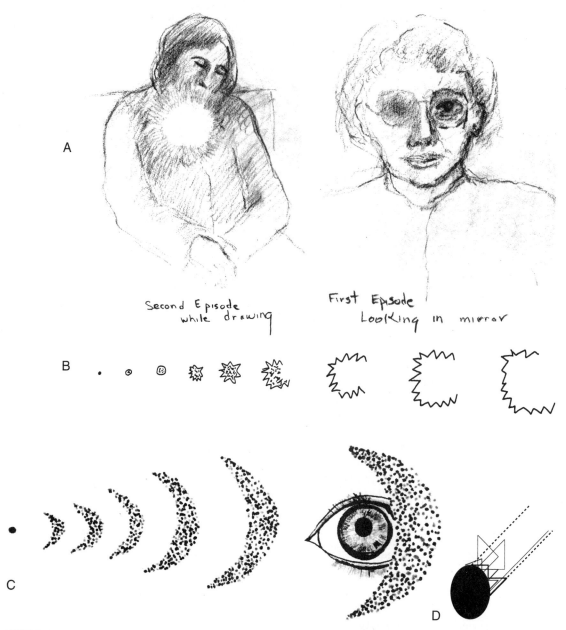

FIGURE 9–2. **A,** These drawings by a migraine patient show the typical visual obscurations of a *scotoma* that precedes her migraine headache. In both cases, a small circular area near the center of vision is lost entirely or reduced in clarity. Even though the aura is gray and has a relatively simple shape, she is captivated by it. Surprisingly, in view of the impending headache, such visual hallucinations mesmerize patients. **B,** The patient who drew this aura, a *scintillating scotoma,* wrote, "In the early stages, the area within the lights is somewhat shaded. Later, as the figure widens, you can sort of peer right through the area. Eventually, it gets so wide that it disappears." The scotoma is typical. It consists of an angular, brightly lit margin and an opaque interior that begins as a star and expands into a crescent. It scintillates at 8 to 12 Hz. Angular auras are sometimes called *fortification scotomas* because of their similarity to military fortresses. **C,** A 30-year-old woman artist in her first trimester of pregnancy had several classic migraine headaches that were heralded by this scotoma. It began as a blue dot and, over 20 minutes, enlarged to a crescent of brightly shimmering, multicolored dots. When the crescent's intensity was at its peak, she was so dazzled that she lost her ability to see and think clearly. **D,** Having patients draw visual hallucinations has great diagnostic value. One patient, who had no artistic talent, reconstructed this "visual hallucination" using a computer drawing program. Children might provide similar valuable diagnostic information if they are asked to draw what they "see" before a headache.

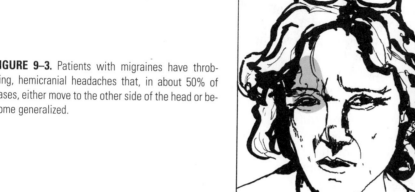

FIGURE 9–3. Patients with migraines have throbbing, hemicranial headaches that, in about 50% of cases, either move to the other side of the head or become generalized.

Common Migraine (Migraine without Aura)

The *common variety*, which affects about 75% of migraine patients, has no aura. The headache, which typically lasts 4 to 24 hours, is initially throbbing or pulsating, hemicranial (felt on one side of the head), and predominantly temporal, retro-orbital (located behind the eye), or periorbital (around the eye). In about 50% of patients, the headache moves to the opposite side or becomes generalized (Fig. 9–3). When migraines occur frequently, pain evolves into dull, symmetric, and continual headache that mimics a tension-type headache.

Accompanying nonheadache symptoms are characteristic: sensory hypersensitivity, autonomic dysfunction, and disability. In common terms, people want to go to bed; they are nauseated if not vomiting; and they seek dark, quiet places.

In conjunction with seclusive behavior, patients often have episodic mood changes that can mimic depression, partial complex seizures, and other neurologic disturbances (Table 9–4). Although some patients with migraines may become feverishly active and work excessively, most become despondent, feel dysphoric, and try to escape from other people, light, smells, and noise. If unable to find solitude, they may become distraught. Partly because of autonomic dysfunction, they tend to drink large quantities of water and crave food or sweets, particularly chocolate. Some chil-

TABLE 9–4. *Common Neurologic Causes of Transient or Recurrent Altered Mental Status*

Drugs
  Illicit
  Medicinal
Metabolic aberrations, e.g., hypoglycemia
Migraines
Seizures (see Chapter 10)
  Absence
  Partial complex
  Frontal lobe
Sleep attacks, e.g., narcolepsy, sleep apnea naps (see Chapter 17)
Transient global amnesia (see Chapter 11)
Transient ischemic attacks (TIAs; see Chapter 11)

dren become confused and overactive. After a migraine clears, especially when it ends with sleep, people sometimes sense a remarkable tranquillity or even euphoria.

As with tension-type headaches, both classic and common migraines occur more frequently in women than in men and tend to affect more than one family member. In contrast to tension-type headaches, migraines begin in the early morning rather than the afternoon. In women, they tend to start at menarche, recur premenstrually, and be aggravated by some oral contraceptives. During pregnancy, about three-quarters of women with migraines experience a dramatic relief; however, the remainder either have no improvement or an exacerbation. Some women develop their very first migraine during the first trimester. In men and women, migraines tend to arise during REM sleep (see Chapter 17), sometimes exclusively *(nocturnal migraines)*.

Another important characteristic of migraines is that they can be precipitated—especially in susceptible individuals—by certain factors or "triggers," such as skipping meals or fasting on religious holidays, too little or excessive sleep, menses, psychologic or occupational stress, overexertion, head trauma, and alcoholic drinks. (Alcoholic drinks can also provoke cluster headaches [see below].) According to common belief, red wine and brandy are the alcoholic drinks most likely to trigger migraines, and vodka and white wine the least likely. Alternatively, cheap wine may be more likely than fine wine to cause headaches. In any case, alcoholic drinks tend to ameliorate tension-type headaches.

To the chagrin of migraine patients, weekends and the start of a vacation appear to precipitate migraines. Too many factors come into play to assign sole responsibility. The *relief* of obvious work-related stress, a "letdown," may provoke a migraine. Alternatively, leisure periods carry their own psychologic stresses. Also, too little sleep or sleeping later than usual into the morning—especially if a customary cup of coffee is skipped (see below)—can precipitate a migraine. Weekend or vacation eating, which typically may include alcoholic drinks and foods spiced with monosodium glutamate (MSG), often lead to migraines.

Psychiatric Comorbidity

Contrary to old, elitist views, migraines are not especially prevalent among people in upper-income brackets or among those who are rigid, perfectionist, and competitive. The familiar "migraine personality" is now an outmoded concept.

However, certain personality traits or psychiatric disturbances do co-exist with migraines at a greater than expected frequency. A statistically significant association, *comorbidity,* may indicate that one disorder causes the other (causal relationship) or merely that both have the same cause (shared etiology).

Neuroticism in females is comorbid with migraines. It frequently precedes development but does not correlate with frequency or severity. The comorbidity, which persists even after controlling for major depression and anxiety, makes neuroticism a risk factor for migraines.

Migraines are also comorbid with major depression, anxiety, panic attacks, and, less so, bipolar disorder. When depression is comorbid with migraines, timing and perhaps other aspects are bidirectional: migraines can develop before or after depression. In addition, comorbid depression places the migraine patient at risk for attempting suicide.

Comorbidity can obscure some issues. Depression, for example, can be overlooked because common symptoms, such as mood disturbances, can be attributed to migraine. Subtly extracting psychiatric diagnoses from the complex clinical picture of migraines aids treatment of each condition. Also, some medications will help both conditions, but others may be inadvisable.

The most common therapy for patients with migraine and comorbid depression should include simple behavioral advice, such as getting sufficient sleep on a regular schedule, exercising moderately, and avoiding alcohol and drugs. As with tension-type headaches, neither insight-oriented psychotherapy nor psychoanalysis has been shown in adequately controlled studies to reduce migraines (although they may facilitate treatment). Cognitive-behavioral therapy, as an adjunct to medication, may be effective.

For patients with migraine and comorbid major depression, effective treatment requires medications. Tricyclic antidepressants are effective for both conditions. In contrast, selective serotonin reuptake inhibitors (SSRIs) seem generally less effective than tricyclic antidepressants in treating migraines with or without depression. Moreover, when used concurrently with serotonin agonists, such as sumatriptan (Imitrex) and dihydroergotamine (DHE), SSRIs carry the risk of producing the serotonin syndrome (see Chapters 6 and 21). When migraines are comorbid with bipolar disorder, divalproex (Depakote) may be effective for both conditions. Of course, propranolol (Inderal) and other β-adrenergic blockers used in prophylactic treatment for migraines should be avoided in migraine patients with depression because they may cause depression.

Recognizing the neurologic basis of migraines, the *Diagnostic and Statistical Manual of Mental Disorders-IV (DSM-IV)* would include headaches on Axis III. Psychiatric disorders comorbid with migraines, such as depression and anxiety, remain on Axis I, that is, migraines with comorbid depression would not be considered a single condition but two separate disorders. Alternatively, if psychologic factors were judged to play an important role in individuals' migraines, their illness could rise to the level of a *Pain Disorder Associated with Both Psychologic Factors and a General Medical Condition.* In the rare situation where patients fabricate reports of severe, intractable migraines to sustain a narcotic addiction, the diagnosis would be *Malingering.*

Migraine Varieties.   *Childhood migraines* are not simply the same illness in "short adults." The headache component of childhood migraine is less likely to be unilateral (only one-third of cases) and is briefer (frequently less than 2 hours) but—according to patients' descriptions—more severe. More important, associated, non-headache components, such as nausea, are more prominent. Migraine typically makes children confused, incoherent, or distraught or may produce a cyclic pattern of incapacitating nausea and vomiting. Children also are more susceptible to migraine variants, such as basilar artery, ophthalmoplegic, and hemiplegic migraines.

In *basilar migraines,* headaches are accompanied or even overshadowed by symptoms—ataxia, vertigo, dysarthria, and diplopia—that reflect dysfunction in the basilar artery distribution: the cerebellum, brainstem, and posterior cerebrum (see Fig. 11–2). Thus, when basilar migraines impair the posterior cerebrum, which contains the temporal lobes, patients may have memory impairment (e.g., transient global amnesia [see Chapter 11]).

Hemiplegic migraines are characterized by combinations of various grades of hemiparesis, hemiparesthesia, and aphasia preceding or accompanying otherwise typical migraines. The hemiparesis may occasionally develop without an associated headache. In *familial hemiplegic migraine,* patients develop transient hemiparesis, which often represents the aura, preceding or following the headache. This rare variety's main feature is its genetic basis. Transmission in almost all cases is in an autosomal dominant pattern on chromosome 19. As a *complication of migraine,* hemiplegic migraine deficits become permanent, that is, migraines are a risk factor for stroke.

Most important, in evaluating a patient who has had transient or prolonged hemiparesis, the physician must consider hemiplegic migraines along with transient ischemic attacks (TIAs), a stroke, postictal (Todd's) hemiparesis, and conversion disorder.

Migraine-Like Conditions: Food-Induced Headaches.   Certain foods and medications can cause nonspecific headaches. In susceptible individuals, they can trigger a migraine. However, other than alcohol, the role of foods and chocolate is overemphasized: food precipitates migraines in only about 15% to 20% of patients.

The clearest examples of headaches precipitated by foods are the *Chinese restaurant syndrome*, where the offending agent is MSG, and the *hot dog headache*, where the offending agent is the nitrite in processed meats. Another example is the *ice cream headache*, which is triggered by any very cold food that overstimulates the pharynx. Some people, but fewer than generally assumed, develop migraine-like headaches after eating tyramine-containing foods, such as ripened cheese, or phenylethylamine-containing foods, notably chocolate.

In the opposite situation, people deprived of regular, daily caffeine intake—coffee, for example—develop a *caffeine-withdrawal syndrome* that consists of moderate to severe headache accompanied often by anxiety, depression, and lethargy. Although this syndrome is almost synonymous with coffee deprivation, it can be precipitated by withdrawal of other caffeine-containing beverages or medications (Table 9–1 and Chapter 17). Caffeine-withdrawal headaches pose a dilemma for heavy coffee drinkers. Excessive coffee leads to irritability, palpitations, and gastric burning, but foregoing it results in headaches, anxiety, and other symptoms.

Medication-Induced Headaches.   Antianginal medicines, such as nitroglycerin or isosorbide (Isordil), probably because they contain nitrites or dilate cerebral as well as cardiac arteries, cause headaches. Elderly patients who have cerebrovascular atherosclerosis are particularly vulnerable. Curiously, whereas some calcium channel blockers, such as nifedipine (Procardia), trigger headaches, others, such as verapamil (Calan), may prevent them. For the psychiatrist, the most notorious iatrogenic headache, which is often complicated by cerebral hemorrhage, is produced by the interaction of monoamine oxidase inhibitor (MAOI) antidepressants with other medications or foods (see below).

Sex-Related Headaches.   Sexual activity, whether intercourse or masturbation, with or without orgasm, may trigger a migraine-like *headache associated with sexual activity*, which was previously termed *coital cephalgia* or *orgasmic headache*. Sex-related headaches, which are especially common in individuals with migraines, typically last for several minutes to several hours. Pain may be severe and incapacitating, but the neurologic problem is almost always benign. Nevertheless, before dismissing severe headaches occurring during sexual activity or any vigorous activity, physicians might consider intracerebral or subarachnoid hemorrhage (see below). When the diagnosis of sex-related headaches has been assured, taking propranolol or indomethacin before sex can usually prevent the ensuing headache.

Proposed Causes of Migraines.   A long-standing but possibly outdated theory is that constriction of cerebral arteries in the carotid system (see Fig. 11–1) causes the migraine aura. When constriction fatigues and changes to dilation, unsuppressed pulsations pound the arteries and produce the headache. An alternative hypothesis suggests that the aura is caused by "neuronal depression" (impaired metabolism of cerebral neurons that spreads in an orderly fashion over the cerebral cortex). Decreased cerebral metabolic requirements, rather than vasoconstriction, reduce cerebral blood flow.

An important aspect of these theories is that the trigeminal nerve, which supplies the meninges and large blood vessels in the head, releases neuropeptides and other neurotransmitters, such as substance P and neurokinin A. These neurotransmitters incite painful vasodilation and perivascular inflammation.

Other theories postulate faulty serotonin (5-hydroxytryptamine [5-HT]) neurotransmission. Although no single serotonin mechanism has been proven, several observations are important. Most serotonin-producing neurons are in the brainstem's dorsal raphe nuclei. During a migraine, platelet serotonin concentration falls, but urinary serotonin and its metabolite (5-HIAA) concentrations increase. Reserpine, which depletes serotonin, induces migraines. Sumatriptan and the other "triptans" (Table 9–1) act primarily as agonists to serotonin receptors (5-HT$_{1D}$) in the trigeminal nerve endings in the cerebral vessels. On the other hand, methysergide (Sansert), which is a prophylactic medication, is essentially a serotonin receptor (5-HT$_2$) antagonist.

Whatever the biochemical mechanism, undoubtedly genetic predisposition to migraines exists. The genetic basis of hemiplegic migraine is well established. Overall, about 70% of migraine patients have a close relative with migraines, and studies of twins found a high concordance. Risk of migraines is 50% or greater in relatives of a patient than those of controls, and risk to relatives increases with severity of migraines in the patient.

Treatment: Abortive Therapy. In attempting to identify migraine triggers, neurologists usually suggest that patients create a "headache diary" to record headache days, medications, diet, menses, school examinations, and other potential precipitants. If triggers cannot be avoided, at least they can be anticipated. Patients are generally advised to obtain regular and sufficient sleep, follow a steady exercise routine, and adhere to other common approaches to good health. For some individuals, biofeedback or relaxation techniques are helpful, but usually only when used in conjunction with medications.

For almost all patients, successful treatment of migraines requires medications. As with tension-type headache, medications are given primarily to abort or prevent migraines. For abortive treatment of occasional, mild to moderate migraines, simple analgesics and NSAIDs may be sufficient and produce minimal side effects (Table 9–1). If those medications do not relieve migraines in progress, neurologists usually prescribe more potent drugs that might be administered by injection, nasal spray, or sublingual wafer.

The triptans and dihydroergotamine are abortive for moderate to severe attacks. Although they affect different receptors, they both produce vasoconstriction. Injections, sublingual wafers, and nasal sprays deliver effective treatment fastest, but, whichever administration route is used, medications should be given as soon as the headache has begun. However, for menstruation-related migraine, taking a triptan for several days before menses may prevent the headache and other symptoms.

Potent abortive migraine medications have worrisome side effects. Excessive ergotamine use can lead to a chronic daily headache or *ergotism* (spasm of coronary or limb arteries that might be severe enough to cause angina or gangrene). Sumatriptan can also precipitate myocardial infarctions in patients with coronary artery disease. Also, because MAO metabolizes them, these medicines should not be given to patients receiving MAOIs. Similarly, administering a SSRI concurrently with these serotonin agonists might lead to the serotonin or neuroleptic malignant syndrome, as well as hypertension.

Sometimes nausea and vomiting are migraine's main symptoms. Even when minor, they preclude orally administered medications. They may also represent a side effect of DHE or other abortive medication. Rectal or intravenous antiemetics are extraordinarily helpful in this situation and are administered as the sole medication in some patients or, more commonly, concurrently with migraine medications. One caveat is that dopamine-blocking antiemetics may cause acute dystonic reactions identical to those caused by antipsychotics (see Chapter 18).

Treatment: Prophylactic Therapy. Prophylactic therapy is indicated if headaches occur more than four times a month, cause 3 to 4 days of disability per month, or abortive medicines are ineffective or are taken excessively. β-blockers are widely used for migraine prophylaxis, as well as for treatment of angina, hypertension, and essential tremor (see Chapter 18).

Tricyclic antidepressants, particularly amitriptyline, act effectively in migraine prophylaxis to reduce severity, frequency, and duration of migraines. Apart from any elevation of mood, antidepressants may be useful because they decrease or alter REM sleep, during which some migraine headaches develop, and are analgesic (see Chapter 14). As mentioned previously, when depression is comorbid with either migraine or tension-type headache, tricyclics may alleviate both conditions. SSRIs are no better than tricyclic antidepressants in preventing migraines. Also, in view of the possibility of their leading to a serotonin syndrome, administering serotonin agonists as abortive medications to someone taking an SSRI must be done cautiously.

Calcium channel blockers, such as verapamil (Calan), are also widely used and effective in migraine prophylaxis. Although their benefit cannot be reliably predicted, they have a relatively low incidence of side effects.

Methysergide (Sansert), a congener of LSD that blocks certain serotonin receptors ($5\text{-}HT_2$), is an effective prophylactic medicine but may induce mood changes. Most worrisome, if methysergide is taken for longer than 6 months, it may cause retroperitoneal, pleural, and endocardial fibrosis.

Antiepileptic medications have long been used for trigeminal neuralgia, other painful conditions (see Chapter 14), and affective disorders, as well as for epilepsy. Divalproex (Depakote), a well-established antiepileptic medication, is an effective prophylactic medication for migraines in individuals with or without affective disorders. It may act by reducing 5-HT neurons firing in the dorsal raphe nucleus or by altering trigeminal $GABA_A$ receptors in the meningeal blood vessels. In addition to providing prophylaxis, divalproex is indicated when epilepsy or bipolar disorder is comorbid with migraines.

Other Strategies.   Whether tension-type headaches and migraines are actually separate illnesses or not, physicians should estimate what portion of their patients' headaches are migraines. If the headaches are at some time unilateral, throbbing, accompanied by nausea, precipitated by menses, or preceded by the other known migraine triggers, a working diagnosis of migraine is appropriate. Physicians should institute migraine treatment without requiring patients to have the full array of symptoms.

Patients with chronic daily headache (see below) who have been overmedicated might be considered to have drug addiction. The offending medications will determine the rapidity of a withdrawal and the need for alternate analgesics, vasoconstrictors, NSAIDs, or antidepressants.

Under certain circumstances, headache patients should be hospitalized. Patients with migraines lasting for more than 3 days *(status migrainosus)*, prostration, or nausea and vomiting that has led to dehydration would benefit from hospitalization for parenteral medication, intravenous fluids, antiemetics, and a quiet, dark refuge. In addition, abuse of over-the-counter medications as well as narcotics may require hospitalization for withdrawal. Patients with ergotism often require hospitalization.

Chronic Daily Headaches

Many people who have had migraines and medication overuse experience "chronic daily headaches" (CDH). These headaches have most of the characteristics of tension-type headaches and often carry an overtone of depression. Only a minority has any further defining characteristic, such as a throbbing sensation, nausea, or hypersensitivity to light or sound. Underlying organic disease and head trauma precludes diagnosis of CHD.

One of the most common etiologies of CHD is migraine that, over many years, has increased in frequency, decreased in severity, and lost the impact of associated features. In this situation, *transformed migraine*, patients have daily headache with superimposed episodes of migraine without aura. In a related situation, CDH may result from a combination of migraine and tension-type headaches that blend, vary, and recur (Table 9–5). Although usually portrayed as separate entities, migraine and tension-type headaches may represent different manifestations of an underlying disorder.

Many other cases of CDH are ironically attributable to daily or near daily use of antimigraine medications, particularly aspirin-butalbital-caffeine compounds (e.g., Fiorinal), benzodiazepines, ergotamine, and narcotics. Although almost any anti-headache medication might cause CDH, the least likely are the NSAIDs. CDH probably results from medication dependency, withdrawal, or *rebound* from either vasoconstriction or pain. Treatment may require intravenous DHE three times daily to reinstitute a near normal degree of vasoconstriction.

Cluster Headaches

Cluster headaches occur in groups (clusters) of one to eight times daily for a period of several weeks to months. Many patients have a cyclic pattern that occurs most often in the spring. Cluster-free intervals range from a few months to several years.

Each headache consists of sharp, nonthrobbing pain that most often bores into one eye and adjacent areas for one-half to 3 hours. Suffering from repetitive bouts of agitating and excruciating pain, patients speak of wanting to kill themselves. The pain is accompanied by ipsilateral eye tearing, conjunctival injection, nasal congestion, and a partial Horner's syndrome (Figs. 9–4 and 12–15).

During a cluster period, headaches can occur randomly throughout the day and can be precipitated by alcoholic drinks, but they often occur with stereotyped regularity, especially during REM sleep. Compared to the symptoms of a migraine, a cluster headache is simply extraordinary pain. It is not preceded by an aura or other warning, unaccompanied by nausea, not alleviated by bedrest or seclusion, and not associated with mental changes.

Demography is also unique. Cluster headaches affect men six to eight times more commonly than women. In addition, unlike migraines, cluster headaches typically have no familial tendency. They typically begin in individuals aged 20 and 40 years. More than 80% of patients smoke and 50% drink alcohol excessively.

Cause and Treatment.   A different form of cerebrovascular dysfunction than migraines probably causes cluster headaches. Nevertheless, because the two probably

TABLE 9–5. *Comparison of Tension-type and Migraine Headaches*

	Tension-type	Migraine
Location	Bilateral	Hemicranial*
Nature	Dull ache	Throbbing*
Severity	Slight–moderate	Moderate–severe
Associated symptoms	None	Nausea, hyperacusis, photophobia
Activity	Continues working	Seeks seclusion
Effect of alcohol	Reduces headache	Worsens headache

*In approximately one half of patients, at least at onset.

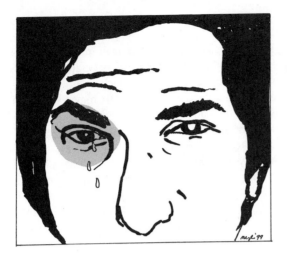

FIGURE 9–4. As with this 43-year-old man, patients with cluster headaches usually have unilateral periorbital pain accompanied by ipsilateral tearing and nasal discharge, along with ptosis and miosis (a partial Horner's syndrome). He has a right-sided partial Horner's syndrome, tearing, and a typical instinctual compensatory elevation of the right eyebrow to uncover the right eye.

result from cerebrovascular dysfunction and share several features (episodic, unilateral pain), both are called "vascular headaches."

Abortive medicines are relatively ineffective for cluster headaches because of each headache's abrupt, unexpected onset and relatively short duration. However, sumatriptan injections and, in a unique treatment, oxygen inhalation at 8 to 10 L/min may interrupt them. Prophylactic medicines include lithium and those useful for migraines. (Lithium was introduced because cluster headaches, like manic-depressive episodes, are cyclic and afflict middle-aged individuals. Neurologists prescribing divalproex for cluster headache may tacitly accept that concept.)

TRIGEMINAL NEURALGIA

Formerly called *tic douloureux, trigeminal neuralgia* is a chronic, recurring condition more accurately classified as a "cranial neuralgia," rather than a "chronic recurring headache." Patients, for whom that distinction is of no importance, suffer from dozens of brief, 20- to 30-second jabs of excruciatingly sharp pain that extend along one of the three divisions of the trigeminal nerve. The division most often affected is V_2 (see Fig. 4–11). Unlike all other headaches, stimulating the affected area can provoke the pain. These regions, *trigger zones*—when stimulated by eating, touch, brushing teeth, or drinking cold water—evoke a dreadful shock. Patients in the midst of a severe attack hesitate to eat, brush their teeth, and speak. Fortunately, in a characteristic reprise, trigeminal neuralgia abates at night, allowing the patient a full night's sleep. Trigeminal neuralgia typically develops after age 60 years, making it one of the most important causes of headache in the elderly (Table 9–6).

TABLE 9–6. *Conditions That Cause Headaches Predominantly in the Elderly*

Brain tumors: glioblastoma, metastases
Cervical spondylosis
Vasodilators and other medications
Postherpetic neuralgia
Subdural hematomas after little or no trauma
Temporal arteritis (giant cell arteritis)
Trigeminal neuralgia

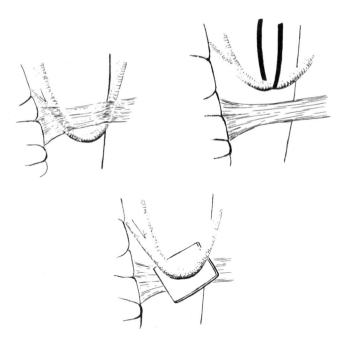

FIGURE 9–5. *Top left,* Microscopic vascular decompression to alleviate trigeminal neuralgia is a major neurosurgical advance. As pictured through an operating microscope, the brainstem is on the left side of the field, and the trigeminal nerve lies horizontally to the right. A large, aberrant artery compresses the nerve from below. *Top right,* A surgical loop plucks the artery out from beneath the trigeminal nerve. *Bottom,* The artery is then placed over a barrier that protects the nerve.

Cause and Treatment. In most cases, the cause is an aberrant superior cerebellar artery or other cerebral blood vessel compressing the trigeminal nerve root as it emerges from the brainstem. Tumors of the cerebellopontine angle may have the same effect. When trigeminal neuralgia develops in young adults, a multiple sclerosis plaque that irritates the trigeminal nerve nucleus may be responsible.

Treatment is usually begun with carbamazepine (Tegretol) and may proceed to other, newer antiepileptic medications. In the majority of patients, in whom an aberrant vessel is responsible for the neuralgia, an effective, although highly invasive, procedure is a craniotomy that places a barrier between the vessel and trigeminal nerve (Fig. 9–5). Less risky procedures are percutaneous glycerol injections and placing radiofrequency or gamma knife lesions in the root of the trigeminal nerve.

HEADACHES SECONDARY TO ORGANIC DISEASE

Temporal Arteritis

Temporal arteritis is a disease of unknown etiology in which the temporal and other cranial arteries become inflamed. Because histologic examination of affected arteries reveals giant cells, the condition is properly called *giant cell arteritis.*

Patients are almost always older than 55 years. They usually have a dull, continual headache in one or both temples. Almost pathognomic, but rare, is increasing jaw pain on chewing ("jaw claudication"). In advanced cases, the temporal arteries are red and tender. Temporal arteritis is often accompanied by signs of systemic illness, such as malaise, low-grade fever, and weight loss. It may be only one aspect of polymyalgia rheumatica or other rheumatologic disorder.

Because untreated arterial inflammation leads to arterial occlusion, serious complications may develop when the diagnosis is delayed. The two most important complications are ophthalmic artery occlusion, which will cause blindness, and cerebral artery occlusion, which will cause cerebral infarctions. In over 90% of cases, an erythrocyte sedimentation rate (ESR) above 40 mm supports the diagnosis. A temporal artery biopsy is the definitive test, but it is often unnecessary, hazardous, or impractical. Timely treatment with high dose steroids will relieve the headaches and prevent complications.

Intracranial Mass Lesions

Brain tumors and subdural hematomas often induce persistent or progressively severe headaches as their first or most bothersome symptom (see Chapters 19 and 20). Headaches that result from brain tumor most often mimic tension-type headaches because they are bilateral, dull, and less intense than vascular headaches. They worsen when intracranial pressure is raised, as when people bend over, cough, or strain at stool, and during early morning REM sleep. Although brain tumors notoriously begin during sleep and awaken patients, that pattern is present in less than half the patients, and numerous other headache conditions display the same course: migraines, cluster headaches, carbon dioxide retention, sleep apnea, and caffeine withdrawal.

Brain tumor–induced headaches are usually accompanied by at least subtle cognitive and personality changes. If not present initially, lateralized signs usually develop within 8 weeks. However, evidence of increased intracranial pressure—papilledema and stupor—may be late or absent. Neurologists tend to order computed tomography (CT) or magnetic resonance imaging (MRI) in almost all patients with unexplained progressive headaches and, in those with the onset of headaches after 55 years, an ESR.

Chronic Meningitis

Chronic meningitis usually produces a dull, continual headache accompanied by cognitive impairment, behavioral changes, and symptoms of a systemic illness. In addition, the meningeal inflammation at the base of the brain chokes various cranial nerves. Most often, patients with chronic meningitis develop facial palsy (from 7th cranial nerve injury), hearing impairment (8th nerve), or extraocular muscle palsy (3rd, 4th, or 6th nerves).

Lyme disease can cause a chronic meningitis (see Chapter 5). Chronic meningitis from *Cryptococcus* usually develops in patients who have impaired immune systems, including the elderly, those taking steroids, and those with AIDS, who are particularly susceptible. CT or MRI, which should be performed before a lumbar puncture (LP), may show communicating hydrocephalus. The LP will yield cerebrospinal fluid (CSF) that has a lymphocytic pleocytosis, low glucose concentration, elevated protein concentration, and often specific antigens. Because fungi and tubercle bacilli may take weeks to culture (see Chapter 20), the diagnosis is usually based on the clinical evaluation and preliminary CSF results.

Pseudotumor Cerebri

Pseudotumor cerebri (benign or idiopathic intracranial hypertension), which stems from idiopathic cerebral edema, occurs predominantly in young, obese women who have menstrual irregularities. Some cases have been attributed to excessive vitamin A use and outdated tetracycline. Whatever the cause, intracranial hypertension gives rise to papilledema and a dull, generalized headache. Many patients with moderately severe headaches show a surprising discrepancy between florid papilledema and an otherwise unremarkable examination. In particular, despite marked, generalized cerebral edema, patients have no alteration in their intellect or mood.

CSF pressure can reach levels over 400 mm H_2O. Papilledema may lead to blindness from optic atrophy (see Chapter 12). Treatment usually consists of diuretics, carbonic anhydrase inhibitors, dieting, repeated LPs to drain CSF, or steroids. In refractory cases, surgeons decompress the system by installing CSF shunts or performing an optic nerve sheath fenestration.

Bacterial Meningitis, *Herpes,* and Subarachnoid Hemorrhage

Commonly occurring, life-threatening, headache-producing illnesses are bacterial meningitis and subarachnoid hemorrhage. Bacterial meningitis is usually caused by *meningococcus* or *pneumococcus* that often spreads in epidemic fashion among young adults in confined areas, such as dormitories or military training camps. It causes a rapidly developing, severe headache accompanied by photophobia, malaise, fever, and nuchal rigidity. When bacterial meningitis is suspected, the CSF must be examined and treatment started with penicillin or another antibiotic.

Viral infections of the brain *(encephalitis)* or meninges *(meningitis)* cause headaches. These conditions are usually nonspecific clinically and more benign than bacterial infections. They are diagnosed by an LP, CT or MRI, and sometimes an electroencephalogram (EEG).

In contrast to almost all other forms of encephalitis, *Herpes simplex* encephalitis has distinct clinical findings. This virus, which is the most frequent cause of serious, nonepidemic encephalitis, has a predilection for the inferior surface of the frontal and temporal lobes. It causes fever, somnolence, and delirium and, because the temporal lobe is infected, partial complex seizures and memory impairment (amnesia). Bilateral temporal lobe damage in some patients has led to the human variety of the Klüver-Bucy syndrome (see Chapter 16).

The other important acutely occurring headache is the *subarachnoid hemorrhage* from a ruptured cerebral aneurysm. Cerebral artery aneurysms—often shaped like "berries" *(berry aneurysms)*—usually develop in the arteries that comprise the circle of Willis (see Fig. 11–2 and Chapter 20). If the arteries are incompletely fused in utero, the weak junctions eventually form an aneurysm. If an aneurysm ruptures, blood spurts into the brain and subarachnoid space, which normally contains clear CSF. After a subarachnoid hemorrhage, blood can be seen on a CT or MRI and in the CSF.

A subarachnoid hemorrhage typically causes a severe headache, prostration, and nuchal rigidity—symptoms similar to those in bacterial meningitis. However, sentinel bleeds ("leaks") or otherwise atypical subarachnoid hemorrhages are not as dramatic. Subarachnoid hemorrhages often occur during exertion, including exercise, straining at stool, and sexual intercourse. They are sometimes misdiagnosed as a common migraine or tension-type headache. If the CSF is examined several days after a subarachnoid hemorrhage, it will usually be xanthochromic (yellow) from blood breakdown products.

Although an LP, which may be performed for any of several reasons, provides important diagnostic information, it frequently leads to a severe headache called the "post-LP headache." As though withdrawal of CSF lets the brain "bounce" unprotected against the inside of the skull, sitting upright, or even rapidly turning the head and neck, exacerbates the headache. Post-LP headache often radiates to the back of the neck and is accompanied by nausea. Recommended treatments have included intravenous fluid infusions, bed rest, caffeine, and, to stop CSF leaks from the LP site, instillation of a blood patch.

MAOIs and Hemorrhage.   A variation of the ruptured congenital aneurysm that is almost peculiar to psychiatric practice is the striking iatrogenic intracerebral or subarachnoid hemorrhage induced by a hypertensive reaction to MAOI and antidepressants. If patients taking these medicines eat tyramine-containing foods or receive particular medications, the interaction can precipitate severe hypertension, excruciating headache, and hemorrhage. High tyramine foods that must be avoided are aged cheese, pickled herring, Chianti, beer with and without alcohol, and numerous other spicy, tasty, and seemingly innocuous staples and appetizers. The medicines that must not be administered with MAOI antidepressants are ones often used by neurologists and psychiatrists: sumatriptan, meperidine (Demerol), L-dopa (as in Sinemet), sympathomimetics, such as amphetamines, and the entire class of dibenzepin derivatives, which includes carbamazepine (Tegretol) and the tricyclic antidepressants.

Commonly used MAOI antidepressants—isocarboxazid (Marplan), pargyline (Eutron), phenelzine (Nardil), and tranylcypromine (Parnate)—normally cause an accumulation of epinephrine, norepinephrine, and serotonin. Hypertensive reaction should be treated by intravenous phentolamine (Regitine), which is an α-adrenergic blocking agent. Substitutes, which are possibly more readily available, are chlorpromazine and propranolol.

REFERENCES

Abramowicz M (ed): New "triptans" and other drugs for migraine. Med Lett *40:* 97–100, 1998

Akpunonu BE, Ahrens J: Sexual headaches: Case report, review, and treatment with calcium blocker. Headache *31:* 141–145, 1991

Becker WJ: Use of oral contraceptives in patients with migraines. Neurology *53* (Suppl 1): S19–S25, 1999

Boyle CAJ: Management of menstrual migraine. Neurology *53* (Suppl 1): S14–S18, 1999

Breslau N, Chilcoat HD, Andreski P: Further evidence on the link between migraine and neuroticism. Neurology *47:* 663–667, 1996

Breslau N, Schultz LR, Stewart WF, et al: Headache and major depression: Is the association specific to migraine? Neurology *54:* 308–313, 2000

Finelli PF: Coital cerebral hemorrhage. Neurology *43:* 2683–2685, 1993

Forsyth PA, Posner JB: Headaches in patients with brain tumors: A study of 111 patients. Neurology *43:* 1678–1683, 1993

Headache Classification Committee of the International Headache Society: Classification and diagnostic criteria for headache disorders, cranial neuralgias and facial pain. Cephalalgia *8* (Suppl 7): 1–96, 1988

Jensen R, Brink T, Olesen J: Sodium valproate has a prophylactic effect in migraine without aura. Neurology *44:* 647–651, 1994

Kaufman DM, Solomon S: Migraine visual auras: A medical update for the psychiatrist. Gen Hosp Psychiatry *14:* 162–170, 1992

Lipton RB, Stewart WF: Migraine headaches: Epidemiology and comorbidity. Clin Neurosci *5:* 2–9, 1998

Littlewood JT, Glover V, Davies PTG, et al: Red wine as a cause of migraine. Lancet *1:* 558–559, 1988

Mathew NT: Chronic refractory headache. Neurology *43* (Suppl 3): S26–S33, 1993

Maytal J, Young M, Shechter A, et al: Pediatric migraine and the International Headache Society (IHS) criteria. Neurology *48:* 602–607, 1997

Ostergaard JR, Kraft M: Benign coital headache. Cephalalgia *12:* 353–355, 1992

Raieli V, Raimondo D, Cammalleri R, et al: Migraine headaches in adolescents. Cephalalgia *15:* 5–12, 1995

Rasmussen BK: Migraine and tension-type headache in a general population: Precipitating factors, female hormones, sleep pattern and relation to lifestyle. Pain *53:* 65–72, 1993

Richards W: The fortification illusions of migraines. Sci Am *224:* 89–96, 1971

Sacks OW: Migraine: Revised and Expanded. Berkeley, University of California Press, 1992

Silberstein SD: The role of sex hormones in headache. Neurology *42* (Suppl 2): 37–42, 1992

Silberstein SD: Comprehensive management of headache and depression. Cephalalgia *21:* 50–55, 1998

Silverman K, Evans SM, Strain EC, et al: Withdrawal syndrome after the double-blind cessation of caffeine consumption. N Engl J Med *327:* 1109–1114, 1992

Solomon S, Lipton RB, Newman LC: Clinical features of chronic daily headache. Headache *32:* 325–329, 1992

Tenser RB: Trigeminal neuralgia: Mechanisms of treatment. Neurology *51:* 17–19, 1998

The Subcutaneous Sumatriptan International Study Group: Treatment of migraine attacks with sumatriptan. N Engl J Med *325:* 316–321, 1991

The Subcutaneous Sumatriptan International Study Group: Treatment of acute cluster headache with sumatriptan. N Engl J Med *325:* 322–326, 1991

Ziegler DK, Hurwitz A, Preskorn S, et al: Propranolol and amitriptyline in prophylaxis of migraine. Arch Neurol *50:* 825–830, 1993

QUESTIONS and ANSWERS: CHAPTER 9

1–4. A 17-year-old Marine recruit has developed a severe generalized headache, lethargy, and nuchal rigidity.

1. What disease must be considered first?

2. What diagnostic procedure must be performed first?

3. What would the typical result be?

4. What is the therapy?

> **ANSWERS:** Acute bacterial meningitis, particularly meningococcal meningitis, is a common, often fatal disease in military recruits, schoolchildren, and other young people brought into confined areas. The possibility of bacterial meningitis merits immediate investigation with a lumbar puncture (LP) for cerebrospinal fluid (CSF) analysis. With bacterial meningitis, the CSF reveals a low glucose concentration (0–40 mg/100 ml), high protein concentration (greater than 100 mg/100 ml), and a polymorphonuclear pleocytosis (over 100/ml). Although alternatives have been suggested, penicillin, 20 million U/day intravenously, remains the standard treatment.

5–9. A 45-year-old man has had moderate bitemporal headaches and then the gradual onset of stupor over 5 days. He has episodes of unusual, repetitive behavior, describes having unusual smells, and photophobia. He has fever, delirium, mild nuchal rigidity, and bilateral Babinski signs.

5. What might the episodic behavioral disturbances indicate?

6. What do the delirium and Babinski signs suggest?

7. What is the most common cause of sporadic (nonepidemic) encephalitis?

8. What areas of the brain are particularly susceptible?

9. What are the major sequelae of this infection?

> **ANSWERS:** He is having partial complex seizures that usually originate in the temporal lobes. He probably has cerebral as well as meningeal involvement. *Herpes simplex* encephalitis is the most common, nonepidemic encephalitis. *Herpes simplex* encephalitis has a predilection for the temporal lobes, which include portions of the limbic system. Temporal lobe inflammation may cause partial complex seizures and, because of the limbic system involvement, profound memory impairment (amnesia). In rare cases, it may produce a human form of the Klüver-Bucy syndrome (see Chapter 16).

10. A young hypertensive woman suddenly develops severe right retro-orbital pain, prostration, a right third cranial nerve palsy, and nuchal rigidity. What is the most likely cause?

a. An aneurysm of a portion of the circle of Willis
b. An ocular migraine
c. An ophthalmoplegic migraine
d. None of the above

> **ANSWER:** a. Although there are many causes of severe retro-orbital pain, a third nerve palsy indicates that a posterior communicating artery aneurysm has ruptured and caused a subarachnoid hemorrhage.

11. A middle-aged hypertensive man has the sudden onset of the worst headache of his life while watching television. Although he has nausea and vomiting, he is able to speak coherently. What are the likely possible causes?

a. An intracranial hemorrhage
b. Migraine headache
c. Seizure
d. Brain tumor

> **ANSWER:** a. The symptom, "the worst headache of my life," indicates a cerebral or subarachnoid hemorrhage. Migraine or cluster headaches, which may appear in middle age, might be considered; however, they should be entertained only when headaches

have become a chronic illness (often requiring months of observation) and when potentially fatal conditions have been excluded.

12. An elderly, depressed man has a moderately severe generalized headache and decreased attention span, but no "hard" findings. What entities should be given special consideration?

ANSWER: Although elderly people are subject to most forms of headaches, they are prone to develop giant cell arteritis, falls leading to head trauma and thus subdural hematomas, and side effects of medications. Of course, headaches may be a symptom of depression.

13. What medicines are known to cause headaches?

ANSWER: Nitroglycerin, long-acting vasodilators (e.g., Isordil), and several other antianginal medications cause headaches. Reserpine and hydralazine cause a dull frontal pain and nasal stuffiness. The monamine oxidase (MAO) inhibitors cause hypertensive headaches when foods containing tyramine are eaten. Birth control pills can trigger or exacerbate migraines.

14–25. Match the disease (Questions 14–25) with the characteristic symptoms (a–l):

14. Tic douloureux

15. Bell's palsy

16. Pseudotumor cerebri

17. Basilar migraine

18. Subarachnoid hemorrhage

19. Temporal arteritis

20. Angle-closure glaucoma

21. Subdural hematoma

22. Postconcussion headache

23. Medulloblastoma

24. Viral meningitis

25. Hemiplegic migraine

a. Severe ocular pain, "red eye," decreased vision
b. Papilledema, generalized headache, obesity, and menstrual irregularity
c. Mastoid pain followed by facial palsy
d. Lancinating pain in the jaw
e. Moderate headache, focal seizures, and fever
f. Mild headache and hemiparesis after a fortification scotoma
g. Chronic pain, depressed sensorium
h. Temporal pain, malaise, jaw claudication, high sedimentation rate
i. Daily dull headaches, inattention, and insomnia
j. Generalized headache, nuchal rigidity
k. Horner's syndrome
l. Headache, nausea, vomiting, diplopia, and ataxia

ANSWERS: 14-d; 15-c; 16-b; 17-l; 18-j; 19-h; 20-a; 21-g, i, or l; 22-i; 23-l; 24-j; 25-f

26. What features of a headache suggest that it is a migraine?

ANSWER: Typically, a migraine is unilateral (in 50%), pulsating, and accompanied by autonomic nervous system dysfunction (e.g., nausea, vomiting, fatigue, and diaphoresis). Migraine with aura (classic migraine), which is relatively infrequent (only 15% of migraine sufferers have this variety), is preceded by visual scotoma or other hallucinations.

27. What are common triggers of migraine headaches?

ANSWER: Menses, glare, alcohol, missing meals, REM sleep, too much as well as too little sleep, and relief of stress may precipitate migraines. REM sleep, however, is more closely associated with the development of cluster headaches.

28. How do migraine headaches in children differ from those in adults?

ANSWER: Although patients of all ages may have autonomic dysfunction, these symptoms may be the primary or exclusive manifestation of migraines in children. Children are also more prone than adults to develop ophthalmoplegic and basilar artery migraine. They are also more likely to have behavioral disturbances, such as agitation or withdrawal. They are particularly prone to have cyclic vomiting and abdominal pain as a manifestation of migraine.

29. Which neurologic disorders cause visual hallucinations?

ANSWER: Migraines with auras (classic migraines), seizures originating in the temporal or occipital lobes, narcolepsy, hallucinogens (PCP and LSD), and alcohol withdrawal (DTs) all may precipitate visual hallucinations.

30. In which parts of the brain are serotonin-containing neurons concentrated?

a. Limbic system
b. Frontal lobes
c. Dorsal raphe nucleus
d. Cerebellum

ANSWER: c

31. Concerning migraine, to which process does "cortical depression" refer?

a. The organically based changes in affect that accompany migraines
b. The wave of neuron hypometabolism that causes or at least precedes the migraine
c. The inability of the cortex to respond to stimulate during the migraine
d. The comorbid depressive disorder

ANSWER: b

32. Which of the following is not indicated by xanthochromic CSF?

a. The CSF is yellow.
b. Subarachnoid bleeding that probably occurred within the previous several days.
c. The serum bilirubin concentration or CSF protein concentration may be highly elevated.
d. The CSF is opaque.

ANSWER: d

33. Which one of the following is not a sign of acute *Herpes simplex* encephalitis?

a. Partial complex seizures
b. Amnesia
c. Klüver-Bucy syndrome
d. Hemorrhagic lesions in the temporal lobes
e. Myoclonus

ANSWER: e. The *Herpes simplex* virus, which is the most common cause of nonepidemic encephalitis, invades the undersurface of the brain where it invades the temporal and frontal lobes. Damage to those regions, which is hemorrhagic, causes seizures, limbic system impairment, and occasionally changes in sexuality, oral behavior, and aggressiveness (the Klüver-Bucy syndrome).

34–37. Does sleep ameliorate these headaches? (Yes/No)

34. Classical migraine

35. Trigeminal neuralgia

36. Cluster

37. Temporal arteritis

ANSWERS: 34-Yes. Sleep typically relieves migraines, but it may trigger them. 35-No. Sleep has no effect on trigeminal neuralgia, but this headache does not disturb sleep. 36-No. In fact, REM sleep typically precipitates cluster headaches. 37-No. Temporal arteritis is independent of sleep.

38–44. Which of these headaches typically awaken patients from sleep?

38. Migraine

39. Sleep apnea

40. Brain tumor

41. Subdural hematoma

42. Tension-type

43. Cluster headaches

44. Chronic obstructive pulmonary disease

ANSWERS: 38-Yes, 39-Yes, 40-Yes, 41-Yes, 42-No, 43-Yes, 44-Yes

45. In what stage of sleep do migraine and cluster headaches begin?

a. REM
b. NREM
c. Slow-wave
d. None of the above

ANSWER: a

46. What common laboratory tests are abnormal with migraine headaches?

a. CT
b. MRI
c. EEG
d. None of the above

ANSWER: d. None. The EEG is often abnormal and epilepsy is comorbid with migraine; however, EEGs do not show changes that are characteristic of migraine.

47. A group of many severe periorbital headaches occurs every winter when the patient goes to Miami. Of which kind of headache is this pattern typical?

a. Depression-induced headaches
b. Tension-type
c. Migraine
d. Cluster
e. Trigeminal neuralgia
f. Giant cell arteritis

ANSWER: d. Cluster headaches are indicated by their temporal grouping. Alternatively, migraines may be precipitated by going on vacation.

48. Of the following, which two conditions cost industry the largest number of hours?

a. Low back pain
b. Epilepsy
c. Headache
d. Cerebrovascular disease
e. Brain tumors
f. Neck pain

ANSWER: a and c

49–51. Which of the following headaches follow family patterns? (Yes/No)

49. Migraine headaches

50. Cluster headaches

51. Tension-type headaches

ANSWERS: 49-Yes, 50-No, 51-Yes

52. A 35-year-old man who suffers several migraines a year developed a uniquely severe headache during sexual intercourse. He described it as "the worst headache of his life." Two evenings later, this headache recurred during masturbation. Which is the most likely variety of his headache?

a. Psychogenic
b. Cluster
c. Coital
d. Tension-type

ANSWER: c. Most likely, he has sex-induced, benign headaches, which are common and fall into the realm of coital migraine or "headache associated with sexual activity." However, the development of a uniquely severe headache, especially when it occurs during vigorous activity, usually requires further evaluation. In particular, a subarachnoid or intracerebral hemorrhage must be considered. A CT, MRI, or lumbar puncture, depending on the circumstances, is usually performed because the possibility of a potentially fatal subarachnoid hemorrhage should be considered when confronted with a patient with the "worst headache" of his or her life.

53. Which statement is false regarding psychiatric conditions comorbid with migraine?

a. They occur together more frequently than statistics would predict.
b. Comorbid conditions must have a causal relationship.
c. Depression, anxiety, and panic attacks are comorbid with migraine.
d. The temporal relationship has to be constant, such as migraines always preceding depression.

ANSWER: b. Comorbid conditions, which do not necessarily have a constant temporal relationship, may have a common cause or different but related causes, as well as one causing the other.

54. Which two of the following are not causes of "chronic daily headache" (CDH)?

a. Transformed migraine
b. Analgesic abuse
c. Ergotism
d. Depression
e. Narcotic abuse
f. Vasoconstrictor rebound
g. Trigeminal neuralgia
h. Cluster headache·

ANSWER: g, h

55. Which cranial nerve innervates the meninges?

a. Olfactory
b. Oculomotor
c. Trigeminal
d. Facial

ANSWER: c

56. Which one of the following statements concerning serotonin is false?

a. Serotonin (5HT) is metabolized to 5-hydroxyindoleacetic acid (5HIAA).
b. Platelet 5HT concentration falls at the onset of migraines.
c. Sumatriptan, dihydroergotamine, and ergotamine all act on serotonin receptors.
d. Serotonin-containing neurons are concentrated in the dorsal raphe.
e. During a migraine, urinary serotonin and 5-HIAA concentrations fall.

ANSWER: e

57–60. Match the adverse effects with the following medications:

57. Methysergide (Sansert)

58. Propranolol (Inderal)

59. Cafergot

60. Aspirin

a. With prolonged use, vascular spasm, claudication, and muscle cramps
b. Retroperitoneal, pleural, and cardiac fibrosis
c. Painful gastric distress, gastroduodenal bleeding, and easy bruisability
d. Bradycardia, asthma, and fatigue
e. None of the above

ANSWERS: 57-b, 58-d, 59-a (ergotism), 60-c

61. Which headache variety usually is cyclic or periodic, develops predominately in men, and responds to lithium treatment?

a. Migraines
b. Cluster headaches
c. Trigeminal neuralgia
d. Giant cell arteritis

ANSWER: b. Cluster headaches were initially treated with lithium, which is effective, because their periodicity is similar to manic-depressive illness.

62. A 40-year-old woman has had migraines since adolescence and depression for 10 years. Her psychiatrist changed her antidepressant to a serotonin reuptake inhibitor that initially seemed to reduce her headaches and improve her mood. However, after 1 month, her headaches returned in even greater severity. She is brought to the emergency room with agitated confusion and tremulousness. Her blood pressure is 110/70 and her temperature, 100°F. Her urine contains a small quantity of myoglobin. Of the following, which is the most likely cause of her condition?

    a. Neuroleptic malignant syndrome
    b. SSRI overdose
    c. Serotonin syndrome
    d. A monoamine oxidase (MAO) inhibitor crisis

> *ANSWER:* c. She has the serotonin syndrome because she undoubtedly took an antimigraine serotonin agonist, such as sumatriptan, in addition to her SSRI. Tricyclic antidepressants are usually preferable to SSRIs for depression comorbid with migraines. She lacks the muscle rigidity and high temperature of neuroleptic malignant syndrome. MAO metabolizes sumatriptan and related medications. However, an MAO inhibitor crisis is unlikely in this case because she is not hypertensive.

63. Which headache variety is most often associated with a mood change?

    a. Cluster
    b. Trigeminal neuralgia
    c. Giant cell arteritis
    d. Migraine
    e. Pseudotumor cerebri

> *ANSWER:* d

64. Which headache variety occurs more often in men than women?

    a. Classic migraine
    b. Common migraine
    c. Pseudotumor cerebri
    d. Trigeminal neuralgia
    e. Tension-type headaches
    f. Cluster headaches

> *ANSWER:* f

65. Which two CNS structures are pain-sensitive?

    a. Optic nerves
    b. Meninges
    c. Cerebral neurons
    d. Ventricles

> *ANSWER:* a, b

66–73. Match the headache (Questions 66–73) with its most likely cause (a–k):

66. Tic douloureux

67. Hot dog headache

68. Sinusitis with seizures

69. Pseudotumor cerebri

70. Temporal arteritis

71. Chinese restaurant syndrome

72. Nocturnal migraine

73. Antianginal medication-induced headaches

    a. Giant cell inflammation of extra- and intracranial arteries
    b. Autonomic nervous system dysfunction
    c. Vascular compression of the trigeminal nerve
    d. Nitrites
    e. Monosodium glutamate (MSG)
    f. Cerebral edema
    g. Nightmares
    h. REM sleep
    i. NREM sleep
    j. Spread of infection to cause meningitis or a brain abscess
    k. Cerebral artery as well as coronary artery effects

> *ANSWERS:* 66-c, 67-d, 68-j, 69-f, 70-a, 71-e, 72-h, 73-k

74. Which one of the following is an invalid explanation for tricyclic antidepressants (TCAs) helping people with migraine headaches who do not have overt depression?

a. TCAs improve sleep patterns.
b. TCAs increase the concentration of serotonin, which is analgesic.
c. TCAs themselves are analgesic.
d. TCAs are endorphins.
e. Depression is often comorbid with migraines.

ANSWER: d

75. Which of the following headaches switches the side of the head it affects during and between attacks?

a. Migraine
b. Trigeminal neuralgia

c. Cluster
d. Pseudotumor

ANSWER: a. Migraines are predominately unilateral and on the same side most of the times, but they tend to generalize and switch sides during and between attacks. Trigeminal neuralgia and cluster are unilateral and on the same side as virtually a life-long affliction. The headache in pseudotumor is generalized, bilateral.

76. Which of the following is not an indication for changing a strategy from abortive to prophylactic migraine therapy?

a. More than four migraines monthly
b. Tinnitus from aspirin-containing medications
c. Ergotism
d. Habitual narcotic use
e. Once monthly migraine with aura (classic migraine)

ANSWER: e

77. Which two conditions do not occur on a familial basis?

a. Temporal arteritis
b. Tuberous sclerosis
c. Multiple sclerosis
d. Migraines
e. Absence (petit mal) seizures

f. Cluster headaches
g. Frontotemporal dementia
h. Tension-type headaches
i. Tourette's syndrome

ANSWER: a, f

78. When are women's migraines exacerbated?

a. Premenstrual days
b. Menopause
c. Taking oral contraceptives

d. Menarche
e. All of the above

ANSWER: e

79. Which type of headache do brain tumors most often mimic?

a. Tension-type
b. Migraine
c. Cluster

d. Subarachnoid hemorrhage
e. Trigeminal neuralgia

ANSWER: a

10

Seizures

Seizures are characterized by specific clinical features and electroencephalographic (EEG) patterns. They have distinctive etiologies and onset ages, and specific medical treatments (anticonvulsants or antiepileptic drugs [AEDs]). A tendency to have recurrent seizures, *epilepsy*, affects about 6 of every 1,000 people.

In addition, seizures can mimic psychiatric disturbances, have prominent cognitive and affective components, and be precipitated by psychotropic medicines. The EEG, which is the most specific laboratory test for seizures, also assists in diagnosis of several other neurologic conditions.

ELECTROENCEPHALOGRAM (EEG)

Normal and Abnormal

The routine EEG records cerebral electrical activity detected by "surface" or "scalp" electrodes (Fig. 10–1). Four frequency bands of cerebral activity, represented by Greek letters, emanate from the brain (Table 10–1).

EEG readers first determine the display of the electrodes (the EEG *montage*). They also note the time scale, which is determined by vertical lines on the EEG paper or displayed as a 1-second horizontal bar (Fig. 10–1). Although approaches vary, most readers then determine the EEG's *dominant* or *background rhythm* (see below), organization, and symmetry. Abnormal patterns, especially if they occur in paroxysms, are accorded special attention. EEG readers judge all these features in relation to whether the patient is awake, asleep, unresponsive, or having observable seizure activity.

The normal dominant or background EEG activity is in the *alpha* range of 8 to 13 cycles-per-second, or Hertz (Hz), and is detectable over the occipital region (Fig. 10–2). Alpha activity is prominent when individuals are relaxed with their eyes closed, but it disappears if they open their eyes, concentrate, or become anxious. Because alpha activity reflects an anxiety-free state, it represents the goal in "alpha training," biofeedback, and other behavior modification techniques. Alpha activity also disappears when people fall asleep or take medicines that affect mental function. The background rhythm typically slows below the alpha range in the elderly and in al-

TABLE 10–1. *Common EEG Rhythms*

Activity	Hz (cycles/sec)	Usual Location
Alpha	8–13	Posterior
Beta	>13	Anterior
Theta	4–7	Generalized*
Delta	1–3	Generalized*

*May be focal.

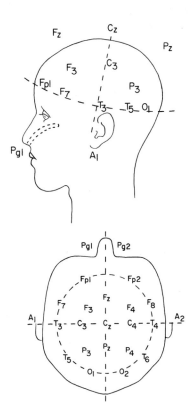

FIGURE 10–1. In the standard array of scalp electrodes, most are named for the underlying cerebral region (e.g. frontal, central, parietal, and occipital). Odd-numbered ones are on the left and even-numbered ones on the right. The P_g electrodes are from the nasopharyngeal leads and the A electrodes, the ears (aural leads).

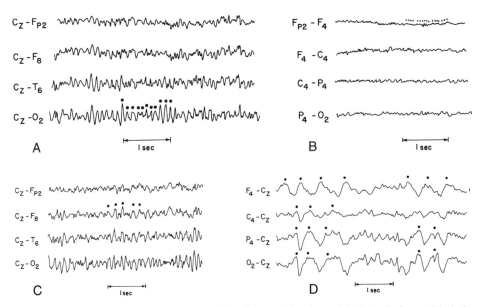

FIGURE 10–2. A, *Alpha* activity is the regular 11-Hz activity overlying the occipital lobe. **B,** *Beta* activity is the low-voltage, irregular 17-Hz activity overlying the frontal lobe. **C,** *Theta* activity is the 5-Hz activity overlying the right frontal lobe. **D,** *Delta* activity is the high-voltage 2- to 3-Hz activity present over the entire hemisphere.

most every neurologic illness that affects the brain. However, in the early stages of Alzheimer's disease, the background activity, although slower than normal, often remains in the alpha range.

Beta activity, frequencies faster than 13 Hz, usually has low voltage and overlies the frontal lobes. Beta activity replaces alpha activity when people concentrate, become anxious, or have taken benzodiazepines.

Theta (4 to 7 Hz) and *delta* (1 to 3 Hz) activities are normally prominent in children, in all people as they enter deep sleep, and in many with trivial disturbances, but are usually absent in healthy, alert adults. When present over the entire brain, theta or delta activity may indicate a degenerative illness or metabolic derangement. In a different situation, continuous focal slow activity with *phase reversal* in bipolar montages (Fig. 10–3) suggests an underlying cerebral lesion; however, its absence certainly does not exclude one.

Unusually pointed waves—"sharp waves" or "spikes"—may suggest a cerebral lesion and a predisposition to seizures. When they are phase-reversed in bipolar montages, they even more strongly indicate an irritative focus with potential to produce a seizure. However, this EEG abnormality alone does not prove that a patient has epilepsy.

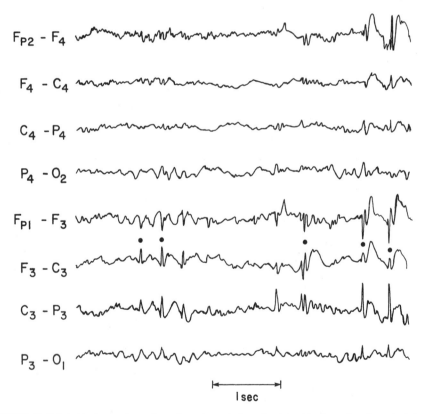

FIGURE 10–3. This in bipolar montage shows four channels from the right side above four from the left. Each side progresses from the frontal to the occipital region.

On at least five occasions (marked by dots), sharp waves and spikes, in *phase reversal*, appear to point toward each other. They originate from the F_3 electrode, which is over the left frontal lobe. A finding of such isolated, phase-reversed sharp waves is associated with seizures but, without additional clinical or EEG evidence, it is insufficient for diagnostic purposes.

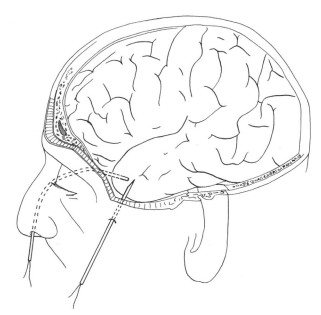

FIGURE 10–4. *Nasopharyngeal electrodes,* which are inserted through the nostrils, reach the posterior pharynx. There, separated by the thin sphenoid bone, they are adjacent to the temporal lobe's medial surface, which is the focus or origin of about 80% of partial complex seizures. (Refer to figures in Chapter 20 to see the relatively great distance between the temporal lobe's medial surface and the scalp and the close relationship between the temporal lobe and the sphenoid bone.) *Sphenoidal* electrodes are inserted through the skin to reach the lateral, external surface of the sphenoid wing. Electrodes in this location are near the temporal lobe's inferior surface. (However, specially placed scalp electrodes, new arrays, electronic filters, and critical reading of the EEG may be just as accurate.)

Seizures

During a seizure *(ictus),* the EEG reveals *paroxysmal* EEG activity that usually consists of bursts of spikes, slow waves, or complexes of spike-and-waves or polyspike-and-waves. However, muscle or movement artifacts may obscure the ictal EEG abnormalities. After the seizure, in the *postictal period,* EEGs usually show only slow, low-voltage activity, *postictal depression,* often followed by diffuse high-voltage slowing.

EEGs obtained between seizures, in the *interictal period,* contain abnormalities that support—but do not prove—a diagnosis in up to 80% of epilepsy patients. On the other hand, because about 20% of epilepsy patients have normal interictal EEGs, normal interictal EEGs cannot exclude a diagnosis of seizures. Their value is further confused by the finding that about 15% of the normal population has nonspecific EEG changes, such as a slow wave or an occasional sharp wave or spike. These same nonspecific EEG changes also confound studies of patients with various neurologic, psychiatric, or medication-induced disorders.

In patients suspected of having epilepsy, several maneuvers are used to evoke characteristic EEG abnormalities. These patients are usually asked to hyperventilate for 3 minutes or to look toward a stroboscopic light while an EEG is obtained.* If these maneuvers fail to yield diagnostic information and a strong suspicion of seizures persists, an EEG is repeated after sleep deprivation. In about 15% of epileptic patients, a *sleep-deprived EEG* reveals abnormalities not apparent in routine studies.

In some epilepsy patients, specially placed electrodes will reveal abnormalities undetectable by ordinary scalp electrodes. For example, anterior temporal scalp, nasopharyngeal, or sphenoidal electrodes can detect discharges from the temporal lobe's inferior-medial (mesial or medial) surface (Fig. 10–4). Electrodes surgically implanted in the dura, subdural space, or cerebral cortex can pinpoint an epileptic focus and also show that a seizure focus seen on scalp electrodes may only be a reflection ("mirror") of the actual focus.

---

*Children with sickle cell disease should not be asked to hyperventilate because that maneuver might precipitate a sickle crisis. Similarly, patients likely to have cerebrovascular disease are not asked to hyperventilate because it might induce cerebral ischemia.

Intensive EEG-video monitoring consists of several days of continuous, split-screen videotaped clinical and EEG recordings of seizures, changes in behavior, and effects of sleep. Serum AED concentrations and various physiologic data can be monitored and correlated with seizures. EEG-video monitoring has become the gold standard for diagnosing, classifying, and determining the frequency of seizures; evaluating patients for epilepsy surgery; treating patients who seem to suffer from *refractory seizures* (frequent seizures that do not respond to AEDs); and identifying disorders that mimic seizures, particularly pseudoseizures (see below).

Quantitative EEG analysis (QEEG), often referred to as *EEG brain mapping*, consists of topographic displays and comparisons of a patient's EEG to normal EEG data. This technique, used mostly in research, remains too unreliable for clinical evaluation of patients with minor and moderate head injury, postconcussive syndrome, learning disabilities, attention deficit-hyperactivity disorder, and psychiatric illnesses. Its fledging status should preclude introduction in litigation.

(With children, an evaluation could actually begin with parents' videotaping their child during suspected seizures or almost any episodic disturbance, including temper tantrums, breath-holding spells, sleep disorders, and movement disorders. The parents and physicians could then review the videotape.)

Toxic-Metabolic Encephalopathy

During the initial phase of toxic-metabolic encephalopathy or "delirium," when patients have only subtle behavioral or cognitive disturbances, the EEG loses alpha activity and develops generalized theta and delta activity. In addition, hepatic and uremic encephalopathy characteristically produce *triphasic waves* (Fig. 10–5). In hepatic failure, triphasic waves may appear before the bilirubin levels rise. Equally valuable, a normal EEG virtually excludes a toxic-metabolic encephalopathy.

Dementia

In early Alzheimer's disease, the background alpha activity usually slows from about 10 to 12 Hz down to 8 Hz. This decrease is subtle and, especially for people

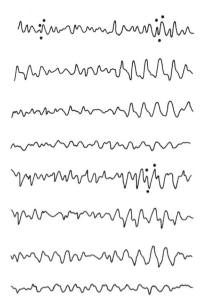

FIGURE 10–5. This EEG obtained from a patient with hepatic encephalopathy reveals typical *triphasic waves,* which can be seen in the first and fifth channel. There is also a lack of organized background activity—ordinarily seen clearly in the lowermost channels—consisting of medium-voltage alpha frequency over the occipital lobes.

100μV ⌊___
1 sec

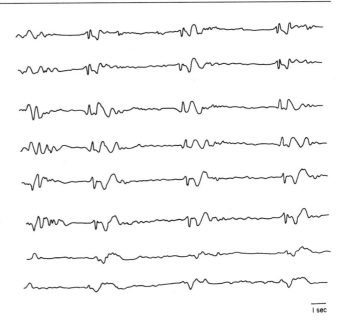

FIGURE 10–6. *Periodic complexes* are seen in all channels as four fairly regular bursts of electrical activity followed by minimal activity, which is termed "burst-suppression." Periodic complexes are associated with myoclonic jerks, and together they are cardinal features of two illnesses characterized by dementia: subacute sclerosing panencephalitis (SSPE), which occurs in children, and Creutzfeldt-Jakob disease, found in the elderly (see Chapter 7).

older than 65 years, remains within the normal range. In moderately advanced Alzheimer's disease, however, the background EEG is unequivocally slow. Eventually the EEG becomes disorganized.

Multi-infarct (vascular) dementia also induces EEG abnormalities. However, the EEG cannot reliably differentiate multi-infarct dementia from Alzheimer's disease dementia (see Chapters 7 and 11). It could be helpful, at best, when asymmetric EEG changes suggest infarctions rather then Alzheimer's disease.

In contrast, the EEG is almost definitive in diagnosing subacute sclerosing panencephalitis (SSPE) and Creutzfeldt-Jakob disease (see Chapter 7). In these conditions—characterized by dementia and myoclonic jerks—the EEG shows *periodic complexes* (Fig. 10–6). However, new variant Creutzfeldt-Jakob disease ("mad cow") fails to produce these EEG changes.

The EEG is also effective in distinguishing between *pseudodementia* and dementia (see Chapter 7). In pseudodementia, the EEG remains normal or has only slightly slowed background activity. In advanced dementia from almost any cause, it shows theta and delta activity. In the many patients who have a mixture of depression and mild dementia, the EEG cannot measure each condition's relative contribution.

With few exceptions, neurologists do not perform an EEG in the routine evaluation of a patient with dementia. However, EEGs are indicated when Creutzfeldt-Jakob disease or a related illness is suggested by the onset of dementia in less than 3 months or by the development of myoclonus; when seizures or metabolic encephalopathy are suggested by fluctuations in the patient's behavior or level of consciousness; or when a diagnosis of dementia is equivocal.

Structural Lesions

The EEG does not reliably detect or exclude structural lesions that cause seizures, such as brain tumors, abscesses, strokes, or subdural hematomas. In fact, it is normal in many of these conditions. When abnormal, it cannot distinguish among them. Computed tomography (CT) and especially magnetic resonance imaging (MRI) are the standard tests that, despite expense, are cost-effective in detecting structural lesions, whether or not they cause seizures. The CT is usually satisfactory. However, for detecting mesial temporal sclerosis, which underlies many partial complex seizures, MRI is superior (see below).

Altered States of Awareness

The EEG shows distinctive changes during normal sleep's progressively deeper stages and dreaming. Coupled with monitors of ocular movement and muscle activity in the polysomnogram (PSG), the EEG is critical in diagnosing sleep disturbances (see Chapter 17).

The EEG is also useful in diagnosing the *locked-in syndrome,* a condition in which patients might appear to be comatose but are actually fully alert and cognizant (see Chapter 11). Usually because of infarctions in their pons or medulla, patients in the locked-in syndrome cannot speak or move their trunk or limbs. However, with their cerebral hemispheres and upper brainstem intact, they remain alert with normal cerebral activity, including cognitive function. Thus, they have a normal EEG.

The locked-in syndrome must be differentiated from the *persistent vegetative state,* which typically follows cerebral cortex anoxia from cardiac arrest, drug overdose, or carbon monoxide poisoning. Because these insults lead to extensive cerebral cortex injury, patients have profound dementia accompanied by an inability to speak or move. Their "vegetative functions," such as breathing and digesting food, continue. Their eyes open and close, but mostly spontaneously or in response to light. As would be predicted, extensive cerebral cortical damage leads to a markedly abnormal—slow and disorganized—EEG.

Finally, if the EEG detects no electrical activity *(electrocerebral silence),* in most circumstances, it can be instrumental in declaring brain death. Making that determination before the heart stops beating permits harvesting organs for transplant. However, the exceptions are important: hypothermia or barbiturate overdose precludes a diagnosis of brain death based on an EEG. People routinely fully recover after barbiturate overdoses or drowning in icy water that initially left them with no obvious sign of life and a "flat" EEG.

Psychiatric Disturbances and Psychotropics

Although the EEG was developed as an aid in diagnosing psychiatric illness, that role has never been realized. Obtaining EEGs on a routine basis on psychiatric patients is not warranted. Most such EEGs are normal. When abnormal, the changes are typically minor and nonspecific, such as excessive beta or theta activity. Moreover, there is simply no consensus as to the nature or frequency of various EEG patterns in psychiatric illnesses.

To further confound any potential diagnostic value, psychotropic medications induce EEG abnormalities. Although psychotropic-induced EEG changes are usually minor and nonspecific, some may be prominent and persist for up to 2 months after medications are withdrawn.

There are few guidelines in assessing psychotropics' EEG effects. Most produce intermittent or continuous background slowing with theta or even delta activity. Benzodiazepines and barbiturates typically produce beta activity, which is sometimes a telltale sign of their surreptitious use. Phenothiazines also produce sharp waves, even at therapeutic serum concentrations. Lithium at toxic levels causes spikes and sharp waves. Phencyclidine (PCP) and other excitatory drugs cause generalized, paroxysmal discharges.

Electroconvulsive therapy (ECT) also induces EEG changes. During and immediately after ECT, EEG changes resemble those of a generalized tonic-clonic seizure and its aftermath. After a course of ECT, EEG slow-wave activity persists over the frontal lobes or entire cerebrum for up to 3 months. When ECT is unilateral, EEG slowing is generally less pronounced and more restricted to the treated side. ECT-induced EEG slowing is associated with memory impairment but with more effective treatment of depression.

Antipsychotic-Induced Seizures.   Antidepressants and antipsychotics often do more than produce EEG changes. Depending on whether patients take an overdose or therapeutic doses, the route of administration, and patient history, many precipitate seizures.

Seizures induced by antipsychotic medications are associated with high dose or parenteral administration of the medication, definable brain damage underlying the psychiatric illness, or, in most cases, pre-existing epilepsy. Of those individuals with pre-existing epilepsy, antipsychotic-induced seizures are closely associated with polypharmacy or noncompliance with an AED regimen. Seizures follow antipsychotic drug overdose in only about 1% of cases.

In therapeutic doses, of the older antipsychotic agents, chlorpromazine carries the highest seizure risk. Haloperidol, thioridazine, and fluphenazine carry a relatively low risk. With bupropion (Wellbutrin) treatment, the seizure incidence rises almost tenfold as dose increases from 450 mg to 600 mg daily. In routine dosage, however, it does not pose a significant risk for seizures.

Of the atypical antipsychotic agents in routine dosages, olanzapine (Zyprexa), risperidone (Risperdal), and quetiapine (Seroquel) have an incidence of seizures of less than 1%. On the other hand, clozapine (Clozaril) induces generalized tonic-clonic seizures in about 4% of patients taking high doses ($\geq$600 mg/day), although in only 1% of those taking low doses (<300 mg/day). Patients who experienced a seizure at the lower dose usually had pre-existing epilepsy. Most patients who had an antipsychotic-induced seizure were able to tolerate a reintroduction of the medication if the dose were raised slowly, an AED were added to the regimen, or the AED dose were increased.

Antidepressant-Induced Seizures.   Physicians frequently encounter patients who have had a seizure following antidepressant overdose because deliberate overdose of these medicines is a frequently used method in suicide attempts and between 4% and 20% of antidepressant overdoses are complicated by seizures. The incidence of seizures following overdoses of amoxapine and maprotiline (Ludiomil) is greater than following overdoses of tricyclic antidepressants, which is about 8%. Seizures rarely complicate overdose of selective serotonin reuptake inhibitors (SSRIs). Whichever antidepressant is used, seizures usually occur within the first 8 hours of the overdose.

With antidepressants in therapeutic doses, risk factors for seizures are a personal or family history of seizures, abnormalities on a pretreatment EEG, underlying brain damage, prior ECT, and drug or alcohol use or withdrawal. Seizures induced by antidepressants usually occur in the first week of treatment and are related to excessive or sudden elevations in serum antidepressant concentration and to use of multiple medications.

Antidepressants lower the seizure threshold and readily precipitate seizures in epileptic individuals. In high enough doses or under certain circumstances, antidepressants can cause seizures in depressed nonepileptic individuals. However, when patients develop seizures, physicians must guard against reflexively blaming medications. Structural lesions, such as a brain tumor, might be the cause of both depression and seizure. Moreover, seizures in depressed patients may result from a deliberate drug overdose, and some seizurelike episodes might actually be pseudoseizures.

TABLE 10–2. *International Classification of Epilepsies (Modified Version)*

Partial (or focal) epilepsies
    Partial seizures with elementary symptomatology: *Without* impairment of consciousness
    Partial seizures with complex symptomatology: *With* impairment of consciousness
    Partial seizures with secondary generalization
Generalized epilepsies
    Primary generalized epilepsies
        Absences (petit mal)
        Tonic-clonic (grand mal)

Tricyclic antidepressants are associated with a seizure in about 1% or less of patients. For example, depending on dose, imipramine has a seizure rate of 0.1% to 1.1% and amitriptyline a rate of approximately 0.9%. The heterocyclic maprotiline had a high rate of seizures until recommended doses were reduced.

Clomipramine (Anafranil) has led to seizures in 1.5% of patients taking 300 mg or less per day. This relatively high rate of seizures represents clomipramine's most significant adverse reaction. Moreover, this risk does not diminish over time, as with most other antidepressants.

Especially compared to the tricyclic and heterocyclic antidepressant therapy, SSRI therapy is almost never complicated by seizures. The following SSRIs have an incidence of less than 0.3%: citalopram, fluoxetine, fluvoxamine, mirtazapine, nefazodone, paroxetine, sertraline, and venlafaxine

Despite their other hazards, monoamine oxidase inhibitors (MAOIs) carry only a minute risk of seizures—less than 0.012%. In fact, MAOIs may possess antiepileptic activity.

Alprazolam and lithium carry a low incidence of seizures. However, abrupt withdrawal from any benzodiazepine notoriously leads to seizures and even status epilepticus.

ECT in epilepsy patients who are depressed can be beneficial. (The treatment originated in neuropsychiatrists' observing that depressed epileptic patients' mood improved after a seizure.) Although ECT may be complicated by prolonged seizures, that complication is rare and readily treated.

SEIZURE VARIETIES

The two major seizure categories are *partial seizures* and *primary generalized (generalized) seizures*. Most partial seizures are classified either as *partial with elementary symptoms* or *partial with complex symptoms*. Most generalized seizures are classified as either *absences* or *tonic-clonic seizures* (Table 10–2).

Partial seizures are said to have *elementary* symptoms when their clinical manifestations consist of only a particular movement or sensation without alteration in consciousness. Impaired consciousness, with or without psychologic abnormalities, constitutes a *complex* symptom. Both varieties of partial seizures originate from paroxysmal electrical discharges in a discrete region of the cerebral cortex—the *focus*. For example, partial seizures with motor symptoms are attributable to a focus in the contralateral frontal lobe. These and other seizures consist of similar, *stereotyped* symptoms for each patient in almost every episode. Thus, variable symptoms suggest a nonepileptic disorder.

Most partial seizures last between several seconds and several minutes. However, in a condition known as *epilepsia partialis continua* or *focal status epilepticus*, they continue for many hours or days. As long as the discharge remains confined to its focus, the original symptoms persist. Patients with partial complex status epilepticus may remain alert and ambulatory but usually very dull and immobile. The seizures, continuing without intermission, interfere with complex mental and physical activity; however, patients can continue to perform routine *despite* the seizure.

More often, however, the cerebral cortex discharges spread in a slow, brush-fire-like manner to adjacent cortical areas. Including more of the cortex usually produces additional symptoms. Then discharges can spread over the entire cortex. Sometimes they travel directly through the corpus callosum to the contralateral cerebral hemisphere. If the entire cerebral cortex is engulfed *(secondary generalization)*, patients lose consciousness, develop bilateral motor activity, and have generalized EEG abnormalities. Despite the seizure's final, all-encompassing nature, it would still be called a partial seizure with secondary generalization because nomenclature is based on initial manifestations.

In primary generalized seizures, the thalamus or other subcortical structure generates discharges. They immediately spread upward to excite the entire cerebral cortex. Primary generalized seizures are bilateral, symmetric, and without focal clinical or EEG findings.

Usually caused by a genetic propensity (from one or more genes) or a metabolic aberration, primary generalized seizures are characterized by unconsciousness and generalized EEG abnormalities; however, they do not necessarily generate gross motor activity. Generalized seizures can persist for many hours, in which case they become a life-threatening condition, *generalized status epilepticus.*

PARTIAL ELEMENTARY SEIZURES

Partial seizures with elementary *motor* symptoms, formerly called focal motor seizures, usually consist of rhythmic jerking (clonic movement) of a body region that may be as limited as one finger or as extensive as an entire side (Fig. 10–7). These

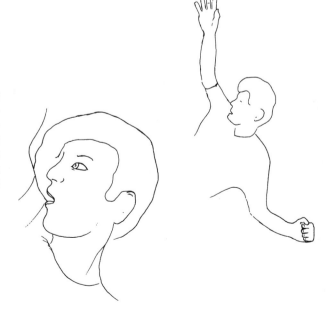

FIGURE 10–7. In a patient having a partial seizure with motor symptoms, his head, neck, and eyes deviated toward the right, his right arm extended, and his left flexed. This entire "adversive posture" results from a focal epileptic discharge in the contralateral left frontal lobe.

seizures can develop into focal status epilepticus or undergo secondary generalization. Sometimes, in a "Jacksonian march," a seizure discharge spreads along the motor cortex, and movements that began in one finger extend to the entire arm and then the face. After a partial motor seizure, affected muscles may be weakened. A postictal *(Todd's)* monoparesis or hemiparesis may persist for up to 24 hours. Thus, the differential diagnosis of transient hemiparesis includes transient ischemic attacks (TIAs), hemiplegic migraines, conversion disorder, and Todd's hemiparesis.

Seizures with elementary *sensory* symptoms, which usually are attributed to a focus in the parietal lobe's sensory cortex, typically consist of tingling or burning paresthesias in body regions with extensive cortical representation, such as the face. Sometimes sensory loss, a "negative symptom," might be a seizure's only manifestation.

Partial elementary seizures with "special sensory" symptoms consist of specific simple auditory, visual, or olfactory sensations. Although these symptoms are so vivid that they can be described as "hallucinations," patients readily recognize them as manifestations of cerebral dysfunction rather than actual events.

Auditory symptoms, which are attributable to temporal lobe lesions, usually consist of repetitive noises, musical notes, or single, meaningless words. Visual symptoms, which are attributable to occipital lesions, usually consist of relatively simple or elementary bright lines, spots, or splotches of color that move slowly across the visual field or, like a view through a kaleidoscope, stars rotating around the center of vision. In contrast, elaborate visual seizure phenomena, alone or combined with other sensory symptoms or emotional changes, are complex symptoms that must be differentiated from other visual hallucinations (see Table 12–1).

Olfactory symptoms classically consist of smelling vaguely recognizable odors, such as the frequently cited one of burning rubber. However, contrary to popular belief, these odors are not necessarily repugnant. Because olfactory hallucinations usually result from discharges in the amygdala or the *uncus* (the anterior inferior tip of the temporal lobe), partial seizures with olfactory symptoms are often called *uncinate seizures* or *fits.* As with sensory symptoms, olfactory hallucinations are actually the initial phase of the seizure rather than merely a warning of one. If discharges spread from those regions to engulf a larger area of the temporal lobe, they trigger partial complex seizures.

EEG and Etiology

During partial elementary seizures, EEGs show spikes, slow waves, or spike-wave complexes overlying the seizure focus. For example, during seizures with motor symptoms, EEG abnormalities may be prominent in channels over the frontal lobe (Fig. 10–8) and, during the interictal period, EEGs may still show occasional spikes in the same channels.

Depending mostly on the patient's age at seizures' onset, particular lesions may be suspected. When young children develop partial seizures, typical causes are congenital cerebral injuries (see below), neonatal meningitis, and neurocutaneous disorders (see Chapter 13).

In young adults, common causes of partial elementary seizures are head trauma, arteriovenous malformations (AVMs), and previously asymptomatic congenital injuries. Posttraumatic seizures are associated not with trivial head injuries but with trauma causing more than 30 minutes of unconsciousness, a depressed (not just linear) skull fracture, an intracranial hematoma, or a penetrating wound. Young adults with major psychiatric disturbances, particularly autism, are prone to seizures. Also, genetic disorders can cause both partial and generalized seizures.

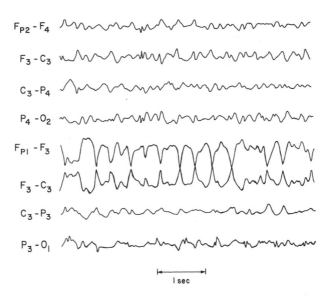

$F_{P2}-F_4$

F_3-C_3

C_3-P_4

P_4-O_2

$F_{PI}-F_3$

F_3-C_3

C_3-P_3

P_3-O_I

I sec

FIGURE 10–8. This EEG obtained during a partial seizure with motor symptoms contains a paroxysm of 4-Hz sharp-wave activity with phase reversals referable to the F_3 electrode. Because this electrode overlies the left frontal region, the seizure probably consists of right face or arm motor activity and, in 50% of cases, a deviation of the head and eyes to the right.

Drug and alcohol abuse carries multiple neurologic ramifications and should be considered in young adults presenting with seizures. Especially when seizures are accompanied by psychotic or otherwise abnormal behavior, physicians should suspect cocaine, PCP, and amphetamine intoxication. Cocaine reduces seizure threshold, causes strokes, leads to noncompliance with established AED regimens, and is associated with inadequate nutrition and sleep. Seizures induced by these drugs occur immediately or soon after use.

Withdrawal from benzodiazepines (especially alprazolam) and daily high alcohol consumption also produces seizures after several days to a week. Most cases of benzodiazepine-withdrawal seizures are associated with prescription medications rather than "street" drugs. Withdrawal seizures often evolve into status epilepticus.

A seizure associated with drug or alcohol abuse does not necessarily constitute epilepsy but can reveal dependency or addiction. Moreover, they may have been caused by an acute, life-threatening neurologic complication rather than the drug itself. For example, cocaine routinely causes cerebral hemorrhages that in turn cause seizures. Similarly, heroin and other drugs, which themselves usually do not cause seizures, can lead to bacterial endocarditis, acquired immune deficiency syndrome (AIDS), hepatitis, and vasculitis, which all cause seizures.

Adults aged 40 to 60 years develop seizures most often because of a structural lesion, typically a primary or metastatic brain tumor. Older people are more likely to have a stroke rather than a tumor. In South and Central Americans, cysticercosis infection is the most common structural lesion that induces seizures; in young adults with AIDS, it is cerebral toxoplasmosis.

PARTIAL COMPLEX SEIZURES

Usually, partial complex seizures begin between patients' late childhood and early 30s. Affecting about 65% of epilepsy patients, they are the most common seizure variety. EEG-video monitoring studies have defined ictal and postictal seizure manifestations and separated them from nonepileptic disturbances. Still unclear, however, is the genuineness of patients' reports of a broad range of ictal symptoms, including violence. Another puzzle is epilepsy's relationship to interictal personality traits, violence, and cognitive impairment.

Before discussing partial complex seizures, however, a note on nomenclature must be inserted. The older literature used the less accurate titles, *psychomotor seizures* and *temporal lobe seizures* or *epilepsy (TLE)* to name these disturbances. "Psychomotor seizures" is properly applied only to the rare partial complex seizures with exclusively behavioral abnormalities. Likewise, TLE is inappropriate because the seizure focus in about 10% of cases is not located in the temporal lobe (see below, Frontal Lobe Seizures). TLE is also inconsistent with the current classification of seizures according to symptoms rather than anatomic origin.

Symptoms of partial complex seizures in about 10% of patients include a characteristic premonitory sensation, an *aura*. Not merely a warning, it constitutes the first part of the seizure.

During most of a partial complex seizure, patients usually display only a blank stare and are inattentive and uncommunicative. They always (by definition) have impaired consciousness. In most cases, they also have partial or complete memory loss, *amnesia*, presumably because the limbic system in the temporal lobe is beset with seizure discharges. The amnesia is so striking that it may seem to be a patient's only symptom. (Partial complex seizures, therefore, must be strongly considered among the neurologic causes of the *acute amnestic syndrome* [see Table 7–1].)

Physical manifestations of partial complex seizures usually consist of only simple, repetitive, purposeless movements *(automatisms)* of the face and hands. Present in more than 80% of these seizures, common automatisms include repetitive swallowing, kissing, lip-smacking, fumbling with clothing, scratching, and rubbing the abdomen (Fig. 10–9). Other physical manifestations are simple actions, such as standing, walking, and pacing, or even driving; however, sometimes these actions are simply ingrained tasks that continue despite the seizure. In addition, about 25% of patients utter brief phrases or unintelligible sounds.

Many times the environment triggers actions and words. For example, a child may clutch and continually stroke a nearby stuffed animal while repeating an endearing phrase. What would distinguish this activity from normal behavior would be impaired consciousness, apparent self-absorption, and subsequent failure to recall the event.

Symptoms might occasionally be elaborate visual or auditory hallucinations accompanied by appropriate emotions. Although often dramatic, these symptoms are rare.

Similarly, the various "experiential phenomena," such as *déjà vu*, *jamais vu*, dreamlike states, mind-body dissociations, and floating feelings, cannot automatically be accepted as seizure symptoms. They are rarely associated with other clinical or EEG

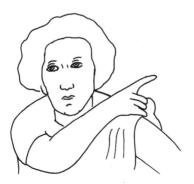

FIGURE 10–9. During partial complex seizures, patients are typically dazed. They perform rudimentary, purposeless actions, such as pulling on their clothing, paying little or no attention. Their hands and fingers are clumsy and often misdirected. Repetitive, simple body movements, *automatisms*, such as lip smacking, are present in 80% of cases.

evidence of seizures. Experiential phenomena are not only nonspecific, they have also been so popularized that they have virtually no diagnostic value.

Another frequently encountered symptom with a dubious association with partial complex seizures is the *rising epigastric sensation.* It consists of a sensation of swelling in the abdomen that, as if progressing upward within the body, turns into tightness in the throat and then suffocation. Although it could be an aura, the rising epigastric sensation has a striking similarity to a panic attack and *globus hystericus,* a common psychogenic disturbance in which people also feel tightening of the throat and an inability to breathe.

After an actual partial complex seizure, which usually has a duration of 2 to 3 minutes, patients characteristically experience postictal confusion, clouding of the sensorium, disorientation, a flat affect, and sleepiness. Postictal confusion may be intensified if a seizure involves the brain's language arc and causes transient aphasia (see Chapter 8). Similarly, if the seizure focus includes the corticospinal tract, patients may have a Todd's hemiparesis. For 15 to 30 minutes after the seizure, at least 40% of patients have an elevated serum prolactin concentration. They may also have focal postictal EEG depression.

Most partial complex seizures eventually undergo secondary generalization. Thus, a guideline for differentiating them from a recurring psychogenic event is that at least every 1 to 2 years a partial complex seizure will evolve into a generalized seizure.

Another important complication of partial complex seizures is *partial complex status epilepticus.* In the absence of automatisms or other movements, when manifestations are exclusively psychological aberrations or a change in sensorium, it may be referred to as *nonconvulsive status epilepticus.* Despite the prevalence of such a disorder in popular literature as a cause of bizarre behavior, it is rare in neurologic practices. Patients in partial complex status epilepticus experience up to 24 hours of confusion accompanied by thought and language disorders, automatisms, or other purposeless motor activity. Episodes may mimic schizophrenia and occasionally merit their description, *ictal psychosis.*

Otherwise, partial complex seizures and psychotic episodes are unlikely to be mistaken for each other. Partial complex seizures last only a few minutes, are stereotyped, necessarily include impaired consciousness, and have a postictal period characterized by sleepiness, amnesia, and often behavioral changes and thought disturbances. Patients gradually return to their interictal personality, which admittedly might be abnormal. Psychotic episodes, in contrast, are often triggered by the environment, have a duration of at least several days, vary greatly in their manifestations, which often include hypervigilance, and are not followed by sleepiness and amnesia.

Frontal Lobe Seizures

Seizures that originate in the frontal lobe, *frontal lobe seizures,* constitute a distinct, important variety of partial complex seizures. Compared to conventional partial complex seizures, their manifestations more often consist of abrupt, aura-less onset of vocalizations, bilateral complex movements, relatively short duration (less than 1 minute), and little or no postictal confusion. In addition, frontal lobe seizures tend to begin in adult years, occur relatively frequently (several times a month), develop predominantly during sleep, and produce discharges difficult to detect by conventional EEG.

With their manifestations so bizarre and paroxysmal changes so rarely detectable on a routine EEG, frontal lobe seizures mimic *pseudoseizures* (psychogenic seizures, a variety of nonepileptic seizures, see below). Also, when they begin exclusively during sleep, frontal lobe seizures mimic sleep disorders (see Chapter 17).

Ictal Sex

During a seizure, patients commonly fumble with buttons or tug at their clothing, and thus may seem to undress partially, but they are not exposing themselves or attempting to engage in sex. Less common seizure activity with sexual overtones includes rudimentary masturbatory movements and scratching of the perineum. Except for rare instances, seizures are unaccompanied by erotic or interactive sexual behavior. Most seizurelike symptoms, particularly hyperventilation, that develop during sexual activity are simply manifestations of anxiety.

Ictal Violence and Aggression

EEG-video monitoring has demonstrated that *ictal* violence usually consists only of random shoving, pushing, kicking, or verbal abuse, such as screaming. This behavior is fragmented, unsustained, and, most important, unaccompanied by rage or anger. Less than 0.1% of seizures include violence. Moreover, it is virtually never the sole manifestation of a partial complex or any other type of seizure.

Another type of violence associated with seizures, *resistive violence*, occurs when patients are restrained during the ictal or postictal period. It naturally occurs much more frequently than ictal violence and stems, in part, from patients' naturally fighting off people who attempt to restrain them or give them injections. Family members, as well as health care workers, can provoke it.

Seizure-related violence, and possibly violence in general, must be distinguished from aggression (see below, episodic dyscontrol syndrome). Although violence injures people or damages property, it is not consciously directed and does not result from anger. Neither ictal nor resistive violence is directed or purposefully destructive.

Aggression, on the other hand, encompasses not only deliberately offensive destruction and injury but also threats or seizing control. It is accompanied by a consistent affect and has a conscious or unconscious rationale. Aggression is a prerequisite for violent crimes.

During seizures, patients cannot engage in sequential activities, premeditated actions, or meaningful interactions with other people. They cannot operate mechanical devices. These limitations preclude violent crimes either in the midst of a seizure or as a manifestation of a seizure. Most neurologists believe violence may be accepted as a rare manifestation of seizures, but aggression and performing criminal activities cannot be attributed to seizures.

Interictal Mental Abnormalities

Personality Traits.   Classic studies by Bear, Fedio, and others described temporal lobe epilepsy patients as distinctively circumstantial, hyposexual, humorless, "sticky" in interpersonal relations, and overly concerned with general philosophic and religious questions, such as the order of the universe. They often would write excessively and compulsively *(hypergraphia)*. Supporting studies suggested that these and other emotional traits depended on whether the seizure focus was in the right or left temporal lobe. Right-sided foci supposedly predisposed a patient to anger, sadness, and elation but left-sided ones to ruminative and intellectual tendencies.

Recent studies, based on EEG-video monitoring and strict methodology, have either not corroborated those personality traits or found them in as little as 7% of patients with partial complex seizures. In fact, these same traits were found in patients without epilepsy. For example, hypergraphia can be a symptom of schizophrenia or bipolar disorder. The studies also found no difference in personality traits when foci are in different temporal lobes or even other brain areas and no difference in personality traits among patients with different varieties of epilepsy.

As a general rule, personality changes and cognitive impairment—to the extent that they exist—are associated with other markers of extensive brain damage, such as the onset of seizures in childhood, episodes of status epilepticus, multiple seizure types, need for two or more AEDs, and abnormalities on the neurologic examination, CT, or MRI.

In view of the underlying brain damage, previous editions of the *Diagnostic and Statistical Manual of Mental Disorders (DSM)* have classified personality traits associated with epilepsy, in view of the underlying brain damage, with the well-known term "organic personality disorder." In *DSM-IV*, they are classified—in equally broad terms—as constituting a *Personality Disorder NOS* or a *Personality Change Due to a General Medical Condition.*

"Schizophreniform Psychosis." Partial complex seizures are associated in up to 10% of patients with schizophrenia-related symptoms (subsumed in Slater and Beard's term "schizophreniform psychosis"), such as hallucinations, paranoia, and social isolation. However, unlike typical schizophrenic patients, seizure patients' affect is relatively normal, they do not deteriorate, and their families do not have an increased incidence of schizophrenia. The schizophrenia-related symptoms arise, on the average, when patients are 30 years old and when epilepsy began in childhood, especially between ages 5 and 10 years.

Pathologic studies show that epilepsy patients with psychosis, compared to those without psychosis, have larger cerebral ventricles, greater periventricular gliosis, and increased focal damage. In contrast, multiple sclerosis (MS) patients, despite having equally extensive cerebral damage, rarely have schizophrenic symptoms.

Many studies have reported that psychosis complicates epilepsy when seizures are frequent. Sometimes—as in *postictal psychosis*—psychotic behavior or thoughts begin after a flurry of seizures. Occasionally, in the opposite situation, vigorous AED suppression of seizures ("forced normalization," see below) seems to precipitate psychosis or, less often, depression.

In treating acute schizophreniform psychosis or other psychoses in epileptic patients, routine psychiatric medications can be added, but AEDs should remain the mainstay of treatment. In addition, the physician must keep in mind that haloperidol, chlorpromazine, and other antipsychotic agents may either directly precipitate seizures or adversely interact with AEDs.

Distinguishing features of psychosis arising in epileptic patients are mostly neurologic and epidemiologic and do not constitute a distinct psychiatric symptom complex. In *DSM-IV*, the psychosis associated with epilepsy should be included in the category of *Psychosis Due to a Medical Condition (Epilepsy).*

Cognitive Impairment. Many individuals have a combination of epilepsy, mental retardation, and congenital neurologic deficits, that is, static encephalopathy or cerebral palsy (see Chapter 13). In them, incidence of epilepsy, which usually becomes evident before age 5 years, increases in proportion to physical and intellectual impairments. In addition, some of these individuals with little or no mental retardation have been uneducated. Overall, 10% to 20% of individuals with either mental retardation or cerebral palsy have epilepsy. Of mentally retarded individuals in institutions, 40% have epilepsy.

Whether their cause is static or progressive brain injury, seizures are deleterious because they disrupt normal biochemical and physiologic processes, lead to head trauma, and may cause cerebral anoxia. In addition, seizures from mesial temporal sclerosis progressively damage the surrounding limbic system, which is the basis of the memory circuit. Seizures also require AED treatment that places another burden on cognitive function.

When the brain damage underlying seizures is progressive—as in tuberous sclerosis—seizure control, cognitive capacity, and motor function decline. Conversely, progressive cognitive decline or increasingly refractory seizures suggests a progressive rather than a static neurologic disorder.

Cognitive decline must also be distinguished from development of depression and other psychiatric complications. These problems, which can develop separately or together, may result from the underlying neurologic disorder, the seizures, or AEDs.

Crime and Interictal Violence.   Although incidence of epilepsy is at least four times as great among men in prison as in the general population, crimes of epileptic prisoners are no more violent than those of nonepileptic ones. Conversely, prevalence of epilepsy is the same in nonviolent as violent criminals. Also, EEG abnormalities do not correlate with violent offenses. Among neurologists, consensus is that epilepsy does not cause either crime or violence. Instead, epilepsy, head trauma, and congenital or acquired brain injury lead to poor impulse control, lower socioeconomic status, and other conditions that steer people to crime.

Interictal rather than ictal violence tends to occur in epilepsy patients who are schizophrenic or mentally retarded. Underlying neurologic, psychiatric, and social disorders alone—without epilepsy—are sufficient to account for interictal violence and aggressive personality traits.

Depression.   Depression is more prevalent in epilepsy patients than in those with comparable disabilities. It occurs particularly in epilepsy patients who have partial complex seizures, are male, or require multiple AEDs. Unlike the risk factors for schizophreniform psychosis, depression is not related to the duration of epilepsy, seizure frequency, or a family history of depression. Also, epilepsy-associated depression is rarely bipolar.

Suicide occurs four to five times more frequently in epilepsy patients, particularly those with partial complex seizures, than in the general population. In such instances, it is more likely to be a manifestation of psychotic behavior or a borderline personality disorder than a result of depression. (Other neurologic illnesses associated with an increased incidence of suicide are MS, Huntington's disease, spinal cord transection, and AIDS dementia.)

Another aspect of depression may be refractory seizures. Sometimes depressed epilepsy patients are neglectful or surreptitiously noncompliant with their AED regimen. Also, they may consciously or unconsciously superimpose pseudoseizures on epileptic seizures. Also, depression-associated behavior, such as sleep deprivation or drug or alcohol abuse, may precipitate seizures.

Treatment of depression in epileptic patients should rest less on psychotherapy and more on psychopharmacology, which often produces better control of epilepsy, as well as improvement in mood. Nevertheless, antidepressants must be given cautiously in epilepsy patients because they can interact with AEDs. As discussed previously, even by themselves at therapeutic concentrations, antidepressants can produce seizures.

Confusion.   The most common cause of confusion and related disturbances in epilepsy patients is simply a prolonged postictal period. During this time, patients may be disoriented, amnestic, and possibly aphasic. Their affect is typically flat, and they may have paranoid delusions and hallucinations. They might act in an irrational, agitated, and belligerent manner that suggests a serious psychiatric illness.

Another cause of confusion in epilepsy patients is AED intoxication inadvertently induced by changes in a medication regimen, including adding psychotropics and another AED. For example, the addition of lamotrigine to valproate (valproic acid/divalproex) readily precipitates toxicity. In addition, occasionally patients deliberately induce intoxication by taking an AED in excessive quantities or mixing it with alcohol or illicit drugs.

Confusion may also be produced by prolonged seizures—partial complex or absence status epilepticus ("nonconvulsive status epilepticus"). Such seizures may cause mental changes without overt physical abnormalities. Seizures also lead to head trauma that can be further complicated by intracranial bleeding.

A rare and controversial cause of confusion and other mental impairments is *forced normalization*. In this condition, after AEDs have controlled an epileptic patient's seizures and "forced" the EEG to be normal, the patient develops psychotic behavior or, in some cases, depression. The usual explanation is that the seizures had suppressed a psychosis or mood disorder. In any case, physicians should closely monitor patients who suddenly achieve complete seizure control.

At the other extreme, a flurry of seizures or even status epilepticus may result from abruptly withdrawing AEDs. The risk is especially great after withdrawal of benzodiazepines and phenobarbital. In an important variation of that theme, *withdrawal-emergent psychopathology*, discontinuing AEDs produces or unmasks anxiety, depression, and other psychiatric disorder in about a third of patients. In general, the AEDs presumably had a soporific effect on the patient's psychiatric disorder, as well as the epilepsy. In particular, an AED might have been vital to a patient with bipolar disorder. Withdrawal-emergent psychopathology is apparently analogous to *withdrawal emergent dyskinesia*, in which tardive dyskinesia-like movements appear after withdrawal of antipsychotic agents (see Chapter 18).

Testing During and After Partial Complex Seizures

EEG. During a partial complex seizure, the EEG ideally shows paroxysms of spikes, slow waves, or other abnormalities in channels overlying the temporal or frontotemporal region. Even though a seizure focus may be unilateral, bilateral EEG abnormalities may be present because of additional foci, interhemispheric projections, or "reflections."

In the interictal period, the routine EEG contains spikes or spike and slow-wave complexes over the temporal lobes in about 40% of cases. When accompanied by an appropriate history, these EEG abnormalities are specific enough to corroborate the diagnosis. Looking at the situation in reverse, about 90% of persons with anterior temporal spikes on the EEG will have partial complex seizures. Nevertheless, diagnosis of seizures should not be based only on EEG spikes. Diagnosis of partial complex or other seizures requires correlation of EEG abnormalities with symptoms and signs.

If diagnosis remains a problem, especially where episodic behavioral abnormalities are believed to result from seizures, EEG-video monitoring should be used. EEG corroboration of partial complex seizures should rely first on routine EEG, which has a 40% yield; EEG during sleep and wakefulness or following sleep deprivation; and, finally, EEG-video monitoring, with virtually a 100% yield. To determine origin and other facts about individual cases of partial complex seizures, neurologists sometimes use nasopharyngeal and other specially placed leads (Fig. 10–10).

Other Tests. Because partial elementary and partial complex seizures usually originate from structural lesions, neurologists routinely order a CT or MRI (see Chap-

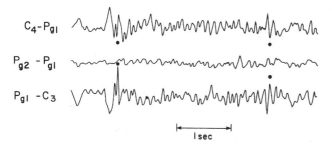

FIGURE 10–10. An interictal EEG with nasopharyngeal electrodes (Pg_1 and Pg_2) shows phase-reversed spikes that routine scalp electrodes may not detect.

ter 20). These tests may reveal clinically unsuspected temporal lobe atrophy, tuberous sclerosis nodules, strokes, and AVMs. In partial complex epilepsy, an MRI with thin cuts through the temporal lobes is preferable to a CT. An MRI can more readily detect the common underlying structural abnormalities, such as mesial temporal lobe sclerosis, minute vascular malformations, or other cryptic lesions. Moreover, it offers greater resolution and freedom from artifacts produced by the bones surrounding the middle fossa (see Fig. 20–20).

A CT or MRI is also performed for tonic-clonic seizures because clinical and EEG data may not be able to distinguish between primary generalized seizures and partial seizures with secondary generalization. With drug- or alcohol-withdrawal seizures and absences (see below), these scans may be unnecessary.

Positron emission tomography (PET) has been used to study cerebral metabolism in epilepsy and to plan surgery in epilepsy patients with partial complex seizures. With those seizures, PET studies interictally show that the affected temporal lobe—a region usually far larger than the actual focus—is hypometabolic. However, PET's relatively low resolution does not permit further localization.

Magnetoencephalography (MEG) provides a plot of magnetic fields. Its equipment, which is as expensive and complex as MRI equipment, can be coupled with the EEG to combine electric and magnetic images. MEG by itself is not yet useful in the diagnosis or treatment of epilepsy or any other illness.

Etiology

Lesions that cause partial complex seizures include temporal lobe hamartomas, astrocytomas, mesial temporal sclerosis, and those that cause partial elementary seizures (see above). Mesial temporal sclerosis, probably the most common cause of partial complex seizures, is characterized by sclerosis of the hippocampus and temporal lobe atrophy.

Except in about 10% of cases, the lesion is within the temporal lobe. Like other seizures, partial complex seizures may be precipitated by menses, sleep deprivation, intercurrent illness, and low AED serum concentration. (Almost 80% of women with epilepsy report an increase in seizure frequency before menses.)

AEDs

Usually the first and only treatment for epilepsy consists of AEDs (Table 10–3). They are also widely used for other neurologic disorders, including migraines, trigeminal neuralgia, various painful conditions (chronic pain, neuropathic pain, and painful diabetic polyneuropathy [see Chapter 14]). The mechanism of AEDs' action is largely unknown; however, several AEDs increase gamma-aminobutyric acid (GABA), which is an inhibitory neurotransmitter.

Clinical experience provides several reliable guidelines. Treatment with a single AED, *monotherapy,* is preferable to treatment with two or more, *polypharmacy.* Monotherapy minimizes side effects, noncompliance, and, in most cases, cost.

Moreover, except in an emergency, AEDs must be introduced slowly. Because AEDs are most often metabolized primarily in the liver, they may alter the metabolism of various psychotropics and each other. For example, phenytoin lowers the effectiveness, usually by reducing the serum concentration, of haloperidol, clozapine, methadone, and oral contraceptives. Beginning to treat a patient who takes daily methadone with phenytoin, in other words, will precipitate a narcotic withdrawal syndrome unless the methadone dose is raised. Similarly, if a woman who takes birth-control pills begins to take phenytoin, carbamazepine, phenobarbital, or topiramate, the efficacy of the contraceptive may be reduced so much that she may conceive. Moreover, the fetus will be exposed to the potential teratogenic effects of the AED. On the other hand, physicians may safely discontinue an AED in many patients, especially children, if they can provide careful planning, slow withdrawal, and subsequent monitoring.

Mental Side Effects. In general, excessive concentrations of AEDs cause cognitive impairment, confusion, lethargy, and, in extreme cases, stupor or coma. Cognitive impairment typically consists of memory difficulties, intellectual dulling, and inattention. AEDs can superimpose this burden not only on individuals already coping with neurologic deficits but also on psychiatric patients.

Cognitive impairment from AEDs usually results from polypharmacy, excessive medication concentration, too rapid introduction of the medication, or use of phenobarbital or primidone. Impairment from phenytoin is partly attributable to slowed motor activity that impairs performance on timed psychologic tests. Carbamazepine, on the other hand, produces a beneficial effect that probably results from its structural similarity to the tricyclic antidepressants. Phenytoin, carbamazepine, and valproate—the older AEDs—otherwise do not create significant differences in incidence or type of cognitive impairment. Preliminary information on the newer AEDs indicates that gabapentin and lamotrigine produce only minimal impairments but that topiramate may initially impair attention and word fluency.

AEDs also can produce severely disordered thinking and personality changes that can rise to the level of a psychosis. The primary example, although rare, is psychosis

TABLE 10–3. *Commonly Used AEDs*

AED	Usual Daily Dose (mg)	Therapeutic Serum Concentration (µ/ml)*
Carbamazepine (Tegretol)†	600–1200	5–12
Divalproex (Depakote)	1500–2000	50–100
Ethosuximide (Zarontin)	2000	40–100
Gabapentin (Neurontin)	900–1800	
Lamotrigine (Lamictal)	100–500	
Phenytoin (Dilantin)	300–400	10–20
Topiramate (Topamax)	400	

*Recommended concentrations vary and should be altered by the clinical situation. Often a "subtherapeutic level" is sufficient, and increasing the dose will create side effects without improving seizure control.

†To reach a steady state, five "half-lives" are required (e.g., carbamazepine 4–6 days; phenytoin 5–10 days; and valproate 3–6 days).

N.B.: These AEDs have mostly replaced phenobarbital and its closely related AED, primidone (Mysoline), which both cause inordinate sedation and cognitive impairment. Also, barbiturates, particularly when used in children and adults with brain damage, may produce a "paradoxical reaction" of excitement and hyperactivity rather than sedation.

precipitated by AEDs suddenly stopping seizures, that is, "forced normalization" (see above). In general, patients most apt to develop AED-induced behavioral changes are those with a history of epilepsy that has had an onset in early life, secondarily generalized seizures, and EEGs showing bilateral changes. Iatrogenic behavioral changes are also apt to develop in epilepsy patients with a history of an affective disorder or, less so, psychosis.

Physical Side Effects.   Even at therapeutic levels, most AEDs can cause liver abnormalities and bone marrow suppression. While frequent, those side effects are usually self-limited and harmless. Use of many AEDs involves checking patients' white blood count and liver function tests, as well as the serum AED concentration. Individual AEDs may also require evaluation of other organs.

Phenytoin (hydantoin or diphenylhydantoin [Dilantin]) intoxication causes a well-known combination of nystagmus, ataxia, and dysarthria. Many AEDs can induce a benign rash shortly after they are initiated. More important, but rarely and unpredictably, they cause a fulminant, potentially fatal mucocutaneous allergic reaction, the *Stevens-Johnson syndrome* (erythema multiforme). This condition, which begins as a rash, consists of blisters on the mouth, eyes, and skin that are often weeping and confluent. The disrupted skin and mucus membranes leak serum, fluid, and electrolytes and allow bacteria to invade the bloodstream.

AEDs and Pregnancy.   Apart from a fetus' exposure to AEDs, epilepsy itself carries a teratogenic risk. For mothers with epilepsy, the rate of fetal malformations—exclusive of AED-induced malformations—is approximately 5%. That rate is approximately twice that for nonepileptic mothers. If only the father has epilepsy, there is still an increased but lesser teratogenic risk. Other risk factors for fetal malformations in mothers with epilepsy include a low socioeconomic status, older age, and a family history of fetal malformations.

AEDs increase the rate of fetal malformations, some of which are devastating. No AED is risk-free, and none exclusively induces a particular malformation. Phenobarbital and phenytoin carry only slightly greater risk of major congenital malformations than other AEDs.

Malformations associated with AEDs are probably induced during the first trimester when organs, particularly the CNS, are formed. The most serious—*meningomyelocele* and other *neural tube defects* (see Chapter 13)—have been closely but not exclusively associated almost equally with both carbamazepine (0.5%) and valproate (1%). AEDs also increase the rate of cleft lip, cleft palate, and ventricular septal defect.

Less severe fetal malformations are likewise not exclusively associated with any specific AED. In particular, *fetal hydantoin syndrome*, which includes craniofacial abnormalities and limb defects, is clearly not peculiar to hydantoin (phenytoin).

AEDs can also induce CNS abnormalities later in life. For example, hydantoin therapy begun before puberty may retard normal cerebellar growth. Through their effect on the hepatic cytochrome P-450 oxidases, AEDs can also increase or decrease concentration of other medications and thus have wide-ranging unexpected or unintended consequences. Carbamazepine, phenytoin, and phenobarbital induce P-450 enzymes but valproate inhibits them. Gabapentin and several other newer AEDs have little or no effect.

Several strategies have been proposed to reduce AEDs' teratogenic potential. Preconception planning should attempt to taper and discontinue the AED before conception through at least the first trimester, if not the entire pregnancy. If AEDs must be continued, the patient should take just one (monotherapy). Physicians should perform clinical evaluations and blood testing to assure the lowest dose that will suppress seizures.

Particularly to reduce the risk of neural tube defects, women should take folic acid before conception and during the pregnancy. Also, pregnant women taking valproate or carbamazepine should undergo tests to detect neural tube defects, such as ultrasound examination and serum α-fetoprotein determination. Because some AEDs (including phenobarbital, primidone, phenytoin, and carbamazepine) produce a deficiency in vitamin K–dependent clotting factors that can lead to intracerebral hemorrhage, obstetricians administer vitamin K in the third trimester to both mother and infant.

Surgery

When partial complex seizures are refractory to AEDs, surgical removal of a seizure focus with or without a surrounding portion of the brain may be highly beneficial. Approximately two-thirds of patients enjoy a virtually complete cessation of seizures. Another quarter has a major reduction in frequency. In addition, if only by reducing the need for multiple or high doses of AEDs, surgery often improves mental function.

Surgical candidates, who may be children or adolescents, as well as adults, ought to have a single frontal or temporal lobe lesion that is clearly identifiable on clinical, EEG, and radiographic testing. They must often undergo a Wada test (see Chapter 8) or substitute study to determine if surgery would likely be complicated by postoperative aphasia, amnesia, or other neuropsychologic problems. (If the dominant frontal or temporal lobes were injured during surgery, aphasia might result [see Chapter 8]. If both temporal lobes were damaged, from birth or during surgery, patients might also suffer from permanent amnesia and the Klüver-Bucy syndrome [see Chapters 12 and 16].)

Most patients also eventually enjoy a marked improvement in their psychosocial status after surgery, but that improvement may require many years and remains uncertain. Also, schizophreniform psychosis persists. Behavioral and cognitive capacity of less than 8% of patients deteriorates. These complications occur in spite of (or possibly because of) greater seizure control. Nevertheless, epilepsy surgery has been a major medical advance.

Under rare circumstances, individuals with intractable bilateral frontal seizures or infants with atonic seizures ("drop attacks") might benefit from a *commissurotomy* or *corpus callosotomy*. In this procedure, a neurosurgeon longitudinally splits the anterior two-thirds or entire corpus callosum, interrupting the spread of discharges between cerebral hemispheres. Despite its extent, postoperative deficits are so subtle that special neuropsychologic tests are required to demonstrate its major consequence, *split-brain syndrome* (see Fig. 8–8).

Vagus Nerve Stimulation

A newly introduced technique for reducing refractory seizures consists of an implanted pacemaker-like device that stimulates the vagus nerve in the neck, where it emerges from the base of the skull. The device sends electric impulses that ascend the vagus nerve, which is the tenth cranial nerve, into the medulla. The stimulation may suppress epileptic activity in the brainstem or spread to suppress cerebral cortical activity. This technique helps children and adults and suppresses generalized as well as partial seizures. It produces seizure suppression at least as effectively as the new AEDs but not as much as resection of a seizure focus.

Rolandic Epilepsy

Another variety of partial seizures is *rolandic epilepsy (benign childhood epilepsy with centrotemporal spikes)*. Virtually always beginning between ages 5 and 9 years, occurring predominantly in boys, and remitting by puberty, rolandic epilepsy is the most common partial epilepsy of childhood.

Rolandic seizures consist of unilateral paresthesias, movements of the face, and speech arrest. They tend to undergo secondary generalization during sleep. Interictal EEG changes—high-voltage spikes in the central temporal region (Rolandic spikes)—occur during sleep. AEDs readily suppress the seizures.

Unlike other partial epilepsies, this condition is restricted to childhood, not associated with an underlying structural lesion, and inherited (in an autosomal dominant pattern). Unlike children with absences (see below), those with rolandic epilepsy are not at risk of eventually developing other varieties of epilepsy.

GENERALIZED SEIZURES

Immediate loss of consciousness accompanied by bilateral, symmetric, synchronous, paroxysmal EEG discharges characterizes generalized seizures. These seizures are usually the result of either an autosomal dominant genetic disorder, a physiologic disturbance, or a metabolic aberration, including drug and alcohol withdrawal. In contrast to partial seizures, generalized seizures lack an aura, lateralized motor or sensory disturbances, and focal EEG abnormalities. Also, true generalized seizures, as opposed to secondary generalized seizures, practically never result from brain tumors, cerebral infarctions, or other structural lesions. Most generalized seizures are of either the absence *(petit mal)* or tonic-clonic *(grand mal)* variety.

Absences

Absence (petit mal) seizures usually begin between ages 4 and 10 years and disappear in early adulthood. The seizures, which can occur many times daily, consist of 2- to 10-second lapses in attention accompanied by automatisms, subtle clonic limb movements, or blinking (Fig. 10–11). The blinking sometimes occurs rhythmically at 3 Hz, which is the frequency of the associated EEG abnormality. During the seizure, children maintain muscle tone and bladder control, but their mental and physical activity is interrupted. After the seizure, as though it had never occurred, they have no retrograde amnesia, confusion, agitation, or sleepiness.

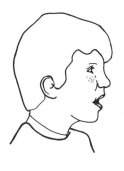 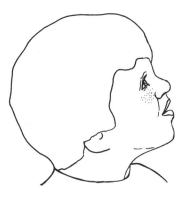

FIGURE 10–11. This 8-year-old boy talking to his parents suddenly, during an absence, has a 1- to 3-second staring spell. During the seizure, he becomes glassy-eyed and mute. He rolls his eyes upward and blinks at 3 Hz. Although he loses consciousness, he maintains bodily tone and does not become incontinent. Absence seizures and the accompanying EEG abnormality (Fig. 10–12) may be precipitated by having him slowly count numbers while hyperventilating. Typically, his seizures begin when the counting pauses. At the end of his seizure, he resumes talking to his parents.

TABLE 10–4. *Comparison of Partial Complex and Absence Seizures*

Feature	Partial Complex	Absence
Aura	Often	Never
Consciousness	Impaired	Lost at onset
Movements	Usually simple, repetitive but may include complex activity	Blinking and facial and finger automatisms
Postictal behavior	Amnesia, confusion, and tendency to sleep	No abnormality, except amnesia for ictus
Frequency	1 to 2 per week	Several daily
Duration	2 to 3 minutes	1 to 10 seconds
Precipitants		Hyperventilation, photic stimulation
EEG	Spikes and polyspike and waves, usually over both temporal regions	Generalized 3-Hz spike-and-wave complexes
AEDs	Carbamazepine, phenytoin	Ethosuximide, valproate

Children with unrecognized absences may be misdiagnosed as inattentive, dull, or even mentally retarded. Their seizures may be mislabeled as partial complex seizures, but the two conditions can be differentiated and treated differently (Table 10–4).

On occasion, *absence status epilepticus* leads to a several-hour episode of apathy, psychomotor retardation, and confusion. This condition usually typically develops in children and young adults, with a history of absences or other seizures, who have suddenly stopped taking their AEDs. Occasionally, children with absences can grow up to be adults with absences who are liable to develop absence status epilepticus. Absence status epilepticus in any age group may appear as an acute psychosis. If an EEG confirms a clinical diagnosis, intravenous benzodiazepine will abort an attack.

EEG, Etiology, and Treatment.   During an absence, the EEG shows synchronous 3-Hz spike and slow-wave complexes in all channels (Fig. 10–12). Even in the interictal period, an EEG reveals occasional asymptomatic bursts of 3-Hz spike and slow-wave complexes lasting 1 to 1.5 seconds. In patients with absences, either hyperventilation or photic stimulation can precipitate the characteristic clinical and EEG abnormalities. Just as the EEG abnormality is generalized, PET scans performed during absences show increased metabolism in the thalamus and entire cerebral cortex.

Patients' relatives often also have absences or 3-Hz spike and slow-wave complexes that can be precipitated by hyperventilation. This finding supports the hypothesis that a predisposition to absences is inherited in an autosomal dominant pattern. In contrast to tonic-clonic seizures, absences are not associated with drug withdrawal, metabolic aberrations, or structural lesions. Therefore, CTs and MRIs are usually not required.

Absences are treated with ethosuximide, valproate, or occasionally clonazepam. Most children readily respond to one or another of these AEDs. About two-thirds of children, as if "growing out of" epilepsy, enjoy a permanent remission during adolescence. In them, AEDs can be discontinued. In other children, tonic-clonic or other generalized seizures develop as a replacement or in conjunction with the absences.

Tonic-Clonic Seizures

Unlike absences, tonic-clonic seizures begin at any age after infancy, persist into adult life, and cause massive motor activity and profound postictal residua. Although

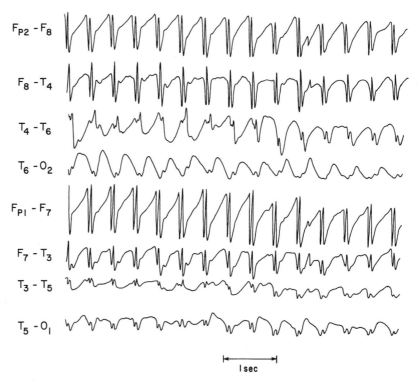

FIGURE 10–12. During an absence, the EEG characteristically shows regular, symmetric, and synchronous 3-Hz spike-and-wave complexes. The discharge arises from and returns to a normal EEG background.

patients may have a prodrome of malaise or a depressed mood, tonic-clonic seizures are usually an unheralded explosion. The initial tonic phase forces patients to lose consciousness; roll their eyes upward; and extend their neck, trunk, and limbs as if to form an arch. Immediately afterwards, in the dramatic clonic phase, the seizure violently and symmetrically jerks patients' limbs, neck, and trunk (Fig. 10–13).

A potential diagnostic problem is that during this terrible episode of tonic-clonic activity, the primary generalized seizure appears similar to a partial seizure that has undergone secondary generalization. Often only a detailed history, a trained observer, or an intraictal EEG can distinguish between them.

During the tonic phase, if the superimposed muscle EEG artifact can be eliminated by electronic filters, the EEG shows repetitive, increasingly higher amplitude spikes occurring with increasing frequency in all channels. In the clonic phase, the spikes, which become less frequent but greater in amplitude, are interrupted by slow waves (Fig. 10–14).

After the clonic phase, the EEG shows postictal depression. The postictal EEG is often the only one available, but it can confirm the diagnosis. Similarly, after ECT, the EEG is slow. After either a tonic-clonic seizure or ECT-induced seizure, the serum prolactin level rises for 15 to 30 minutes in many patients. After a pseudoseizure, in contrast, the EEG is relatively normal, and the prolactin level remains at baseline.

About 20% to 30% of patients with tonic-clonic seizures have interictal asymptomatic, brief bursts of spikes, polyspikes, or slow waves. Photic stimulation or hyperventilation may precipitate seizures and accompanying EEG abnormalities.

Etiology. Many cases of tonic-clonic epilepsy are the result of an autosomal dominant trait expressed between the ages of 5 and 30 years. In many cases, patients

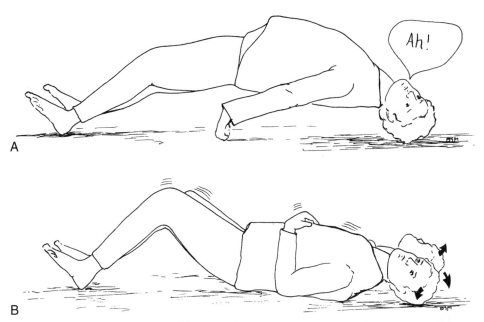

FIGURE 10–13. **A,** This patient in the tonic phase of a tonic-clonic seizure arches his torso and extends his arms and legs. He assumes this position because of the relatively greater strength of the extensor muscles compared to the flexor muscles. Simultaneous diaphragm, chest wall, and laryngeal muscle contractions force air through a tightened larynx and produce the shrill, epileptic cry. During this phase, patients often bite their tongue and involuntarily force urine out of their bladder. **B,** In the clonic phase, the patient's head, neck, and legs contract symmetrically and forcefully for about 10 to 20 seconds. Saliva, which becomes aerated and often blood-tinged from tongue lacerations, froths from his mouth. His pupils dilate, and he sweats profusely. Finally, his muscular contractions become progressively less frequent and weaker. The seizure usually ends with a sigh, followed by stertorous breathing. In the immediate postictal period, patients are unresponsive. Before regaining consciousness, patients may pass through a state of confusion and agitation, loosely called "postictal psychosis."

FIGURE 10–14. During a tonic-clonic seizure, the EEG ideally shows paroxysms of spikes, polyspikes, and occasional slow waves in all channels; however, muscle artifact can obscure this pattern. The interictal background EEG activity usually contains multiple bursts of generalized spikes. In contrast to occasional temporal lobe spikes, this is a pattern that confirms a diagnosis of epilepsy.

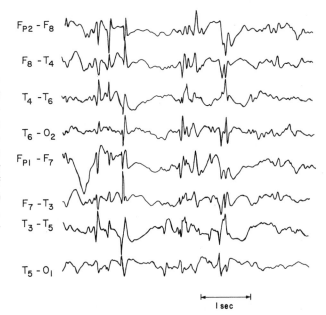

have a history of childhood absences. Sleep deprivation is another common precipitant. For example, medical house officers who have worked all night are susceptible to tonic-clonic seizures during the next day.

With or without sleep deprivation, non-rapid eye movement (NREM) sleep, particularly stages 1 and 2, precipitate tonic-clonic seizures in epileptic patients (see Chapter 17). Rapid eye movement (REM) sleep, in contrast, is relatively seizure-free. Many epileptic patients have seizures predominantly or exclusively during sleep, but some patients have them virtually only on awakening. (To avoid a diagnostic error, physicians should evaluate these patients for a sleep disorder masquerading as epilepsy [see below and Chapter 17]).

Alcohol can precipitate seizures in cases of profound intoxication, alcohol-induced hypoglycemia, or sleep deprivation. Abrupt withdrawal from chronic, excessive alcohol consumption produces alcohol-withdrawal seizures, which usually occur after 1 to 3 days of abstinence. Although the clinical and EEG manifestations of these seizures are similar to those in genetically determined seizures, the interictal EEG is normal.

A small group of children, adolescents, and some adults have absences or tonic-clonic seizures in response to particular sensory stimulation, *reflex epilepsy*. In its most common variety, *photosensitive* or *photoconvulsive epilepsy*, seizures are triggered by specific visual stimuli, such as discotheque stroboscopes, television pictures that have lost their vertical stability, televised cartoons, or video games. Even stationary patterns of certain letters, words, or figures may trigger seizures. Likewise, particular musical passages may trigger seizures.

Treatment. AEDs commonly used for tonic-clonic seizures are valproate, phenytoin, and carbamazepine. As in treatment of partial seizures, neurologists usually attempt control with monotherapy.

Febrile Seizures

Febrile seizures, which occur at least once in 2% to 4% of all children, are the most common variety of childhood seizure. "Simple" febrile seizures usually last less than 30 seconds, lack focal findings, and constitute more than 80% of cases. Because they do not lead to epilepsy, they are considered benign. On the other hand, "complex" febrile seizures, which are more prolonged or include focal findings, are associated with subsequent development of epilepsy. Moreover, because mesial temporal sclerosis has followed unusually severe febrile seizures, some authors suggest a causal relationship between complex febrile seizures and subsequent partial complex epilepsy.

Daily phenobarbital had been given as a prophylactic AED or administered at the onset of fever. However, it notoriously impairs cognitive function, produces hyperactivity, and provides little protection. To prevent recurrent febrile seizures, some neurologists recommend oral or rectal diazepam when fevers develop.

RELATED ISSUES

Driving

Patients with epilepsy might have seizures while driving. In addition, their AEDs can make them sleepy enough to cause a traffic accident. Epilepsy patients have increased rates of traffic violations, including driving under the influence of alcohol or drugs, as well as of accidents. As in the general population, automobile accidents are closely associated with drivers who are male and younger than 25 years.

Almost all states require a waiting period for a driving license after having a seizure, but modifications are sometimes allowed for seizures that arose from an isolated medical illness, such as hypoglycemia, and for seizures with a prolonged aura. Most states set a waiting period of 3 to 6 months, but several, including New York, California, and New Jersey, require 12 months. Patients are usually required to reveal any history of seizures or loss of consciousness (for any reason) to a state's motor vehicle department. In addition, several states require physicians to report drivers with seizures.

Pseudoseizures

The category of *nonepileptic seizures* includes both psychogenic and physiologic seizure-like events. *Pseudoseizures* or *psychogenic seizures* are psychogenic seizurelike episodes. They were originally classified as a sign of a conversion disorder, but now they are seen as a manifestation of a wide range of psychiatric disorders, including depression, anxiety, psychosis, somatoform disorder, personality disorder, factitious disorder, and posttraumatic stress disorder. Pseudoseizures, which are frequently superimposed on a history of childhood sexual abuse, are more prevalent in women, children, and adolescents.

Like epileptic seizures, pseudoseizures tend to be stereotyped for each individual. In contrast, however, they typically develop slowly with prominent flailing, struggling, agitation, alternating limb movements (asymmetric or out-of-phase clonic movements), and rhythmic side-to-side head movements. They often include characteristic sexually suggestive pelvic thrusting. As fatigue ensues, the movements decline in intensity and regularity, but characteristically resume after rest. Duration—typically 2 to 5 minutes—exceeds that of the average epileptic seizure.

Also in contrast to epileptic seizures, pseudoseizures usually have no tonic phase or incontinence. Sometimes pseudoseizure patients bite their lip or tip of their tongue, rather than the side of the tongue, as in epilepsy. Most striking, despite the apparent generalized nature of pseudoseizures, consciousness is preserved. After a pseudoseizure, patients have no postictal symptoms, such as confusion, headache, or retrograde amnesia.

If electronic filters can eliminate muscle artifact, an EEG obtained during a pseudoseizure would be normal. An EEG performed after the episode, which is more feasible, would not show postictal depression. The serum prolactin concentration after an episode, which often rises 30 to 45 minutes after a generalized or partial complex seizure, would remain at the baseline after a pseudoseizure.

If routine testing fails to provide a diagnosis, EEG-video monitoring would probably be helpful. It can readily differentiate pseudoseizures from epileptic seizures. The portion of the EEG monitoring obtained during sleep would be especially important because epileptic seizures—not pseudoseizures—arise from genuine sleep. (To reiterate the caveat: Sleep disorders can be mistaken for seizures [see below].)

Several other diagnostic pitfalls remain. Although the extremes are readily identifiable, even experienced clinicians find many episodes problematic. Pseudoseizures can be convincing because they can closely mimic epileptic seizures, include urinary incontinence, and, in as many as 20% of cases, deliberately or inadvertently produce self-injury. Applying only clinical criteria, the distinction between pseudoseizures and epileptic seizures in most studies is no more reliable than 80% to 90%.

One source of confusion and concern is that about 25% to 40% of patients with pseudoseizures also have epileptic seizures. Moreover, pseudoseizures in epilepsy patients mimic their epileptic seizures so closely that EEG-video monitoring is required. The combination of pseudoseizures and epileptic seizures can be responsible for "refractory epilepsy." Another difficulty is that some seizures, particularly frontal lobe seizures, produce such bizarre behavior that they are liable to be dismissed summarily as pseudoseizures or other psychogenic disturbance.

Episodic Dyscontrol Syndrome/Intermittent Explosive Disorder

The episodic dyscontrol syndrome—roughly equivalent to the *DSM-IV* condition *Intermittent Explosive Disorder*—consists of violently aggressive, primitive outbursts that injure people or destroy property. Outbursts are usually provoked by minor stimuli, such as verbal threats, anger, or frustration, especially after consuming even small amounts of alcohol. (If the episodes are caused by alcohol, however, they cannot be classified, using the *DSM-IV,* as an Intermittent Explosive Disorder.)

In contrast to violent partial complex seizures (see above), which are rare, these episodes are nonstereotyped, provoked by external factors, at least momentarily purposeful and directed (aggressive), and include overwhelming emotional component. Most often the episodes are preceded and then accompanied by a highly charged affect. After barbaric screaming, punching, wrestling, and throwing bottles, patients typically claim either repentance or amnesia.

The attacks are aggression, not merely violence. They occur almost exclusively in young men who have congenital or traumatic brain injury, borderline intelligence, or minor physical neurologic abnormalities. Because of these neurologic injuries, many have epilepsy and interictal EEG abnormalities that undoubtedly account for some reports of aggression in seizures. Suggested medical treatments, in addition to prohibiting alcoholic beverages, have included mood stabilizers and AEDs.

Cerebrovascular Disturbances

TIAs resemble partial seizures because both may involve momentarily impaired consciousness and physical deficits (see Chapter 11). In general, however, TIAs have a slower onset, rarely cause loss of consciousness, and tend to begin only when the patient is standing upright.

Of the various cerebrovascular disturbances that can mimic partial complex seizures, the most important is *transient global amnesia* (*TGA,* see Chapter 11). During an episode of TGA, which is a frequent cause of transient amnesia (see Table 7–1), patients cannot remember new information, such as the date, location, and examining physicians; however, they retain basic memories, such as their and their spouse's names, address, and telephone numbers. This discrepancy separates TGA from psychogenic amnesia, in which the amnesia seems to wipe out basic as well as new information.

During a TGA, the EEG shows spikes but not paroxysmal bursts. TGA is probably caused by vascular insufficiency of the temporal lobes that leads to ischemia of the limbic system. It may be diagnosed, although with some difficulty, from the clinical features.

Migraines, another vascular disturbance, may induce episodes of confusion and personality change followed by a tendency to sleep (see Chapter 9). Migraines also mimic seizures because they lead to transient hemiparesis and abnormal EEGs. In fact, the incidence of seizures in migraine patients is greater than in the general population, making migraines a risk factor for epilepsy. The correct diagnosis, which is frequently difficult, relies on the patient's history and response to medications.

Sleep Disorders

Bizarre behavior during the night might be a sleep disorder (see Chapter 17) rather than a nocturnal seizure. For example, children may be having *parasomnias,* particularly night terrors. Older adults are liable to develop *REM behavior disorder.* These conditions so closely mimic seizures in certain respects that polysomnography or EEG-video monitoring may be required to distinguish them.

An alternative diagnosis to seizures in unresponsive patients is the *narcolepsy-cataplexy syndrome,* which includes momentary loss of body tone (cataplexy), irresistible sleep (narcolepsy), and dreamlike hallucinations (see Chapter 17). Unlike seizures, this disorder has no aura, motor activity, incontinence, or subsequent symptoms. Moreover, an EEG or polysomnogram during an attack displays REM activity.

Metabolic Aberrations

Of the various metabolic aberrations that can mimic seizures, reactions to medicines are probably the most common. Many medicines, including even some administered as eyedrops, produce transient mental and physical alterations. However, they practically never induce movements or stereotyped thoughts.

Hyperventilation commonly induces giddiness, confusion, and other psychologic symptoms that can be confused with seizures (see Chapter 3). Prolonged, deep hyperventilation can precipitate seizures, but probably only in epileptic individuals.

Hypoglycemia, which can result from excessive insulin, alcohol intoxication, skipping meals, and prediabetic states, can induce symptoms of anxiety attacks, as well as of seizures. Similar symptoms occur with excessive coffee intake. Although the severity and frequency of hypoglycemia's symptoms are probably overestimated, small, frequent meals along with reduction of caffeine consumption should remedy most cases.

REFERENCES

AEDs and Surgical Treatment

Alldredge BK: Seizure risk associated with psychotropic drugs. Neurology *53* (Suppl 2): S68–S75, 1999

Bourgeois BFD: New antiepileptic drugs. Arch Neurol *55*: 1181–1183, 1998

Dodrill CB, Troupin AS: Neuropsychological effects of carbamazepine and phenytoin: A reanalysis. Neurology *41:* 141–143, 1991

Eliashiv SD, Dewar S, Wainwright I, et al: Long-term followup after temporal lobe resection for lesions associated with chronic seizures. Neurology *48:* 621–626, 1997

Fisher RS, Handforth A: Reassessment: Vagus nerve stimulation for epilepsy: A report of the Therapeutics and Technology Subcommittee of the American Academy of Neurology. Neurology *53:* 666–669, 1999

Gallassi R, Morreale A, DiSarro R, et al: Cognitive effects of antiepileptic drug discontinuation. Epilepsia *33* (Suppl 6): S41–S44, 1992

Ketter TA, Malow BA, Flamini R, et al: Anticonvulsant withdrawal-emergent psychopathology. Neurology *44:* 55–61, 1994

Krystal AD, Coffey CE: Neuropsychiatric considerations in the use of electroconvulsive therapy. J Neuropsychiatry *9:* 283–292, 1998

Martin R, Kuzniecky R, Ho S, et al: Cognitive effects of topiramate, gabapentin, and lamotrigine in healthy young adults. Neurology *52:* 321–327, 1999

Mattson RH, Cramer JA, Collins JF, et al: A comparison of valproate with carbamazepine for the treatment of complex partial seizures and secondarily generalized tonic-clonic seizures in adults. N Engl J Med *327:* 765–771, 1992

Meador KJ, Loring DW, Allen ME, et al: Comparative cognitive effects of carbamazepine and phenytoin in healthy adults. Neurology *41:* 1537–1540, 1991

Morrell MJ: The new antiepileptic drugs and women. Epilepsia *37* (Suppl 6): S34–S44, 1996

Olafsson E, Hallgrimsson JT, Hauser WA, et al: Pregnancies of women with epilepsy. Epilepsia *39:* 887–892, 1998

Quality Standards Subcommittee of the American Academy of Neurology: Practice parameter: Management issues for women with epilepsy. Neurology *51:* 944–948, 1998

Samren EB, van Duijin CM, Koch S, et al: Maternal use of antiepileptic drugs and the risk of major congenital malformations. Epilepsia *38:* 981–990, 1997

Trimble MR: Antiepileptic drugs, cognitive function, and behavior in children: Evidence from recent studies. Epilepsia *31* (Suppl 4): S30–S34, 1990

Wyllie E, Comair YG, Kotagal P, et al: Seizure outcome after epilepsy surgery in children and adolescents. Ann Neurol *44*: 740–748, 1998

Interictal Disorders

Bear DM, Fedio P: Quantitative analysis of interictal behavior in temporal lobe epilepsy. Arch Neurol *34*: 454–467, 1977
Bruton CJ, Stevens JR, Frith CD: Epilepsy, psychosis, and schizophrenia. Neurology *44*: 34–42, 1994
Devinsky O, Kelly K, Yacubian EMT, et al: Postictal behavior: A clinical and subdural electroencephalographic study. Arch Neurol *51*: 254–259, 1994
Flor-Henry P: Psychosis and temporal lobe epilepsy. Epilepsia *10*: 363–395, 1969
Hansotia P, Broste SK: The effect of epilepsy or diabetes mellitus on the risk of automobile accidents. N Engl J Med *324*: 22–26, 1991
Kanner AM, Nieto JCR: Depressive disorders in epilepsy. Neurology *53* (Suppl 2), S26–S32, 1999
Mendez MF, Doss RC, Taylor JL, et al: Interictal violence in epilepsy: Relationship to behavior and seizure variables. J Nerv Ment Dis *181*: 566–569, 1993
Mendez MF, Grau R, Doss RC, et al: Schizophrenia in epilepsy: Seizure and psychosis variables. Neurology *43*: 1073–1077, 1993
Morrell MJ, Sperling MR, Stecker M, et al: Sexual dysfunction in partial epilepsy: A deficit in physiologic arousal. Neurology *44*: 243–247, 1994
Pillmann F, Rohde A, Ullrich A, et al: Violence, criminal behavior, and the EEG. J Neuropsychiatry Clin Neurosci *11*: 454–457, 1999
Pincus JH: Violence: The neurologic contribution. Arch Neurol *49*: 595–603, 1992
Rodin E, Schmaltz S: The Bear-Fedio personality inventory and temporal lobe epilepsy. Neurology *34*: 591–596, 1984
Sachdev P: Schizophrenia-like psychosis and epilepsy: The status of the association. Am J Psychiatry *155*: 325–336, 1998
Slater E, Beard AW: The schizophrenic-like psychosis of epilepsy. Br J Psychiatry *109*: 95–150, 1963
Trimble MR: The Psychoses of Epilepsy. New York, Raven Press, 1991
Whitman S, Coleman TE, Patmon C, et al: Epilepsy in prison: Elevated prevalence and no relationship to violence. Neurology *34*: 775–782, l984

Seizures and Epilepsy

Alper K, Devinsky O, Perrine K: Nonepileptic seizures and childhood sexual and physical abuse. Neurology *43*: 1950–1953, 1993
Engle J, Pedley TA: Epilepsy: A Comprehensive Textbook. Philadelphia, Lippincott-Raven, 1997
Lesser RP: Psychogenic seizures. Neurology *46*: 1499–1507, 1996
Goossens LAZ, Andermann F, Andermann E, et al: Reflex seizures induced by calculation, card or board games, and spatial tasks: A review of 25 patients and delineation of the epileptic syndrome. Neurology *40*: 1171–1176, 1990
Laskowitz DT, Sperling MR, French JA, et al: The syndrome of frontal lobe epilepsy: Characteristics and surgical management. Neurology *45*: 780–787, 1995
Manford M, Fish DR, Shorvon SD: An analysis of clinical seizure patterns and their localizing value in frontal and temporal lobe epilepsies. Brain *119*: 17–40, 1996
Pacia SV, Devinsky O: Clozapine-related seizures: Experience with 5,629 patients. Neurology *44*: 2247–2249, 1994
Sackheim HA, Prudic J, Devanand DP, et al: Effects of stimulus intensity and electrode placement on the efficacy and cognitive effects of electroconvulsive therapy. N Engl J Med *328*: 839–846, 1993
Saygi S, Katz A, Marks DA, et al: Frontal lobe partial seizures and psychogenic seizures. Neurology *42*: 1274–1277, 1992

Testing

Hughes JR: A review of the usefulness of the standard EEG in psychiatry. Clin Electroencephalogr *27*: 35–39, 1996
Therapeutics and Technology Assessment Subcommittee of the American Academy of Neurology: Assessment of digital EEG, quantitative EEG, and EEG brain mapping. Neurology *49*: 277–292, 1997
Therapeutics and Technology Assessment Subcommittee of the American Academy of Neurology: Assessment: Magnetoencephalography (MEG). Neurology *42*: 1–4, 1992

QUESTIONS and ANSWERS: CHAPTER 10

1–4. Read the EEG and match it with the interpretation (see pages 258–259).

1. Fig. EEG-A

2. Fig. EEG-B

3. Fig. EEG-C

4. Fig. EEG-D

a. Spike and polyspike and wave
b. 3-Hz spike and wave

c. Normal
d. Temporal spike focus

   ANSWERS: 1-c, 2-d, 3-b, 4-a

5–8. Match the EEG abnormality with its associated seizure.

5. Interictal temporal lobe spikes

6. Generalized 3-Hz spike and wave

7. Generalized spike and polyspike and wave

8. Occipital spike and wave

a. Tonic-clonic (grand mal)
b. Partial elementary

c. Partial complex
d. Absence (petit mal)

   ANSWERS: 5-c, 6-d, 7-a, 8-b

9–16. Match the EEG pattern with its most likely cause (a–j).

9. Delta activity, phase reversed over left posterior cerebrum

10. Bifrontal beta activity

11. Alpha rhythm

12. Triphasic waves

13. Rapid extraocular movement artifact

14. Periodic complexes

15. Unilateral cerebral theta and delta activity

16. Electrocerebral silence

a. Normal resting state
b. Hepatic encephalopathy
c. Use of benzodiazepines
d. Occipital lobe tumor
e. Cerebral death

f. Dream-filled sleep
g. Unilateral ECT
h. Psychoses
i. Creutzfeldt-Jakob disease
j. Barbiturate overdose

   ANSWERS: 9-d; 10-c; 11-a; 12-b; 13-f (REM sleep); 14-i; 15-d, g; 16-e, j

17. In which five conditions will an EEG be helpful in making a specific diagnosis?

a. Cerebral tumor
b. Hepatic encephalopathy
c. Neurosis
d. Huntington's disease
e. Cerebral abscess
f. Creutzfeldt-Jakob disease
g. Psychogenic seizures
h. Manic-depressive illness

i. Cerebellar tumor
j. Subacute sclerosing panencephalitis (SSPE)
k. Psychoses
l. Multiple sclerosis
m. Early Alzheimer's disease
n. Pseudodementia

   ANSWER: b, f, g, j, n

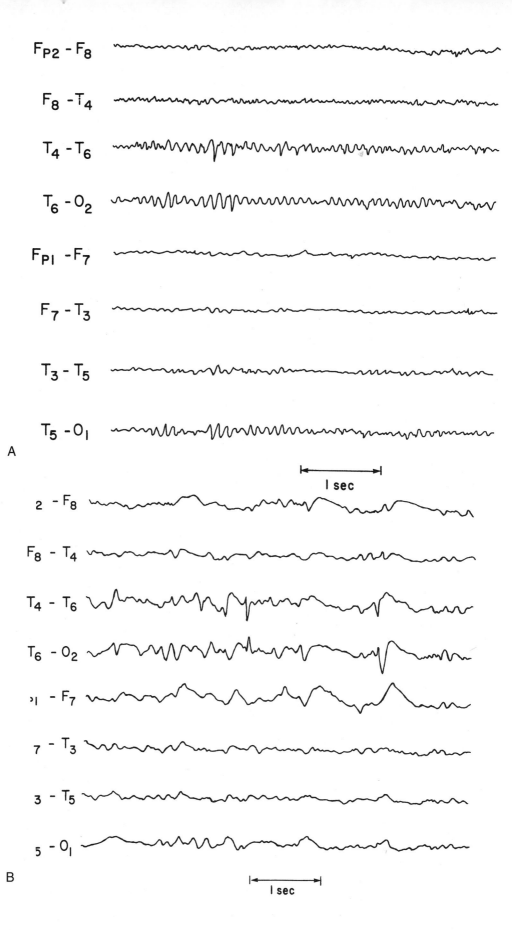

A

1 sec

B

1 sec

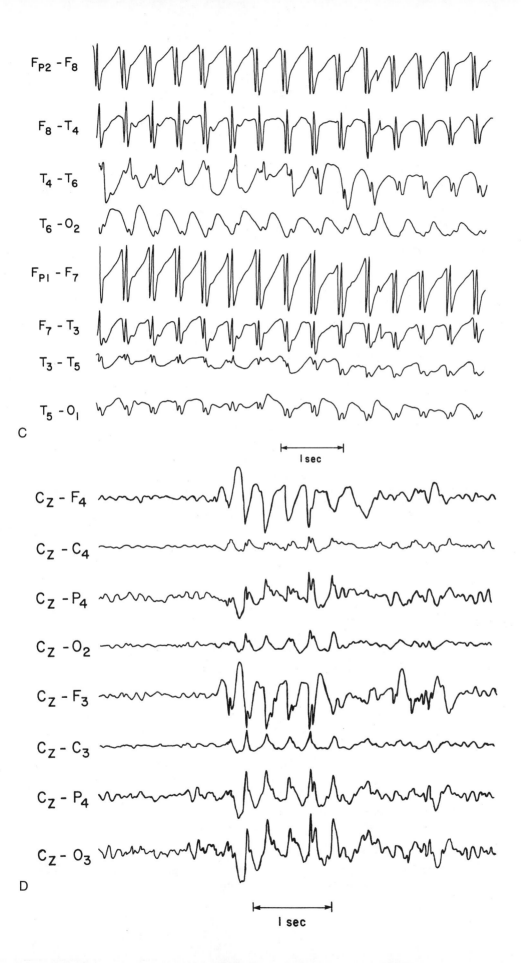

$F_{P2} - F_8$

$F_8 - T_4$

$T_4 - T_6$

$T_6 - O_2$

$F_{P1} - F_7$

$F_7 - T_3$

$T_3 - T_5$

$T_5 - O_1$

C

1 sec

$C_Z - F_4$

$C_Z - C_4$

$C_Z - P_4$

$C_Z - O_2$

$C_Z - F_3$

$C_Z - C_3$

$C_Z - P_4$

$C_Z - O_3$

D

1 sec

18–20. Match the rare but serious complication of treatment with antiepileptic drugs (AEDs)—previously known as anticonvulsants—with its definition.

18. Stevens-Johnson syndrome

19. Forced normalization

20. Paradoxical hyperactivity

    a. Conversion to a normal EEG and suppression of seizure activity that purportedly may trigger a psychosis
    b. Frequently fatal allergic reaction that primarily involves the gastrointestinal mucosa
    c. Psychosis as an allergic reaction
    d. Excitement instead of sedation, especially with phenobarbital in children and brain-damaged adults

    ANSWERS: 18-b, 19-a, 20-d

21–24. Identify the following statements as true or false.

21. Use of the EEG in the diagnosis of psychiatric illness is complicated by drug-induced EEG changes.

22. Diazepam (Valium), meprobamate (Miltown), and barbiturates induce rapid (beta) EEG activity.

23. Tricyclic antidepressants and phenothiazines may induce nonfocal sharp-wave EEG activity.

24. The major tranquilizers, antidepressants, and lithium may cause slowing of EEG background activity.

    ANSWERS: 21-True, 22-True, 23-True, 24-True

25. Carbamazepine (Tegretol) is often used in the treatment of epilepsy patients who are depressed. Which of the following medications has the chemical structure that is the closest to carbamazepine?

    a. Lithium
    b. Phenytoin
    c. Imipramine
    d. Haloperidol
    e. Phenelzine
    f. Tranylcypromine

    ANSWER: c. Carbamazepine is a structural cogener of imipramine.

26. For which condition is quantitative EEG (QEEG) accepted as a clinical test?

    a. Attention deficit hyperactivity disorder
    b. Postconcussive syndrome
    c. Head trauma
    d. Depression
    e. Epilepsy
    f. Learning disabilities

    ANSWER: e. QEEG remains an "investigational" diagnostic procedure for almost all conditions except epilepsy, which requires sophisticated data analysis.

27. Which application of electroconvulsive (ECT) therapy is least likely to produce amnesia?

    a. Unilateral, nondominant hemisphere
    b. Unilateral, dominant hemisphere
    c. Bilateral
    d. Each pattern will produce similar incidence and severity of amnesia.

    ANSWER: a. Although it might be least effective in reversing depression, application of ECT in a unilateral pattern over the nondominant hemisphere will produce the least amnesia.

28. Compared to other partial complex seizures, which features indicate a frontal lobe seizure?

a. Childhood onset
b. Readily detectable frontal lobe EEG paroxysms
c. Absence of an aura, duration of less than 1 minute, and little postictal symptomatology
d. The ability of sleep to suppress these seizures.

ANSWER: c. Frontal lobe seizures, unlike other partial complex seizures, tend to develop in adults and consist of numerous, relatively brief episodes of bizarre activity devoid of aura, automatisms, and postictal confusion. These seizures develop predominantly during sleep. A routine EEG is often unable to assist in the diagnosis.

29. A 28-year-old man was admitted following several seizures. He denied prior seizures, head trauma, use of illicit drugs and alcohol, and systemic symptoms. He had been maintained in a methadone program for narcotic addiction. The seizure was finally attributed to a congenital cerebral injury. He was treated with phenytoin and the methadone was continued. Several days later he began to develop agitation, anxiety to the point of incoherence, diaphoresis, and tachycardia. Which should be the consulting psychiatrist's first step?

a. Administer a tranquilizer
b. Administer an SSRI
c. Administer an atypical neuroleptic
d. None of the above

ANSWER: d. Phenytoin decreases methadone activity. As in this case, initiating phenytoin treatment precipitated narcotic withdrawal. To avoid this problem, physicians should increase the dose of methadone rather than stopping the phenytoin, which might precipitate one or more seizures, even status epilepticus. Changing the AED would require 5 to 7 days.

30. What is the effect of carbamazepine and phenytoin on oral contraceptives?

a. These AEDs increase the contraceptive's effectiveness, permitting lower estrogen preparations to be effective.
b. These AEDs decrease the contraceptive's effectiveness, risking conception.
c. These AEDs have no effect on a contraceptive's effectiveness.
d. In contrast to these AEDs having a teratogenic effect, other AEDs have been shown to be risk-free.

ANSWER: b

31. In which phase of sleep is a seizure least likely to occur?

a. Stage 1 or 2 NREM
b. REM
c. Sleep following sleep deprivation
d. Awakening from sleep

ANSWER: b. Sleep and sleep deprivation lower the seizure threshold. In about 10% of all epilepsy patients, seizures occur only during sleep. In addition, children with rolandic epilepsy have seizures predominantly during sleep. Epilepsy patients are most vulnerable during stage 1 or 2 NREM sleep, sleep following sleep deprivation, and awakening. They are less vulnerable during REM sleep.

32. Which statement is true regarding the incidence of depression in epilepsy patients?

a. The seizure frequency is proportionate to the incidence of depression.
b. The seizure frequency is inversely proportionate to the incidence of depression.
c. Compared to the naturally occurring condition, epilepsy-induced depression is more often bipolar.
d. ECT is contraindicated in epilepsy.

ANSWER: b. Depression is more prevalent in epilepsy patients than in individuals with comparable neurologic conditions. Epilepsy patients with infrequent seizures have a higher incidence of depression than epilepsy patients with frequent seizures. Depression occurs particularly in epilepsy patients who have partial complex seizures, are male, or require multiple AEDs.

33. Which statement is false regarding the schizophreniform psychosis that develops in epilepsy?

a. It is associated with intractable epilepsy.
b. Epileptic patients who develop schizophreniform psychosis, compared to those who do not, have larger cerebral ventricles and more cerebral damage.

c. The incidence of schizophrenia in first-degree relatives of epilepsy patients with schizophreniform psychosis is similar to the incidence of schizophrenia in first-degree relatives of schizophrenia patients.

d. Butyrophenones are preferred over chlorpromazine for treatment of acute psychosis in epileptic patients.

ANSWER: c. In contrast to the first-degree relatives of nonepileptic, schizophrenic patients having an increased incidence of schizophrenia, first-degree relatives of epileptic patients with schizophreniform psychosis have no increased incidence of schizophrenia. Chlorpromazine, more so than the butyrophenones, precipitates seizures in epileptic patients.

34–43. The patient's age when partial (elementary or complex) seizures begin suggests the cause. Match the seizure cause with the age(s) when it is likely to first appear.

34. Head injury

35. Congenital cerebral malformation

36. Arteriovenous malformation

37. Glioblastoma multiforme

38. Metastatic brain tumor

39. Cocaine use

40. Cerebrovascular accident

41. Pseudoseizure

42. Medial temporal sclerosis

43. Perinatal cerebral hypoxia

a. Childhood, e.g., 3–8 years
b. Adolescence, e.g., 13–21 years
c. Middle age, e.g., 45–65 years

ANSWERS: 34-b; 35-a; 36-a, b; 37-c; 38-c; 39-b; 40-c; 41-b; 42-a, b; 43-a

44–46. A 60-year-old man, who has been previously healthy, is brought to the emergency room in a state of confusion and excitement. Examination reveals that he has poor memory for recent and past events, but he can recall his own and his wife's name and their address. His judgment, language, and other cognitive processes are slow but intact. There are no physical abnormalities. He gradually improves during 2 hours.

44. What is the name of this condition?

a. Delirium
b. Dissociative fugue (formerly psychogenic fugue)
c. Acute amnestic syndrome
d. Dissociative amnesia (formerly psychogenic amnesia)

ANSWER: c. Preserved personal information distinguish an acute amnestic syndrome from dissociative (psychogenic) states. The lack of traveling distinguishes an amnestic syndrome from dissociative (psychogenic) fugue.

45. Which one of the following is *not* an acceptable explanation?

a. Partial complex seizures
b. Wernicke-Korsakoff syndrome
c. Psychogenic disturbances
d. Medications
e. Transient global amnesia
f. AED intoxication

ANSWER: f. AED intoxication can cause delirium and cognitive impairment, but not so selective an impairment as amnesia. The other conditions are capable of impairing memory and sparing other cognitive functions.

46. Dysfunction of which area of the brain is most likely responsible?

a. Temporal lobe
b. Entire cerebrum
c. Thalamus
d. Frontal lobe

ANSWER: a

47. A 6-year-old boy has absence seizures with paroxysms of 3-Hz spike-and-wave EEG activity. He was unable to tolerate ethosuximide (Zarontin). Which AED should then be given?

a. Phenytoin (Dilantin)
b. Carbamazepine (Tegretol)
c. Divalproex (Depakote) or valproic acid
d. Phenobarbital

ANSWER: c. Absences with 3-Hz spike-and-wave activity are usually first treated with ethosuximide (Zarontin), but valproic acid is appropriate if ethosuximide is unacceptable or if grand mal seizures accompany the absence seizure.

48. A 23-year-old medical student was experimenting with smoking marijuana. Its effect, which was completely different than anticipated, was anxiety and fear. The student was brought to the emergency room with hallucinations, agitation, fever, and nystagmus. Increasing mental and physical agitation culminated in a seizure. Of the following, which is the most likely culprit?

a. Marijuana
b. Phencyclidine (PCP)
c. Cocaine
d. Demerol

ANSWER: b. PCP, even in minute amounts, can cause hallucinations and seizures. It is sometimes mixed with marijuana and smoked. Large doses of cocaine are required to produce these effects. When cocaine is taken in higher amounts, it often causes cerebral hemorrhage, stroke, or vasculitis. Although PCP and Demerol use among medical students is rare, when health care personnel develop seizures, the treating physicians should consider drug abuse.

49. After developing lethargy and confusion, a 30-year-old woman who has a history of partial complex seizures is brought to the emergency room. Which of the following conditions is the most likely cause?

a. Expansion of a temporal lobe tumor
b. Development of a subdural hematoma from head trauma
c. Partial complex status epilepticus
d. AED intoxication
e. Development of a systemic disorder, such as renal failure

ANSWER: d. All these causes must be considered; however, in the majority of such cases, the cause is AED intoxication. If the intoxication is profound or represents one of several episodes, the physician should consider the possibility that the episode was a deliberate overdose.

50. Which six of the following physical signs may indicate AED intoxication?

a. Hemiparesis
b. Ataxia of gait
c. Nystagmus
d. Aphasia
e. Dysarthria
f. Lethargy or stupor
g. Dysmetria on heel-shin testing
h. Tremor on finger-nose testing
i. Papilledema

ANSWER: b, c, e, f, g, h

51. In which part of the skull is the temporal lobe located?

a. Sella
b. Anterior fossa
c. Posterior fossa
d. Middle fossa

ANSWER: d

52. What is the duration of the serum prolactin level elevation after a generalized tonic-clonic or partial complex seizure?

a. 24 hours
b. 12 hours
c. 2 hours
d. 1 hour or less

ANSWER: d. Determining the serum prolactin level after a seizurelike episode may help distinguish a pseudoseizure from generalized tonic-clonic or partial complex seizure.

53. Which of the following statements are true? (1) Epileptic people are more likely than nonepileptic people to be convicted of a crime and sent to prison. (2) Epileptic criminals are no more likely than other criminals to have committed a violent crime.

ANSWER: 1-True, 2-True

54. Which one of the following statements concerning neural tube defects is false?

a. Meningomyeloceles may be induced by AED treatment of pregnant women.
b. The incidence of neural tube defects is reduced by folic acid diet supplements.
c. The neural tube is derived from the endoderm.
d. The neural tube forms the brain, as well as the spinal cord.

ANSWER: c. Soon after conception, well within the first trimester, the ectodermal layer of the embryo invaginates to form the neural tube.

55. Seizures induced by antipsychotic medications are associated with each of the following except:

a. Pre-existing epilepsy
b. Polypharmacy
c. Noncompliance with AED regimen
d. Left-sided rather than right-sided temporal lesions

ANSWER: d

56. If a medication that inhibited CYP 3A4 metabolic enzymes were administered to an individual taking carbamazepine, what would happen to the carbamazepine plasma concentration?

a. The plasma concentration of carbamazepine would increase.
b. The plasma concentration of carbamazepine would decrease.
c. The plasma concentration of carbamazepine would remain unchanged.
d. None of the above.

ANSWER: a. Medications, including erythromycin and fluoxetine, that inhibit CYP 3A4 enzymes raise the plasma concentration of carbamazepine, possibly to toxic levels.

57. If a medication that induced CYP 3A4 metabolic enzymes were administered to an individual taking carbamazepine, what would happen to the carbamazepine plasma concentration?

a. The plasma concentration of carbamazepine would increase.
b. The plasma concentration of carbamazepine would decrease.
c. The plasma concentration of carbamazepine would remain unchanged.
d. None of the above.

ANSWER: b. Medications, including phenobarbital, phenytoin, and carbamazepine itself, that induce CYP 3A4 enzymes decrease the plasma concentration of carbamazepine, possibly to subtherapeutic levels. In the case of carbamazepine therapy, increasing doses are often required to maintain a therapeutic concentration. Moreover, carbamazepine-induced enzymes decrease plasma concentrations of alprazolam, clozapine, haloperidol, oral contraceptives, and valproate.

58. Compared with absence seizures (petit mal seizures), partial complex seizures (e.g., psychomotor seizures), possess all the following qualities except which one of the following?

a. Longer in duration
b. More likely to be suppressed by carbamazepine
c. Associated with an aura and postictal confusion
d. Induce retrograde amnesia
e. Likely to disappear in young adult life

ANSWER: e

59. Which three conditions are causes of electrocerebral silence despite a regular sinus rhythm on the electrocardiogram?

a. Psychogenic unresponsiveness
b. Depression
c. Brain death
d. Barbiturate overdose
e. Hypothermia
f. Locked-in syndrome

ANSWER: c, d, e. Before declaring brain death on the basis of an EEG, the physician must be assured that the patient's body temperature is near normal and that blood tests do not detect barbiturates.

60. Which is the best test for demonstrating mesial temporal sclerosis?

a. MRI of the head
b. SPECT of the head
c. CT of the head
d. CT of the head with contrast
e. EEG
f. EEG with nasopharyngeal leads

ANSWER: a

61. Which one of these relationships between the EEG and ECT treatment is false?

a. When unilateral, right-sided ECT is administered, the EEG changes are found predominantly over the right hemisphere.
b. Generalized EEG changes after ECT are associated with more successful treatment of depression.
c. Generalized EEG changes after ECT are associated with greater amnesia.
d. ECT can precipitate status epilepticus in patients with epilepsy or a structural lesion.
e. Especially when the EEG has a slow background rhythm, ECT is contraindicated in Parkinson's disease patients.

ANSWER: e

62. Regarding the normal EEG, which statement is false?

a. Becoming anxious or concentrating on a simple problem will abolish alpha activity.
b. Hyperventilation will produce slow waves or slow the background activity.
c. The normal background activity is low voltage and "fast."
d. Becoming drowsy will slow the background activity.
e. Stroboscopic lights may capture cerebral activity.

ANSWER: c. The normal background activity is alpha activity, which is 8–12 Hz and medium in voltage. Beta, which is faster and lower in voltage, replaces alpha when the patient has anxiety, preoccupation, or concentrates on mental activities.

63. An alcoholic man who has epilepsy treated with phenytoin presents with confusion, nystagmus, and ataxia. He has alcohol on his breath. After a routine medical and neurologic evaluation, what should be the two first steps?

a. Determine the blood alcohol concentration
b. Obtain an EEG
c. Administer more phenytoin
d. Administer thiamine

ANSWER: a, d. Many alcoholic individuals have epilepsy. When inebriated, they pose several dilemmas. Wernicke-Korsakoff syndrome, hypoglycemia from liver disease, or head trauma each could cause confusion and obtundation. Although he has the signs, phenytoin intoxication is unlikely because alcoholics during binges usually do not take their medications, which might include insulin and antihypertensives, as well as AEDs.

64–65. A 32-year-old left-handed woman has had partial complex seizures since she was 14 years old. Her seizures have been refractory to monotherapy. She usually required two or more AEDs in high doses, which often caused intoxication. EEG-video monitoring documented that her seizures were partial complex, they occurred when appropriate AED concentrations were therapeutic, and their focus was in her left anterior temporal lobe.

64. In contemplating surgery, what test should be performed next?

a. Amobarbital interview
b. Withdrawal of AEDs
c. PET scan
d. Wada test

ANSWER: d. The patient, who may be right-hemisphere dominant, might be well advised to undergo a partial or complete left temporal lobectomy. However, if that temporal lobe were dominant, she would be able to withstand only a limited resection.

65. Provided that surgery can be safely performed, what is the likelihood of her achieving a complete or near-complete remission in her seizures from a temporal lobectomy?

a. 25%
b. 50%
c. 75%
d. Almost 100%

ANSWER: c. Epilepsy surgery has been a major medical advance.

66. Which of the following statements is true regarding rolandic epilepsy?

a. It is also called benign childhood epilepsy with centrotemporal spikes.
b. The most common cause is mesial temporal sclerosis.
c. When children with the condition become adults, they are prone to develop other varieties of seizures.
d. The diagnosis of rolandic epilepsy often requires EEG-video monitoring, and if a single focus were identified, a partial lobectomy would be indicated.

ANSWER: a. Rolandic epilepsy, an inherited condition, is restricted to the childhood years. It is readily responsive to AEDs. EEGs performed during sleep may be necessary for diagnosis, but elaborate monitoring is rarely necessary. Unlike generalized absences where about one-third of children later develop tonic-clonic or other seizures, rolandic epilepsy usually remits in adolescence.

67–71. Match the condition with its closest description.

67. Nonconvulsive status epilepticus

68. Activity under conscious control that mimics seizures

69. Activity not under conscious control that mimics seizures

70. Withdrawal emergent psychopathology

71. Forced normalization

a. Psychiatric disturbances, including psychotic behavior, after control of seizures
b. Psychiatric disturbances, especially anxiety and depression, after the complete withdrawal of AEDs
c. Pseudoseizures
d. Repetitive or prolonged seizures that cause mental impairment as the primary or exclusive symptom

ANSWERS: 67-d, 68-c, 69-c, 70-b, 71-a

72. Which two statements are true regarding the relationship of interictal violence to epilepsy?

a. Violence is associated with epileptic patients using two or more AEDs.
b. Violence tends to occur in epileptic patients who are schizophrenic or mentally retarded.
c. Crimes of adult epileptic incarcerated criminals (prisoners) are no more violent than those of nonepileptic ones.
d. The prevalence of epilepsy is no greater in prisoners than in the general population.

ANSWER: b, c

73. Which variety of seizure is most apt to be misdiagnosed as a pseudoseizure?

a. Partial complex seizure that originates in the temporal lobe
b. Partial complex seizure that originates in the frontal lobe
c. Febrile seizure
d. Absence
e. Drug withdrawal seizure

ANSWER: b. A partial complex seizure that originates in the frontal lobe can induce behavior that is bizarre and contain characteristics of pseudoseizures, such as pelvic thrusting, flailing limb movements, and alternating head movements.

74. Which finding is associated with postictal EEG depression?

a. Vegetative symptoms
b. Tendency toward suicide
c. Sleep-wake disturbances
d. Slow, low-voltage EEG activity

ANSWER: d. Postictal EEG depression is a term applied to the slow, low-voltage EEG patterns detected after seizures, including those induced by ECT. This pattern is not detectable after many focal seizures or after a pseudoseizure. It is often associated with a transient rise in the serum prolactin concentration.

75. A commercial airliner from South America crashed in New York after exhausting its fuel supply. About 1 hour after arriving in the hospital, a young man with blunt abdominal trauma became agitated, incoherent, diaphoretic, and hypertensive. During an evaluation, which showed no signs of abdominal or head injuries, he developed status epilepticus and unstable vital signs. During one seizure, he passed through his rectum several condoms filled with white powder and several that had ruptured. What is the cause of his seizures?

a. An epidural hematoma
b. Cysticercosis
c. An isodense subdural hematoma
d. Cocaine overdose
e. Hypoxia

ANSWER: d. Smuggling cocaine and other contraband into the United States by swallowing numerous substance-filled condoms is a common but hazardous practice. If one breaks, enough cocaine, heroin, or other illicit drug is absorbed by the intestines to cause an overdose. In this case, a cocaine overdose caused psychosis, cardiac instability, and seizures. In addition to stabilizing vital functions, treatment includes intravenous benzodiazepine or phenytoin for control of seizures.

76. Which of the following is least likely to be associated with AED use in women of childbearing age?

a. Thinning of the scalp hair
b. Polycystic ovaries with hyperandrogenism
c. Unplanned pregnancy
d. Neural tube defects
e. Coarsening of facial hair
f. Infertility

ANSWER: f. Polycystic ovaries with hyperandrogenism is associated with valproate. Phenytoin and carbamazepine reduce the effectiveness of oral contraceptives. Carbamazepine and valproate increase the risk of neural tube defects. Valproate may cause transient thinning of hair. Phenytoin usually causes increased facial hair. Nevertheless, AEDs are effective and relatively safe.

77. Which one of the following statements does not describe Todd's paralysis?

a. Todd's paresis is apparent only during the first 24 hours following a seizure.
b. Todd's hemiparesis can follow any seizure.
c. Todd's hemiparesis may be accompanied by other lateralized deficits, such as aphasia.
d. Todd's paralysis suggests a partial rather then a generalized seizure disorder.

ANSWER: b. Todd's paralysis, which is typically transient postictal hemiparesis rather than quadriparesis or paraparesis, usually follows partial motor seizures. It does not follow absences or several other seizure varieties.

11

TIAs and Strokes

Transient ischemic attacks (TIAs), cerebrovascular accidents (CVAs or strokes), and multi-infarct (vascular) dementia cause certain temporary or permanent neuropsychologic and physical deficits. Well-informed psychiatrists should be able to recognize common TIAs and strokes, localize the lesion, and predict its physical and neuropsychologic manifestations, including aphasia, dementia, confusion, and amnesia.

TRANSIENT ISCHEMIC ATTACKS (TIAs)

As their name suggests, TIAs are temporary interruptions in cerebral circulation that give rise to constellations of deficits. TIAs typically last from 30 to 60 minutes, but about 10% last up to 4 hours. Most result from platelet emboli that arise from the inner surface of atherosclerotic, stenotic, and ulcerated plaques in the *extracranial arteries:* the carotid and vertebral arteries and the aorta. When an embolus courses through a cerebral artery, it interrupts circulation and induces ischemia. Cardiac arrhythmias and other causes of hypotension also produce TIAs.

Not only do TIAs cause neurologic deficits, they also indicate underlying atherosclerotic cerebrovascular disease and increased risk of sustaining stroke. TIAs lead to strokes when atherosclerotic plaques give rise to large emboli that permanently block a cerebral artery or plaques grow large enough to occlude the extracerebral vessel. Following a TIA, about 4% of individuals develop a stroke within the month and 12% during the year.

TIAs mimic other transient neurologic conditions, particularly partial seizures, postictal confusion and (Todd's) hemiparesis, migraine, and metabolic aberrations. In addition, when they produce aphasia or another neuropsychologic deficit but no physical deficit, they mimic psychogenic episodes.

Carotid Artery TIAs

Platelet emboli that form on plaques at the common carotid artery bifurcation (Fig. 11–1) lead to cerebral hemisphere TIAs. These TIAs are characterized by (contralateral) hemiparesis, hemisensory loss, paresthesias, or hemianopsia. In addition, because the ophthalmic artery is the first branch of the internal carotid artery, carotid artery emboli that flow into the ophthalmic artery cause several minutes of visual obscuration or blindness in that eye. Patients with the distinctive symptom of transient monocular blindness, *amaurosis fugax,* typically describe a "blanket of gray" descending slowly in front of one eye (Table 11–1).

Between TIAs, patients are typically normal. However, a harsh systolic sound (bruit) over the carotid artery bifurcation suggests atherosclerotic cerebrovascular disease without necessarily confirming the presence of carotid stenosis. Retinal emboli

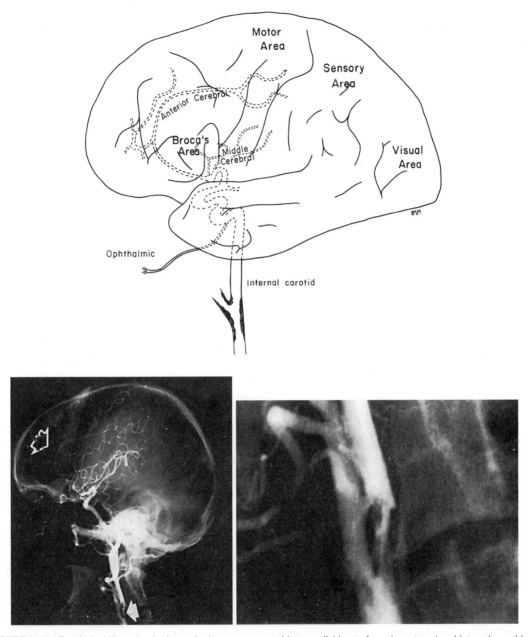

FIGURE 11–1. *Top,* At its bifurcation in the neck, the common carotid artery divides to form the external and internal carotid arteries. Within the skull, the internal carotid artery gives rise to the ophthalmic artery, and then it branches into the anterior and middle cerebral arteries. It also gives rise to the posterior communicating artery—not the posterior cerebral artery. Thus, each internal carotid artery perfuses the ipsilateral eye and most of the ipsilateral cerebral hemisphere.

Each *middle cerebral artery* supplies the deep and midsection of the hemisphere that contain most of the motor cortex, sensory cortex, and, in the dominant hemisphere, the language arc (see Fig. 8–1). Each anterior cerebral artery supplies the frontal lobe, including the medial surface of the motor cortex, which contains the motor innervation for the leg (see Fig. 7–6). The *posterior cerebral arteries* (not pictured) originate from the basilar artery and supply the occipital and most of the temporal lobes.

Bottom left, An arteriogram of the carotid artery and its branches prominently displays the bifurcation *(closed arrowhead),* the typical "candelabra" of branches of the middle cerebral artery rather than a single vessel, and a faint anterior cerebral artery that sweeps from anterior to posterior *(open arrowhead).*

Bottom right, A magnification of the bifurcation shows that an extensive circumferential plaque constricts the internal carotid artery. The remaining blood flow appears as an "apple core." The rough interior surface of the artery gives rise to retinal and cerebral emboli.

TABLE 11–1. *Carotid Artery TIAs*

Symptoms
    Contralateral hemiparesis, hemianopsia, hemisensory loss
    Aphasia
    Ipsilateral amaurosis fugax
Associated findings
    Carotid bruit
    Retinal artery emboli
Tests
    Ultrasonography (carotid Doppler and duplex studies)
    Magnetic resonance imaging angiography (MRA)
    Cerebral arteriography
Therapy
    Medical: platelet inhibitors (e.g., aspirin)
    Surgical: carotid endarterectomy, if stenosis >70% and symptomatic

(Hollenhorst plaques) of atheromatous material, which are observable on funduscopy, also imply carotid artery stenosis.

Carotid artery TIAs often induce neuropsychologic aberrations. Dominant hemisphere TIAs may cause suddenly occurring but transient aphasia. Similarly, nondominant hemisphere TIAs may cause brief hemi-inattention and related neuropsychologic deficits (see Chapter 8). In both situations, the deficits, which may not be accompanied by hemiparesis, can induce or mimic amnesia, confusion, or agitation.

TIAs in patients with preexisting Alzheimer's disease or multi-infarct dementia may convert a mild, compensated intellectual impairment into a marked confusional state. A similar deterioration may develop when both cerebral hemispheres derive their blood supply from one carotid artery through the circle of Willis (Fig. 11–2, top right) because the other carotid artery has been occluded by years of atherosclerosis. In this case, emboli from the patent artery lead to generalized cerebral ischemia.

Laboratory Tests.   Because TIAs are a precursor for strokes, neurologists test patients for highly stenotic atherosclerotic plaques that might be amenable to surgery (see below). Ultrasound (Doppler and duplex) studies, which can measure blood flow and portray artery structure, are a generally reliable technique for revealing or excluding carotid artery stenosis. The traditional, definitive diagnostic procedure has been arteriography. However, because it requires catheterization of an artery followed by injection of a "contrast agent," this procedure may cause a stroke or other serious complications. Magnetic resonance imaging angiography (MRA), which will supplant traditional arteriography (angiography) when its resolution improves, readily permits noninvasive observation of extra- and intracerebral vessels (see Chapter 20).

A computed tomography (CT) or magnetic resonance imaging (MRI) is almost always performed to exclude strokes and cerebral mass lesions. A routine evaluation for transient neurologic deficits sometimes includes an electrocardiogram (ECG), a 24-hour study of the cardiac rhythm (Holter monitor), and blood glucose determinations. Neurologists order an electroencephalogram (EEG) if the patient is likely to be having seizures.

Therapy.   Preventive measures for strokes are aimed primarily at risk factors that can be modified and require treatment in their own right. For example, antihypertensive therapy has been instrumental in lowering incidence of stroke. Likewise, neurologists urge that patients with atrial fibrillation, mitral stenosis, and certain other

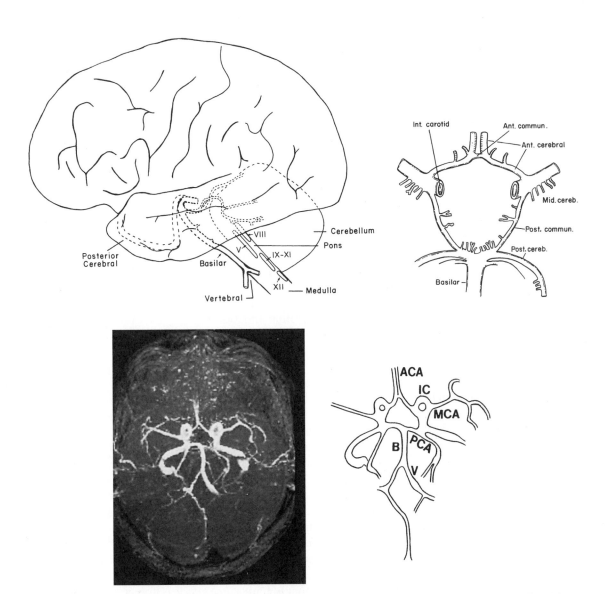

FIGURE 11–2. *Top left,* After ascending encased in the cervical vertebrae, the two vertebral arteries enter the skull. They join to form the basilar artery at the base of the brain. Small, delicate branches from the basilar artery supply the brainstem. (The Roman numerals refer to cranial nerve nuclei.) Large branches, as if wrapping their arms around the brainstem, supply the cerebellum and posterior portion of the cerebrum (i.e., the occipital lobes and inferomedial portions of the temporal lobes). The posterior cerebral arteries are, for practical purposes, the terminal branches of the basilar artery. They supply the occipital cortex and the posterior, inferior aspect of the temporal lobes.

Top right, The circle of Willis, the "great anastomoses," is completely patent in only about 20% of people. It is formed by connections between the basilar and internal carotid arteries and gives off the anterior, middle, and posterior cerebral arteries. The circle also potentially provides anastomoses between anterior-posterior and right-left cerebral circulations. Although the circle confers advantages, junctions of the arteries are weak spots. Defects may balloon outward, form berry aneurysms, rupture, and produce subarachnoid hemorrhages.

Bottom left, An MRA-generated axial view of the vertebral arteries shows them merging to form the basilar artery. The basilar artery terminates by dividing into the posterior cerebral arteries.

Bottom right, This sketch of the MRA shows the basilar (B) and internal carotid (IC) arteries. The circle gives rise to the anterior (ACA), middle (MCA), and posterior (PCA) cerebral arteries. (Communicating arteries are not labeled.)

cardiac conditions be given an anticoagulant, such as warfarin (Coumadin). Optimizing patients' diet, exercise, and other habits may be helpful for cerebrovascular disease, as well as coronary artery disease.

One commonly used approach in attempting to prevent TIAs and strokes is inhibiting platelet aggregation. Common aspirin (one 81-mg tablet daily) remains the most effective platelet aggregation inhibitor, but similar medicines, such as clopidogrel (Plavix), may hold some advantages.

Carotid endarterectomy is a surgical procedure in which the carotid artery is briefly opened for the removal of atherosclerotic plaque. It is a delicate procedure because the cerebral blood supply may be briefly interrupted or pieces of the plaque may fly off and lodge in the brain. Nevertheless, carotid endarterectomy, under ideal conditions, is currently the best treatment for patients with carotid artery TIA symptoms who have at least 70% carotid artery stenosis. Carotid endarterectomy for asymptomatic individuals with carotid stenosis may also be indicated, but the criteria remain uncertain. Surgery is not feasible for complete occlusion of the carotid artery.

A proposed alternative to carotid endarterectomy is intravascular insertion of perforated tubes (stents) that are expanded at atherosclerotic obstructions (see Fig. 20–22). This procedure, which is performed under local anesthesia, is much less invasive than an endarterectomy. Stents have already been widely used in coronary artery disease and expanding abdominal aneurysms.

Basilar Artery TIAs

The two vertebral arteries join to form the basilar artery at the undersurface of the brain. This group of vessels, which is usually called the *vertebrobasilar system* or simply the *basilar artery,* supplies the brainstem, cerebellum, and the posterior-inferior portion of the cerebrum (the occipital and medial-inferior portion of the temporal lobes [Fig. 11–2]). Emboli-generating plaques tend to develop at the origin of the vertebral arteries (in the chest) and at their junction. In these locations, plaques are inaccessible to surgeons.

Symptoms and signs of basilar artery TIAs, which usually result from patchy brainstem ischemia, are distinctly different from those of carotid artery TIAs (Table 11–2). Typical symptoms include tingling around the mouth (circumoral paresthesias), dysarthria, nystagmus, ataxia, and vertigo. On rare occasions, when all blood flow through the basilar artery is momentarily interrupted, the entire brainstem becomes ischemic. The generalized brainstem ischemia impairs consciousness and body tone, which causes patients to collapse, that is, have a *drop attack.* (Drop attacks appear similar to cataplexy [see Chapter 17].)

TABLE 11–2. *Vertebrobasilar Artery TIAs*

Symptoms	Tests
Vertigo, vomiting, tinnitus	Ultrasonography (transcranial Doppler studies)
Circumoral paresthesias or numbness	
Dysarthria, dysphagia	Magnetic resonance imaging angiography (MRA)
Transient global amnesia	
Drop attacks	Cerebral arteriography
Associated findings	Therapy
Nystagmus	Medical: platelet inhibitors (e.g., aspirin)
Ataxia	Surgical: none
Cranial nerve abnormalities	

Vertigo, one of the most characteristic symptoms of basilar artery TIAs, should be diagnosed only when a patient has a sensation of either revolving in space or feeling that the surroundings are revolving. The thoughtful physician should accept no other descriptions. In particular, the common complaint of "dizziness" has no clinical value because it can also mean lightheadedness, giddiness, anxiety, confusion, or imbalance.

As in a carotid artery evaluation, ultrasound examination, MRA, and conventional arteriography can show the vertebral arteries and their blood flow pattern. In addition, a transcranial Doppler examination, which can penetrate the skull, may portray the vertebrobasilar system's architecture. Neurologists rely on the same medications used for carotid artery TIAs. Because the usual sites of vertebrobasilar stenosis remain shielded by the vertebrae and skull, an endarterectomy would not be feasible. However, stents can be inserted through critical stenoses and then expanded to restore normal blood flow.

Transient Global Amnesia

Although seizures, migraines, metabolic aberrations, and other conditions have been suggested as etiologies for *transient global amnesia (TGA)*, basilar artery TIAs are its most likely cause. In this scenario, TIAs impair circulation in the artery's terminal branches, the posterior cerebral arteries, which supply the temporal lobes (Fig. 11–2). Because the temporal lobes contain portions of the limbic system (see Fig. 16–5), temporal lobe ischemia induces temporary amnesia and personality change.

During a TGA attack, patients cannot memorize or learn new information, such as a sequence of digits, that is, they have *anterograde amnesia*. Also, they cannot recall recently acquired information, such as the events of the last several hours or days, that is, they have *retrograde amnesia*. Typically, patients do not know how they came to the physician's office or the emergency room. Their recall of other recent events is also filled with gaps. They lose track of their responses during an interview by a physician, who may have to be reintroduced several times during the examination. As a secondary aspect, some patients understandably become perplexed or even agitated. Some, as if recoiling, become apathetic and immobile.

In contrast to their impaired memory for recently learned facts, TGA patients characteristically retain their general knowledge and fundamental personal information. For example, they are typically able to recite their name, address, telephone number, and occupation. Their retention of fundamental personal information distinguishes them from individuals with a nonneurologic amnesia (see below). TGA patients may also be able to perform complex tasks that were learned before the TGA. (All this preserved memory contradicts the term *global* in TGA.)

Despite their amnesia, TGA patients do not confabulate in the manner of Wernicke-Korsakoff patients. Because their motor system is completely spared, they walk and talk normally—making TGA a prime example of a transient mental disturbance unaccompanied by physical deficits.

TGAs typically occur in middle-aged and older individual in the midst of exertion, particularly sexual activity, which might erroneously lead to various psychologic interpretations. After an abrupt onset, the TGA lasts for several hours, with its intensity most pronounced during the initial 1 to 2 hours. By definition, the total duration must not exceed 24 hours. The recurrence rate is about 10%.

TGAs are a frequently cited cause of acutely occurring amnesia and transiently altered mental status. Unlike other conditions that produce amnesia, TGAs strike individuals who are apt to have cerebrovascular disease. Of the conditions that most closely mimic TGAs, partial complex seizures differ by producing dulling of the sensorium, simple repetitive actions, epileptiform EEG changes, and a high rate of recurrence (see Chapter 10).

"Psychogenic amnesia" is a loosely defined neurologic description applied to people who seem to have forgotten their fundamental personal information. Loss of that information distinguishes psychogenic amnesia from TGA, Wernicke-Korsakoff syndrome, or other neurologic form of amnesia.

Dissociative Amnesia, as described in the *Diagnostic and Statistical Manual of Mental Disorders, Fourth Edition (DSM-IV)*, consists of one or more episodes of amnesia for fundamental personal information "usually of a traumatic or stressful nature." The amnesia might be highly selective regarding prior events and not include an anterograde component. Individuals who just survived a devastating earthquake might develop dissociative amnesia.

In a related *DSM-IV* disorder, *Dissociative Fugue,* previously called *Psychogenic Fugue,* individuals travel away from home or work. Sometimes they assume a new identity. As a secondary aspect of this disorder, they seem to be amnestic for personal information concerning their past life. In contrast to their retrograde amnesia, they do not seem to have anterograde amnesia. In other words, once their new location or personality is established, they are able to recall the new relevant information.

STROKES (CEREBROVASCULAR ACCIDENTS)

Strokes cause permanent physical and neuropsychologic deficits. Most result from an arterial thrombosis, embolus, or hemorrhage that disrupt cerebral blood flow. Predisposing or merely associated conditions, *risk factors,* are numerous and sometimes avoidable.

The greatest risk factor is age. The incidence of strokes rises almost exponentially after the age of 65 years, but about 25% of stroke victims are younger than 65 years. Hypertension, the other major risk factor, leads to strokes in middle-aged, as well as older individuals. It is probably the cause of most cases of multi-infarct dementia (see below). Both systolic and diastolic hypertension are associated with thrombotic and hemorrhagic strokes. A steady decline in the incidence of deaths from strokes in the United States since 1915 is mostly attributable to widespread treatment of hypertension. (On the other hand, antihypertensive medications may have bothersome side effects [see below].)

Various cardiac conditions—valvular disease, acute myocardial infarction, and atrial fibrillation—comprise another risk factor. These conditions tend to produce thromboses on the endocardial surface that embolize to the brain. Diabetes mellitus is risk factor for stroke but an even greater risk factor for myocardial infarction.

Cigarette smoking conveys a grave risk for stroke that has been overshadowed by its other hazards. Compared to nonsmokers, smokers have a fourfold greater risk of stroke; ex-smokers still have almost a twofold greater risk; and, most striking, smokers who are hypertensive have a 20-fold greater risk. In addition, although judicious alcohol drinking (one drink daily to weekly) provides a slight protective effect, heavy alcohol intake is a risk factor.

Migraines are a risk factor for stroke and may be the cause of 25% of strokes in young adults. Other causes in young adults include drug abuse, sickle-cell disease, cardiac disease, and vasculitis.

Drug abuse causes strokes frequently through intravenous injection of particulate material, episodes of anoxia and hypotension, bursts of hypertension, and cerebral vasculitis. In particular, cocaine alkaloid ("crack") causes cerebral hemorrhage (see Chapter 21).

Older studies implicated oral contraceptives and pregnancy as risk factors for stroke. In contrast, recent studies have found that any danger from oral contraceptives is probably restricted to the original, relatively high-dose estrogen preparations. Currently available low-estrogen preparations do not predispose women to stroke. Similarly, pregnancy represents a minimal risk factor.

Other conditions no longer considered risk factors for stroke include "Type A" personality and stress. Despite the popular appeal of the concept, scientific studies have not shown that stress or other psychologic factors pose risk for strokes.

Thrombosis and Embolus

The majority of strokes are caused by a thrombosis that propagates within an atherosclerotic extracranial or intracerebral (cerebral) artery and simply occludes it. This process, which comprises the vast majority of strokes, is technically an *ischemic stroke*.

Another cause is an embolus from a carotid artery lodging in a cerebral artery, that is, an *arterial-arterial embolus*. Similarly, an embolus from the heart's endocardial surface may lodge in a cerebral artery. Other causes of thrombosis and embolism are vasculitis, drug abuse, sickle-cell disease, and other blood dyscrasias. In short, the usual causes of strokes are usually abnormalities of the heart, blood vessels, or blood.

Cell death in these strokes may be from an accumulation of excitatory, neurotoxic neurotransmitters, such as *glutamate*. For example, during a stroke, the *N*-methyl-D-aspartate *(NMDA)* receptors, which normally bind glutamate to open calcium channels, are overstimulated and allow fatal concentrations of calcium to flood the cells.

Infarctions in the Carotid Artery Distribution.   Cerebral artery thrombosis and embolism produce cerebral infarction in the distribution of the artery and patterns of clinical deficits (Fig. 11–1 and Table 11–3).

TABLE 11–3. *Strokes or Cerebrovascular Accidents (CVAs)*

Carotid artery
  Anterior cerebral
    Contralateral lower extremity paresis
    Mutism, apathy, pseudobulbar palsy*
  Middle cerebral
    Contralateral hemiparesis
    Hemisensory loss
    Aphasia
    Hemi-inattention
  Posterior cerebral
    Contralateral homonymous hemianopsia
    Alexia without agraphia
Vertebrobasilar system
  Basilar artery
    Total occlusion
      Coma
      Locked-in syndrome[†]
    Occlusion of branch
      Cranial nerve palsy with contralateral hemiparesis[†]
      Internuclear ophthalmoplegia[†]
  Vertebral artery
    Lateral medullary (Wallenberg's) syndrome[†]

*With bilateral infarctions.
[†]No cognitive impairment.

- *Anterior* cerebral artery infarction damages the anterior and medial aspects of the frontal lobe. It typically causes paresis and apraxia of the contralateral leg. With bilateral anterior cerebral artery infarctions, the resulting extensive frontal lobe damage causes pseudobulbar palsy, apathy, mutism, and the other signs of the "frontal lobe syndrome" (see Chapter 7), along with motor impairments of both legs.

- *Middle* cerebral artery infarction, which is the most common, results in contralateral hemiparesis, hemisensory loss, aphasia with dominant hemisphere lesions, and hemi-inattention with nondominant hemisphere strokes (see Fig. 20–8).

Cerebral emboli-induced infarctions develop suddenly and painfully as the embolus lodges in a cerebral vessel. Cerebral thromboses, in contrast, generally develop slowly or intermittently, begin during sleep, and are relatively painless. In both cases, the region surrounding the infarction becomes edematous. When edema is most severe, during the third to fifth days, the deficits are most pronounced. Some clinical recovery occurs as the edema resolves; however, the infarction remains a functionless scar that can produce seizures (see Chapter 10).

Infarctions in the Basilar Artery Distribution. Infarctions in the basilar artery distribution cause brainstem, cerebellar, or posterior cerebral injuries. In contrast to cerebral hemisphere infarctions, brainstem infarctions generally do not cause language or intellectual impairment (Table 11–3). Small brainstem infarctions usually cause constellations of cranial nerve injuries and hemiparesis. Large ones usually cause coma, if not immediate death.

The posterior cerebral arteries, as previously noted, are really branches of the basilar artery. Infarction of a posterior cerebral artery causes a contralateral homonymous hemianopsia and occasionally alexia without agraphia (see Chapters 8 and 12). Bilateral posterior cerebral artery TIAs or strokes can lead, respectively, to transient or permanent (cortical) blindness. As previously noted, these TIAs can also lead to TGA.

Precise localization of small brainstem infarctions is often desirable for both practical and academic reasons. Lesions of the midbrain cause ipsilateral oculomotor nerve and contralateral paresis (see Fig. 4–8). Pontine lesions cause ipsilateral abducens nerve and contralateral paresis (see Fig. 4–10). Midline pons or midbrain infarctions cause the medial longitudinal (MLF) syndrome (see Chapters 12 and 15). Finally, lateral medullary infarctions, which are the most common brainstem infarction, cause ipsilateral limb ataxia, palatal paresis, Horner's syndrome, and alternating hypalgesia (see Wallenberg syndrome, Fig. 2–10).

One clinical implication of localization is that once it is known that the lesion is situated in the brainstem, the physician can surmise that the patient's mental function is intact. For example, a patient with right hemiparesis and a left sixth cranial nerve palsy is unlikely to have aphasia.

Hemorrhages

Cerebral hemorrhages are most often the result of hypertension and erupt in the basal ganglia, thalamus, pons, and cerebellum (see Figs. 18–1 and 20–8). They typically occur abruptly and, because of the increased intracranial pressure, produce headaches, nausea, and vomiting. Patients usually lose consciousness and have profound neurologic deficits.

Although cerebral hemorrhage patients are usually sent immediately to neurologists, psychiatrists should be able to identify several varieties of cerebral hemorrhage. They should recognize a hemorrhage induced by certain monamine oxidase inhibitors, especially because an antihypertensive medication might attenuate it (see Chapter 9). The *cerebellar hemorrhage*, which can be diagnosed by its clinical characteristics—occipital headache, gait ataxia, dysarthria, and lethargy—should usually be immediately evacuated as a life-saving step.

Subarachnoid hemorrhage (SAH), usually the result of a ruptured berry aneurysm (a balloonlike arterial dilation), most often causes a prostrating headache and nuchal rigidity but not necessarily any physical deficits. Sexual activity and other exertion can precipitate a SAH. Sometimes a SAH mimics coital cephalalgia or a migraine (see Chapter 9). However, when an aneurysm ruptures, the CT or MRI will usually reveal blood in the subarachnoid space at the base of the brain or within the ventricles, and the lumbar puncture will yield bloody or xanthochromic cerebrospinal fluid (CSF).

STROKES AND COGNITIVE CHANGES

Dementia

Multi-infarct dementia (*Vascular Dementia* in the *DSM-IV* [see below]) has been cited as one of the most common causes of dementia, but the incidence of Alzheimer's disease and its relative, diffuse Lewy body disease (see Chapter 7), is actually much greater. In addition, many, if not most, individuals with multi-infarct dementia also have underlying or coexistent Alzheimer's disease.

Multi-infarct dementia can result from several mechanisms. The most common is simply multiple cerebral cortical infarctions that obliterate large chunks of brain tissue. Another common one is hypertension-induced multiple small subcortical strokes or *lacunes*. This condition, *état lacunaire* and *Binswanger's disease*, essentially consists of numerous 0.5 to 1.5 cm scars in the white matter. Alternatively, in critical areas only a few small strokes can produce marked cognitive impairment.

Multi-infarct dementia is more closely associated with left-sided than right-sided lesions, even allowing for aphasia. Otherwise, location or severity of strokes has little effect on the development of dementia.

The clinical hallmarks of multi-infarct dementia are the accompanying *focal neurologic deficits*, such as hemiparesis, dysarthria, clumsiness, and gait impairment. Signs of frontal lobe injury—apathy, emotional instability, impaired executive ability, incontinence, and pseudobulbar palsy—often predominate. Of the various physical deficits, gait impairment is so prominent that it places most cases of multi-infarct dementia in the subcortical dementia category.

Another important, although not pathognomonic, feature is that neurologic function deteriorates stepwise. An irregular succession of strokes presumably adds various physical and cognitive impairments.

Certainly more than the quality of cognitive impairment, physical deficits distinguish multi-infarct dementia from Alzheimer's disease. Cognitive impairment in both conditions is complicated by delusions and, less frequently, hallucinations. However, depression is more common in multi-infarct dementia than Alzheimer's (see below).

In evaluating a patient for dementia or to assess the damage following a stroke, CT and MRI can reveal cerebral infarcts and other signs of cerebrovascular changes in multi-infarct dementia. Although rarely necessary clinically, positron emission tomography (PET) and single positron emission computed tomography (SPECT) shows multiple, almost random hypometabolic regions. (In contrast, hypometabolism in Alzheimer's disease involves the temporal and parietal association cortex regions and eventually the frontal lobes.)

As noted earlier, multi-infarct dementia is included in the *DSM-IV* as *Vascular Dementia*. Dementia in *Vascular Dementia* is diagnosed by the same criteria as the dementia in Alzheimer's disease and other illnesses (see Chapter 7). The *DSM-IV* criteria also require focal neurologic signs or laboratory evidence, presumably by CT or MRI, that indicates cerebrovascular disease causally related to the cognitive impairment. Unlike the criteria in previous editions, vascular dementia's characteristic stepwise, often abrupt, course is no longer required.

Other Mental Changes

Well-known, stroke-induced neuropsychologic disturbances include aphasia, Gerstmann's syndrome, apraxia, and hemi-inattention. In addition, strokes may also cause partial complex and other seizures because about 5% of cerebral infarctions become irritative, that is, their scars have epileptogenic potential. Therefore, in patients with cerebrovascular disease, brief, generalized confusion may result from TIAs, transient global amnesia, or partial complex seizures.

Other, more extensive or more variable neuropsychologic deficits result from infarctions of the large areas of the cerebral cortex tenuously perfused at the periphery of the cerebrovascular perfusion network, the *watershed areas*. These areas are vulnerable because of their tenuous blood supply by delicate terminal branches of the cerebral arteries. Episodes of severe anoxia, hypotension, carbon monoxide poisoning, or similar insult, often produce a *watershed infarction*. Depending on its extent and severity, patients are often left with dementia, a persistent vegetative state, cortical blindness, or, because the perisylvian language arc is relatively well-perfused, isolation aphasia (see Chapter 8).

Depression

Following a stroke, from 30% to 50% of patients display symptoms of depression ranging from apathy to a sense of complete worthlessness. These patients have been loosely diagnosed as having *post-stroke depression*. (The comparable *DSM-IV* term is Mood Disorder Due to a General Medical Condition.)

The classic association of depression and strokes in the left frontal lobe has been challenged by several recent studies. In them, depression has been correlated with lesions in the right as well as the left cerebral hemispheres; basal ganglia, thalamus, and other subcortical, as well as cortical, lesions; and other regions besides the frontal lobes.

In contrast to anatomic correlates, the clinical correlates of post-stroke depression are reliable and practical. In these, post-stroke depression is associated with older patient age, greater functional disability, aphasia, cognitive impairment, and subsequent mortality. Depression is also likely in stroke patients recovering more slowly than expected or "underachieving" in rehabilitation programs. However, physicians must bear in mind other stroke-induced conditions that can mimic, induce, or coexist with depression, such as aphasia, frontal lobe syndromes, dementia, pseudobulbar palsy, and aprosody.

Antidepressants may help, but lack of thorough studies does not permit neurologic guidelines. In general, however, partly because patients with post-stroke depression have lost cerebral tissue, they usually require small doses of antidepressants. Stroke patients older than 65 years are relatively resistant to antidepressants. Neurologists tend to treat many individual symptoms, such as insomnia and anxiety, with specific medications rather than antidepressants. Although electroshock therapy may cause more confusion than usual, it is safe in post-stroke depression.

Alternatively, some mood changes can be induced by medications that stroke patients are apt to be taking. For example, many antihypertensives, such as propranolol

(Inderal), impair mentation by reducing cerebral blood flow, acting as false neuro-transmitters, or otherwise interfering with neuronal metabolism. When diuretics reduce serum sodium concentration below 125 mEq/ml, they can cause confusion and seizures. Antihypertensives can lead to orthostatic hypotension, lightheadedness, vertigo, and, when patients suddenly stand upright, loss of consciousness.

Locked-In Syndrome

Among the innumerable patients who have sustained multiple strokes and appear demented, mute, and quadriplegic, physicians should search for the patient who has the *locked-in syndrome.* In this rare but important condition, mute, quadriplegic patients have *intact cognitive capacity* and, if only by moving their eyes, some ability to communicate.

The locked-in syndrome usually results from an infarction of the base or ventral surface of the pons (basis pontis, see Fig. 2–9) or medulla (bulb) when a branch of the basilar artery is occluded (Fig. 11–3). Patients are mute because of complete bulbar palsy and quadriplegic because of interruption of the corticospinal tract. They usually require tracheostomy and ventilator support because of the bulbar palsy. The locked-in syndrome can also develop as a result of peripheral nervous system diseases in which the cranial as well as the peripheral nerves are affected. It has complicated the course of myasthenia gravis, amyotrophic lateral sclerosis, and the Guillain-Barré syndrome (see Chapters 5 and 6).

The upper brainstem, bulb's dorsal surface, and connections with the cerebral cortex are all intact. Thus, patients are alert and retain normal cognition, affective capacity, and, given sufficient clues, a sleep-wake cycle. Otherwise almost totally paralyzed, they can still purposefully move their eyes and eyelids. By closing their eyes in a "yes" or "no" pattern, patients can communicate by answering questions. Their EEGs are relatively normal because the physiologic connections between the thalamus and cerebral cortex are preserved.

The medical, social, and legal management of locked-in syndrome patients should be based on their being cognizant. They can understand people talking and reading to them, and they can accurately convey their wishes, including decisions regarding their care. Although patients who have suffered a brainstem infarction occasionally

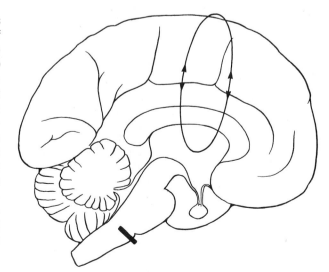

FIGURE 11–3. The locked-in syndrome usually results from an infarction of the ventral or basilar portion of the lower brainstem, typically at the basis pontis (see Fig. 2–9). A lesion in this area (indicated by the bar) would sever the corticospinal tracts and directly injure cranial nerves IX through XII. However, it would not damage several vital systems: (1) the brainstem's reticular activating system; (2) the cerebral hemispheres, particularly the cerebral cortex; and (3) the cerebral and brainstem system that governs ocular movement (see Fig. 12–12). This lesion, which is nowhere near the cortex, would not affect the brain's cognitive, language, or visual centers. The EEG is relatively normal because the reverberating circuits between the thalamus and the cerebral cortex (indicated by the loop), which generate the organized, relatively regular background EEG activity, are also unharmed.

partially recover, overall prognosis is poor. On the other hand, those debilitated from peripheral nervous system illnesses often totally recover.

An examination for locked-in syndrome might be undertaken in patients who are unable to speak or move their limbs but can voluntarily look from side to side. The physician should ask these patients to blink a certain number of times. If they respond, a system of communication can be developed. (One patient communicated freely using eyelid blinks in Morse code.) If patients can blink meaningfully, the physician should test their ability to see and calculate. Afterward, detailed status testing can be undertaken.

Persistent Vegetative State

A massive cerebral injury or progression of a neurologic degenerative disease may result in a *persistent vegetative state (PVS)*. Both children and adults may develop PVS, which is much more common in both than locked-in syndrome. Patients in PVS are completely unaware of either themselves or their surroundings, devoid of cognitive capacity, and unable to interact or communicate in any manner (Fig. 11–4). While patients can retain a sleep-wake cycle, breathe without respirators, withdraw a limb from noxious stimulation, and maintain hypothalamic and brainstem reflexes (vegetative functions), they are bedridden with quadriparesis and incontinence (Fig. 11–5). Their eyes, moving spontaneously and randomly, may momentarily fix on a face or, in a reflex, turn toward sounds, including voices. Unfortunately, these eye movements may be misinterpreted by relatives as the patient appreciating their presence or understanding their words. Patients are neither in suspended animation, temporary unconsciousness, nor in a prolonged sleep. Their vegetative activity and seeming wakefulness are rudimentary.

The PVS is usually caused by massive cerebral insults, such as major head trauma, cerebral anoxia from cardiac arrest, profound hypoglycemia, and massive strokes. After these insults, most patients are comatose for days or weeks and then enter the PVS. Alternatively, patients with degenerative illnesses, such as Alzheimer's disease or childhood-onset metabolic disorders, slip into the PVS without first being comatose. School-aged children and teenagers sustain cerebral injuries—usually from motor vehicle and other accidents, drug overdoses, or suicide attempts—that produce this

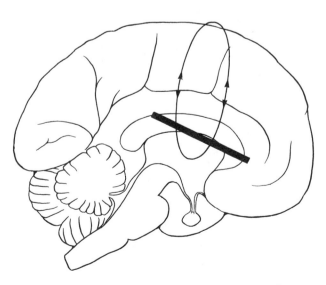

FIGURE 11–4. The persistent vegetative state, which can be caused by cerebral anoxia or numerous other conditions, results from extensive damage to the cerebral cortex or the tissue immediately underlying it (indicated by the bar). These injuries impair all cerebral functions, including cognitive ability, purposeful motor activity, vision, and speech. The brainstem, being relatively unaffected by these conditions, becomes independent of cerebral control. It then operates by reflex to regulate the body's vegetative functions: swallowing, digestion, breathing, metabolism, and temperature regulation. The EEG is abnormal because the cerebrum and its interactions with the brainstem (indicated by the loop) are damaged.

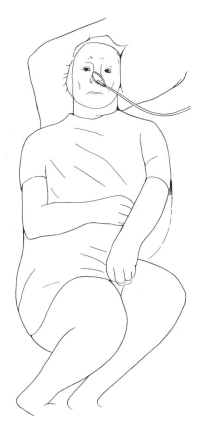

FIGURE 11–5. Patients in the persistent vegetative state tend to assume a decorticate (flexed or fetal) posture because of extensive cerebral damage. Although they are awake, have roving eye movements, retain a sleep-wake cycle, and usually do not require a respirator, they are mute, virtually motionless, and unable to respond to visitors or examiners. Patients are almost always dependent on combinations of nasogastric tubes, intravenous lines, urinary catheters, tracheostomies, and other mechanical devices. Being immobile, they are vulnerable to aspiration pneumonia, urinary tract infections, and pressure sores.

hopeless state. Once patients have been in PVS from head trauma for 1 year or from degenerative illness for 3 months, there is almost no chance of recovery.

Beyond its heart-wrenching neurologic aspects, PVS raises important ethical and legal considerations. Many patients may have directed that they "not live like a vegetable," and their relatives have sought to discontinue nutrition, as well as artificial supports. Several legal cases have explored the limits of maintaining PVS patients according to or against their wishes. The role of the psychiatrist in this grim situation might be to assess cognitive function; confirm that the patient does not have a toxic-metabolic encephalopathy, the locked-in syndrome, or a correctable cause of dementia; and discuss the prognosis with colleagues and family members. The psychiatrist might also help the patient's family and primary physicians write orders, if the need were to arise, for administration or withdrawal of medications, including oxygen, intravenous solutions, and blood products; renal dialysis and other mechanical, "life-sustaining" procedures; and resuscitation procedures.

MANAGING STROKE

Laboratory Tests

In most cases, diagnosis of stroke is based on clinical evaluation and confirmed by CT or MRI. The most common alternative diagnoses are structural lesions, such as a brain tumor, abscess, or subdural hematoma, and systemic illnesses with neurologic complications, such as vasculitis and temporal arteritis. Either type of scan will indicate the presence and location of almost all strokes, except those that are fresh or small. Skull x-rays and EEGs are superfluous. MRA is often performed to visualize the cerebral arteries. Arteriography is performed only in selected cases to diagnose carotid stenosis, cerebral aneurysms, and vascular malformations.

Examination of the CSF through a lumbar puncture (LP) is used to diagnose a subarachnoid hemorrhage and infections, such as meningitis and encephalitis that might mimic stroke. However, an LP is unnecessary for a routine stroke and should be avoided when an intracranial mass lesion is present (see Transtentorial Herniation, Chapter 19).

Therapy

For strokes judged to be ischemic, neurologists have been able to administer thrombolytic agents, such as tissue plasminogen activator (TPA), with the expectation that cerebral arterial occlusions will be at least partly dissolved and cerebral blood flow restored. As could be expected, TPA is potentially complicated by cerebral hemorrhage. Because TPA is dangerous, as well as beneficial, it must be administered by neurologists following a demanding set of guidelines, including administration within 3 hours after stroke onset and a CT showing no blood. Research is developing other thrombolytic agents, which are administered by angiography directly to an occlusion, and "neuroprotective agents" (medications that preserve ischemic brain tissue). Steroids, oxygen, and vasoactive medicines have no proven benefit.

Medical and nursing care is directed at preventing complications: aspiration pneumonia, decubitus ulcers, and urinary tract infections. If the patient is not alert or the gag reflex is diminished, medications and nutrition must be given intravenously or by a nasogastric tube. To prevent decubiti, which are unsightly, malodorous, and liable to lead to sepsis, physicians usually order air mattresses, sweat-absorbent bed surfaces (e.g., artificial sheepskins), and elbow and heel cushions for paretic limbs. Since urinary incontinence adds to the likelihood of developing a bed sore, makes patients cold and wet, and creates repugnant odors, physicians generally order catheters.

The patient's bed should be placed against the wall so that all visitors and staff must approach the patient from the side without perceptual impairment. For example, a patient with a left hemiparesis and a *left* homonymous hemianopsia should be placed with his or her *left* side against the wall so that people approach from the *right*, and important objects (e.g., call-buttons, television controls, clock, and pictures) can be seen and grasped.

In the initial phase, relatives who act as caregivers of stroke patients can be helpful by orienting the patient and bringing a luminous dial clock, a calendar, and pictures; repositioning the patient and moving paretic limbs to avoid contractures; and locating appropriate rehabilitation facilities. Eventually they may have greater difficulty in coping with the patient's mental than physical impairments. Caregivers are subject to depression at about three times the expected rate.

Physical therapy will often maintain the patient's muscle tone, forestall decubitus ulcers, and prevent contractures. It will usually help patients with simple hemiparesis to regain ability to walk, circumvent some impediments, and avoid maladaptive but expeditious physical compensations. Speech therapy may help with dysarthria and offer patients encouragement. Cognitive and perceptual skill training for impaired mentation, sensory impairment, and visual loss remains without proven value.

Hemi-inattention and anosognosia resolve over a period of 1 to 3 weeks. However, aphasias usually improve to almost their fullest extent in 4 to 6 weeks, after which deficits are usually permanent. Poor prognostic factors for recovery—as any physician might sense—are advanced age, dementia, persistent hemi-inattention, incontinence, bilateral brain damage, and prior strokes.

REFERENCES

Abramowicz M (ed): Alteplase for thrombolysis in acute ischemic stroke. Med Letter *38:* 99–100, 1996

Abramowicz M (ed): Clopidogrel for reduction of atherosclerotic events. Med Letter *40:* 59–60, 1998

Astrom M, Adolfsson R, Asplund K: Major depression in stroke patients. Stroke *24:* 976–982, 1993

Barnett HJM, Taylor DW, Eliasziw M, et al: Benefit of carotid endarterectomy in patients with symptomatic moderate or severe stenosis. N Engl J Med *339:* 1415–1425, 1998

House A: Depression associated with stroke. J Neuropsychiatry *8:* 453–457, 1997

Inzitari D, Pantoni L, Lamassa M, et al: Emotional arousal and phobia in transient global amnesia. Arch Neurol *54:* 866–873, 1997

Kaufman D, Lipton R: The persistent vegetative state: An analysis of clinical correlates and costs. NY State J Med *92:* 381–387, 1992

Lyden PD, Grotta JC, Levine SR, et al: Intravenous thrombolysis for acute stroke. Neurology *49:* 14–29, 1997

The Multi-Society Task Force on PVS: Medical aspects of the persistent vegetative state. N Engl J Med *330:* 1499–1508, 1572–1579, 1994

Petiti DB, Sidney S, Bernstein A, et al: Stroke in users of low-dose oral contraceptives. N Engl J Med *335:* 8–15, 1996

Quality Standards Subcommittee of the American Academy of Neurology: Practice parameters: Assessment and management of patients in the persistent vegetative state. Neurology *45:* 1015–1018, 1995

Tatemichi TK, Desmond DW, Paik M, et al: Clinical determinants of dementia related to stroke. Ann Neurol *33:* 568–575, 1993

Wannamethee SG, Shaper AG, Whincup PH, et al: Smoking cessation and the risk of stroke in middle-aged men. JAMA *274:* 155–160, 1995

QUESTIONS and ANSWERS: CHAPTER 11

1–10. Match the neurologic deficit (1–10) with the most likely artery of infarction (a–k).

Deficit

1. Left hemiparesis with relative sparing of the leg

2. Left lower extremity monoparesis

3. Monocular blindness from optic nerve ischemia

4. Left homonymous hemianopsia

5. Left palate paresis, left limb ataxia

6. Right third cranial nerve palsy with left hemiparesis

7. Right hemiparesis with aphasia

8. Quadriplegia and mutism with intact mentation

9. Left sixth and seventh cranial nerve palsy with right hemiparesis

10. Coma, quadriparesis

Artery

a. Right posterior cerebral
b. Left posterior cerebral
c. Right anterior cerebral
d. Right middle cerebral
e. Left anterior cerebral
f. Left middle cerebral
g. Ophthalmic
h. Vertebral or posterior inferior cerebellar
i. Perforating branch of basilar
j. Anterior spinal
k. Basilar

    ANSWERS: 1-d; 2-c; 3-g; 4-a; 5-h; 6-i; 7-f; 8-i, k; 9-i; 10-k

11–20. Match the type of transient neurologic deficit with the artery involved (carotid [a], basilar [b], both, or neither).

Deficit

11. Transient global amnesia

12. Monocular amaurosis fugax

13. Paresthesias of right arm and aphasia

14. Vertigo, nausea, nystagmus, and ataxia

15. Migraines

16. Locked-in syndrome

17. Diplopia

18. Cortical blindness

19. Transient hemiparesis

20. Quadriparesis and anesthesia below the chest but preserved position and vibration sensation

Artery

a. Carotid
b. Basilar

ANSWERS: 11-b; 12-a (ophthalmic artery); 13-a; 14-b; 15-a usually, but sometimes b; 16-b; 17-b; 18-b; 19-Both; 20-Neither. Occlusions of the anterior spinal artery, which is an occasional complication of surgery involving the aorta, injure the entire spinal cord except for the posterior columns.

21–30. A 74-year-old man has had a steadily worsening left-sided headache for 7 days, a nonfluent aphasia, right hemiparesis with hyperreflexia, a Babinski sign, and right homonymous hemianopsia. Which of the following should be considered as likely possibilities?

21. Cerebral hemorrhage

22. Subarachnoid hemorrhage

23. Brain tumor

24. Subdural hematoma

25. Basilar artery occlusion

26. Carotid artery occlusion

27. Brain abscess

28. Toxoplasmosis

29. Cerebral embolus

30. Multiple sclerosis

ANSWERS:

21. No. Cerebral hemorrhages usually are suddenly occurring catastrophic processes.
22. No. The headaches would also be sudden and incapacitating. Nuchal rigidity would be present.
23. A good choice. With the relatively short history and extensive deficits, only a rapidly growing brain tumor, such as a metastasis or glioblastoma, would be possible.
24. Unlikely. Although the headache and hemiparesis are consistent, the aphasia and hemianopsia are rare with masses outside the brain substance (i.e., extra-axial lesions).
25. No. He would be comatose.
26. Good choice. This is a typical story of progressive carotid stenosis leading to occlusion.

27. Another good choice.
28. Unlikely. Toxoplasmosis is found virtually only as a complication of AIDS. Moreover, because toxoplasmosis typically produces multiple infections, it rarely causes such a localized, unilateral constellation of symptoms.
29. No. Although the deficits are compatible, emboli occur suddenly.
30. No. The headache, extent of the lesion, and his age are inconsistent.

31–36. After a stroke, a 65-year-old man is alert, but he is mute and unable to move his palate, arms, or legs. He has bilateral hyperreflexia and Babinski signs. He responds to verbal and written questions by blinking his eyelids.

31. Does this man have a fluent, nonfluent, or global aphasia?

32. Is his vision impaired?

33. Is there evidence of cerebral damage?

34. How would the EEG appear?

35. What is this syndrome called?

36. Where is the lesion?

ANSWERS:

31. No. There is no evidence of aphasia. He can understand spoken language and respond appropriately.
32. No. He can read written questions.
33. No. The palate weakness and other motor pareses may be the result of brainstem damage. Cortical functions seem to be intact.
34. The EEG might appear normal because cortical functions are intact.
35. It is called the locked-in syndrome.
36. The lesion is in the ventral surface of the lower brainstem (i.e., the base of the pons or basis pontis).

37–41. A 64-year-old man who had sustained a right cerebral infarction the previous year is admitted after the sudden, painless onset of right hemiparesis and mutism. He now has bilateral paresis and no verbal output. Although his eyes are frequently open, he fails to respond to either voice or gesture. He seems to have normal sleep-wake cycles.

37. Where is the probable site of the recent injury?

38. What is the probable cause?

39. Would the EEG be normal?

40. If he were not paralyzed, would he be able to write?

41. Would he have bulbar or pseudobulbar palsy?

ANSWERS:

37. The new lesion is in the left (dominant) hemisphere. With the history of a prior right cerebral infarction, he now has bilateral infarctions.
38. The sudden, painless onset suggests a thrombotic or embolic stroke.
39. The EEG will be abnormal because of extensive cerebral damage.
40. No. Aphasic patients generally have difficulty in all modes of communication. Moreover, as the result of extensive cerebral cortex damage, he probably has dementia (i.e., multi-infarct [vascular] dementia).
41. He would probably have pseudobulbar palsy because, in the setting of bilateral cerebral infarctions, he is mute, bilaterally weak, and unresponsive to voice but has open eyes and a discernible sleep-wake cycle. Moreover, because he has evidence of no cognitive function and the EEG is abnormal, he is vegetative. If he makes no improvement in 1 month, he will probably evolve into a persistent vegetative state.

42–52. A 20-year-old woman awakens from sleep and finds that she has a mild left hemiparesis. Which are the possible causes of her deficit?

42. Cerebral thrombosis associated with high-dose estrogen oral contraceptives

43. Cerebral vasculitis from lupus or drug abuse

44. Cerebral embolus from mitral stenosis

45. Cerebral embolus from drug abuse

46. Septic cerebral embolus from bacterial endocarditis

47. Cerebral embolus from an atrial myxoma

48. Cerebral toxoplasmosis from a previously undiagnosed HIV infection

49. Infarction from sickle cell disease

50. Migraine-induced transient paresis (i.e., hemiplegic migraine)

51. A prolonged postictal (Todd's) paresis

52. Multiple sclerosis

> *ANSWERS:* All yes. Strokes in young people are the result of diseases of the heart, blood, or blood vessels. The other processes (48, 50–52), although not strictly strokes, may mimic them.

53–56. A 20-year-old woman is brought to the emergency room by her family because she is suddenly unable to speak or move her right side. She looks directly forward, but does not follow verbal requests. On inspection of her fundi, her eyes constantly evert. She seems to respond to visual images in all fields. The right arm and leg are flaccid and immobile, but her face is symmetric. Deep tendon reflexes (DTRs) are symmetric, and no pathologic reflexes are elicited. She does not react to noxious stimuli on the right side of her face or body.

53. Where is the apparent lesion?

54. (a) What pathologic features usually found with such a lesion are not present in the patient? (b) What non-neurologic features are present?

55. What is the most likely origin?

56. What readily available laboratory tests would lend great support to the diagnosis?

> *ANSWERS:*
>
> 53. A patient who seems to have global aphasia and a right hemiparesis would usually have a left hemisphere lesion.
> 54. (a) She does not have the usual paresis of the lower (right) face, asymmetrical DTRs, Babinski signs, or a right homonymous hemianopsia. (b) Eversion of the eyes during inspection is almost always a voluntary act. Inability to perceive noxious stimuli is rare in cerebral lesions. Likewise, a sharply demarcated sensory loss (splitting the midline) is not neurologic.
> 55. A psychogenic disturbance is the most likely cause.
> 56. A normal EEG, CT, or MRI would support the diagnosis.

57–61. A 70-year-old man has the sudden onset of an occipital headache, nausea, vomiting, and an inability to walk. He has no paresis but a downward drift of the right arm and symmetrically active DTRs with normal plantar response. He has dysmetria on right finger–nose and heel-shin movements. His gait is so ataxic that he must be supported when he attempts to walk.

57. Where is the lesion?

58. Which side?

59. What is its origin?

60. What is the consequence of increased size of the lesion?

> *ANSWERS:*
>
> 57. The lesion is in the cerebellum.
> 58. Abnormal cerebellar findings are referable to the ipsilateral hemisphere, which is the right side in this case.
> 59. In view of the patient's age and the sudden onset, a stroke is most likely. Because it is painful, a cerebellar hemorrhage must be given first consideration.

60. If the hemorrhage were to expand, it would compress the fourth ventricle and cause obstructive hydrocephalus. With further expansion, the hemorrhage would compress the brainstem. Coma and death would follow.

61. Which one of the following is a typical finding in a 65-year-old man with transient global amnesia (TGA)?

a. Retaining ability to recall his name and address
b. Having underlying psychopathology
c. Having several prior episodes
d. Ability to perform mathematics

> **ANSWER:** a. Patients with TGA, despite gross amnesia otherwise, can typically state their own name and several other personal identifying facts. Their problem is recalling recently acquired information. Preservation of their identity characteristically sets TGA apart from many psychogenic disturbances. In addition, unlike partial complex seizures, TGA episodes rarely recur.

62–65. A 75-year-old man has had 5 days of moderately severe, unremitting left-sided headaches and then right-sided hemiparesis with hyperreflexia and a Babinski sign. On admission, he has neither aphasia nor visual field loss. During the initial 3 days in the hospital, however, he develops stupor with a dilated, unreactive left pupil and bilateral Babinski signs.

62. Where is the lesion?

63. What are the possible causes?

64. Which would be the most appropriate diagnostic test?

65. What is the origin of the pupillary abnormality?

> **ANSWERS:**
>
> 62. In view of the left-sided headaches and contralateral hemiparesis, the lesion would be on the "left side" of the CNS, but the physician cannot initially be certain that the deficit is referable to the cerebral hemisphere rather than the brainstem because the patient has no language or visual disturbance. The development of transtentorial herniation, however, makes it clear that the lesion had been in the left supratentorial (cerebral) compartment.
> 63. The rapid demise with transtentorial herniation suggests that a mass lesion continued to expand. A subdural hematoma is most likely, but an occlusion of the internal carotid artery with subsequent cerebral swelling and herniation is possible. Tumors, arteriovenous malformations, and abscesses are less common, nonvascular causes (see Chapter 19).
> 64. The most appropriate diagnostic test would be a CT or MRI. Presumably, a routine history, physical examination, and initial hematologic and chemistry tests would have been done on admission. By the time he "herniates," however, emergency measures must be instituted and those preliminary studies postponed.
> 65. The dilation and unreactivity of the left pupil are caused by mass lesion's compressing the third cranial nerve between the temporal lobe and the tentorial notch.

66–67. Found wandering about in a confused manner, a 45-year-old woman is brought to the emergency room. She is lethargic, inattentive, and confused. She has word-finding difficulties, but she is not aphasic. Her pupils are equal and reactive, and her fundi are normal. Extraocular movements are full. All her extremities move well. She has hyperactive DTRs and bilateral Babinski signs.

66. Where is the lesion?

67. What is the most likely cause?

> **ANSWERS:**
>
> 66. Since the woman has no lateralizing signs or indications of increased intracranial pressure, a physician cannot say that she has a "lesion." She is more likely to have a toxic-metabolic encephalopathy (delirium).
> 67. Causes of diffuse neurologic dysfunction are most often metabolic alterations (uremia, hypoglycemia), postictal confusion, infectious processes (encephalitis), intoxications (medications, alcohol, drugs, barbiturates), and head trauma.

68. Which of the following varieties of strokes most often appears as patients awaken in the morning?

a. Cerebral hemorrhage
b. Cerebral thrombosis
c. Cerebral embolus
d. Subarachnoid hemorrhage

ANSWER: b

69. Which of the varieties of strokes described in Question 68 most often develops during sexual intercourse?

ANSWER: d

70. Of the following, which is the most important stroke risk factor?

a. "Type A" personality
b. High cholesterol diet
c. Obesity
d. Cigarette smoking
e. Hypertension
f. Lack of exercise

ANSWER: e

71. Which of the following is the standard therapy for vertebrobasilar artery TIAs?

a. Endarterectomy
b. Surgical anastomosis
c. Coumadin
d. Aspirin

ANSWER: d

72. Which of the following is the most important cause of multi-infarct (vascular) dementia?

a. Carotid bifurcation atherosclerosis
b. Cerebral emboli
c. Generalized atherosclerosis
d. Hypertension causing small vessel disease

ANSWER: d

73. Which is aspirin's mechanism of action in reducing TIAs?

a. It interferes with platelet adhesion.
b. It retards prostaglandins production.
c. It inactivates the NMDA receptor.
d. It is a vasodilator.

ANSWER: a

74. A 28-year-old man has had a 3-day history of increasing left arm weakness and clumsiness and a mild generalized headache. Examination reveals only hyperactive DTRs in the mildly paretic left arm. Routine medical evaluation reveals no abnormalities. Both CTs and MRIs show about five large ring-enhancing cerebral lesions. Of the following, which is the most likely cause of his neurologic difficulties?

a. Cerebral infarction
b. Cerebral hemorrhage
c. Toxoplasmosis
d. Glioblastoma
e. Meningioma

ANSWER: c. The most common cause of multiple ring-enhancing cerebral lesions in young adults is toxoplasmosis, which is a typical manifestation of AIDS. Cerebral lymphoma is another complication, but it usually causes only a single lesion. Cerebral cysticercosis (not offered as a choice) causes focal signs and multiple cerebral lesions, but this condition develops insidiously and usually presents with a seizure. Cerebral infarction in a 28-year-old man, in the absence of a predisposing condition, is rare. With cerebral infarctions, the scans usually show a "pie-shaped" pattern. Cerebral hemorrhage is typically a sudden event, associated with blood-density on scans. A glioblastoma would also be rare in a 28-year-old individual, and the scans would have indicated an infiltrating tumor. A meningioma is likewise rare in young adults. When it does occur, a meningioma is extra-axial and slowly growing.

75–86. Match the sign (75–86) with the condition (a–b), both, or neither.

75. Mutism

76. Quadriparesis

77. Voluntary eye movement

78. Results from cerebral hypoxia

79. Sleep-wake cycles may be preserved

80. Electrocerebral silence

81. Cognitive capacity intact

82. Cognitive capacity lost

83. Due to lesion in base of pons that spares reticular activating system

84. Due to lesions that damage virtually all of cerebral cortex

85. May be caused by Guillain-Barré syndrome or myasthenia gravis

86. Can be caused by insulin injections, as in attempted murder

a. Locked-in syndrome
b. Persistent vegetative state

ANSWERS: 75-Both, 76-Both, 77-a, 78-b, 79-Both, 80-Neither, 81-a, 82-b, 83-a, 84-b, 85-a, 86-b

87. Which of the following characteristics most reliably distinguishes multi-infarct (vascular) dementia (MID) from Alzheimer's dementia?

a. Stepwise development
b. MRIs that show atrophy
c. Aphasia
d. Focal physical findings
e. Greatest cognitive deficit is loss of memory

ANSWER: d. Focal physical findings, such as hemiparesis, homonymous hemianopsia, and pseudobulbar palsy, which are manifestations of infarctions of the cerebrum, cerebellum, or brainstem, characterize multi-infarct (vascular) dementia. A stepwise development of multi-infarct dementia is frequent but this is not the most characteristic aspect. Moreover, a stepwise onset is typical, but it is no longer a requirement in *DSM-IV* for the diagnosis of vascular dementia. Both multi-infarct and Alzheimer's disease dementias follow progressive as well as a stepwise pattern. Atrophy is seen in both conditions. However, in multi-infarct dementia, infarctions are often visible on an MRI or CT. Aphasia is a characteristic finding of multi-infarct dementia, but anomic aphasia is also sometimes found in Alzheimer's disease. Loss of memory is a common feature and diagnostic criteria for both conditions.

88. In patients with symptomatic carotid stenosis, what degree of stenosis justifies surgery?

a. 50%
b. 60%
c. 70%
d. 80%
e. 90%
f. 100%

ANSWER: c. A 70% or greater stenosis of the suspected carotid artery in a symptomatic individual justifies surgery, provided that it can be performed with little risk (i.e., 3% or less). Arteries with 100% stenosis (total occlusion) are inoperable. The data is less clear on the severity of carotid stenosis in an asymptomatic individual.

89. Which pattern is most likely found on positron emission tomography (PET) and single positron tomography (SPECT) in an individual with multi-infarct (vascular) dementia?

a. Multiple, scattered hypometabolic regions
b. Hypometabolism in the temporal and parietal association cortex
c. Hypometabolism in the frontal lobes
d. None of the above

ANSWER: a. The multiple discrete areas probably reflect the underlying strokes. Alzheimer's disease scans show hypometabolism in the temporal and parietal association cortex and eventually hypometabolism in the frontal lobes.

90. Which are the following characteristics of the *N*-methyl-D-aspartate receptor?

a. It is usually called the NMDA receptor.
b. It regulates calcium channels.
c. Excitatory neurotransmitters, such as glutamate, bind onto this receptor.
d. Overstimulation of the receptor leads to cell death by calcium flooding.
e. All of the above.

ANSWER: e

91. A 73-year-old woman arises from a vigorous hair washing at her local beauty parlor and finds that she is vertiginous and nauseated. A physician detects nystagmus and ataxia of her limbs and trunk. Her symptoms and signs resolve over 1 hour. What is the most likely cause of her disturbance?

a. Carotid artery TIA
b. Vertebrobasilar artery TIA
c. A chemical in the hair wash
d. Ordinary lightheadedness

ANSWER: b. She probably has had hyperextension (excessive backward bending) of her neck that crimped her vertebral arteries and caused a vertebrobasilar artery TIA. This condition is most common in elderly people who have vertebral osteophytes that press against the vertebral arteries as they pass upward through the cervical spine. This disorder is sometimes called the *vanity syndrome* because it was first described in patrons of beauty parlors who had their hair washed in basins (vanities).

92. In which groups of patients is post-stroke depression least likely to be found?

a. Patients older than 75 years
b. Patients younger than 55 years
c. Patients with a high mortality rate
d. All of the above

ANSWER: b. Post-stroke depression is most common in elderly patients. It carries an increased risk of morbidity and mortality.

93. With which disability is post-stroke depression least associated?

a. Functional disability, particularly hemiplegia
b. Aphasia
c. Cognitive impairment
d. Bulbar palsy

ANSWER: d. Post-stroke depression is associated with physical, language, cognitive deficits, and pseudobulbar palsy. In other words, when asked to evaluate a stroke victim for depression, the conscientious psychiatrist should seek these neurologic disorders that can mimic, precipitate, or coexist with a stroke.

94. A variety of studies have shown that post-stroke depression arises from lesions in the left frontal lobe. (True/False)

ANSWER: False. Although classic studies reported an association of post-stroke depression with lesions in the left frontal lobe, newer studies have implicated the right cerebral hemisphere, other lobes, and subcortical structures, such as the basal ganglia and thalamus.

Visual Disturbances

Visual disturbances are frequent and complex. This chapter describes several common neuro-ophthalmologic problems likely to occur in psychiatric patients, including decreased visual acuity, visual field loss, glaucoma, and visual hallucinations (Table 12–1). It also describes several ophthalmologic causes of visual impairment in the elderly (Table 12–2).

EVALUATING VISUAL DISTURBANCES

After determining the patient's specific visual symptom, the physician's initial examination typically includes inspecting the globe or "eyeball" (Fig. 12–1); assessing visual acuity, visual fields, and optic fundi; and testing pupil reflexes and ocular movement. Subsequent examinations are required for psychogenic blindness, visual agnosia, and other perceptual disturbances (see below).

Physicians routinely measure visual acuity by having the patient read from either a Snellen wall chart or a handheld card (Fig. 12–2). A person with "normal" visual acuity can read $\frac{3}{8}$-inch letters at a distance of 20 feet. This acuity, which is the refer-

TABLE 12–1. *Common Neurologic Causes of Visual Hallucinations*

Blindness
    Blindness with hearing impairment (e.g., sensory deprivation)
    Palinopsia
    Sudden blindness, including Anton's syndrome
Delirium tremens
Dementia-producing diseases
    Alzheimer's
    Lewy body
    Parkinson's
Intoxications
    Alcoholic hallucinosis
    Hallucinogens: Phencyclidine (PCP, angel dust), lysergic acid diethylamide (LSD),
        mescaline, amphetamines
    Medicines: L-dopa, scopolamine, atropine, penicillin
Migraine with aura (classic migraine)
Narcolepsy: Hypnopompic (awakening) and hypnagogic (falling asleep) hallucinations
    (see Chapter 17)
Peduncular hallucinosis
Seizures (see Chapter 10)
    Frontal lobe
    Elementary (visual)
    Complex partial

TABLE 12–2. *Common Causes of Visual Impairments in Individuals Older than 65 Years*

Presbyopia and other accommodation problems
Cataracts
Macular degeneration
Glaucoma
Temporal (giant cell) arteritis
Visual agnosia and cortical blindness from multiple infarctions or Alzheimer's disease

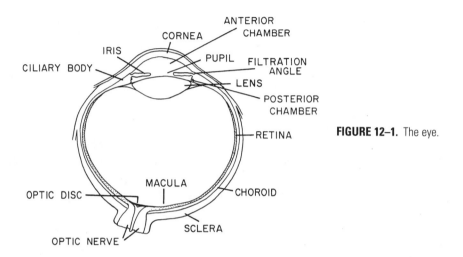

FIGURE 12–1. The eye.

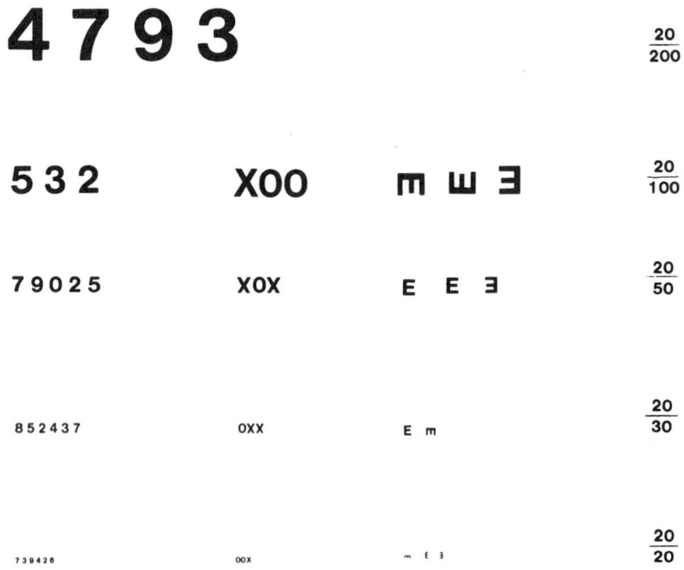

4 7 9 3
$\frac{20}{200}$

5 3 2   **XOO**   **ⱶ ш Ǝ**
$\frac{20}{100}$

7 9 0 2 5   **XOX**   **E   E   Ǝ**
$\frac{20}{50}$

852437   OXX   E ɯ
$\frac{20}{30}$

739426   OOX
$\frac{20}{20}$

FIGURE 12–2. This handheld visual acuity chart should be held 14 inches from the patient. The acuity is that line that can be read without a mistake. Each eye should be tested individually. For neurologic evaluations, patients should wear their glasses or contact lenses.

ence point of the system, is designated 20/20. People with 20/40 acuity must be as close as 20 feet to see what a normal person can see from a distance of 40 feet.

Optical Disturbances

In *myopia*, usually because of either too "thick" a lens, too "long" a globe, or other optical abnormality, people have increasingly blurred vision at increasingly greater distances (Fig. 12–3). Myopia first becomes troublesome during adolescence when it causes difficulty with seeing blackboards, watching movies, and driving. Because reading and other close activities are unimpaired, people with myopia are said to be nearsighted.

In its counterpart, *hyperopia* or hypermetropia (farsightedness), the lens is usually too "thin" or the globe too "short." The refractive strength of the lens is insufficient. People with hyperopia have increasing visual difficulty at increasingly shorter distances. In *presbyopia*, older individuals are unable to focus on closely held objects because their relatively inelastic and dehydrated lenses cannot properly change shape. With their impaired near vision, people with hyperopia and those with presbyopia tend to hold newspapers and sew with needles at arms' length. Reading glasses usually can compensate for the problem by bringing the focal point into the proper working distance.

In addition to these naturally occurring conditions, use of certain medications can interfere with the *accommodation reflex*. Normally, when a person looks at a closely held object, the accommodation reflex, which is parasympathetic-mediated, contracts the ciliary body muscles. The accommodation reflex thickens the lens to focus the image on the retina, causes miosis, and increases convergence muscle tone. For example, when a person begins to read a newspaper, the eyes slightly converge, the pupils constrict, and the lens thickens to provide greater refraction of the closely held newsprint on the retina.

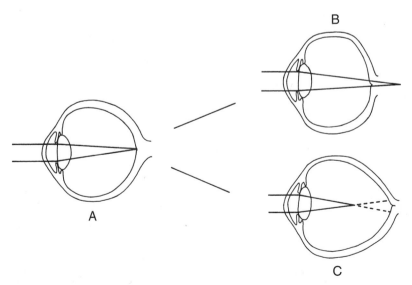

FIGURE 12–3. Image focusing in hyperopic and myopic eyes. **A,** In normal eyes, the lens focuses the image on to the retina. **B,** In hyperopic eyes, the shorter globe or improperly focusing lens causes the image to fall behind the retina. **C,** In myopic eyes, the longer globe or improperly focusing lens causes the image to fall in front of the retina. Lenses correct the refractive errors of hyperopia and myopia. In addition, surgical "flattening" of the lens corrects myopia in many individuals.

In *drug-induced accommodation paresis*, patients have visual acuity impairment for closely held objects (Fig. 12–4). The serotonin reuptake inhibitors and clozapine, as well as the tricyclic antidepressants, which have well-known anticholinergic properties, all produce blurred vision as a relatively common side effect. For example, venlafaxine (Effexor) causes paresis of accommodation in 9% of patients taking 75 mg daily, and sertraline (Zoloft) and paroxetine (Paxil) causes blurred vision in approximately 4% of patients. These medicines can impair accommodation without producing other anticholinergic effects, such as dry mouth, constipation, and urinary hesitancy.

Abnormalities of the Lens, Retina, and Optic Nerve

Cataracts (loss of lens transparency) result from complications of old age (senile cataract), trauma, diabetes, and myotonic dystrophy (see Chapter 6). In prolonged, high doses, phenothiazines produce minute lens opacities, but they rarely impair vision. Preliminary data also suggests that quetiapine (Seroquel) causes cataracts.

Pigmentary changes in the retina can be a manifestation of congenital injuries, degenerative diseases, diabetes, or the use of massive doses of phenothiazines (Fig. 12–5). In addition, acquired immune deficiency syndrome (AIDS) leads to opportunistic retinal infections.

In 25% or more of Americans older than 65 years, the cells of the retina's pigment epithelium, mostly in the macula, degenerate through a variety of mechanisms, including proliferation of the underlying blood vessels. When this condition involves the macula, *macular degeneration*, it impairs patients' fine, critical central vision. Some peripheral vision is spared. Patients characteristically lose their reading ability and have distorted images of friends' and relatives' faces. Despite those devastating losses, because some side vision remains, they can negotiate around their living

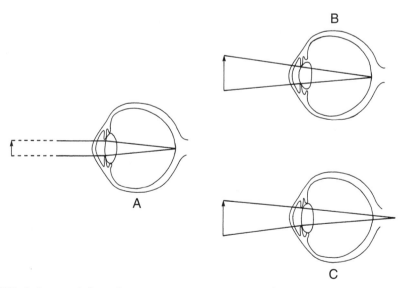

FIGURE 12–4. Accommodation and accommodation paresis. **A,** When looking at a distant object, parallel light rays are refracted little by a relatively flat lens onto the retina. **B,** Accommodation: when looking at a closely held object, ciliary muscle contraction increases the curvature of the lens, greatly refracting the light rays. **C,** Accommodation paresis: if the ciliary muscles are paretic, the lens cannot form a rounded shape. Its weakened refractive power can only focus the light rays from closely held objects behind the retina; however, parallel light rays from distant objects are still focused on the retina. Therefore, with accommodation paralysis, closely held objects will be blurred, but distant ones will be distinct.

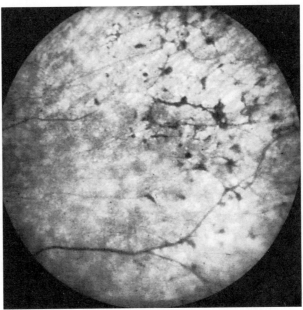

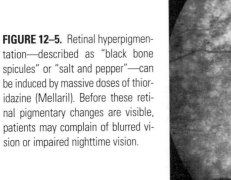

FIGURE 12–5. Retinal hyperpigmentation—described as "black bone spicules" or "salt and pepper"—can be induced by massive doses of thioridazine (Mellaril). Before these retinal pigmentary changes are visible, patients may complain of blurred vision or impaired nighttime vision.

areas. Following a course of insidiously increasing, although painless, functional impairment, patients often develop complete blindness. More so than younger individuals who become blind, those older than 65 years who lose their sight are liable to lose their self-sufficiency, develop visual hallucinations (especially if they have hearing or cognitive impairments [Table 12–1]), and appear to have greater cognitive impairment.

Optic Nerve. Optic nerve injuries generally produce marked visual loss, optic nerve atrophy, and impairment of the afferent limb of the light reflex (see Chapter 4). Unless a "common denominator" has also affected the cerebrum, illnesses that injure the optic nerves do not produce mental aberrations. Conditions injuring both areas include storage diseases, multiple sclerosis (MS), methanol and other intoxications, and chronically increased intracranial pressure, as with pseudotumor cerebri.

A classic example of combined injury, which is usually painless and insidious, is olfactory groove or sphenoid wing *meningioma*. This tumor both compresses the adjacent optic nerve (see Chapters 19 and 20) and burrows into the frontal or temporal lobe. It can then induce intellectual and personality changes and trigger partial complex seizures, while causing blindness in one eye. Other examples are pituitary tumors, such as *adenomas* or *craniopharyngiomas*, which can slowly grow upward to compress the optic chiasm and hypothalamus and downward to infiltrate the pituitary gland (see Fig. 19–4). Long-standing compression of the optic chiasm causes optic atrophy and bitemporal hemianopsia. Compression of the hypothalamus and pituitary causes headache, decreased libido, diabetes insipidus, and loss of secondary sexual characteristics.

Inflammation of the optic nerve, *optic* or *retrobulbar neuritis*, causes a distinctive sudden, painful visual loss in one eye (Fig. 12–6). One aspect of the loss is that patients perceive the color red as less intense or "desaturated." For example, they "see" red in the American flag in less intense color and less vivid hues than normal. The pupil usually has a preserved but diminished reaction to light (reactivity). In addition, normal movement of the eye, probably because it applies a little traction on the optic nerve, is painful.

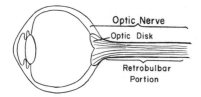

FIGURE 12–6. The long segment of the optic nerve behind the eye, the *retrobulbar* portion, is subject to multiple sclerosis and other inflammatory conditions. The resulting condition, called *optic* or *retrobulbar neuritis,* causes pain and loss of vision (see Fig. 15–2). However, in the early stages, optic neuritis does not cause any observable change in the optic disk, which is the *bulbar* portion of the nerve.

The usual treatment for optic neuritis consists of high-dose, intravenous steroids. However, this treatment can produce mental aberrations, which often include euphoria and sometimes psychosis. In fact, optic neuritis patients might be misdiagnosed as suffering from a psychogenic disturbance (see Chapter 3). Because they are usually young adults and otherwise in good health, the optic disk may appear normal, their pupils remain reactive, and the treatment might be causing mental side effects. At least one third of optic neuritis patients—depending on the presence of other lesions—ultimately develop MS (see Chapter 15). With recurrent optic neuritis attacks, whatever their origin, the optic nerve becomes atrophic, the pupil unreactive, and the eye blind.

An inflammatory condition of the arteries that supply the optic nerve, *temporal* or *giant cell arteritis,* often leads to ischemia of the optic nerves. Moreover, the arteritis potentially spreads to the cerebral arteries (see Chapter 9). Typically affecting only people older than 65 years, temporal arteritis often first causes a nonspecific subacute headache and systemic symptoms, such as malaise, polyarthralgia, and weight loss. The combination of these initial symptoms—prolonged aches, pains, and headache in an older individual—understandably may give the appearance of depression. However, physicians should avoid being diverted because, unless it is promptly treated with steroids, temporal arteritis can cause blindness and strokes.

Although it does not cause mental aberrations, *Leber's hereditary optic atrophy,* a recently elucidated disorder, causes blindness because of a point mutation in mitochondrial DNA. As with the muscle mitochondria disorders (see Chapter 6) and possibly Parkinson's disease, Leber's atrophy is an example of genetically determined energy production abnormalities causing progressive, severe neurologic illness.

GLAUCOMA

In most cases, glaucoma is elevated intraocular pressure resulting from obstructed outflow of aqueous humor through the *filtration angle* of the anterior chamber of the eye (Fig. 12–7). Two common varieties—*open-angle* and *angle-closure*—are recognized, and the angle-closure variety occasionally results from psychotropic medications. If glaucoma remains untreated, it damages the optic nerve, causes visual field impairments, and eventually leads to blindness.

Open-Angle Glaucoma

Open-angle or *wide-angle glaucoma* occurs seven times more frequently than closed-angle glaucoma. People at greatest risk are older than 65 years, diabetic, myopic, and relatives of glaucoma patients. Because symptoms are usually absent at the onset, glaucoma might be diagnosed only by an ophthalmologist detecting elevated intraocular pressure, certain visual field losses, or changes in the optic nerve. Later, when central vision or acuity is impaired, the optic cup is abnormally deep and permanently damaged. Lack of symptoms in the initial phase of open-angle glaucoma is the best reason for routine ophthalmologic examinations.

Open-angle glaucoma usually responds to topical medications (eye drops), laser therapy, or surgery. Psychotropic medications do not precipitate open-angle glaucoma. In general, patients with open-angle glaucoma may be given antidepressants and other psychotropic medications provided that their glaucoma treatment is continued.

Angle-Closure Glaucoma

In *angle-closure glaucoma*, which is also called *closed-angle* or *narrow-angle glaucoma*, intraocular pressure is usually raised by impaired aqueous humor outflow at the filtration angle. In one variety, the fluid becomes trapped behind the iris. Patients with narrow-angle glaucoma, like those with open-angle glaucoma, usually are older than 40 years and often have a family history, but they also have had a history of hyperopia and long-standing narrow angles. Few have had symptoms, such as seeing halos around lights, preceding an attack of angle-closure glaucoma. In contrast to the relatively normal appearance of the eye in open-angle glaucoma, in acute angle-closure glaucoma the eye is red, the pupil dilated and unreactive, and the cornea hazy. Moreover, the eye and forehead are painful, and vision is impaired.

Angle-closure glaucoma is sometimes iatrogenic. For example, when pupils are dilated for ocular examinations, the "bunched-up" iris can block the angle. Likewise, angle-closure glaucoma can be precipitated by medications with anticholinergic properties, probably because they dilate the pupil.

Despite the attention to the potential problem, the complication rate of glaucoma with tricyclic antidepressant use is low and, with selective serotonin reuptake inhibitors (SSRIs), almost nonexistent. With the shift to SSRIs, physicians are liable to dismiss the potential problem of tricyclic antidepressants inducing glaucoma; however, with tricyclics prescribed for increasingly numerous, mostly neurologic conditions—chronic pain, urinary incontinence, headache, and diabetic neuropathy—many patients remain vulnerable.

Whatever the cause, prompt treatment of angle-closure glaucoma is mandatory. Topical and systemic medications open the angle (by constricting the pupil) and also reduce aqueous humor production. Laser iridectomy immediately and painlessly creates a passage directly through the iris to drain aqueous humor.

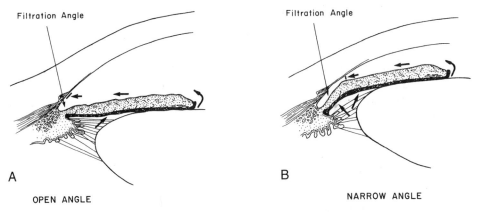

FIGURE 12–7. A, Open-angle glaucoma: the aqueous humor is not drained despite access to the absorptive surface of the angle. Impaired flow from the eye leads to gradually increased intraocular pressure (glaucoma). B, Narrow-angle glaucoma: when the iris is pushed forward, as may occur during pupil dilation, the angle is narrowed or even closed. Obstruction of aqueous humor flow, which usually occurs suddenly, leads to angle-closure glaucoma.

Because glaucoma poses such a threat, individuals older than 40 years should have intraocular pressure measured every 2 years and those older than 65 years, every year. Most patients who are under treatment for either form of glaucoma may receive psychotropic medications. Glaucoma medications, such as pilocarpine, and ophthalmic beta-blockers, such as timolol (Timoptic), may be absorbed into the systemic circulation and create cardiovascular and psychologic side effects. Their absorption can cause orthostatic lightheadedness, bradycardia, and even heart block. Not surprisingly, elderly patients who use beta-blocker eyedrops sometimes experience brief periods of confusion.

Children are also particularly susceptible to systemic absorption. For example, when given scopolamine or other atropine-like eye drops for ocular examination, they frequently develop agitation. On the other hand, marijuana, despite claims of its enthusiasts, is no more effective than standard medications for treating glaucoma.

CORTICAL BLINDNESS

Bilateral occipital cortex damage can produce visual impairment called *cortical blindness*. The cause is usually bilateral posterior cerebral artery occlusion or occipital head trauma. Blindness can also result from extensive brain injury from anoxia, multiple infarctions, or MS. Because of the cerebral damage that underlies cortical blindness, the electroencephalogram (EEG) characteristically loses the normal 8–12 Hz (alpha) rhythms detectable over the occipital lobes. Whether the cortical blindness results from limited or generalized cortex injury, the pupils are normal in size and reactivity to light because the optic nerves and brainstem remain intact.

Anton's Syndrome

Cortical blindness may be complicated by the dramatic neuropsychologic phenomenon of *Anton's syndrome*, in which patients, believing that their vision is intact, deny blindness. With little prompting, they confabulate by "describing" their room, clothing, and various other objects. In addition, they sometimes behave as though they had normal vision and proceed to stumble about their room.

Many cases of Anton's syndrome are accompanied by other signs of generalized cerebral cortex injury, especially delirium and dementia. When posterior cerebral injuries are its cause, Anton's syndrome may accompany anosognosia for other deficits (from right-sided parietal lobe injury) or amnesia (from bilateral temporal lobe injury). For example, a 76-year-old man, who had just sustained a right-sided posterior cerebral artery infarction and had a left posterior cerebral infarction the previous year, first blamed his inability to see the examiner's blouse on poor lighting and then claimed to be disinterested in it. When pressed, still denying his blindness, he confabulated by calmly describing the blouse as "lovely" and "becoming," at times elaborating that it was "obviously made from fine material."

VISUAL PERCEPTUAL DISTURBANCES

Visual perceptual disturbances usually consist of impaired processing of visual information or inability to integrate visual information with other neuropsychologic information. Beware that, although these fascinating disturbances seem to be neatly defined, they are usually incomplete and their elements overlap. In addition, patients may actually have some underlying visual loss. Most important, visual impairments are often inextricably combined to a certain extent with other neuropsychologic disorders, such as dementia, aphasia, and apraxia. In these cases, patients' problems more than coexist: they are multiplicative.

Palinopsia

Palinopsia (Greek, *palin*, again; *opsis*, vision), which may be likened to "visual perseveration," consists of recurrent images, which are technically hallucinations, that usually appear within an area of incomplete visual loss in the left lateral field. Patients with palinopsia reexperience images of objects, scenes, or family members. Sometimes several afterimages appear in rapid succession as "visual echoes," but sometimes hours or days elapse. Because most images are duplicates of common inanimate objects, which have just been seen, palinopsia usually does not elicit an emotional response.

Both the left lateral visual impairment and superimposed hallucinations stem from right-sided cerebral lesions that affect the occipital and parietal lobes. In some cases, palinopsia has coincided with focal EEG seizure activity, in which case it may represent an inability of the malfunctioning cortex to capture only a single image. When images recur following a long interval from the exposure, they are often manifestations of a seizure.

Agnosia

Another visual perceptual disturbance, *visual agnosia*, consists of an inability to appreciate the meaning of an object by sight, despite an intact visual system and the absence of aphasia and dementia. Patients with visual agnosia simply cannot comprehend what they see. An example would be a man shown a stop sign describing it and even reading it but being unable to explain what action must be taken.

With visual agnosia, unlike aphasia, when vision is bypassed (as when patients touch objects), language function is normal. The lesion causing visual agnosia is not clearly established—certainly not as well as for aphasia (see Fig. 8–1). However, it can be envisioned as a disconnection of the occipital visual cortex from cognitive centers. Although localization cannot be definitely established, etiology is most often cerebral infarctions or Alzheimer's disease.

Visual agnosia is also a major aspect of the infamous, although relatively rare, *Klüver-Bucy syndrome*, a behavioral disorder produced in monkeys by resection of both temporal lobes, which contain the amygdalae and components of the limbic system (see Chapter 16). The limbic system damage results in visual agnosia so severe that the monkeys not only touch all objects but they also identify objects by putting them into their mouth ("psychic blindness"). Their behavior can be repetitive, compulsive, and indiscriminate.

When the Klüver-Bucy syndrome occurs in humans, it includes a toned-down version of psychic blindness, *oral exploration*. This aspect of the syndrome consists of patients' placing inedible objects in their mouth but only intermittently, briefly, partly, and absent-mindedly.

Color agnosia is a particular inability to identify colors by sight. The affected individual's problem is not common color blindness, which is a sex-linked inherited retinal abnormality, or aphasia. The real problem is that patients cannot identify (by speech or writing) the name of colors. When shown painted cards, for example, they cannot say the name of the colors. In striking contrast, they behave as though they appreciate colors. Patients can typically match pairs of cards of the same color, read Ishihara plates (pseudoisochromatic numbered cards), and recite the colors of well-known objects, such as the sky.

In a related impairment, *prosopagnosia*, patients cannot recognize *familiar faces* (Greek, *prosopon*, face, person; *agnosia*, lack of knowledge). However, they can identify the same people by their voice, dress, and mannerisms. Prosopagnosia is often accompanied by an inability to identify objects out of their usual (visual) context, such as a shirt pocket cut from a shirt. It is usually attributed to bilateral occipitotemporal injury but sometimes to Alzheimer's disease. In a variation, patients with right cerebral lesions are unable to match pairs of pictures of *unfamiliar* faces. This impairment probably reflects visual-spatial impairments from nondominant parietal lobe lesions.

Balint's Syndrome

Balint's syndrome consists of three elements, each of which is complex: *psychic paralysis of fixation, optic ataxia, and simultanagnosia*. Psychic paralysis of fixation is the psychologic inability of a patient to shift attention by looking away from one object to another, which is located in the periphery of vision. Patients behave as though they were mesmerized by the original object or as a radar system that has locked onto an approaching hostile aircraft. Their gaze can be shifted by briefly closing the eyes, which momentarily interrupts attention.

Optic ataxia, another element of Balint's syndrome, is the inability to look or search in a deliberate pattern. A common example is patients' inability to read in methodical visual sweeps. The third element, simultanagnosia, which is related to impaired double simultaneous stimulation, consists of being able to attend only to objects immediately in the center of vision. When simultaneously confronted with objects in the center and in the periphery of vision, the patient will invariably ignore the one in the periphery even though it might be important or attractive. Balint's syndrome has been attributed to bilateral parietal lobe damage from infarctions or Alzheimer's disease.

Psychogenic Blindness

Cases of *psychogenic blindness* that convincingly mimic true blindness are rare. People do not have an intuitive knowledge of visual pathways, psychogenic blindness is burdensome and incapacitating, and even bedside testing can easily reveal its spurious nature.

When it does occur, psychogenic blindness' most common patterns are complete loss (or generalized impairment), blindness in the eye ipsilateral to a psychogenic hemiparesis, and *tubular* or *tunnel vision* (Fig. 12–8). The unilateral visual loss defies the laws of neuroanatomy: the division of optic pathways at the optic chiasm provides that hemiparesis is accompanied by hemianopsia—not monocular blindness. Similarly, loss of vision in a tubular pattern defies the laws of optics: the visual area

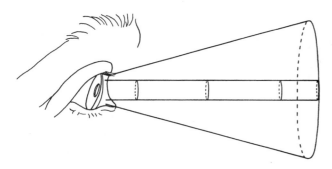

FIGURE 12–8. The area seen by a person normally increases conically in proportion to the distance from the object. In *tubular* or *tunnel vision,* which defies the laws of optics, the visual area is constant despite increasing distance.

expands with increasing distance. (An important exception to this law, however, sometimes occurs in migraine with aura [see Chapter 9], in which patients have the perception of peripheral vision constriction.) Uncommon but relatively sophisticated patterns of psychogenic blindness are homonymous hemianopsia and combinations of monocular loss and a contralateral hemianopsia.

To unmask most varieties of psychogenic blindness, an uninhibited examiner simply might make childlike facial contortions or ask the patient to read some four-letter words. The patient's reaction to these provocations would reveal ability to see. When only one eye is affected by psychogenic blindness, fogged, colored, or polarized lenses will often confuse (or fatigue) a patient into revealing that vision is present. Repeated testing in cases of tubular vision may reveal a spiral pattern of loss that eventually recedes.

Another technique is to spin a vertically striped cylinder (drum) in front of a person with questionable visual loss. The drum will elicit *opticokinetic* nystagmus in individuals with normal vision, even those too young to speak. Likewise, having patients look at a large, moving mirror forces those with normal vision to follow their own image.

A useful test is to have patients wear lenses with negligible optical value to reveal normal vision. As an added benefit, it permits patients to extract themselves without embarrassment from psychogenic blindness.

If clinical tests are inconclusive, EEG and other electrophysiologic testing may help. An intact visual system would be indicated by alpha rhythm on the EEG of patients at rest with eyes closed and loss of that rhythm when they open their eyes. However, a confounding problem would be that alpha rhythm is suppressed if patients are anxious or concentrating. In addition, with an impaired visual system, visual evoked response (VER) testing produces abnormal potentials (see Chapter 15).

Visual Hallucinations

Unlike auditory hallucinations, visual hallucinations *in adults* almost always indicate neurologic dysfunction. (They are, however, a frequent symptom of childhood schizophrenia.) Visual hallucinations can originate in the frontal lobe, temporal lobe, or cerebral peduncles, as well as the occipital cortex. They can be manifestations of problems as diverse as toxic-metabolic encephalopathy, dementia-producing diseases, medication side effects, structural lesions, and physiologic disturbances (Table 12–1). Despite varied etiologies, certain clinical features provide diagnostic clues.

Tumors, strokes, and other structural lesions can produce partial elementary, frontal lobe, or complex seizures—all of which can produce visual symptoms (see Chapter 10). These hallucinations, which tend to be stereotyped, are "seen" in both eyes and can even appear in an hemianopic area. They range from simple geometric forms in partial elementary seizures to detailed visions accompanied by sounds, thoughts, emotions, and, characteristically, impairment of consciousness, in partial complex seizures.

Migraines with aura (classic migraine) also produce stereotyped visual hallucinations (Fig. 9–2). Typically, distinctive crescent scotomata or scintillating fortification spectra usually move slowly across the visual field for 1 to 20 minutes before yielding to a hemicranial headache. In a potentially confusing situation, visual auras sometimes are the sole manifestation of a migraine.

As an element of narcolepsy-cataplexy (see Chapter 17), visual hallucinations intrude into a patient's partial consciousness. Like dreams, they are composed of variable, unpredictable—not stereotyped—intricate visions accompanied by rich thoughts and strong emotions. They tend to occur while patients fall asleep (hypnagogic hallucinations) or awaken (hypnopompic hallucinations). As with normal dreams, these hallucinations are associated with flaccid, areflexic paresis and rapid eye movements (REMs).

A different sleep-related visual hallucination is peduncular hallucinosis, a condition caused by infections or vascular injuries of the midbrain and pons. (This portion of the brainstem contains the cerebral peduncles [Fig. 4–4], connections to the limbic system, and pathways involved in REM.) Peduncular hallucinations are typically accompanied by somnolence and oculomotor nerve palsies. Although the visual disturbances might mimic those seen in other conditions, the underlying illnesses are not likely to be confused.

Visual hallucinations are a hallmark of diseases that cause dementia, particularly Alzheimer's, Lewy body, and Parkinson's diseases (see Chapters 7 and 18). Patients, who usually have reached the point of dementia, tend to have visual hallucinations, often with a paranoid element, that occur at night. In a strong diagnostic clue, in Lewy body disease, compared to Alzheimer's disease, visual hallucinations occur earlier in the course and more frequently. Hallucinations in Parkinson's disease are usually partly medication-induced.

Many classes of medications, in addition to anticholinergics or dopamine enhancers, and illicit drugs may be responsible. Even withdrawal from alcohol and other substances can cause visual hallucinations. The best-known example is *delirium tremens (DTs)*. In most patients with DTs, varied hallucinations often stem from the environment and are accompanied by agitation, confusion, sweating, and tachycardia. Sometimes patients, petrified by the hallucinations, become reticent and immobile.

Finally, visual hallucinations can be produced by any visual loss. Palinopsia and cortical blindness (see above) induce hallucinations. With palinopsia, they may be stereotyped. Sudden blindness from ocular injury may have the same effect as from cortical injury. For example, soldiers with blinding eye wounds have periods of "seeing" brightly colored forms and even entire scenes. Similarly, eye surgery in the elderly is occasionally followed by visual hallucinations along with disorientation and agitation. Thus, elderly patients should not undergo simultaneous bilateral ophthalmologic surgical procedures.

Whether acute or chronic, visual loss represents sensory deprivation. Especially when superimposed on hearing and cognitive impairments, it is a well-known cause of visual hallucinations and other mental aberrations. Many elderly patients with visual impairments who are not demented or otherwise psychologically abnormal frequently have picturesque colored or black-and-white hallucinations of benign, familiar objects. The hallucinations, which are certainly not stereotyped, have a duration of minutes to several hours. In this condition, the *Charles Bonnet syndrome,* elderly, visually handicapped patients sit and have quiet, harmless hallucinations that they disclose only reluctantly.

VISUAL FIELD LOSS

The patterns of visual loss (Fig. 12–9) are a reliable guide to localization and diagnosis. In general, the following guidelines apply:

Monocular quadrantanopsias, hemianopsias, scotomata, and blindness are the result of optic nerve injury.

Homonymous quadrantanopsias and hemianopsias almost always result from visual tract injuries between the optic chiasm and the occipital cortex (see Fig. 4–1). The most common situation is a middle cerebral artery infarction that results in a contralateral homonymous hemianopsia accompanied by hemiparesis and hemisen-

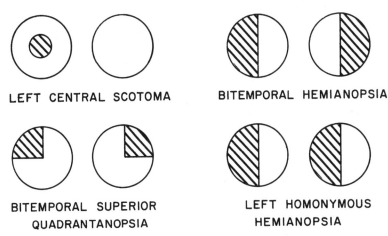

LEFT CENTRAL SCOTOMA　　　　BITEMPORAL HEMIANOPSIA

BITEMPORAL SUPERIOR　　　　LEFT HOMONYMOUS
QUADRANTANOPSIA　　　　　　　HEMIANOPSIA

FIGURE 12–9. Uniocular *central scotomata* may be caused by migraine attacks, optic neuritis, or other ipsilateral optic nerve injuries. *Bitemporal superior quadrantanopia* is usually caused by lesions of the optic chiasm, such as pituitary adenomas or craniopharyngiomas. *Bitemporal hemianopsias* are caused by more advanced compression of the optic chiasm by the same lesions. *Homonymous hemianopsias*, with or without macular sparing, are most often caused by contralateral cerebral lesions, such as infarctions.

sory loss. A homonymous superior quadrantanopia (Fig. 12–10), although rare, is important because it may be the only physical manifestation of a contralateral temporal lobe lesion that produces partial complex seizures. It also results from epilepsy surgery that amputates a portion of the temporal lobe. Another noteworthy pattern is a homonymous hemianopsia that excludes the center of vision (macular sparing) because it indicates an occipital lobe lesion.

The visual field loss most commonly associated with mental aberrations is the left homonymous hemianopsia. Left sensory inattention, visual-spatial impairments, and anosognosia (see Chapter 8) often accompany it.

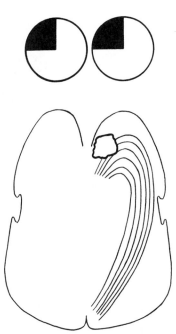

FIGURE 12–10. A large lesion or a surgical resection of the temporal lobe may interfere with forward sweeping optic tract fibers. Such damage may cause contralateral superior quadrantanopsia, as well as partial complex seizures.

Bitemporal quadrantanopsias and hemianopsias indicate a lesion at the optic chiasm. The vast majority are pituitary adenomas, which, as discussed previously, compress the optic chiasm, cause optic atrophy, and lead to hypopituitarism with an elevated serum prolactin level.

CONJUGATE OCULAR MOVEMENT

Both eyes normally move together in a paired, coordinated *(conjugate)* manner so that people can look *(gaze)* laterally and follow *(pursue)* moving objects. Conjugate movement is generated by a succession of cerebral and brainstem *gaze centers* that receive cerebellar modulation and visual feedback. Because these centers innervate pairs of oculomotor, trochlear, and abducens cranial nerve *nuclei*, conjugate movements are *supranuclear.*

Conjugate movement originates in each frontal lobe's *cerebral conjugate gaze center.* When a person is at rest, each cerebral center continuously emits impulses that go through a complicated pathway to "push" the eyes contralaterally. With the counterbalancing effect of each center, the eyes remain midline (Fig. 12–11). When a person wants to look to one side, the contralateral cerebral gaze center increases activity. For example, when someone wants to look toward a water glass on the right, the left cerebral gaze center activity increases, and, as if pushing the eyes away, the eyes turn to the right. If this person wished to reach for the glass, the left cerebral corticospinal center, which originates adjacent to that gaze center, would mobilize the right arm.

Partial seizures also increase activity of the conjugate gaze center. They push the eyes contralaterally and, because they usually envelop the adjacent corticospinal tract, they push the head and neck contralaterally and produce tonic-clonic activity of the contralateral arm and leg.

In contrast, when patients have unilateral destructive cerebral injuries, such as large strokes, the activity of the gaze center on that side is abolished. The activity of the other center, being unopposed, pushes the eyes toward the injured side. (The eyes "look toward the stroke.") For example, with a left cerebral infarction, the eyes deviate toward the left. Also, because the corticospinal tract is generally involved, the right side of the body is paralyzed. (Here the saying is "When the eyes look away from the paralysis, the stroke is cerebral.")

When intact, each cerebral gaze center produces conjugate eye movements by stimulating a contralateral *pontine gaze center,* which is also called the *pontine paramedian reticular formation (PPRF).* In contrast to the cerebral center, each pontine center *pulls* the eyes toward its own side (Fig. 12–12). A unilateral pontine infarction allows the eyes to be pulled toward the opposite side. For example, if the right pontine gaze center were damaged, the eyes would deviate to the left. Also, because the right pontine corticospinal tract would be damaged, the left arm and leg would be paralyzed. Thus, with a pontine lesion, the eyes "look toward the paralysis."

After the pontine gaze centers receive impulses from the contralateral cerebral conjugate gaze center, each pontine gaze center stimulates the adjacent abducens (sixth cranial nerve) nucleus and, through the *medial longitudinal fasciculus (MLF),* the contralateral oculomotor (third cranial nerve) nucleus (see Figs. 15–3 and 15–4). Innervation of one abducens nucleus and the contralateral oculomotor nucleus is necessary for conjugate lateral eye movement. If both abducens nuclei were stimulated simultaneously, both eyes would turn outward. If both oculomotor nuclei were simultaneously stimulated, both eyes would turn inward.

When the MLF is injured, as often occurs in MS and brainstem strokes, the *MLF syn-*

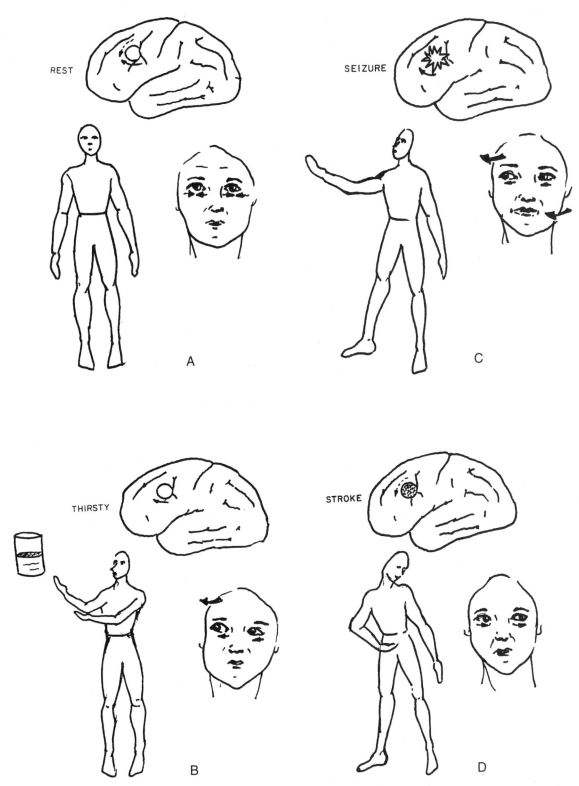

FIGURE 12–11. **A,** At rest, the eyes are midline because the impulses of each frontal lobe conjugate gaze center are balanced, each "pushing" the eyes contralateral. Visual fixation is an active process. **B,** Voluntarily increased activity of the left cerebral gaze center drives the eyes to the right (contralateral). **C,** Involuntarily increased cerebral activity also drives the eyes contralateral. Also, with left cerebral seizure activity, the right arm and leg develop tonic-clonic activity. **D,** A stroke destroys the left cerebral gaze center, permitting the right center to push the eyes toward the lesion. It also destroys the cerebral motor strip, causing contralateral paresis. The eyes "looking" away from the hemiparesis characterize this common stroke.

drome or *internuclear ophthalmoplegia (INO)* develops. In this condition, the cranial nuclei and nerves are normal, but the eyes cannot move conjugately (see Chapter 15).

Another important ocular movement is *nystagmus* (rhythmic horizontal, vertical, or rotatory eyeball oscillation). Nystagmus is caused by various central nervous system (CNS) injuries, including MS, brainstem infarctions, and Wernicke-Korsakoff syndrome. It may be the most prominent physical finding in the abuse of diazepam, barbiturates, or alcohol, and with excessive concentrations of antipsychotic and antidepressant medications. Nystagmus is routinely found in seizure patients who take therapeutic doses of phenytoin (Dilantin) or phenobarbital: its absence even suggests noncompliance with an anticonvulsant regimen.

Although typically a sign of CNS injury, nystagmus may be a normal variant. When many normal individuals look to the extreme of lateral gaze, they have horizontal nystagmus (end point nystagmus). Some have congenital nystagmus, which may be disconcerting to people looking at them, but it does not interfere with their vision. Their nystagmus is usually pendular, direction changing, and absent when they look toward a particular point (the null point). Lacking CNS involvement, predominantly horizontal nystagmus is often caused by labyrinthitis, in which case it is associated with vertigo, nausea, and vomiting.

Saccades and Pursuit Movement

Under ordinary circumstances, when an object enters the periphery of the visual field, the eyes tend to dart toward it to redirect the line of sight and refocus attention. The eyes rotate conjugately, rapidly, smoothly, and without disturbing the eyelids or head. These movements, *saccades*, are characterized by rapidity, which may exceed 700 degrees per second. Saccades are examined in patients by asking them to stare at an object 45 degrees to one side and suddenly to shift their gaze to a different object 45 degrees to the other. At the bedside, slowness is the primary abnormality. Other abnormalities are overshooting or undershooting (hypermetria and hypometria), irregular or jerky movements, and—a subtle one—initiating the saccade by blinking or a head jerk.

Many conditions, including stroke, MS, tumor, and degenerative illness, can damage the intricate mechanisms that generate and govern saccades. Moreover, lesions located in the cerebellum, pons, or occasionally elsewhere can impair them. Extensive cerebral cortex injury, as occurs in Alzheimer's disease and multiple infarctions, may also be responsible. Abnormal saccades are most notably associated with Huntington's disease (see Chapter 18), where they may be detected early and characteristically. Depending on the task used to demonstrate saccades, schizophrenics may or may not have an abnormality.

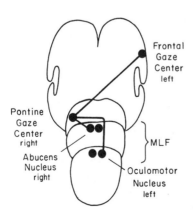

FIGURE 12–12. When looking to the right, the left frontal conjugate gaze center stimulates the right (contralateral) pontine gaze center, which is also called the *pontine paramedian reticular formation (PPRF)*. The pontine center, in turn, stimulates the right (adjacent) abducens nerve nucleus and, through the left medial longitudinal fasciculus (MLF), the left (contralateral) oculomotor nerve nucleus.

TABLE 12–3. *Common Causes of Smooth Pursuit Abnormalities*

Dementia-producing diseases
   Alzheimer's
   Huntington's
   Multiple
   Parkinson's
Medications
   Antiepileptic drugs
   Barbiturates and benzodiazepines
   Neuroleptics
Psychiatric illnesses
   Affective disorders
   Attention deficit hyperactivity disorder
   Borderline personality disorder
   Obsessive-compulsive disorder
   Schizophrenia

Pursuit or *smooth pursuit,* the counterpart of saccades, is the continual, relatively slow ocular tracking of a moving object, such as a bird in flight. The bedside test consists of asking the patient to gaze at the examiner's finger as it moves horizontally at about 30 degrees per second. The eyes should remain on the target and smoothly follow it. The primary abnormality would be a slow or jerky path instead of a rapid smooth curve or straight line.

Parietal, temporal, or occipital cortex lesions; brainstem lesions; numerous medications; and various illnesses—even fatigue and inattention—impair smooth pursuit. Several neurologic and psychiatric illnesses impair smooth pursuit, usually by slowing it (Table 12–3). In particular, schizophrenia patients' smooth pursuit eye movements are characteristically slow, jerky, and interrupted. This abnormality is detectable early in the disorder and serves as a neurophysiologic marker. It is also detectable in many schizophrenics' asymptomatic family members. Schizophrenia is more closely linked to abnormalities in smooth pursuit than in saccades.

However, abnormal smooth pursuit movement is not specific enough to be diagnostic of schizophrenia. Smooth pursuit abnormalities are also found, although less frequently, in individuals with other psychiatric disturbances, as well as in those with various neurologic illnesses. They improve with successful treatment of depression.

DIPLOPIA

Diplopia ("double vision") perceived with one eye (monocular diplopia) is usually the result of either ocular abnormalities, such as a dislocated lens, or psychogenic factors. Individuals with monocular diplopia, whatever the cause, will have diplopia when covering the unaffected eye. In addition, their diplopia will usually persist in all directions of gaze.

Those with the usual form of diplopia—binocular diplopia—usually have it only in certain directions of gaze and covering either eye will abolish it. This diplopia is almost always caused by lesions in the brainstem or further "down" the neurologic ladder: internuclear ophthalmoplegia (INO) and other brainstem syndromes, oculomotor or abducens cranial nerve injury, neuromuscular junction disorders, or extraocular muscle paresis. Often fatigue, as occurs during long nighttime drives, causes enough muscle weakness to produce diplopia. In contrast, lesions above the brain-

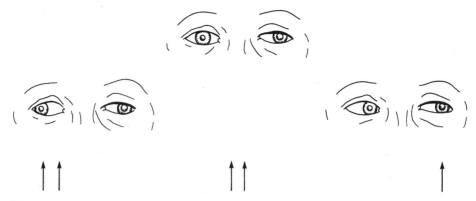

FIGURE 12–13. Left oculomotor (third cranial) nerve palsy. In the center picture, a patient looks ahead. The left upper lid is lower, the pupil larger, and the eye deviated slightly laterally. Because the eyes are dysconjugate, the patient sees two arrows (diplopia) when looking ahead. In the picture on the left, the patient looks to the right. Because the paretic left eye fails to cross medially beyond the midline (i.e., it fails to adduct), the eyes are more dysconjugate and there is greater diplopia. In the picture on the right, the patient looks to the left. The eyes are almost conjugate and there is little or no diplopia.

stem—cerebral and other supranuclear lesions—cause conjugate gaze palsies, not diplopia.

Oculomotor (third cranial) nerve injury results in ptosis, lateral deviation of the eye, diplopia that is greatest when the patient looks away from the midline, and, most important, a dilated pupil (Fig. 12–13). However, one important exception is third nerve infarctions from diabetes, where characteristically the pupil is spared. It remains reactive to light and the same size as its counterpart. Abducens (sixth cranial) nerve injury results in medial deviation of the eye and diplopia when looking laterally but in neither ptosis nor pupil abnormality (Fig. 12–14).

When myasthenia gravis, the classic neuromuscular junction disorder, causes diplopia, patients have fluctuating symptoms and asymmetric combinations of ptosis and ocular muscle paresis. However, no matter how severe the diplopia and ptosis, patients' pupils are round, equal, and reactive to light (see Chapter 6).

Although congenital ocular muscle weakness, *strabismus,* causes dysconjugate gaze, children do not have diplopia because the brain suppresses the image from the

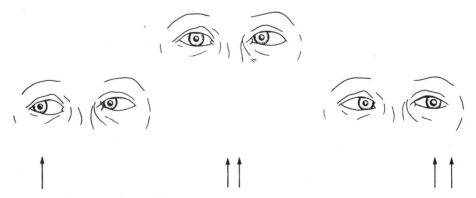

FIGURE 12–14. A left abducens (sixth cranial) nerve palsy. In the center picture, a patient looks ahead. The patient's left eye is deviated medially. The eyes are dysconjugate, and the patient sees two arrows when looking ahead. In the picture on the left, the patient looks to the right. The eyes are conjugate, and the patient sees only a single arrow. In the picture on the right, the patient looks to the left. The paretic left eye fails to cross the midline laterally, that is, it fails to abduct. The exaggeration of the dysconjugate gaze increases the diplopia.

weaker eye. With continuous suppression of vision from one eye, that eye will become almost blind *(amblyopic)*. Thus, babies and children with strabismus often have the "good" eye patched several hours each day, or they undergo various procedures, such as muscle surgery and intramuscular botulinum injections, to stimulate the visual pathways of the weak eye.

Before diagnosing psychogenic diplopia, physicians must not overlook subtle neurologic conditions, especially myasthenia gravis and the MLF syndrome. Psychogenic diplopia is usually intermittent, inconsistent, and present in all directions of gaze. Patients with this condition have no observable abnormality. A common set of tests consists of the patient reading colored or polarized charts using colored or polarized lenses. In another psychogenic disturbance, *convergence spasm*, children or young adults, as if looking at the tip of their nose, fix their eyes in a downward and inward position. This position is a burlesque that can be overcome by inducing opticokinetic nystagmus.

HORNER'S SYNDROME AND ARGYLL-ROBERTSON PUPILS

Contrary to a reasonable expectation that the brain would innervate all eye muscles entirely through a short and direct pathway, the sympathetic tract follows a re-

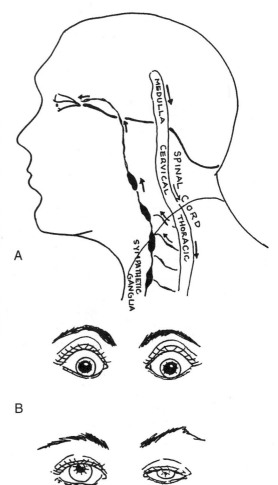

FIGURE 12–15. **A,** The sympathetic nervous system originates in the brainstem, passes through the medulla, and descends into the cervical and then the thoracic spinal cord. Some sympathetic system neurons leave the thoracic spinal cord and, after making a hairpin turn, ascend to form ganglia adjacent to the cervical vertebrae. Postsynaptic neurons ascend further. They are wrapped successively around the common carotid, internal carotid, and then the ophthalmic artery. These neurons, seeming to rise higher than their starting point, innervate the pupil dilator muscles, levator palpebrae (upper eyelid) muscles, and facial sweat glands. **B,** *Top,* Stimulation of the sympathetic nervous system retracts the eyelid, dilates the pupil, and prevents sweating (anhidrosis). These cardinal signs of the flight-or-fright response may also be induced by states of excitement, including amphetamine use. *Bottom,* Sympathetic tract injury causes Horner's syndrome—miosis, ptosis, and anhidrosis—on this patient's left side. An important clue to Horner's syndrome is the eyebrow elevation, which is an unconscious maneuver to uncover the pupil.

markably long and circuitous route (Fig. 12–15, *A*). Injury to the sympathetic tract leads to *Horner's syndrome:* ptosis, miosis (a small pupil), and anhidrosis (lack of sweating; Fig. 12–15, *B*). Given the roundabout course of the sympathetic tract, Horner's syndrome can be found in several widely separate injuries: lateral medullary infarctions (see Wallenberg's syndrome; Fig. 2–10); cervical spinal cord injuries; apical lung (Pancoast) tumors; and, because of a carotid artery abnormality, cluster headaches (see Fig. 9–4).

Horner's syndrome might be confused with an oculomotor nerve injury because ptosis is a prominent, common sign. However, miosis distinguishes Horner's syndrome.

In a different situation, the astute physician confronting a small pupil must also bear in mind that the real problem may be that the contralateral one is abnormally large. Causes of a dilated pupil include, in addition to an oculomotor nerve injury, a congenital variation (Adie's pupil) and accidentally rubbing atropine-like substances into one eye. In a notorious variant, which is a manifestation of Factitious Disorder, people—usually medical personnel—surreptitiously instill such substances. The unilateral dilated pupil triggers a series of investigations that might culminate in cerebral angiography to exclude a posterior cerebral artery aneurysm.

Argyll-Robertson pupils also must be differentiated from oculomotor nerve injury. They are irregular, asymmetric, and small (1 to 2 mm). Moreover, they are characteristically unreactive to light, but constrict normally when patients look at closely held objects (i.e., during accommodation). The impaired light reflex with intact accommodation has given rise to the saying, "Argyll-Robertson pupils are like prostitutes: they accommodate but do not react." Although Argyll-Robertson pupils have historically been a manifestation of syphilis, the majority of cases today result from diabetic autonomic neuropathy and cataract surgery.

REFERENCES

Abramowicz M (ed): Reading machines for the blind. Med Lett *34:* 13–14, 1992

Aldrich MS, Alessi AG, Beck RW, et al: Cortical blindness: Etiology, diagnosis, and prognosis. Ann Neurol *21:* 149–158, 1987

Asaad G: Hallucinations in Clinical Psychiatry, New York, Brunner/Mazel, 1990

Cummings JL, Miller BL: Visual hallucinations: Clinical occurrence and use in differential diagnosis. West J Med *146:* 46–51, 1987

Damasio AR, Damasio H, Hoesen GWV: Prosopagnosia: Anatomic basis and behavioral mechanisms. Neurology *32:* 331–341, 1982

Friedman L, Abel LA, Jesberger JA, et al: Saccadic intrusions into smooth pursuit in patients with schizophrenia or affective disorder and normal controls. Biol Psychiatry *31:* 1110–1118, 1992

Gittinger JW: Functional hemianopsia: A historical perspective. Surv Ophthalmol *32:* 427–432, 1988

Heilman KM, Valenstein E (eds): Clinical Neuropsychology (3rd ed), New York, Oxford University Press, 1993

Keane JR: Neuro-ophthalmologic signs of AIDS. Neurology *41:* 841–845, 1991

Lieberman E, Stoudemire A: Use of tricyclic antidepressants in patients with glaucoma. Psychosomatics *28:* 145–148, 1987

McDaniel KD, McDaniel LD: Anton's syndrome in a patient with posttraumatic optic neuropathy and bifrontal contusions. Arch Neurol *48:* 101–105, 1991

Newman NM: Neuro-Ophthalmology: A Practical Text. Norwalk, CT, Appleton & Lange, 1992

Pomeranz HD, Lessell S: Palinopsia and polyopia in the absence of drugs or cerebral disease. Neurology *54:* 855–859, 2000

Quigley HA: Open-angle glaucoma. N Engl J Med *328:* 1097–1106, 1993

Teunisse RJ, Cruysberg JR, Hoefnagels WH, et al: Visual hallucinations in psychologically normal people: Charles Bonnet's syndrome. Lancet *347:* 397–797, 1996

QUESTIONS and ANSWERS: CHAPTER 12

Answers begin on page 316.

1. Which three findings characterize Argyll-Robertson pupils?

a. Miosis
b. Ptosis
c. Irregular shape
d. Unresponsiveness to light
e. Unresponsiveness to accommodation
f. Failure to dilate with atropine drops

2. Which two medications often produce transient visual impairment because of accommodation paresis?

a. Butyrophenones
b. Amitriptyline
c. Imipramine
d. Phenobarbital
e. Phenytoin

3. Which one of the following does not cause cataracts that interfere with vision?

a. Myotonic dystrophy
b. Diabetes mellitus
c. Ocular trauma
d. Chlorpromazine

4. A 20-year-old soldier develops loss of vision in the right eye. The eye is painful, especially when he looks from side to side. No ocular or neurologic abnormalities are found, except for a decreased light reaction in the right pupil. After 1 week, vision returns, except for a small central scotoma. What illness is he likely to have had?

a. Psychogenic disturbance
b. Optic neuritis
c. Left cerebral infarction
d. Pituitary adenoma

5. Which cells produce the covering of cranial nerve II?

a. Schwann
b. Oligodendroglia
c. Neuron
d. Microglia

6. As individuals age beyond 50 years they typically require reading glasses to discern closely held objects, such as newspapers and sewing. Without their glasses, they must hold such objects at arm's length. What accounts for this visual problem?

a. Cataract formation impairs accommodation.
b. Retinal degeneration prevents accommodation.
c. Their lenses lose elasticity and dehydrate.
d. These visual difficulties are a perceptual problem.

7. A 79-year-old woman who has been blind since cataract surgery 5 years ago discloses that she has been having visual hallucinations. They last several minutes to an hour and occur at any time of the day. She envisions her children as babies, her parents, and various real or imagined scenes. She appreciates that the visions are hallucinations. She is not frightened or inclined to act on them. She has no cognitive impairment or lateralized neurologic signs. What should be the next step?

a. Perform an EEG
b. Obtain an ophthalmology consultation
c. Administer a neuroleptic
d. Administer an antidepressant
e. Obtain an MRI
f. None of the above

8. Which electroencephalogram (EEG) change characterizes blindness?

a. EEG 8–12 Hz rhythms located over the occipital lobes when the patient rests that persist when the eyes open
b. Absence of these rhythms at rest and when the eyes are open
c. Presence of these rhythms when the eyes are open but not at rest
d. None of the above

9. Which one of the following statements is false regarding glaucoma?

a. Serotonin reuptake inhibitors are less likely than tricyclic antidepressants to precipitate glaucoma.

b. Marijuana is more effective and carries fewer potential side effects than traditional glaucoma medications.

c. Beta-blocker topical medications (eyedrops) are often absorbed into the systemic circulation in concentrations great enough to cause episodic mental changes.

d. Patients being treated for glaucoma may reasonably safely be given tricyclic antidepressants.

10–15. Match the usual field loss (10–15) with the underlying illness (a–f) [answers may be used more than once].

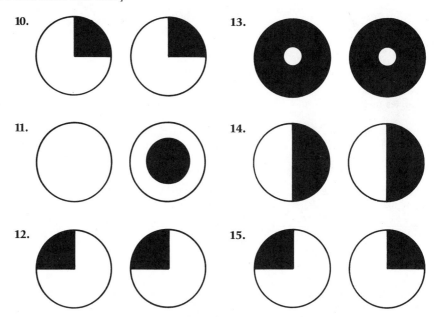

10.

11.

12.

13.

14.

15.

a. A 25-year-old woman has paraparesis and ataxia.

b. A 35-year-old woman has insidious onset of loss of peripheral daytime vision and all nighttime vision. Her mother has a similar illness.

c. A 30-year-old man has episodes of seeing the American flag and hearing the first five bars of "America the Beautiful."

d. A 21-year-old man has loss of bodily hair, gynecomastia, and diabetes insipidus.

e. A 70-year-old man has global aphasia, right hemiplegia, and right hemisensory loss.

f. A 75-year-old man has fluent aphasia.

16–26. Match the characteristics of the visual hallucination with the source (a–c).

a. Seizures that originate in the occipital lobe

b. Seizures that originate in the temporal lobe

c. Migraine with aura (classical migraine)

16. Associated musical hallucinations

17. Flashes of bright lights in the contralateral visual field

18. Associated olfactory hallucinations

19. Rotating blotches of color

20. Formed hallucinations with impaired consciousness

21. Postictal aphasia

22. Throbbing unilateral headache

23. Nausea and vomiting

24. Simple blocks and stars of color

25. Twisting, complicated multicolored lights

26. Faces with distorted features or coloring

27–28. Match the symptom (27–28) with the possible origins (a–d).

a. Left third nerve palsy   c. Right third nerve palsy
b. Left sixth nerve palsy   d. Right sixth nerve palsy

27. Diplopia when looking to the right

28. Diplopia when looking to the left

29–30. Match the actions that cause blindness (29–30) with the outcome (a–c).

a. Methanol-induced optic nerve injury
b. Pigmentary retinal degeneration
c. Retinal burns

29. Staring directly into the sun

30. Drinking nonethanol alcohols

31. What four conditions are common causes of ptosis?

a. Third nerve palsy
b. Sixth nerve palsy
c. Pancoast tumor
d. Multiple sclerosis
e. Myasthenia gravis
f. Psychogenic disturbances
g. Botulinum (Botox) treatment of blepharospasm

32. Which two illnesses cause internuclear ophthalmoplegia?

a. Multiple sclerosis   d. Psychogenic disturbances
b. Poliomyelitis   e. Heroin overdose
c. Muscular dystrophy   f. Brainstem strokes

33. Which abnormality is reported to occur in patients with schizophrenia?

a. Internuclear ophthalmoplegia   d. Conjugate gaze paresis
b. Nystagmus   e. Pursuit abnormalities
c. Ptosis

34. A 70-year-old man awakens with a right hemiparesis, vertigo, and his eyes deviated to the right. Which condition will also be found?

a. Aphasia   c. Dementia
b. Right homonymous hemianopsia   d. Nystagmus

35. Which condition indicates that the dopamine system is involved in conjugate eye movement?

a. Internuclear ophthalmoplegia   c. Pontine gaze center movement
b. Nystagmus   d. Oculogyric crisis

36. Which conditions have a predilection for people older than 65 years?

a. Myopia   e. Temporal or giant cell arteritis
b. Presbyopia   f. Glaucoma
c. Macular degeneration   g. Cataracts
d. Classic migraines   h. Optic neuritis

37. A 70-year-old man sustained a cerebral infarction. He has a right homonymous hemianopsia, right hemisensory loss, and a mild right hemiparesis. Although he can both say and write the names of objects that he feels, he is unable to name objects that he only sees, even when they are presented to his left visual field. What is the name of this condition?

a. Aphasia
b. Hemi-inattention
c. Visual agnosia
d. Gerstmann's syndrome
e. Balint's syndrome
f. Dementia
g. Alexia

38. Match the visual disturbance (1–4) with the etiology (a–e).

1. Psychic blindness
2. Night blindness
3. Cortical blindness
4. Transient monocular blindness

a. Carotid stenosis
b. Occipital infarction (bilateral)
c. Conversion reaction
d. Bilateral temporal lobe injury
e. Vitamin A deficiency

39–46. Match the patient's condition (39–46) with the neuropsychologic disorder (a–j).

a. Cortical blindness
b. Visual agnosia
c. Color agnosia
d. Color blindness
e. Prosopagnosia
f. Anton's syndrome
g. Wernicke-Korsakoff syndrome
h. Alexia without agraphia
i. Congenital cerebral injury
j. Anomia

39. Cannot recognize familiar faces

40. Despite visual loss, willfully but erroneously describes hospital room and physician

41. After cardiac arrest, blindness with intact pupil light reflex. Although alert, mental impairment is prominent

42. Cannot identify a red card, although able to match it to another red card and read a red-colored number on the Ishihara plates

43. Despite only a right homonymous hemianopsia, inability to read. Writing ability is normal

44. Congenital inability to read Ishihara plates

45. Inability to name common objects under any circumstances

46. Cannot name objects when seen, but can name them when described or felt

47. In which conditions are visual hallucinations stereotyped?

a. Partial complex seizures
b. Tonic clonic seizures
c. LSD ingestions
d. Occipital lobe seizures
e. Migraine with aura
f. Migraine without aura
g. Hypnagogic hallucinations
h. Alcohol withdrawal

48. Which two varieties of hallucinations appear predominantly or exclusively in hemianopic areas?

a. Palinopsia
b. Partial seizures
c. Migraines
d. REM-associated dreams
e. LSD intoxication

49. Which of the following is true of slowed smooth pursuit ocular movement?

a. Abnormal saccades are more indicative of schizophrenia.
b. Slowed smooth pursuit is sensitive for schizophrenia but not specific.
c. Slowed smooth pursuit is specific for schizophrenia but not sensitive.
d. When due to neurologic illness, slowed smooth pursuit is highly indicative of basal ganglia disease.

50. Which two of the following statements are true regarding saccades?

a. They are the smooth, steady tracking movements used to follow moving objects.
b. They are the quick, conjugate movements that bring objects from the periphery to the center of vision.
c. They are governed by supranuclear centers.
d. Unlike pursuit movements, they are resistant to structural lesions and degenerative illnesses.

51. Which two of the following statements are true regarding pursuit?

a. They are the smooth, steady tracking movements used to follow moving objects.
b. They are the quick, conjugate movements that bring objects from the periphery to the center of vision.
c. They are governed by supranuclear centers.
d. Unlike saccades, they are resistant to structural lesions and degenerative illnesses.

52. Which two signs are the constituents of Horner's syndrome?

a. Mitosis
b. Miosis
c. Anhidrosis

d. Tearing
e. Third cranial nerve palsy

53. In which four conditions are Horner's syndrome found?

a. Migraine without aura
b. Migraine with aura
c. Cluster headache
d. Trigeminal neuralgia
e. Cervical spinal cord injury

f. Apical lung tumor
g. Pontine CVAs
h. Midbrain CVAs
i. Lateral medullary CVAs

54. Which cerebral artery supplies the occipital lobes?

a. Anterior cerebral
b. Middle cerebral

c. Posterior cerebral
d. None of the above

55. A 33-year-old man claims to have double vision in his right eye after a motor vehicle accident (MVA). When he covers the right eye, the diplopia disappears, but when he covers the left eye, he has persistent diplopia. The visual acuity in the left eye is 20/20 and in the right eye 20/400. Visual fields are normal in the left eye but cannot be determined in the right eye because of the diplopia. Which three statements regarding his situation are true?

a. His symptom is monocular diplopia.
b. With the available information, conclusions cannot be drawn concerning the presence of central nervous system (CNS) injury causing the diplopia.
c. Monocular diplopia is virtually always the result of an ocular injury, such as a dislocated lens or retinal disruption, or psychogenic factors.
d. The first step in determining the cause of diplopia is to establish whether it arises from a single eye. In other words, ask the patient if covering one eye abolishes the diplopia.

56. In which structure is the third cranial nerve nucleus located?

a. Midbrain
b. Pons

c. Medulla
d. Cerebrum

57. In which structure is the fourth cranial nerve nucleus located?

a. Midbrain
b. Pons

c. Medulla
d. Cerebrum

58. In which structure is the sixth cranial nerve nucleus located?

a. Midbrain
b. Pons

c. Medulla
d. Cerebrum

59. A 75-year-old man was shown a picture of his anniversary party that had been held when he was 50 years old. He recognized most friends and family members but could not identify the relationships among them. He could not recall the reason for the party despite a banner wishing them a "Happy 25th Anniversary" in the background. He looked from one person to another, but he failed to survey the scene and was unable to direct his gaze. He was oriented and had good memory and judgment. His visual acuity and visual fields were within normal limits. Which disorder is impairing his ability to comprehend the picture?

a. Dementia
b. Cortical blindness
c. Bilateral hemi-inattention
d. Gerstmann's syndrome
e. Balint's syndrome
f. Depression

60. What is the etiology of *presbyopia*?

a. Relatively inelastic lenses cannot properly expand to permit them to focus on close objects.
b. The macula degenerates.
c. As in farsightedness, the length of the globe is disproportionately short.
d. None of the above

61. During her recovery from a lumbar laminectomy, a 35-year-old nurse complains of the sudden onset of poor vision in her right eye. That eye's pupil is dilated and the intraocular pressure is normal. Pilocarpine eyedrops (1%) fail to constrict the pupil. Her extraocular movements are full and the funduscopic examination reveals no abnormalities. The remainder of the neurologic examination is normal. A CT, MRI, and LP all produce normal results. A similar problem had occurred after her hysterectomy the previous year. What is the most likely cause of her visual impairment?

a. Myasthenia gravis
b. A left-sided Horner's syndrome
c. Spinal cord injury from the laminectomy
d. None of the above

62. A 27-year-old woman has suddenly lost vision in her left eye. The pupils in room light are equal in size. When a light is shone into the left eye, neither pupil constricts; however, when light is shone into the right eye, both pupils constrict. Which portion of the light reflex is impaired?

a. Left afferent
b. Right afferent
c. Left efferent
d. Right efferent

63. In evaluating another patient with an impaired light reflex, the physician finds that when a light is shone into the left eye, only the right pupil constricts. When light is shone into the right eye, only the right pupil constricts. Which portion of the light reflex is impaired?

a. Left afferent
b. Right afferent
c. Left efferent
d. Right efferent

64. Which of the following statements incorrectly describes abnormal smooth pursuit ocular movement?

a. It is found in Huntington's disease as well as a variety of psychiatric disorders.
b. It usually consists of jerky, discontinuous tracking of a slowing moving target.
c. It is highly specific for schizophrenia.
d. Its incidence in schizophrenia patients' family members is greater than in the general population.

ANSWERS

1. a, c, d

2. b, c. The origin of the visual impairment is tricyclic antidepressants' anticholinergic side effects.

3. d

4. b

5. b. Oligodendroglia cells, which produce the myelin that covers the CNS, produce the myelin that covers cranial nerve II. Unlike other cranial nerves, this nerve is actually an extension of the CNS. Schwann cells produce the myelin that covers peripheral nerves and most cranial nerves. Microglia are supporting cells of the CNS.

6. c. Older lenses' loss of elasticity and fluid content prevent them from expanding. Unable to thicken rapidly or fully, the lenses cannot accommodate closely regarded objects.

7. f. She probably has the *Charles Bonnet syndrome,* in which elderly, blind individuals, who are not demented or psychologically disturbed, have frequent benign visual hallucinations. The condition probably results from sensory deprivation. Physicians might monitor her cognitive status, check her hearing, and provide auditory and tactile sensory clues, but diagnostic testing and medication is not warranted.

8. a. These rhythms are normal alpha activity. Individuals at rest with their eyes closed have alpha activity, but when they open their eyes, alpha activity disappears as visual information is transmitted to the occipital lobe. In contrast, if someone is blind, the alpha activity persists because no visual information is transmitted to the occipital lobe.

9. b

10. c. The patient may have partial complex (e.g., psychomotor) seizures and a right superior quadrantanopia as the result of a left temporal lobe lesion. *Or* f. Alternatively, the patient may have a left temporal lobe lesion giving him aphasia and a contralateral superior quadrantanopia. NB: visual fields are drawn from the patient's perspective.

11. a. The patient has spinal cord, cerebellar, and right optic nerve injury, probably as the result of multiple sclerosis.

12. c. The patient may have partial complex seizures and a left superior quadrantanopia as the result of a right temporal lobe lesion.

13. b. The patient and her mother have preservation only of the central vision during daytime. If examination of her fundi showed clumping of retinal pigment, the diagnosis of retinitis pigmentosa would be certain. These visual fields might also be obtained from someone having tunnel vision.

14. e. The patient probably has a dominant hemisphere lesion, such as a cerebrovascular accident or tumor, giving a right homonymous hemianopsia.

15. d. The patient has a large pituitary tumor causing panhypopituitarism and bitemporal hemianopsia.

16. b

17. a, c

18. b, rarely c

19. a

20. b

21. b, rarely c

22. c

23. c

24. a, c

25. b, c

26. b, c

27. a, d

28. b, c

29. c

30. a

31. a, c, e, g. Multiple sclerosis can produce ptosis only if a plaque develops in the midbrain, where it would damage the third cranial nerve. Such a location for a lesion is rare.

32. a, f

33. e. Schizophrenic patients have slow, irregular pursuit movement. They may also have abnormal saccades.

34. d. This patient has an infarction in the left pons. He would have nystagmus because of vestibular nucleus injury. In addition, he might have injury to the left facial and abducens nerve nuclei that would cause left upper and lower facial paresis and medial deviation of the left eye. He would not have signs of cerebral injury, such as aphasia, hemianopsia, or cognitive impairment.

35. d. Oculogyric crises are precipitated by phenothiazines, including those used for nonpsychotic conditions, such as nausea and vomiting.

36. b, c, e, f, g. Moreover, combinations of these conditions may occur together in the same older person. Whatever the cause of a visual impairment, it is a major threat to the mental well-being of people, especially those with other sensory deprivations, such as hearing loss, or cognitive or emotional impairment.

37. c. The patient has visual agnosia, a condition in which patients cannot process visually acquired information. Additional testing might reveal Gerstmann's syndrome or alexia without agraphia (see Chapter 8)—conditions also resulting from posterior dominant hemisphere lesions. His problem is not aphasia because language function is normal as evidenced, once vision is circumvented, by his normal writing and speaking. The lesion causing his visual agnosia is in the left parietal and occipital region.

38. 1-d (Klüver-Bucy syndrome), 2-e, 3-b, 4-a (amaurosis fugax). (Night blindness is also a symptom of retinitis pigmentosa.)

39. e

40. f

41. a

42. c

43. h

44. d

45. j

46. b

47. a, d, e. In primary generalized seizures—petit mal (absences) and tonic-clonic—patients have no aura or visual symptoms. Intoxications and withdrawal cause varied symptoms and, in general, delirium. Hypnagogic and hypnopompic hallucinations are dreams that are highly variable. When migraines have an aura, it is stereotyped.

48. a, b. In palinopsia and partial (elementary and complex) seizures, visual hallucinations are often described exclusively within hemianopsia. Those hallucinations often result from occipital or temporal lobe lesions. Hallucinations related to migraines, dreams, and intoxications occur randomly and do not respect visual fields.

49. b. Slow smooth pursuit ocular movements can result from a wide variety of neurologic diseases, medications, and psychiatric illnesses. This abnormality is a robust neurophysiologic marker of schizophrenia, but it is certainly not specific (see Table 12–3).

50. b, c. Saccades, the high-velocity conjugate gaze movements, are generated by cerebral conjugate gaze centers. They are susceptible to cerebrovascular accidents and other cerebral lesions. Abnormal saccades are one of the first signs of Huntington's disease.

51. a, c. Pursuits, the relatively slow, smooth conjugate gaze movements, are generated mostly by the pontine conjugate gaze centers. They are susceptible to various illnesses and, along with saccades, are abnormal in schizophrenia and, to a lesser extent, affective disorders.

52. b, c. In addition to miosis (small pupil) and anhidrosis (lack of sweating), Horner's syndrome includes ptosis. It results from injury to the sympathetic supply of the face and eye.

53. c, e, f, i. Horner's syndrome may result from lesions in the lower portion of the brainstem (the medulla), upper portion of the spinal cord (the cervical spinal cord), or autonomic nervous system in the chest—anywhere along the circuitous route of the sympathetic innervation of the pupil (see Fig. 12–15).

54. c. The posterior cerebral arteries, which are the terminal branches of the basilar artery, perfuse the occipital lobes. Because the occipital lobes contain the visual cortex, occlusion of both posterior cerebral arteries causes cortical blindness.

55. a, c, d. When the brainstem or cranial nerves III, IV, or VI are injured, patients have diplopia only if both eyes are open. As a general rule, cerebral lesions do not cause diplopia. When diplopia originates from one eye, the patient is said to have monocular diplopia.

56. a

57. a

58. b

59. e. Balint's syndrome is a neuropsychologic syndrome that consists of psychic paralysis of fixation, optic ataxia, and simultanagnosia. The simultanagnosia prevents him from perceiving ("seeing") objects in the periphery, as well as in the center, of his visual fields. The psychic paralysis refers to someone's inability to look from one object to another, as though the first object were overwhelmingly captivating. The simultanagnosia and psychic paralysis inhibit patients from exploring space. Optic ataxia refers to the inability to look directly from one object to another.

60. a. Loss of their elastic qualities prevents the lenses from expanding. Because closely regarded objects' image cannot be focused on the retina, individuals with presbyopia must hold newspapers and sew with needles at arms' length.

61. d. The failure of pilocarpine, a strong miotic agent, to constrict the pupil indicates that she is instilling substances into her eye. Ophthalmologic preparations of cocaine, atropine, or hydroxyamphetamine eyedrops and several readily available chemicals readily dilate a normal pupil. Myasthenia gravis does not affect the pupils. A lumbar laminectomy is performed nowhere near the spinal cord.

62. a. Her left optic nerve has been injured.

63. c. Her left oculomotor nerve or some other portion of the left efferent limb has been injured. Alternatives include ocular trauma and instillation of eye drops.

64. c

Congenital Cerebral Impairments

Several childhood conditions result from perinatal injuries or stem from genetic abnormalities. Children who survive typically have combinations of physical and neuropsychologic impairments that persist into adulthood. Moreover, perinatal cerebral injuries constitute at least a weak risk factor for schizophrenia.

CEREBRAL PALSY

A nonscientific, but generally accepted term, cerebral palsy (CP) describes the permanent, nonprogressive neurologic *motor system* impairments that result from central nervous system (CNS) injuries of the immature brain. The injuries occur *in utero*, around delivery (perinatally), during infancy, or in early childhood.

In cases where cause can be established, prematurity and low birth weights, particularly those less than 1.5 kg, are usually implicated. Other causes or risk factors for CP include a 5-minute Apgar score of less than 4, need for ventilator assistance for more than 48 hours, and perinatal neurologic illnesses, such as meningitis. Over the last 25 years, improved prenatal, obstetric, and postpartum care reduced the incidence of CP to about 0.2% of births. However, it has resisted further reductions sought by a variety of technical devices and public health measures. Despite legal allegations, less than 15% of CP cases result from a preventable obstetric injury, such as anoxia. In fact, more than 70% of cases originate in antepartum factors.

Clinical features of CP are usually so apparent that most cases can be diagnosed "by inspection." However, several conditions mimic CP closely enough to represent diagnostic pitfalls. For example, insidiously advancing leukoencephalopathies (see Chapter 15) can produce spastic paresis that may, during a single examination, be indistinguishable from CP. Similarly, dopa-responsive dystonia (see below and Chapter 18) produces a movement disorder similar to choreoathetotic CP. In fact, the similarity can be so great that neurologists have been urged to treat for dopa-responsive dystonia no matter how unlikely the diagnosis rather than accept the CP diagnosis. Another condition important in evaluating children with permanent (or, more often, progressive) neurologic disabilities is *child abuse* (see Chapter 22).

In diagnosing CP, the two varieties that occur most frequently and have the greatest descriptive value are *spastic paresis* and *extrapyramidal CP (choreoathetosis)* (Fig. 13–1). Each variety has a characteristic motor impairment and predictable association with epilepsy and mental retardation—the major consequences of cerebral injury. Each may also be associated with pseudobulbar palsy, hyperactivity, learning disabilities, hearing impairment, dysarthria, and strabismus.

Neurologists diagnose CP in children who have a "static" or "nonprogressive" motor impairment that has followed a perinatal cerebral injury (Table 13–1). The par-

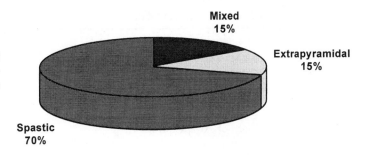

FIGURE 13–1. Most cases of CP are varieties of spastic CP: hemiplegic, diplegic, and quadriplegic. The percent figures are approximations because studies vary.

ticular impairments change little as children grow. Computed tomography (CT), magnetic resonance imaging (MRI), and electroencephalography (EEG) help in identifying etiology and estimating extent of brain damage. However, clinical evaluation remains the basis of diagnosis and prognosis.

Once assured that a child had sustained a static cerebral injury rather than a progressive illness, physicians should concentrate on the problems at hand by evaluating the child or adult's mental and physical abilities and disabilities (Table 13–2). Because approximately 50% of persons with CP have normal intelligence despite major motor deficits, movement disorders, dysarthria, and hearing impairment, physicians should not categorize any child as mentally retarded without a complete, individualized mental status evaluation.

One major, ongoing complication of CP is epilepsy. Like physical impairments and mental retardation, it usually becomes evident before age 5 years. Rates of epilepsy in both spastic and extrapyramidal CP correspond to the magnitude of physical impairments and mental retardation (Fig. 13–2).

TABLE 13–1. *Historical Features of Cerebral Palsy*

Description of deficit
  Motor impairment
    Paresis: extent, degree
    Movement disorder: nature, age of onset
  Delayed acquisition of motor skills
  Associated conditions
    Mental retardation
    Epilepsy
Search for cause
  Maternal health
    Personal or familial neurologic illness
    Prenatal illness or abnormalities
    Drug use
    Amniocentesis
  Delivery
    Prematurity
    Low weight for date
    Prolonged labor, fetal distress
    Obstetric complications
  Neonatal period
    Low Apgar score
    Cyanosis, unresponsiveness
    Sepsis
    Seizures
    Jaundice

TABLE 13–2. *Physical Findings of Cerebral Palsy*

Motor deficits
  Signs of spastic CP
    Gross impairment: paresis/spasticity, growth arrest, pseudobulbar palsy
    Subtle impairment: unequal size of hands or feet, toe walking (from shortened heel
      cords), premature hand preference (e.g., right-handedness) before the age of
      18 months
  Signs of extrapyramidal CP
    Choreoathetosis
Associated conditions
  Mental retardation
  Epilepsy
  Pseudobulbar palsy
  Impairment of special senses
    Visual: strabismus, myopia, blindness (cortical or ocular)
    Auditory: deafness
    Vocal: dysarthria

Not all educational deficiencies in these children result from mental retardation. Many CP and epileptic children, with or without mental retardation, have been unable to attend school. Of children with mental retardation or CP, 10% to 20% have epilepsy. Of mentally retarded children in institutions, 40% have epilepsy.

Spastic CP

The major clinical feature of patients with spastic CP is a combination of paresis and spasticity. The spasticity, which is actually more of an impediment than the paresis, causes slow, clumsy movements that cannot be performed in isolation. It is almost always accompanied by hyperactive deep tendon reflexes (DTRs), clonus, and Babinski signs. In addition, because the cerebral injury occurs before childhood growth, affected limbs have *growth arrest*, that is, the arm, leg, or both are characteristically shortened.

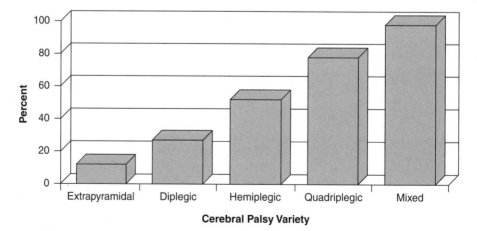

FIGURE 13–2. The proportion of CP patients with mental retardation and epilepsy increases with more extensive *cerebral* disease. The incidence in choreoathetosis or extrapyramidal CP is only approximately 10%; however, the incidence in diplegic CP is 25%; hemiplegic CP 50%; quadriplegic CP 75%; and mixed CP 95%.

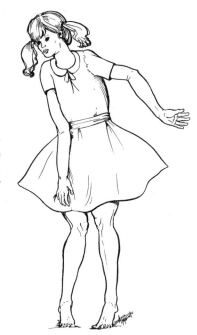

FIGURE 13–3. Spastic diplegia in this 10-year-old girl with low-normal intelligence causes straightening and inturning of the legs, a tiptoe stance, and scissorslike gait. Her uncoordinated, awkward arm movements (posturings) are another but subtler manifestation.

Spastic CP results from necrotic areas in the white matter around the ventricles, *periventricular leukomalacia.* It is detectable by ultrasound examination of an infant's head.

Diplegic CP (spastic diplegia) is symmetric paresis, primarily of the legs (Fig. 13–3). An early sign is that the infants' legs appear straight with the feet pointed downward (extended), drawn together (adducted), and crossed over each other ("scissored"). Without surgical correction, the leg muscles' tendons shorten and hold the knees, ankles, and toes straight, adducted, and extended. When children begin to walk, the spastic diplegia forces them to stand on their toes.

Spastic diplegia is the CP variety most closely related to prematurity. The underlying pathology is *periventricular leukomalacia* that preferentially damages the corticospinal tract fibers destined to innervate the legs (see Fig. 7–7). Because cerebral damage is relatively confined, both epilepsy and mental retardation occur in only about 25% of individuals, which is less frequent than in other forms of spastic CP.

Hemiplegic CP is spastic hemiparesis that affects the face and arm more than the leg (Fig. 13–4). Hemiplegic cerebral palsy patients resemble adults with strokes from middle cerebral artery occlusions, but they have growth arrest of the affected limbs. In particular, their thumb and great-toe nail beds are smaller on the paretic side, and a short Achilles tendon forces them to walk on the toes of the affected foot. Another distinguishing feature is premature hand preference (e.g., right-handedness). Whereas handedness (right or left) normally appears only after 2 years, at a younger age *exclusive* use of one hand suggests palsy of the other.

More important, because the right hemisphere can become dominant when the left is injured in infancy, children who have had congenital left hemisphere damage tend to develop right hemisphere dominance (see Chapter 8). They become left-handed with normal language function, albeit with right hemiparesis. In contrast, adults who sustain left cerebral hemisphere injuries almost always have aphasia in conjunction with right hemiparesis.

The cerebral damage in spastic hemiparesis is generally more extensive than in spastic cerebral diplegia. Thus, in hemiplegia, epilepsy and mental retardation de-

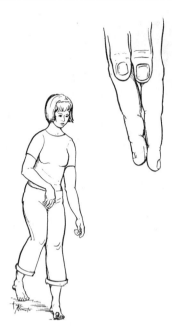

FIGURE 13–4. Spastic hemiparesis since birth in this 28-year-old woman with normal intelligence causes weakness of her right arm and leg. She holds the arm, wrist, and fingers in a flexed posture. Growth arrest of her right hand has led to shortened fingers and, a characteristic finding, a less broad thumb nail bed. The right leg, especially the heel (Achilles) tendon, is also short, causing her to walk on her right toes and circumduct that leg. Her posture and gait are similar to that of adults after a left middle cerebral artery infarction (see Figs. 2–3 to 2–5).

velop frequently (i.e., in 50% of affected children). However, when the damage that causes cerebral diplegia is extensive, children have profound impairments.

Quadriplegic CP is paresis of all four limbs usually accompanied by pseudobulbar palsy. Because it results from extensive cerebral damage, often caused by anoxia during delivery, a large proportion—75%—of these children suffer from epilepsy and mental retardation. In contrast, cervical spinal cord birth injury causes quadriplegia without cerebral damage.

Physical therapy is helpful, and surgery that transposes or lengthens tendons reduces spasticity. Oral antispastic medications may provide some help. Intramuscular injections of botulinum toxin (see Chapter 18) temporarily reduce intense muscle contractions.

Control of epilepsy is difficult, especially in children with mental retardation. It often requires two or more antiepileptic medications, which in turn may produce sedation, paradoxical hyperactivity, and other behavioral disturbances.

Extrapyramidal CP

Extrapyramidal or "dyskinetic" CP is characterized by choreoathetosis, which is involuntary writhing (athetosis) of the face, tongue, hands, and feet punctuated or sometimes overridden by jerking movements (chorea) of the trunk, arms, and legs (Fig. 13–5) (see Chapter 18). Choreoathetosis interferes with fine hand movements, walking, and even sitting still. Involvement of the larynx, pharynx, and diaphragm can lead to incomprehensible dysarthria.

This form of CP must be distinguished from dopamine responsive dystonia, which also produces involuntary movements in young children. Unlike CP, dopamine responsive dystonia is progressive (albeit slowly), has subtle diurnal fluctuations, and responds to small doses of L-dopa (see Chapter 18).

Choreoathetotic CP is usually produced by combinations of low birth weight, anoxia, and neonatal hyperbilirubinemia *(kernicterus)* that damage the basal ganglia and the auditory pathways. Hearing impairment is a frequent complication. Even though the basal ganglia damage usually occurs neonatally, the choreoathetosis

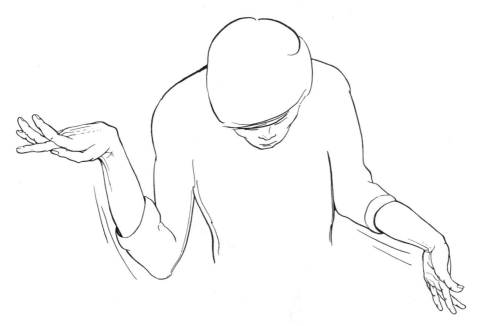

FIGURE 13–5. Choreoathetosis in a 13-year-old girl, obvious only since she was 3 years old, is manifest by slow sinuous movements (athetosis) of the wrists, hands, and fingers. This involuntary movement disorder forces her hands into flexion at the wrist and her fingers into extension with overlapping positions. Intermittent, quick movements (chorea) are often superimposed (also see Fig. 18–13).

might not be apparent until children are 2 years old, by which time they should have developed steady walking and fine motor movements.

Most important, probably because the cerebral cortex can be relatively or entirely spared in kernicterus, choreoathetotic CP is associated with the lowest incidence of epilepsy and mental retardation—10%. Many patients have been able to complete college. Nevertheless, these CP children also are liable to be underrated by a superficial academic or medical evaluation.

Although choreoathetosis is difficult to treat, neuroleptics and sedatives may suppress some movement. Experimental, risky surgical procedures involving ablation of deep cerebral structures reportedly reduce athetosis.

Finally, *mixed forms* of CP—combinations of spastic paraparesis and choreoathetosis—account for about 15% of cases. They reflect the most extensive CNS injury, which is naturally associated with the highest incidence of epilepsy and mental retardation—95%.

NEURAL TUBE CLOSURE DEFECTS

These defects result from defective embryologic development of the CNS. Normally, during the third and fourth weeks of gestation, the dorsal ectoderm invaginates to form a closed midline neural tube that eventually gives rise to the CNS (Fig. 13–6, top). The ectoderm thus forms the CNS, as well as the skin. The mesoderm forms the coverings of the CNS—the meninges, vertebrae, and skull. Defects in neural tube closure, which may spread to include a mesodermal component, are magnified throughout gestation.

Beyond the neurologic issues, neural tube defects create some of the most public, yet privately heart-wrenching, controversies in medicine: harvesting organs in cases

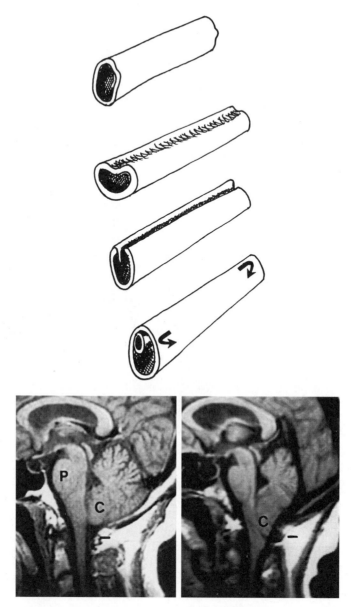

FIGURE 13–6. *Top,* The neural tube's formation takes place during the third and fourth weeks of gestation. It begins when the embryo's external layer, the ectoderm, invaginates to form a distinct, midline neural tube that must close at both ends. Then the embryo begins to bend into a curved, fetal shape with the tube on the convex surface. Failure to complete this process results in "neural tube defects" or "midline closure defects" that are most common at the upper and lower ends of the spinal cord.

Bottom left, The MRI shows the normal relationship of several of the structures contained in the posterior fossa: the pons (P), medulla (unmarked), cerebellum (C), and the fourth ventricle (the black, CSF filled, triangular area between the pons and middle of the cerebellum). Note that the lower portion of the cerebellum is above the level of the foramen magnum (indicated by a short horizontal line).

Bottom right, This MRI shows an Arnold Chiari abnormality. Its primary feature is that the lower portion of the cerebellum, which includes the tonsils, and the medulla have descended below the foramen magnum. In severe cases, the aqueduct is stenotic and hydrocephalus develops.

of anencephaly (see below), parents not consenting to treatment, and the burden of health care costs for infants with a dismal prognosis.

Upper Neural Tube Closure Defects

In an extreme example of a neural tube defect, the entire upper end of the neural tube does not form and the fetus fails to develop a skull and brain. This rare but well publicized condition, *anencephaly,* is invariably fatal within days of birth. The organs are ideal for transplantation.

In an *encephalocele,* a skin-covered brain, meninges, or merely the cerebrospinal fluid (CSF) protrudes through a skull defect. This malformation results from incomplete closure of the mesodermal layers (bone and skin) over the upper neural tube and usually involves the occipital portion of the skull and brain. In a related malformation, *Dandy-Walker syndrome,* which may not be evident when looking at an affected infant, the posterior portion of the upper neural tube fails to develop. Infants are born with only rudimentary posterior brain structures. In particular, the cerebellum and medulla fail to develop beyond an early embryonic stage. As if to fill the empty space, the fourth ventricle grows into a large cyst. As with many other neural tube defects, encephalocele and Dandy-Walker syndrome lead to hydrocephalus and mental retardation.

A variation of upper neural tube closure defects is a group collectively termed *Arnold-Chiari malformation.* Usually not obvious by external appearances, it involves combinations of the medulla and cerebellum being displaced downward through the foramen magnum (see Fig. 20–21), aqueductal stenosis, and overlying skull and cervical spine defects (Fig. 13–6, bottom). Arnold-Chiari malformations are associated with comparable defects in lower neural tube structures, such as *meningomyelocele* (see below).

In older children and adults who may previously have escaped detection, these malformations produce headaches (especially when bending), bulbar palsy, and neck pain. Aqueductal stenosis or blocking by the posterior brain structures of the foramen magnum causes hydrocephalus. Patients typically require neurosurgical insertion of ventriculo-peritoneal shunt or "unroofing" of the upper cervical spine and occipital skull.

Lower Neural Tube Closure Defects

In the most benign and simplest case, *spina bifida occulta,* the spine of the lumbar vertebrae simply fails to fuse. Because both the underlying spinal cord and cauda equina and the overlying skin are intact, this disorder is usually asymptomatic.

In *meningocele,* a more serious problem, the meninges and skin protrude through a lumbosacral spine defect to form a large bulge that is filled with CSF. Although this condition may remain asymptomatic, it usually causes gait impairment, bladder emptying problems, progressive hydronephrosis, and loss of the normal multiple tissue barriers that protect the CNS. To prevent bacteria from entering the CSF and causing meningitis, infants with meningoceles must undergo neurosurgery for repair.

Meningomyelocele or *myelomeningocele,* the worst case, occurs far more frequently than meningocele. This defect consists of a tangle of a rudimentary spinal cord, lumbar and sacral nerve roots, and meninges protruding into a saclike structure overlying the lumbosacral spine (Fig. 13–7). The malformation causes areflexia, paraparesis, and incontinence in infants. In addition, the defective meninges immediately subject neonates to meningitis. Although hydrocephalus is present in only about 25% of infants with meningomyeloceles, it develops in almost all who survive.

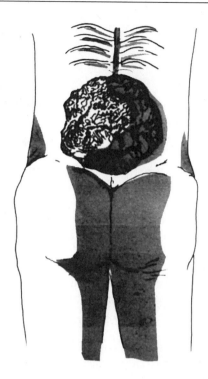

FIGURE 13–7. A newborn infant with a meningomyelocele has a broad-based, loose, translucent sac of thin, friable skin arising from the upper lumbar area that weeps a mixture of serum and CSF. The meningomyelocele contains rudiments of a spinal cord and lumbar and sacral nerves. The infant's legs are weak, flaccid, and areflexic. The bladder is distended.

Meningomyeloceles are repaired in the child's first week, but the clinical deficits usually worsen in childhood and again during adolescent growth spurts. Although high-technology surgery may protect infants from meningitis and reduce the impact of hydrocephalus, almost all survivors are mentally retarded and paraplegic. As children go through the teenage growth spurt, they typically require urinary- and fecal-diversion procedures; revisions of shunts for hydrocephalus; further surgery on the spine; a full array of social, psychologic, and educational support services; and various braces, ramps, and elevators.

Causes

Because a woman who has delivered a baby with meningomyelocele will have a 4% to 10% chance of bearing another baby with a similar abnormality, a tendency toward meningomyeloceles has been attributed to an autosomal recessive genetic abnormality. Meningomyeloceles and other neural tube defects have also been attributed to radiation, folic acid deficiency, and a variety of toxins, including potato blight, vitamin A, and the antiepileptic drugs (AEDs) carbamazepine (Tegretol) and valproate (Depakote). (The relationship between AEDs and meningomyeloceles may be due to the fact that AEDs lower the serum folate level.)

An antenatal diagnosis of meningomyelocele may be made by finding excessive α-fetoprotein in amniotic fluid and maternal serum. Fetal ultrasound examination is a complementary test.

Adequate folic acid intake, by diet or vitamin supplement, before conception and during the first trimester, reduces incidence of neural tube defects. For example, women who eat adequate amounts of fruits and vegetables, which contain folic acids and other nutrients, have as much as a 70% reduction in incidence of neural tube defects in their babies. Based on this evidence, the Food and Drug Administration has ordered that fortified foods, such as pasta and cornmeal, be supplemented with folic acid. Neurologists suggest that women under treatment with carbamazepine or valproate also take vitamins containing folic acid.

NEUROCUTANEOUS DISORDERS

Embryologic defects in the ectoderm also give rise to paired abnormalities of the brain and skin. In addition, these disorders often include abnormalities of other ectoderm and nonectoderm organs. Physicians should be able to deduce the CNS pathology by inspection of these patients.

With at least one exception, the neurocutaneous disorders are inherited largely in an autosomal dominant pattern. They usually remain stable through adult life. However, the cerebral lesions sometimes undergo malignant transformation. This book discusses only major stigmata of the many neurocutaneous disorders.

Tuberous Sclerosis

Tuberous sclerosis usually causes smooth and firm nodules, *adenoma sebaceum* or *facial angiofibromas,* on the malar surface of the face (Fig. 13–8), but this illness-defining abnormality does not appear until adolescence. During infancy and childhood, affected children's skin has characteristic but subtle hypopigmented areas, which in about 20% of cases have a featherlike "ash-leaf" configuration; leathery, scaly lesions on the trunk (shagreen patches); and periungual fibromas of the fingers.

In the classic triad, which actually occurs in the minority of children, epilepsy, which is often intractable, and mental retardation accompany hypopigmented areas or adenoma sebaceum (facial angiofibromas). Many children have delay in speech and language development.

In some children with tuberous sclerosis, additional cognitive impairment develops and their decline eventually reaches the point of dementia. Some have autistic features. However, these manifestations are highly variable, with many affected individuals having only skin or CNS manifestations. The variability is partly attributable to an abnormal gene (TSC1) on chromosome 9 or a related gene (TSC2) on chromosome 16.

The CNS correlate of the skin lesions consists of cerebral *tubers,* which are potato-like brain nodules, 1 to 3 cm in diameter. They grow to compress and irritate the surrounding cerebral cortex and cause the epilepsy and additional cognitive impairment. Although usually benign, the tubers sometimes undergo malignant transformation. Moreover, retinal, renal, and cardiac tumors develop. Because cerebral tubers are relatively large and tend to calcify, CT and MRI readily identify them. They usually cannot be removed because they are too numerous and deeply situated.

Most patients have a relatively benign, stable course with controllable epilepsy and little or no mental retardation. However, combinations of cognitive impairment and epilepsy force many into institutions.

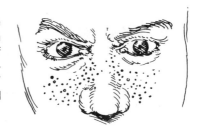

FIGURE 13–8. Adenoma sebaceum (or facial angiofibromas), the cutaneous component of tuberous sclerosis, most prominent in a butterfly distribution on the malar surface of the face, consist of nodules that are several millimeters in diameter, firm, and uniformly pale. They may resemble acne; however, acne "pimples" have a liquid (pus) center that is surrounded by inflammation and accumulate on the trunk, as well as the face.

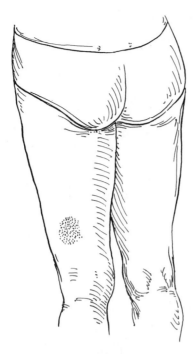

FIGURE 13–9. Café au lait spots are flat, light brown skin lesions. Six or more, each measuring at least 1.5 cm, indicate neurofibromatosis.

Neurofibromatosis

Commonly occurring, classic neurofibromatosis, called *neurofibromatosis type 1 (NF1)*, von Recklinghausen's disease, or "peripheral type" neurofibromatosis, is inherited on chromosome 17 in an autosomal dominant pattern. However, in approximately 50% of patients, it arises sporadically.

A triad of readily identifiable manifestations suggests NF1: multiple *café au lait spots, neurofibromas,* and *Lisch nodules*. Café au lait spots, the signature of neurofibromatosis, are flat and light brown (Fig. 13–9). However, individual café au lait spots are found in at least 10% of normal individuals. What virtually guarantees the diagnosis of neurofibromatosis in adults is the presence of more than six spots, each larger than 1.5 cm.

Neurofibromas are soft, palpable, subcutaneous growths, a few millimeters to several centimeters in size that emerge along peripheral nerves (Figs. 13–10 and 13–11). Sometimes plexiform neuromas induce extraordinary growth of a limb. Neurofibromas can grow large enough to compress the spinal cord, nerve roots, or cauda equina. They occasionally reach grotesque proportions. However, the famous 19th-century

FIGURE 13–10. Neurofibromas often grow to several centimeters of disfiguring protuberances on the face.

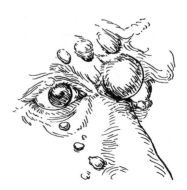

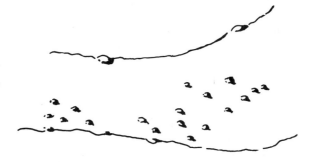

FIGURE 13–11. Neurofibromas are often subtle, multiple, subcutaneous, soft, and typically less than 0.5 cm in size.

"Elephant Man," Joseph Merrick, who was thought to be an example of neurofibromatosis, actually suffered from a related condition, Proteus syndrome.

Lisch nodules are multiple, asymptomatic, macroscopic, yellow to brown nodules (melanocytic hamartomas) situated on the iris (Fig. 13–12). Although a slit-lamp examination may be required to detect and distinguish them from inconsequential pigment collections, Lisch nodules are pathognomonic and the most common manifestation of NF1 in adults.

Excision of neurofibromas, except for those compressing the spinal cord or other key structures, is impractical because NF1 involves innumerable peripheral nerves. Café au lait spots can be blanched by laser treatment.

Although its cutaneous manifestations probably represent the most conspicuous sign of any neurologic disease, NF1 is not entirely peripheral. It induces intracerebral tumors, such as astrocytomas and optic nerve gliomas. Moreover, NF1 has a high association with attention deficit hyperactivity disorder (ADHD) and learning disabilities: depending on tests used, learning disabilities are detectable in one-third to two-thirds of affected children. The average intelligence quotient (IQ) of NF1 patients is about 5 to 10 points lower than average. Mental retardation (IQ two standard deviations below average) occurs in 5% to 8% of patients, which is slightly greater than the incidence in the general population (3%).

Neurofibromatosis type 2 (NF2)—an almost completely different disorder—is characterized by development of bilateral acoustic neuromas that steadily impair hearing until deafness ensues. NF2, also called familial acoustic neuroma or "central type" neurofibromatosis, is inherited on chromosome 22 in an autosomal dominant pattern. It may induce a few neurofibromas and large, pale café au lait spots, but its hallmark remains the acoustic neuromas. In fact, NF2 is usually unrecognized until acoustic neuromas are discovered.

Another manifestation of NF2 is meningiomas. Unless a meningioma compresses a critical area of the brain, this NF2 does not cause mental impairment. Its two neoplastic complications, acoustic neuromas and meningiomas, both "benign," can be

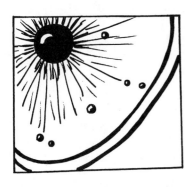

FIGURE 13–12. Lisch nodules, virtually a pathognomonic sign of NF1, are aggregations on the iris that can often be seen with the unaided eye, although a slit-lamp examination may be necessary.

detected with gadolinium enhanced MRIs. Although these tumors can be removed by surgery, sometimes the acoustic or adjacent facial cranial nerve must be sacrificed during the surgery. Alternatively, pinpoint radiation and laser treatment may be able to burn away the tumor and spare the nerves.

Sturge-Weber Syndrome

This syndrome, *encephalo-trigeminal angiomatosis,* consists of vascular malformations of the face *(nevus flammeus)* and underlying cerebral hemisphere. Unlike other the other neurocutaneous disorders, it has no known genetic basis and does not occur in families.

The vascular malformations of the face cause a deep red discoloration (port-wine stain) in the region of one or more divisions of the trigeminal nerve (Fig. 13–13). By contrast, most individuals with small, patchy port-wine stains and infants with small forehead or facial angiomas, such as strawberry nevi, do not have Sturge-Weber syndrome. Whether or not the facial nevus flammeus is a manifestation of Sturge Weber syndrome, it can be bleached by laser treatment.

The cerebral component of the syndrome is a calcified vascular region, accompanied by atrophy, in one cerebral hemisphere. The calcification, which is the major cerebral finding, can be seen on skull x-ray and CT but not on MRI because calcifications, devoid of water, do not emit a signal.

With a variable incidence, patients tend to have mental retardation, learning disabilities, behavioral disturbances, and refractory epilepsy. Depending on the lesion site, they may also have focal physical deficits, such as homonymous hemianopsia and spastic hemiparesis. Recurrent epilepsy and progressively severe sclerosis surrounding the cerebral lesion intensify the neurologic impairments. Sturge-Weber syndrome patients with seizures have a much higher incidence of developmental delay, cognitive impairment, physical deficits, and unemployability.

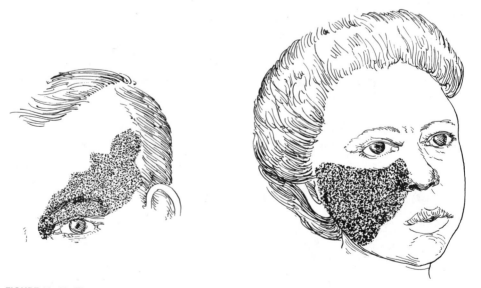

FIGURE 13–13. The cutaneous angiomatosis of Sturge-Weber syndrome involves one or more divisions of the distribution of the trigeminal nerve (see Fig. 4–11). Because the first division is the one most often affected, the most common site includes the anterior scalp, forehead, and upper eyelid. One-third of patients have bilateral involvement.

Ataxia-Telangiectasia

Unlike most other neurocutaneous disorders, ataxia-telangiectasia is inherited in a recessive pattern. It is attributable to a genetic abnormality on chromosome 11 that interferes with DNA repair. The first manifestations, because of associated immunologic deficiency (see below), are chronic sinus and respiratory tract infections. Neurologic manifestations become evident in children 3 to 5 years old when degeneration of the cerebellar vermis gives them a steadily progressive ataxic gait. Subsequently, affected children develop cognitive impairment. The cutaneous component consists of aggregations of small, dilated vessels (telangiectasia) on the conjunctiva, bridge of the nose, and cheeks.

As in few other neurologic diseases, ataxia-telangiectasia is consistently associated with immunodeficiency. Affected children have both cellular immunity impairment and little or no immunoglobulin IgA or IgE. Their immunodeficiency leads to severe sinus and respiratory tract infections and the development of lymphomas and other neoplasms. (The same association of immunodeficiency with lymphoma also occurs in acquired immunodeficiency syndrome (AIDS) and medical immunosuppression for organ transplantation.)

OTHER GENETIC NEUROLOGIC DISORDERS

Neurologists somewhat arbitrarily link several genetic disorders that have a common thread of cognitive impairment and a characteristically abnormal habitus. Aside from changes brought on by puberty, these abnormalities remain stable throughout life. They usually do not cause signs of white matter diseases (leukodystrophies), such as progressive spasticity and blindness, or of metabolic storage diseases, such as progressive cognitive deterioration or hepatosplenomegaly. DNA tests can pinpoint these disorders, but the astute physician should first be able to make a diagnosis by inspection.

Chromosomal Disorders (Autosomal)

Phenylketonuria (PKU) (Chromosome 12).   An autosomal recessive inherited deficiency in *hepatic* phenylalanine hydroxylase produces PKU. The deficiency of this enzyme, which normally converts the amino acid phenylalanine to tyrosine, has three major biochemical ramifications:

1. The deficiency prevents the normal metabolism of phenylalanine to tyrosine. Thus, affected individuals have little or no plasma tyrosine, and untreated individuals have elevated concentrations of plasma phenylalanine.

2. The deficiency prevents the normal synthesis of dopamine, subsequent neurotransmitters, and melanin (see Chapter 21).

$$\text{Phenylalanine} \xrightarrow{\text{phenylalanine hydroxylase}} \text{Tyrosine} \xrightarrow{\text{tyrosine hydroxylase}}$$
$$\text{DOPA} \xrightarrow{\text{DOPA decarboxylase}} \text{Dopamine} \xrightarrow{\text{dopamine }\beta\text{-hydroxylase}}$$
$$\text{Norepinephrine} \xrightarrow{\text{phenylethanolamine }N\text{-methyl-transferase}} \text{Epinephrine}$$

3. The deficiency of the normal metabolic enzyme diverts phenylalanine to metabolism by secondary pathways. These metabolic pathways convert phenylalanine to phenylpyruvic acid and eventually phenylketones, which are excreted in the urine. Untreated patients thus have phenylketonuria.

Until the biochemistry of PKU was elucidated, untreated affected infants, after appearing normal from birth through the next several months, fell behind in all areas of development. Most had blond hair, blue eyes, fair complexion, and eczema owing to reduced melanin pigment production because of the dopamine pathway deficiency. The excreted phenylketones made the urine malodorous.

Cognitive delays appeared as early as 8 months of age, and language development was severely curtailed. In about two-thirds of untreated children, mental retardation was profound. Although children and adults with PKU may have had little or no mental retardation, some were described as having nonspecific, poorly defined "psychiatric illness."

PKU is a model autosomal recessive illness that is transmitted by a defective gene on chromosome 12. In the United States, all infants are supposed to be tested for PKU with screening procedures, such as the Guthrie test, that detect elevated concentrations of plasma phenylalanine. However, these tests may be invalid immediately after birth, when residual maternal enzyme would have metabolized fetal phenylalanine concentration.

Eliminating foods that contain phenylalanine ameliorates the effects of the enzyme deficiency. Most important, adhering to a phenylalanine-free diet prevents mental retardation. Noncompliance with the diet has produced neuropsychologic aberrations in adolescents with PKU and mental retardation in (heterozygote) children of affected women. Physicians should be aware that consuming only phenylalanine-free foods is difficult. The diet, which is devoid of artifical sweeteners, leads to short stature and weight, anemia, and hypoglycemia.

Prader-Willi and Angelman's Syndromes (Chromosome 15).   In an example of *genetic imprinting,* the same autosomal dominant abnormality in chromosome 15 produces a pair of different syndromes in affected children.* The abnormality—a deletion of a segment of chromosome 15—produces Prader-Willi syndrome if the father passes it but Angelman's syndrome if the mother passes it. "Prader-Willi is passed in a paternal pattern" serves as the common mnemonic device. Because the sex of the offspring does not affect the phenotype, boys and girls can be affected by either syndrome.

Most cases of Prader-Willi syndrome are paternally inherited, but some are sporadic. Affected boys and girls have mental retardation and behavior problems, but the distinguishing feature is hyperphagia and obesity that is frequently grotesque (Fig. 13–14). Children with Prader-Willi syndrome have more than a voracious appetite. They compulsively and obsessively eat, frequently grabbing food from family member's plates and even rummaging through garbage cans. Prader-Willi teenagers can take on the demeanor of drug addicts. They search endlessly for food sequestered in their home and, when all else fails, they may steal money to buy it.

Children who inherited the same chromosome abnormality from their mother have Angelman's syndrome, which consists of *severe* mental retardation and microcephaly; stereotyped involuntary movements; jerky-ataxic voluntary movements; a smiling face; and paroxysms of unprovoked laughter. The jerky movements and superficially happy appearance has given rise to the term "happy puppet syndrome." Affected adults require assistance with their daily activities and most have epilepsy.

Girls with Angelman's syndrome may be misdiagnosed as having Rett's syndrome because of common features, including mental retardation, microcephaly, and involuntary movements (see below). They may also be misdiagnosed as being autistic because of inappropriate behavior and movements.

---

*This meaning of "imprinting" has been borrowed from Konrad Lorenz's better-known use in psychology, where it signifies social animals' learning behavior patterns through association with their parents or a substitute.

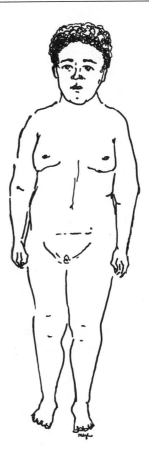

FIGURE 13–14. An 8-year-old boy with Prader-Willi syndrome has the characteristic obesity, small penis and testicles, and short stature, including small hands and short feet. Girls with the syndrome also have hypogonadism: they usually have small labia majora and no labia minora.

Down's Syndrome (Chromosome 21). The most widely known disorder in this group, Down's syndrome, is also, at 1 in 600 births, the most frequently occurring. Affected children are readily recognizable (Fig. 13–15). The syndrome usually causes mild to moderate degrees of mental retardation, with a median IQ of 40 to 50. An unfortunate but extraordinarily important complication of Down's syndrome is that, by the fourth or fifth decade, it uniformly leads to an Alzheimer-like demen-

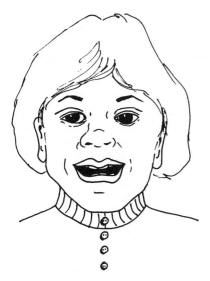

FIGURE 13–15. Children with Down's syndrome are short. Their ears are low-set with small lobes. Their eyes' epicanthal folds are wide, and the lids appear to slant upward—thus the outdated term "Mongolism." The bridge of the nose is depressed. The tongue, which is large, tends to protrude over a slack jaw. Their palms are broad with a single midline crease, and their fingers are short and stubby.

tia (see Chapter 7). In fact, one theory holds that both Down's and Alzheimer's disease result from a common genetic abnormality on chromosome 21.

Down's syndrome children have delayed motor as well as mental development. Their social skills remain intact and are often an asset that compensates for mild mental retardation. Although they do not have psychotic or autistic behavior, Down's syndrome children occasionally have behavior that fulfills criteria for ADHD. Severely affected children may have orofacial dyskinesias unrelated to neuroleptic exposure.

The cause in most children is chromosome 21 trisomy; however, in some the cause is a translocation of that chromosome. (Nevertheless, the translocation variety, because the patients have the same phenotype, is called "trisomy 21" by clinicians.)

The incidence of Down's syndrome is correlated with increasing maternal age (especially older than 40 years). Because a fetus with Down's syndrome can be identified in most cases by a chromosome analysis of amniotic fluid cells, women older than 40 years are urged to undergo amniocentesis. Even though Down's syndrome is genetic, it is not classified as an *inherited* disorder of mental retardation because it is not transmitted from generation to generation. (This subtle consideration allows fragile X syndrome [see below] to be considered the most common form of inherited mental retardation.)

Williams Syndrome (Chromosome 7).   Another autosomal disorder is Williams syndrome. Although the abnormal gene has variable expression, it is probably a recessive trait. The abnormality consists of a minute deletion on chromosome 7, which eventually disrupts the elastic properties of the arteries, root of the aorta (causing supravalular aortic stenosis), skin, and other organs. Individuals with Williams syndrome have a readily identifiable "elfin" facial appearance (Fig. 13–16).

This disease impairs certain neuropsychologic functions, while enhancing others. Williams children have mild to moderate mental retardation with particularly impaired reading and writing skills. They also have a poor sense of visual-spatial relationships and difficulties with nonverbal tasks. Although Williams children do not have gross neurologic abnormalities, such as microcephaly, seizures, or stereotyped movements, they have delayed acquisition of motor milestones and persistent fine and gross motor clumsiness.

In contrast, remarkably and so far inexplicably, Williams syndrome individuals possess extraordinary talents in music and verbal fluency. They are often musically

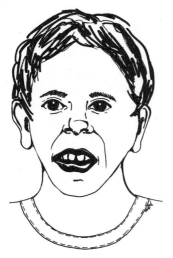

FIGURE 13–16. This 9-year-old girl has the characteristic elfin appearance of Williams syndrome. Her forehead is broad and her cheeks are prominent. Her left eye displays mild esotropia. The nose has a flat bridge, and its nostrils are full and turned slightly upward. Her teeth are hypoplastic and widely spaced. She is short and has supravalvular aortic stenosis.

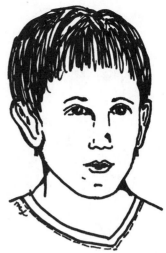

FIGURE 13–17. Boys with the fragile X syndrome tend to have a long, thin face but a prominent forehead and jaw. Another conspicuous feature is their large, everted, low-set, "seashell-shaped" ears. After puberty, their testicles grow to disproportionately larger size *(macro-orchidism)* than their penis. In addition to their having mental retardation, many affected children have autistic behavior, including hand flapping and other stereotypies.

gifted, and their conversations, although devoid of substance, are loquacious, bubbly, and articulate. The discrepancy between their strong language and musical skills and their poor overall cognitive function recalls the distinction between aphasia and dementia (see Chapters 7 and 8). In that dichotomy, patients might be verbal but have marked cognitive impairment (dementia)—or, despite being otherwise cognitively intact, be nonverbal (aphasic).

Chromosomal Disorders (Sex-linked)

Fragile X Syndrome.   The *fragile X syndrome*, like many other genetically determined disorders, is characterized by a combination of mental retardation and prominent, distinctive nonneurologic physical abnormalities (Fig. 13–17). Although this disorder, because it is carried on the X chromosome, is readily expressed in boys, it occasionally develops in girls who inherit the faulty gene. About 70% of boys who inherit the gene have moderate to severe mental retardation. Others have only mild retardation, learning disabilities, or language impairment, but approximately 20% are seemingly normal.

In the usual situation, sex-linked genetic abnormalities, such as hemophilia, color blindness, and Duchenne's muscular dystrophy (see Chapter 6), are not expressed in the female. In contrast, about one-third of females who are carriers of the faulty gene for fragile X syndrome express some of its characteristics. Affected girls often have IQs below 85.

Boys and, to a lesser extent, girls with fragile X syndrome also tend to display behavioral abnormalities, including ADHD. They have excessive rates of learning disability, mood disorder, and repetitive, purposeless, involuntary movements *(stereotypies)*, such as hand flapping or wringing. About 15% of children have been classified as autistic and meet the criteria for Pervasive Developmental Disorder (PDD).

The defective gene consists of excessive repetitions of the CGG trinucleotide in the X chromosome. The DNA abnormality can be easily detected in the blood of affected individuals and, during prenatal screening, in amniotic fluid cells. The normal gene contains 5 to 54 CGG trinucleotide repeats, but the defective gene contains more than 60 repeats. Yet, individuals with 60 to 200 repeats may have few, if any, manifestations. However, those with more than 200 repeats are invariably affected. As with other disorders resulting from excessive trinucleotide repeats, in successive genera-

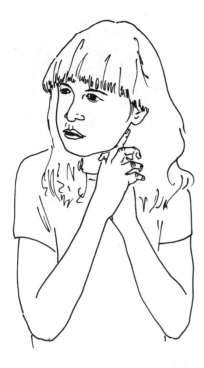

FIGURE 13–18. A 6-year-old girl with Rett's syndrome has developed repetitive hand-washing and clapping movements and acquired microcephaly. Her head circumference is only 48 cm, which would be normal for a 3-year-old girl, but 2 standard deviations below the mean for her age (51 cm). She has progressively lost her ability to speak in a meaningful manner.

tions the size of the genetic abnormality increases, and symptoms both emerge at an earlier age (anticipation) and are more pronounced.*

Unlike Down's syndrome, fragile X syndrome is regularly and predictably transmitted from a parent to one or more children. Occurring in about 1 in 1,500 males and half as frequently in females, it is considered the most common cause of inherited mental retardation and is responsible for as many as 10% of all cases of mental retardation

Rett's Syndrome.   Restricted to girls, *Rett's syndrome* or *disease* starts to appear about 6 months after a normal birth and development when affected baby girls begin to regress in virtually all phases of their psychomotor development. Over several years, they lose their language skills, ability to walk, other learned motor activities, and cognitive capacity. In addition, there is loss of cognitive skills in a pattern similar to developing dementia. Whether the underlying problem is a static encephalopathy or a progressive deterioration, affected children often are left in a state of profound mental retardation. Many victims survive, but their losses, as in CP, persist throughout life.

Rett's syndrome is diagnosed entirely on clinical grounds and only beginning at age 4 to 5 years. Affected girls have two virtually unique physical characteristics: stereotypies and acquired microcephaly (Fig. 13–18). The movements typically consist of incessant hand clapping and wringing. Their microcephaly follows normal head growth from birth to about 6 months. Then the head growth deceleration begins while relatively normal body growth continues. (This pattern contrasts with common cases of congenital microcephaly and mental retardation, as occurs with congenital rubella infections, where the head is small at birth.) In addition, about 50% of the children have seizures.

---

*Excessive trinucleotide DNA repeats produce Friedreich's ataxia and other spinocerebellar degenerations, myotonic dystrophy, and Huntington's disease (see Chapters 2, 6, and 18, respectively), as well as fragile X syndrome (Appendix 3D).

Rett's syndrome has been attributed to a faulty gene on the X chromosome mostly because it only appears in females. Presumably, the same abnormality is lethal in a male fetus.

Loss of language, high incidence of epilepsy, and abnormal behavior in Rett's syndrome mimic autism. However, Rett's syndrome children have a pronounced, progressive loss of motor ability and develop microcephaly. Rett's syndrome also mimics Angelman's syndrome. Aside from the gender differences, Rett's and fragile X have in common mental impairment, behavioral abnormalities, and stereotyped behavior. Overall, Rett's, Angelman's, and fragile X syndromes can reasonably be included in the differential diagnosis of autism.

Turner's Syndrome (XO). Lacking the full complement of both sex chromosomes, females with Turner's syndrome have only 45 chromosomes. Their genotype is designated (XO). From their infancy, Turner's syndrome girls are readily identifiable by their dysmorphic features (Fig. 13–19).

A minority (about 20%) has mild mental retardation. Some have anxiety and depression. In general, they have learning disabilities, attention deficit, and greater impairment on performance than verbal IQ testing. Turner's syndrome may be another example—along with Alzheimer's disease and Williams's syndrome—of preserved verbal ability despite cognitive impairment.

Klinefelter's Syndrome (XXY). With an additional X chromosome, Klinefelter's syndrome boys develop a tall stature, but, failing to mature, they appear eu-

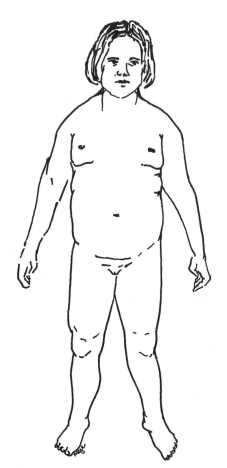

FIGURE 13–19. This 16-year-old girl with Turner's syndrome (XO) has the distinctive short stature and webbed neck. As with other genetic disorders characterized by mental retardation, her ears are low-set, but they are hidden by the low hairline. Her nose is flat and its bridge spreads into broad epicanthal folds. Typically, she has failed to undergo the normal changes of puberty, and lacks breast development and secondary sexual characteristics. Her elbows' carrying angles are poorly accentuated: Her elbows are relatively straight, which is the male pattern. She also has ovarian dysgenesis.

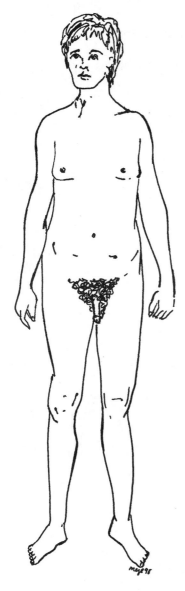

FIGURE 13–20. After a delayed and incomplete puberty, this 30-year-old man with Klinefelter's syndrome (XXY) has typically grown to over 6 feet 2 inches, owing in large part to his disproportionately long legs. His body has assumed a eunuchoid shape with gynecomastia, sparse beard, female pattern of pubic hair, and small testicles. Other conditions characterized by excessive height include the XYY and Marfan's syndromes.

nuchoid after puberty (Fig. 13–20). In fact, Klinefelter's syndrome is most often diagnosed after puberty, particularly during a couple's infertility evaluation, when affected men are discovered to be sterile and have testicular dysgenesis.

In general, Klinefelter's syndrome individuals have a below average IQ, typically between 80 and 90. Only about 25% have some degree of mental retardation, and it is usually mild. They tend to have dyslexia and other learning disabilities. Some clinicians have described Klinefelter's syndrome boys as being passive or as having a decreased libido.

XYY Syndrome.   Men with an additional Y chromosome, as those with an additional X chromosome, are tall—some extremely so—and possess borderline to mildly low intelligence. They also tend to develop severe acne that persists beyond adolescence.

Studies of men with this condition, called "supermales," were originally performed in prisons. The results indicated that the disorder produced deviant, violent, and otherwise aggressive behavior. In retrospect, that location tainted the results with an *ascertainment bias.*

Modern studies have found delays in speech acquisition and other neurodevelopmental milestones, characterologic problems, and psychiatric difficulties, as well as the average to below normal intelligence, as previously noted. These problems were disproportionately greater among men with mental retardation. At this time, both the legal and medical communities have rejected a causal relationship between a XYY karyotype ("supermale syndrome") and violent criminal behavior.

REFERENCES

Botto LD, Moore CA, Khoury MJ, et al: Neural-tube defects. N Engl J Med *341:* 1509–1519, 1999

Coker SB: The diagnosis of childhood neurodegenerative disorders presenting as dementia in adults. Neurology *41:* 794–798, 1991

Creange A, Zeller J, Rostaing-Rigattieri S, et al: Neurological complications of neurofibromatosis type 1 in adulthood. Brain *122:* 473–481, 1999

Crino PB, Henske EP: New developments in the neurobiology of the tuberous sclerosis complex. Neurology *53:* 1384–1390, 1999

Dansky LV, Rosenblatt DS, Andermann E: Mechanisms of teratogenesis: Folic acid and antiepileptic therapy. Neurology *42* (Suppl 5): 32–42, 1992

Denno DW: Legal implications of genetics and crime research. Genetics of Criminal and Antisocial Behavior. New York. John Wiley & Sons, 1996, pp. 248–264

Frank Y (ed.): Pediatric Behavioral Neurology. New York, CRC Press, 1996

Freund LS, Reiss AL, Abrams MT: Psychiatric disorders associated with fragile X in the young female. Pediatrics *91:* 321–329, 1993

Fryns JP, Kleczkowska A, Kubien E, et al: XYY syndrome and other Y chromosome polysomies. Mental status and psychosocial functioning. Genet Couns *6:* 197–206, 1995

Lann LA, den Boer AT, Hennekam RC, et al: Angelman syndrome in adulthood. Am J Med Genet *66:* 356–360, 1996

Lenhoff HM, Wang PP, Greenberg F, et al: Williams syndrome and the brain. Sci Am December, 1997, pp. 68–73

Lindhout D, Omtzigt JGC, Cornel MC: Spectrum of neural-tube defects in 34 infants prenatally exposed to antiepileptic drugs. Neurology *42* (Suppl 5): 111–118, 1992

Miller G, Clark GD: The Cerebral Palsies: Causes, Consequences, and Management. Boston, Butterworth-Heinemann, 1998

Naidu A: Rett syndrome: A disorder affecting early brain growth. Ann Neurol *42:* 3–10, 1997

North KN, Riccardi V, Samango-Sprouse C, et al. Cognitive function and academic performance in neurofibromatosis 1: Consensus statement from the NF1 Cognitive Disorders Task Force. Neurology *48:* 1121–1127, 1997

Rapin I, Katzman R: Neurology of autism. Ann Neurol *43:* 7–14, 1998

Rossen ML, Sarnat HB: Why should neurologists be interested in Williams syndrome? Neurology *51:* 8–9, 1998

Sujansky E, Conradi S: Outcome of Sturge-Weber syndrome in 52 adults. Am J Med Genet *57:* 35–45, 1995

Wald NJ, Watt HC, Hackshaw AK: Integrated screening for Down's syndrome based on tests performed during the first and second trimesters. N Engl J Med *341:* 461–467, 1999

Wiedemann HR, Kunze J: Clinical Syndromes (3rd ed.). London, Times Mirror International Publishers, 1997

QUESTIONS and ANSWERS: CHAPTER 13

1–11. Match the neurocutaneous disorders (a–d) with their primary manifestation (1–11).

a. Tuberous sclerosis
b. Neurofibromatosis type 1 (NF1)

c. Sturge-Weber syndrome
d. Neurofibromatosis type 2 (NF2)

1. Acoustic neuroma

2. Facial lesions vaguely resemble rhinophyma

3. Progressive dementia

4. Neurofibromas

5. Adenoma sebaceum (angiofibromas)

6. Ash leaf, hypopigmented areas

7. Intractable epilepsy

8. Café au lait spots

9. Facial angiomatosis

10. Optic glioma

11. Shagreen patches

ANSWERS: 1-d, 2-a, 3-a, 4-b, 5-a, 6-a, 7-a, 8-b, 9-c, 10-b, 11-a

12–17. Which of the following disorders cause inattention or episodic changes in mood in children? (True/False)

12. Migraines

13. Partial complex seizures

14. Antihistamines

15. Cerebral palsy

16. Sedative medications

17. Absences

ANSWERS: 12-True, 13-True, 14-True, 15-False, 16-True, 17-True

18. In which of the following conditions will CT or MRI provide useful diagnostic information?

a. Attention deficit disorder
b. Absences
c. Migraines
d. Hydrocephalus
e. Sturge-Weber syndrome
f. Learning disabilities
g. Tuberous sclerosis
h. Tourette's syndrome
i. Neurofibromatosis type 2

ANSWER: d, e, g, i (MRI may show acoustic neuromas, the CT cannot)

19. Which is the term for an abnormal gene producing different phenotypes depending on whether the mother or father passed the gene to the offspring?

a. Genetic imprinting
b. Anticipation
c. Sex chromosome (nonautosomal) inheritance
d. Mitochondrial inheritance

ANSWER: a

20. Children who sustain any brain injury until the age of 5 years are eligible for assistance by most programs that serve CP children. (True/False)

ANSWER: True

21. Is the following sentence true or false? "Children with mental retardation because of a genetic abnormality are usually indistinguishable from those with mental retardation for other reasons."

ANSWER: False. They usually have overt physical stigmata, such as low-set ears, that are often specific for a particular genetic abnormality.

22. Which three of the following characteristics of Rett's syndrome children are *not* found in autistic children?

a. Only affects girls
b. Stereotyped behavior
c. Loss of language skills
d. Seizures
e. Acquired microcephaly
f. Ataxia that is progressively more severe

ANSWER: a, e, f

23. Which syndrome carries the lowest incidence of mental retardation?

a. Klinefelter's
b. Trisomy 21
c. Angelman's syndrome

d. Down's
e. Fragile X
f. Prader-Willi

ANSWER: a. Only about 30% of Klinefelter's syndrome men have mental retardation. In addition, when it occurs, their mental retardation is usually mild. Often the disorder remains undetected until they undergo an evaluation for infertility.

24. A one-year-old boy has a stroke because of sickle-cell disease. It results in mild right hemiparesis. Which three of the following conditions will probably be additional consequences?

a. Chorea
b. Aphasia
c. Seizures
d. Spastic cerebral palsy
e. Stunted growth (growth arrest) of right arm

ANSWER: c, d, e. He will probably not have aphasia because his right hemisphere will emerge as dominant for language and motor function.

25–30. Match the disorder (a–d) with its cause (Q25–Q30).

a. Cervical cord injury
b. Kernicterus

c. Cerebral anoxia
d. Stroke in utero

25. Choreoathetosis

26. Spastic quadriplegia

27. Spastic hemiparesis

28. Deafness

29. Seizure disorder

30. Cortical blindness

ANSWERS: 25-b; 26-a or c; 27-d; 28-b; 29-c or d; 30-c

31. Which pair of syndromes represents genetic imprinting?

a. Fragile X and Turner's
b. Alzheimer's disease and trisomy 21

c. Prader-Willi and Angelman's
d. Rett's and Fragile X

ANSWER: c. Prader-Willi and Angelman's syndromes both result from a deletion in chromosome 15. In a prime example of genetic imprinting, the phenotype depends on whether the mother or father passes the abnormal gene to the offspring. When the father passes the gene, the child (boy or girl) may develop Prader-Willi syndrome. When the mother passes the gene, the child (boy or girl) may develop Angelman's syndrome.

32. Regarding phenylketonuria (PKU), which one of the following statements is false?

a. The disease is transmitted in an autosomal recessive pattern.
b. The blood phenylalanine is high and tyrosine is low in affected individuals.
c. When PKU women conceive, their fetus would most likely be heterozygote for the PKU gene and would therefore be unaffected by the mother's diet.
d. Diet sodas and many other "foods" contain phenylalanine, which should be avoided by individuals with PKU.

ANSWER: c. If a pregnant women who has PKU were to disregard her diet restrictions and consume foods with phenylalanine, such as diet soda, the fetus would be damaged by excessive levels of phenylalanine or its metabolic products. The mother with PKU must be homozygote for the PKU gene. Unless the father carried one or two PKU genes, which would be statistically unlikely, the fetus would be heterozygote. Even though the fetus were heterozygote, excessive phenylalanine or its metabolic products might overwhelm its immature enzyme system and cause severe brain damage.

33. An 8-year-old girl has had delayed acquisition of developmental milestones. She has mild mental retardation and especially poor arithmetic and visual-spatial skills. Her handwriting is difficult to read, and she has impaired fine motor skills. However, she is talkative and has learned several foreign languages that she speaks with a natural accent. She also plays two musical instruments and learns new pieces "by ear." Her facial appearance is "elflike." Which is the most likely disorder?

a. Rett's syndrome
b. Turner's syndrome
c. PKU
d. Angelman's syndrome
e. Williams syndrome
f. Klinefelter's syndrome

ANSWER: e. Williams syndrome causes mild mental retardation, with especially poor visual-spatial relationships. Individuals with Williams syndrome often have a outstanding verbal and musical ability and an elflike facial appearance.

34. Which condition is likely to be present in the girl in Question 33?

a. Supravalvular aortic stenosis
b. Microcephaly
c. Stereotypies
d. Hepatosplenomegaly

ANSWER: a. Williams syndrome involves impaired formation of tissue elastin. Microcephaly results from several conditions: Rett's syndrome, Angelman's syndrome, congenital rubella infection, and numerous other disorders. Stereotypies—repetitive, involuntary, meaningless movements, usually of the hands—are characteristic of several neurologic conditions, including Rett's, Angelman's, and fragile X syndromes.

35. Which one of the following statements concerning individuals with the XYY karyotype is false?

a. They are phenotypically male and referred to as "supermales."
b. They are tall, often excessively so, and plagued with severe acne.
c. They frequently have deviant behavior and often commit crimes.
d. Their karyotype is a valid defense against criminal prosecution.

ANSWER: d. These men, who are tall and suffer with acne, often have mild mental retardation and deviant behavior, which may be criminal; however, they are cognizant of their activities and considered culpable if they commit a crime.

36. A 12-year-old girl who has hyperactivity and mild mental retardation has shown a decline in her schoolwork and exhibited behavior problems during the previous 2 months. She has become confrontational and more hyperactive than usual. Of the following disorders that might be superimposed on her preexisting conditions, which is the least likely to be responsible?

a. Multiple sclerosis
b. Sexual abuse
c. Nonsexual abuse
d. Drug abuse

ANSWER: a. Multiple sclerosis rarely develops in adolescents. Moreover, when it develops, the initial symptoms are virtually never behavioral or cognitive. Child abuse, especially in those who are disabled, and drug abuse are relatively common underlying problems in the onset of behavioral disorders.

37. Meningomyelocele is not associated with which of the following conditions?

a. Spastic paraparesis
b. Mental retardation
c. Incontinence
d. Meningitis
e. Flaccid quadriparesis

ANSWER: a. A meningomyelocele is a congenital neural tube closure defect. It causes flaccid, not spastic, paraparesis because the entire junction of the lowest portion of the spinal cord and its emerging nerve roots is malformed. In addition, meningomyeloceles are associated with comparable defects in the upper neural tube. In those cases, meningomyeloceles are typically accompanied by hydrocephalus.

38. Which two neurologic conditions are associated with immunodeficiency?

a. Acquired immunodeficiency syndrome (AIDS)
b. Meningomyelocele
c. Sturge-Weber syndrome
d. Ataxia-telangiectasia

ANSWER: a, d. AIDS is associated with a cellular immunodeficiency and ataxia-telang-iectasia is associated with an IgA and IgE immunoglobulin deficiency as well as cellular immunity impairment. Lymphomas develop in both conditions.

39. Match the condition (a–e) with its clinical feature (1–5).

a. Adrenoleukodystrophy
b. Rett's syndrome
c. Fragile X syndrome
d. Down's syndrome
e. Meningomyelocele

1. In only girls, autistic behavior, repetitive hand slapping, and acquired microcephaly
2. In only boys, progressive deterioration of mental and motor abilities
3. In boys and girls, short stature, prominent epicanthal folds, single crease, low-set ears, and mental retardation
4. In boys and girls with paraparesis, urinary incontinence, hydrocephalus, and mental retardation
5. In boys, but less commonly in girls, mental retardation and large ears; in boys, macro-orchidism

ANSWERS: a-2, b-1, c-5, d-3, e-4

40. Match the structures with their origin in the fetal ectoderm or mesoderm.

a. Brain
b. Scalp and face
c. Dura matter
d. Neural tube
e. Vertebrae
f. Spinal cord
g. Skull

ANSWER: Ectoderm: a, b, d, f. CNS structures, including the neural tube, and skin. Mesoderm: c, e, g. Structural elements, including the skull, dura matter, and vertebrae.

41. Which two parts of the neural tube does the Dandy-Walker malformation affect?

a. The bulb
b. Cerebellum
c. Lower spinal cord
d. The frontal lobes

ANSWER: a, b. In Dandy-Walker malformation, the medulla and cerebellum fail to develop. The fourth ventricle is massively dilated. The malformation usually causes hydrocephalus.

42. Which strategy reduces the incidence of meningomyelocele?

a. Giving the mother thiamine before and during the first trimester
b. Giving the mother vitamin A before and during the first trimester
c. Giving the mother folic acid before and during the first trimester
d. Screening for toxins in the environment

ANSWER: c

43. Match the genetically based disorder (a–c) with all its characteristics (1–11).

a. Rett's syndrome
b. Fragile X syndrome
c. Down's syndrome

1. Repetitive hand movements
2. Acquired microcephaly
3. Associated with trisomy 21
4. Disorder complicated by Alzheimer's diseaselike dementia
5. Associated with excessive trinucleotide repeats
6. A single palm crease is a characteristic
7. Macro-orchidism is a characteristic
8. Autistic behavior is a characteristic
9. Cognitive deterioration beginning in childhood
10. Occurs exclusively in girls
11. Occurs exclusively in males

ANSWERS: 1-a; 2-a; 3-c; 4-c; 5-b; 6-c; 7-b; 8-a, b; 9-a; 10-a; 11-none

44. A 14-year-old girl is short, severely obese, mildly mentally retarded, and has behavioral problems. Her karyotype shows 23 chromosome pairs, including a normal XX, but 15q has a deletion. Which is the most likely syndrome?

a. Angelman's
b. Turner's
c. Fragile X

d. Prader-Willi
e. Down's
f. Trisomy 21

ANSWER: d. All these disorders, including fragile X, can occur in girls and cause mental retardation. Of children with mental retardation, the obesity points immediately to Prader-Willi syndrome, which is confirmed by the deletion in 15q. Angelman's syndrome also results from the deletion in 15q, but its manifestations include severe mental retardation and hyperactivity. Turner's syndrome, which only occurs in girls, results from an absent sex chromosome, that is, XO with only 22 full (autosomal) pairs.

45. How does Angelman's syndrome differ from Prader-Willi syndrome?

a. Angelman's syndrome is inherited from the father.
b. Angelman's syndrome causes greater mental retardation than Prader-Willi syndrome.
c. Angelman's syndrome results from excessive trinucleotide repeats.
d. Angelman's syndrome's genotype is determined by genetic imprinting.
e. Angelman's syndrome, as with autism, has a low incidence of epilepsy.

ANSWER: b. Mental retardation is more pronounced in Angelman's than Prader-Willi syndrome. In addition, epilepsy occurs in 80% of Angelman's syndrome patients, commonly in autistic patients, and rarely in Prader-Willi syndrome patients.

46. Which one of the following statements is true regarding fragile X syndrome?

a. The condition occurs exclusively in girls.
b. When the trinucleotide repeats range from 60 to 200, the individual may be asymptomatic. However, his or her offspring is likely to have a much greater number of repeats and flagrant symptoms.
c. Fragile X syndrome is a rare cause of mental retardation.
d. When it causes mental retardation, the cognitive impairment is unaccompanied by behavioral changes.
e. The condition is restricted to boys.

ANSWER: b. Fragile X syndrome occurs in girls who inherit two abnormal X chromosomes, as well as boys who inherit only one. It is one of the most common, if not the most common, cause of inherited or genetically based mental retardation. Boys with an intermediate number of trinucleotide repeats (60 to 200) may have few if any symptoms, but the abnormal trinucleotide sequence expands with successive generations and their offspring can be predicted to have unequivocal manifestations. The disorder causes hyperactivity and autistic behavior as well as mental retardation.

47. Which of the following syndromes does not produce symptoms that mimic autism?

a. Fragile X
b. Rett's

c. Klinefelter's
d. Angelman's

ANSWER: c

14

Neurologic Aspects of Chronic Pain

Neurologists' informal guidelines for severity and duration of pain from various injuries and illnesses lead them to consider "chronic" any pain, especially when severe, that extends beyond the usual healing process or for 3 to 6 months. Differing from acute, injury-related pain, chronic pain persists through different physiologic mechanisms and requires different treatments. Multidisciplinary teams, which usually include psychiatrists, have come in practice to view chronic pain as a clinical entity rather than a symptom and to emphasize "management"—reducing pain's affective component (suffering) and restoring function—over traditional attempts to diagnose the precise origin of the pain, eradicate it, and distinguish physiologic and psychologic components. Psychiatrists should be aware of modern approaches to pain management; the underlying neuroanatomy; and treatment with opioids (narcotics),* other analgesics, and *adjuvant* (primarily nonanalgesic) medications, such as antidepressants and antiepileptics.

PAIN VARIETIES

In *nociceptive* disorders, specific peripheral nerve pain receptors *(nociceptors)* detect continual tissue damage from common conditions, such as degenerative joint disease, dental infection, or metastases to bone. In these disorders, which are forms of acute pain, the peripheral nervous system (PNS) or certain cranial nerves then transmit the pain stimuli to the central nervous system (CNS) to produce a characteristically dull, aching pain at the site of tissue damage. Removing diseased tissue, reducing inflammation, or administrating analgesics usually alleviates acute pain.

In *neuropathic* disorders, pain arises continually and chronically from direct PNS or CNS *nerve* injury, which may be quiescent rather than active. Some theorize that over time the injury reorganizes CNS processing ("central sensitizing"), causing pain stimuli to be amplified and distorted. (Central sensitization may reflect *plasticity*, a theoretical capacity of the CNS to reorganize its functions. Plasticity is usually beneficial but, as in this case, it may occasionally be detrimental.)

Neuropathic disorders, which include peripheral polyneuropathies, complex regional pain syndrome (reflex sympathetic dystrophy), and thalamic pain, characteristically produces sharp, lancinating, or burning sensations throughout the distribution of the injured nerves, which can extend well beyond the injury site. These

---

*The term "narcotic," literally sleep- or stupor-inducing, is outmoded because people no longer take these medications as sleeping pills (hypnotics). It also carries a popular stigma of illicit drug use. Narcotics are now referred to as "opioids." This term includes certain naturally occurring (endogenous) neurotransmitters, as well as synthetic (exogenous) substances, including medications.

disorders resist treatment. Removing or repairing the injured nerves is rarely feasible. Administering common analgesics, as for acute pain, has little effect; however, administering opioids on a regular basis, which is controversial (see below), or using adjuvant medications may be quite helpful.

The *Diagnostic and Statistical Manual of Mental Disorders-IV (DSM-IV)* approaches pain somewhat differently. Its diagnosis of Pain Disorder requires, in short, that pain is the major symptom of a clinical problem and that it causes distress or functional impairment. The diagnosis excludes pain that is a manifestation of an established mental disorder, such as depression, psychosis, or somatization disorder; an element of dyspareunia; or a factitious disorder. Pain resulting from a neurologic or medical condition, such as headaches, peripheral neuropathy, or low back pain, is classified as a component of the medical condition.

The *DSM-IV* further recognizes *Pain Disorders Associated With Psychological Factors* and *Pain Disorders Associated With Both Psychologic Factors and a General Medical Condition.* In both, psychologic factors are an integral component of the disorder. Also, both are divided into durations shorter (acute) and longer than 6 months (chronic).

The *DSM-IV* labels as Malingering patients who knowingly falsely claim disproportionate great pain or persistence of pain long after a wound has healed. Even though the frequency of Malingering may be less than 1% of cases, the number of such patients is large. Besides financial expectations, incentives to malinger might be freedom from work assignments, attention getting, or retribution.

However, the actual situation is more ambiguous than these definitions suggest. Pain management centers report that as many as 50% of patients with chronic pain have dual diagnoses that include somatoform, personality, substance abuse, and posttraumatic stress disorders. Moreover, chronic pain is inextricably linked to signs of depression, including vegetative symptoms and insomnia, but also a tendency toward drug and alcohol dependency, dysfunctional family relationships, and exaggeration of physical deficits. Similarly, depression lowers the threshold for pain, increases disability from painful injuries, and makes pain refractory to treatment. In many chronic pain patients the sequence of pain and depression is unclear. For many who sustain injuries, the subsequent chronic pain seems to lead to depression. On the other hand, individuals with mood disorders and others psychiatric conditions are prone to develop chronic pain after injuries that normally heal without sequelae.

PAIN PATHWAYS

The function of pain pathways is to bring information rapidly to the brain to identify the pain's nature and location, arouse central mechanisms, and activate the limbic system to respond. These pathways are counterbalanced by pain-relieving *(analgesic)* pathways in the spinal cord and certain brain regions. This neuroanatomy for pain and analgesia provides the framework for many treatment strategies.

Peripheral

Painful bodily injuries, such as contusions, liberate prostaglandins, arachidonic acid, and bradykinin that stimulate nociceptors. While the sensation is still peripheral, pain can be alleviated by medicines that inhibit synthesis of prostaglandins or otherwise reduce tissue inflammation, such as aspirin, acetaminophen, steroids, and nonsteroidal anti-inflammatory agents (NSAIDs).

Unless these medicines interrupt the process, nociceptors transmit pain along two types of PNS small diameter fibers, *A-delta* and *C*. The *A-delta* fibers are covered with a thin sheet of myelin, but C fibers are unmyelinated.

Pain transmission in these fibers may be suppressed by stimulating certain PNS sensory fibers. According to the *gate control theory,* stimulation of large-diameter, heavily myelinated *A-beta* fibers, which ordinarily carry vibration and position sensation, inhibits pain transmission by the A-delta and C fibers, which are thin and have little or no myelin. This theory gave rise to *transcutaneous electrical nerve stimulation (TENS),* in which low-voltage electric current stimulates large fibers to dampen pain transmission by thin fibers (see below).

A more direct way of reducing pain transmission at this level is to block the entire peripheral nerve by injecting it with a local anesthetic. *Nerve blocks* are useful in chest and abdominal pain because the thoracic and lumbar nerve roots can be easily located, as they emerge from the spine. However, this technique is usually not feasible for painful limbs because it often causes paresis, as well as analgesia. Nor is it practical in treating facial pain within the first division of the trigeminal nerve (see Fig. 4–11) because analgesia involving the cornea leads to corneal ulcerations.

Sometimes a sympathetic plexus or ganglia block is helpful. In pancreatic carcinoma, the celiac plexus can be injected with alcohol. In the shoulder-hand syndrome, the stellate ganglion (the sympathetic ganglion adjacent to the upper cervical vertebrae) can be injected with local anesthetics. In complex regional pain syndromes (see below), various sympathetic ganglia can be injected with local anesthetics. When these blocks are administered for complex regional pain syndromes and many other conditions affecting a limb, they are best given in conjunction with physical therapy.

Central

The PNS fibers enter the CNS at the spinal cord's dorsal horn and, either immediately or after ascending a few segments, synapse in its *substantia gelatinosa*. At many of these synapses, the fibers release an 11-amino acid polypeptide, *substance P,* which is the major neurotransmitter for pain at the spinal cord level (Fig. 14–1).

After the synapse, pain sensation "ascends" predominantly within the *lateral spinothalamic tract* to the brain (see Figs. 2–6 and 2–14). This crucial tract crosses from the substantia gelatinosa to the spinal cord's other side and ascends contralateral to the

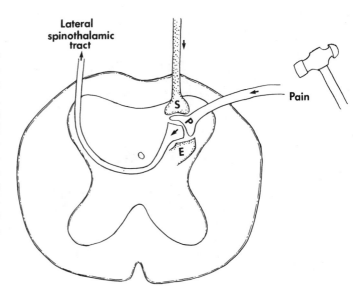

FIGURE 14–1. Painful sensations are conveyed along *A delta* and *C* fibers of the peripheral nerves. These nerves enter the dorsal horn of the spinal cord where, using *substance P (P),* they synapse onto second-order neurons. The second-order neurons cross to the contralateral side of the spinal cord and, comprising the *lateral spinothalamic tract*, ascend to the thalamus. Two powerful pain-dampening or pain-modulating analgesic systems *(stippled)* play upon the dorsal horn synapse. One tract descends from the brain and releases *serotonin (S)*. The other system is composed of spinal interneurons that release *enkephalins (E)*.

TABLE 14–1. *Glossary*

β-endorphin: An endogenous opioid concentrated in the pituitary gland and secreted with ACTH. It consists of amino acid numbers 61–91 of β-lipotropin and gives rise to the enkephalins (see Fig. 14–2).

β-lipotropin: A 91-amino-acid polypeptide, which may be an ACTH fragment. It gives rise to β-endorphin but has no opioid activity itself (i.e., β-lipotropin is not an endogenous opioid).

Endogenous opioids: Polypeptides (amino acid chains) found within the CNS that create effects similar to those of morphine and other naturally occurring opioids. The effects of both endogenous and naturally occurring opioids are characteristically reversed by naloxone.

Endorphins: Endogenous morphinelike substances or opioid peptides. This term is virtually synonymous with endogenous opioids.

Enkephalins: Short (5-amino-acid) polypeptide endogenous opioids that include met-enkephalin and leu-enkephalin. They are found primarily in the amygdala, brainstem, and dorsal horn of the spinal cord.

Naloxone (Narcan): A pure opioid antagonist that reverses the effects of endogenous and exogenous (naturally occurring) opioids.

Substance P: An 11-amino-acid polypeptide that is probably the primary pain neurotransmitter at the first synapse of the primary afferent neuron in the spinal cord.

---

injury to terminate in specific thalamic segments. Additional synapses then relay the stimuli to the somatosensory cerebral cortex, which enables the individual to locate the pain.

A practical application of this knowledge led to a briefly used procedure for patients suffering from intractable cancer-related pain confined to a single limb. In a *cordotomy,* surgeons severed the lateral spinothalamic tract contralateral to the pain and produced moderate analgesia. Unfortunately, the improvement lasted for only several months, possibly because of plasticity of cerebral pain pathways. Also, bilateral cordotomies for extensive pain produced respiratory drive impairment (Ondine's curse) and urinary incontinence.

In another ascending pain pathway, the *spinohypothalamic tract,* fibers travel both ipsilateral and contralateral to their origin and terminate directly in the hypothalamus. This pathway may help explain why pain produces disturbances in temperature regulation, sleep, and other autonomic functions. The spinal cord also transmits pain in other, less well-defined tracts that ascend both ipsilaterally and contralaterally.

In addition to being relayed directly to the thalamus and hypothalamus, pain sensations are eventually conveyed to the entire limbic system, the reticular activating system, and other brainstem regions. This wide dispersal of painful stimuli partially explains why individuals awaken when given a painful stimulus. In cases of chronic pain, it accounts for patients' sleeplessness, loss of appetite, and a tendency to develop depression or anxiety.

ANALGESIC PATHWAYS

A number of pathways suppress pain transmission or release endogenous analgesics. They may be confined to the brain, descend to interfere with spinal cord pain-transmitting pathways, or act within confined spinal cord regions.

Several analgesic pathways originate in the frontal lobe and hypothalamus and pass to the gray matter surrounding the third ventricle and aqueduct of Sylvius (*periaqueductal gray matter,* see Fig. 18–2). These routes contain large amounts of *endoge-*

nous opioids (see the discussion of endorphins below), which are naturally occurring, powerful, narcotic-like analgesics (Table 14–1). When implanted electrodes stimulate the periaqueductal gray matter area, they induce profound analgesia.

Other analgesic pathways originate in the brainstem and descend in the spinal cord's *dorsolateral funiculus.* These pathways provide "descending analgesia" relief of pain by inhibiting spinal cord synapses and the ascending pathways. Unlike most other analgesic pathways, they release *serotonin.*

Short neurons, *interneurons,* which are located entirely within the spinal cord, play on incoming PNS fibers. Among the many neurotransmitters released by these neurons are endogenous opioids that inhibit pain transmission.

ENDOGENOUS OPIOIDS

Often called *endorphins* (*end*ogenous m*orphin*e-like substances), endogenous opioids are naturally occurring amino acid chains (polypeptides) synthesized in the CNS (Fig. 14–2). They bind to receptors in the limbic system, periaqueductal gray matter, spinal cord's dorsal horn, and other CNS sites. Commonly cited examples of endorphins' analgesic effects include "runner's high" and the initial painlessness described by wounded soldiers.

Synthetic or exogenous opioids, particularly morphine, are virtually identical to the endogenous opioids. They bind onto the same CNS receptors and produce the same effects—analgesia, mood elevation (euphoria), sedation, and respiratory depression. *Naloxone* (Narcan) reverses the effects of endogenous, as well as exogenous, opioids. Indeed, naloxone's opioid antagonist effect is so characteristic that *naloxone-reversibility* is a criterion for determining that an analgesic's effect is mediated by the opioid pathways.

TREATMENTS

Physicians can prescribe various medications that can be administered through myriad routes. Combined with physical and psychologic treatments, medicines reduce pain and suffering, increase function, and give patients some control.

Nonopioid Analgesics

Aspirin, other salicylates, NSAIDs, and acetaminophen act predominantly *peripherally* by inhibiting prostaglandin synthesis at the injury site. In addition, NSAIDs and

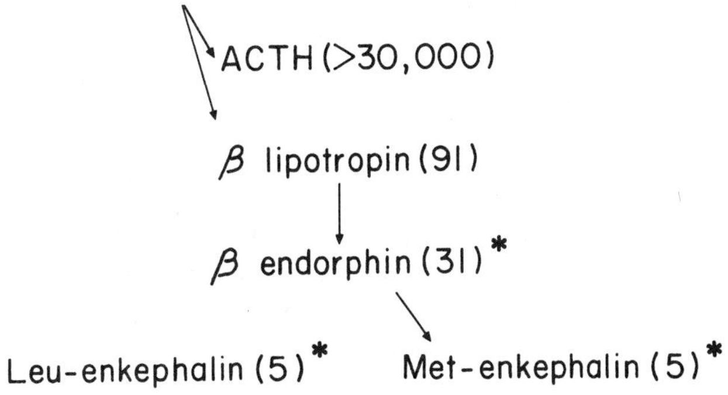

FIGURE 14–2. Endogenous opioids are synthesized and secreted along with adrenocorticotropin (ACTH) from the pituitary gland in people who are under stress or in acute pain. A large precursor molecule (not pictured) gives rise to ACTH and β-lipotropin, which are often released together. β-Lipotropin gives rise to β-endorphin and met-enkephalin, but another precursor gives rise to leu-enkephalin. (The asterisks denote the important endogenous opioids, and the numbers within parentheses are the amino-acid units in the polypeptide chains.)

ACTH (>30,000)

β lipotropin (91)

β endorphin (31)*

Leu-enkephalin (5)*   Met-enkephalin (5)*

TABLE 14–2. *Examples of Nonopioid Analgesics*

Acetaminophen (Tylenol and others)
Aspirin
   Choline magnesium trisalicylate (Trilisate)
   Diflunisal (Dolobid)
Nonsteroidal anti-inflammatory agents
   Celebrex (Celecoxib)
   Ibuprofen (Motrin, Advil, Nuprin)
   Indomethacin (Indocin)
   Ketorolac (Toradol)
   Naproxen (Naprosyn)
   Rofecoxib (Vioxx)

acetaminophen also probably have a central analgesic action. These nonopioid analgesics are effective for mild to moderate acute and chronic pain (Table 14–2). In fact, two tablets (600 mg) of aspirin, which remains the standard, produce approximately the same analgesia as two common opioids: 65 mg of propoxyphene (Darvon) or 50 mg of oral meperidine (Demerol).

In general, NSAID use is uncomplicated by tolerance or dependence: the same dose provides steady analgesia for weeks to months, and withdrawal after a course of treatment does not produce symptoms. Also, they do not induce changes in mood or disruptions in thought.

These medications are more effective if a "loading dose" is taken prophylactically. For example, pain can be partly prevented by taking them before dental procedures or menses. Their analgesic effect is dose-dependent but only up to a point. Once the maximum analgesia has been achieved, greater doses will not increase the benefit (the "ceiling effect"). More important, NSAIDs cause a high incidence of gastrointestinal bleeding that results in considerable morbidity and mortality.

If administered in combination with opioids, which act predominantly *centrally*, these medicines enhance each other's analgesia. Simply taking two tablets of aspirin, for example, will even increase morphine's potency. Likewise, adding NSAIDs to opioids helps alleviate the pain of metastases to bone. When NSAIDs allow a smaller dose of narcotics to be effective, they are said to have an "opioid-sparing effect."

Opioids

The various opioids are indicated for acute, moderate, or severely painful conditions, such as a fracture, myocardial infarction, or surgery (Table 14–3). They are also almost always indicated for cancer pain. In addition, an increasing number of authors suggest that opioids are appropriate for chronic, intractable pain unrelated to cancer, which has been given the possible misnomer "benign pain." This pain typically results from lumbar herniated disks where one or more surgical procedures have not helped, complex regional pain syndrome, and thalamic pain (see below).

Greater doses or more potent preparations of opioids increase the analgesia. Unlike NSAIDs, there is no ceiling effect. Their potency can also be enhanced, without increasing their side effects, by adding NSAIDs or other nonopioid analgesics.

Opioids have usually been administered through traditional routes: oral and intramuscular. Additional routes now available are transdermal (skin patches), intranasal (sprays), rectal (suppositories), continuous intravenous, intrathecal (intraspinal injections), and intra-articular (injections). In a particularly innovative technique, *patient-controlled analgesia (PCA)*, patients regulate continual or intermittent opioid infusions.

Compared to older analgesics, newer opioids, such as fentanyl (Duragesic), provide more rapid onset of action and greater potency because of their biochemical structures and the new routes of administration. Also, those given by parenteral routes maintain analgesia longer, in part because they reduce "first pass" clearance by hepatic metabolism. Some oral analgesics are long-acting because they are embedded in the pill matrix that slowly releases the medicine, not because the medicine is metabolized more slowly. PCA and other analgesic regimens also greatly reduce patients' dependence on hospital staff and family members.

Unless opioids are administered continuously by PCA, patches, or long-acting oral preparations, they should be given on a *regular prophylactic* or *time-dependent* basis, such as every 2 to 4 hours, rather than at the onset of pain. When patients are required to request analgesics only after pain begins, the delay makes pain more difficult to alleviate, creates a pattern of undertreatment and overtreatment, and prevents a restful sleep-wake schedule. Moreover, the patient, fearful about pain recurrence, becomes anxious and preoccupied with obtaining drugs.

Another potential problem is that, because parenteral administration delivers more medication than oral administration, changing the same dose from pill form to either an intramuscular or intravenous injection regimen is likely to produce an overdose. If the situation were reversed, changing the same dose from an intramuscular or intravenous injection regimen to pills is likely to produce undertreatment, which would cause withdrawal symptoms and recurrence of pain.

"Addiction."   One of the most pressing but unresolved issues is whether opioid treatment will lead to addiction. With weeks of opioid treatment, increasingly greater quantities are required to produce the same level of anesthesia *(tolerance)*—as if opioids "up-regulate" the receptors. Similarly, stopping opioid treatment produces unpleasant physical signs *(withdrawal)*. Although tolerance and withdrawal often occur together, each can occur independently.

TABLE 14–3. *Examples of Opioid Analgesics*

For mild to moderately severe pain
    Codeine
    Oxycodone (Percocet)
    Propoxyphene (Darvon)
For moderate to severe pain
    Hydromorphone (Dilaudid)
    Levorphanol (Levo-Dromoran)
    Meperidine (Demerol)
    Morphine
Long-acting oral preparations
    Methadone
    Morphine long-acting (MS Contin, Oramorph SR)
Nasal administration (spray)
    Butorphanol (Stadol)—mixed agonist-antagonist
Transcutaneous administration (skin patches)
    Fentanyl (Duragesic)
Transmucosal administration (lollipops)
    Fentanyl (Fentanyl Oralet)

Physicians have traditionally defined addiction simply as the development of tolerance and withdrawal. Researchers have suggested that it be defined by certain alterations in dopamine receptor activity.

Clinicians, partly from a fear of creating addiction in their patients, tend to underuse opioids. Except for acute, severe pain, they tend to wait until it is incessant or distressing enough to cause suffering, depression, or insomnia, usually restricting opioid treatment to cancer-induced pain. Even then, they tend to withhold opioids, prescribe insufficient doses, and fail to recognize that, as tolerance develops or the underlying disease progresses, more frequent and larger doses are necessary.

In fact, addiction rarely occurs in previously normal individuals who develop a painful illness that requires opioids for several weeks. Moreover, addiction is an irrelevant consideration in seriously ill patients.

In contrast, contemporary physicians who routinely deal with pain management define addiction primarily in behavioral terms, as drug-seeking activity potential harmful to the individual or society. They consider tolerance and dependence physiologic responses, which are often independent of each other and not peculiar to narcotics. Antihypertensive agents, for example, produce tolerance and their withdrawal typically produces undesirable symptoms, such as angina and rebound hypertension. Similarly, withdrawal symptoms almost invariably follow stopping tobacco or coffee.

Other physicians, including many who practice addiction medicine, refer to the patients as clients who are drug users, not drug abusers.

The basic criteria in *DSM-IV* for Substance Dependence (With or Without Physiologic Dependence) and Substance Abuse is substance-induced impairment or distress. Dependence is characterized by leading to socially detrimental drug-seeking behavior and Abuse by leading to illegal, physically hazardous, or otherwise destructive behavior.

Other Side Effects.   For the psychiatric consultant, an important source of potential confusion in this area arises from the similarity of opioid-induced mental status changes to those caused by head trauma, metabolic aberrations, including hypoventilation, and, in cancer patients, cerebral metastases. Respiratory depression or hypoventilation—slow, shallow, insufficient breathing—is almost the only potentially life-threatening problem. It usually results from inadvertent overdose, combinations of medications, or preexisting pulmonary disease.

Constipation, which from many patients' perspective is the most bothersome side effect, can be managed with a combination of laxatives, such as senna (Senokot), and stool softeners, such as docusate sodium (Colace). The underlying illness, radiotherapy, or chemotherapy, as well as the opioids, may themselves cause nausea, often a devastating problem. Patients should be given vigorous, and preferably prophylactic, treatment with antiemetics; however, they should be cautiously prescribed because many contain a phenothiazine or other dopamine-blocking agent that can cause a dystonic reaction or parkinsonism (see Chapter 18). Synthetic marijuana, dronabinol (Marinol), and related preparations, which have been approved as antiemetics, can cause transient mood and thought disorders.

The use of certain opioids is fraught with difficulties. Phenytoin or carbamazepine—whether used for seizure control, mood modulation, or analgesia—accelerate methadone metabolism. Giving them to patients on methadone maintenance may precipitate withdrawal symptoms. The solution is to increase the methadone dose as those medications are added.

Another potential complication of opioids is that meperidine, although one of the most frequently prescribed analgesics, is often surprisingly unsatisfactory. It is especially poorly absorbed when taken orally, and changing its route of administration leads to complications. Moreover, when meperidine is given for several days, especially to patients with renal insufficiency, accumulation of its toxic metabolite, normeperidine, often causes dysphoria, cognitive impairment, delirium, tremulousness, myoclonus, and seizures. When taken with monoamine oxidase inhibitors, including deprenyl, meperidine can cause a potentially fatal hypertensive encephalopathy. With long-term use, it can cause muscle and subcutaneous tissue nodules.

Heroin is also a problematic opioid. Not only is its effectiveness in relieving pain and improving mood no greater than a comparable dose of morphine, but potential for abuse is much greater. Regardless of several medical and nonmedical groups' assertions, from a purely medical standpoint, heroin has no legitimate use that cannot be fulfilled by conventional narcotic medicines.

Finally, opioids with antagonist properties (agonist/antagonist and partial mu agonists), such as pentazocine (Talwin), butorphanol (Stadol), and buprenorphine (Buprenex), have limited usefulness. They were developed, quite rationally, to prevent abuse by incorporating opioid antagonist properties into opioid analgesics; however, they themselves have been abused. In addition, they have psychotomimetic properties, and injections of pentazocine lead to skin and muscle necrosis. Worse, because of their opioid antagonism, a change from a morphinelike opioid to one of these mixed agonist-antagonist drugs will lead to undertreatment and produce withdrawal symptoms and pain recurrence.

As with other medicines, opioids should be discontinued when unnecessary and, in general, tapered rather than stopped abruptly. Sometimes an equivalent dose of methadone can be substituted for another opioid and then tapered. In the final stages of drug withdrawal, patients who agree to a structured program may be given a nonopioid analgesic. If withdrawal symptoms develop, benzodiazepines can somewhat alleviate some of the physical or mental discomfort and clonidine (Catapres) can blunt autonomic nervous system hyperactivity (see Chapter 21).

Adjuvant Medications

Antidepressants. Tricyclic antidepressants (TCAs) are the most widely used adjuvant in chronic benign and malignant (cancer-induced) pain, complementing opioid and nonopioid analgesics. However, by themselves, TCAs are usually insufficient and do not reduce opioid requirements.

Neurologists tend to assume that chronic pain patients have developed depression as a consequence of pain or that previously quiescent depression made the patient vulnerable to pain. They liberally prescribe various TCAs. Evidence of usefulness has been most compelling for amitriptyline and nortriptyline. (Nortriptyline may be preferable because it induces fewer anticholinergic side effects.) TCAs are particularly helpful in treatment of diabetic neuropathy, migraines, thalamic pain, and postherpetic neuralgia. They presumably alleviate pain in these conditions by increasing serotonin concentrations in descending CNS analgesic pathways. In addition to providing analgesia, they help restore a normal sleep-wake schedule and improve a patient's mood.

TCAs, in general, are helpful for patients with chronic pain even without overt depression. For those with pain and depression, TCAs induce analgesia before they improve mood. When used for analgesia, much lower doses of TCAs are required than to treat depression.

Both selective serotonin reuptake inhibitors (SSRIs) and mixed serotonin and norepinephrine reuptake inhibitors have been used to treat chronic pain. SSRIs may not offer pain relief unless the patient also has depression. Unlike the TCAs, the SSRIs may have little primary analgesic effect, which is surprising in view of serotonin's crucial analgesic role. The mixed reuptake inhibitors may have greater potential.

Antiepileptic Drugs.   Antiepileptic drugs (AEDs)—carbamazepine (structurally similar to the TCAs), phenytoin, valproate, gabapentin, and clonazepam—are effective for neuropathic conditions, such as trigeminal neuralgia, diabetic neuropathy, postherpetic neuralgia, and complex regional pain syndrome (see below). For example, carbamazepine relieves trigeminal neuralgia so effectively and predictably that a positive response virtually confirms the diagnosis. Gabapentin also relieves a wide variety of painful disorders.

Not all of AEDs' analgesic effects can be attributed to their anticonvulsant properties. Many have a dual action. For example, structures of carbamazepine and most TCAs, as noted, are similar; valproate modulates patients' mood; and clonazepam is a benzodiazepine.

Other Adjuvant Medications.   Antidepressants and antiepileptics are the mainstay of adjuvant pain therapy; however, if anxiety complicates either acute or chronic pain, as frequently occurs, adding benzodiazepines may produce calm, permit sleep, counteract muscle spasm, and thus indirectly reduce pain and suffering. Physicians should beware of interactions between benzodiazepines and opioids. Neuroleptics are indicated for more severe psychic stress, especially if the illness or its therapies induce nausea.

Finally, many diverse medications may serve as adjuvants. For example, the antihypertensive medication clonidine, which is an alpha-2 adrenergic agonist, purportedly reduces pain in migraine and various chronic neuropathic conditions. (It also may reduce tics [see Chapter 8].) In an apparent paradox, adrenergic alpha-receptor blockers, such as phentolamine, that do not cross the blood-brain barrier have been beneficial for some patients. Even cardiac antiarrhythmics, such as mexiletine, have reduced pain for many patients.

Stimulation-Induced Analgesia

Scientific studies have found that acupuncture is analgesic in some people with mild to moderate pain. For securing analgesia, the "meridians," the traditional regions where needles are placed, have been shown to be less important than dermatomes (see Fig. 16–2). Because acupuncture induces a rise in cerebrospinal fluid (CSF) endorphins and the analgesia is naloxone-reversible, it is presumed to work in part through the endogenous opioid system (Table 14–4).

A frequently used treatment for chronic musculoskeletal disorders is TENS. In this technique, an electric stimulus is applied to the skin just proximal to the painful re-

---

TABLE 14–4. *Analgesics Mediated by the Endogenous Opioid System* *

Acupuncture
Opioids
Placebo
Stimulation[†]
   TENS (transcutaneous electrical nerve stimulation)
   Dorsal column stimulation
   Periaqueductal gray matter stimulation[‡]

---

*Because these analgesics are partially or entirely reversed by naloxone, their effects are considered to be mediated by the endogenous opioid system. In contrast, analgesia induced by tricyclic antidepressants and hypnosis is not reversed by naloxone.
[†]See text regarding efficacy.
[‡]Investigational.

gion. It stemmed from the observation that people instinctually massage a portion of the body proximal to the injury. For example, a person with a sprained ankle will rub the lower leg.

TENS was thought to be analgesic, and the analgesia was believed to result from stimulation of the underlying large, thickly myelinated nerve fibers blocking ascending pain-carrying fibers (gate control) or through the endogenous opioid system. However, subsequent studies have indicated that TENS has no effect, is a placebo, or has another mild, undefinable CNS action. At most, it provides a small degree of analgesia for several weeks.

In *epidural spinal cord stimulation*, electrodes are inserted into the epidural space overlying the spinal cord. Preliminary reports justify its use, despite its potential complications, in carefully selected cases.

In another CNS stimulation technique, neurosurgeons have implanted electrodes into the periventricular and periaqueductal gray matter and adjacent brainstem regions. As noted earlier, stimulation of these sites, which presumably releases stored endogenous opioids, can produce profound analgesia. Despite the strong rationale, the technique remains investigational.

Placebos, Hypnosis, and Behavioral Therapies

Placebos, which are unknowingly given by physicians when they prescribe ineffectual medications or too small doses of potent medications, will produce an unequivocal but brief period of analgesia in at least 30% of patients. They are most effective for acute, severe pain, especially when patients have anxiety, and are least effective for continual, mild pain. Contrary to popular belief, a beneficial response to placebo does not mean that a patient's pain is psychogenic. Because the analgesic effect of placebos is partially naloxone-reversible, placebos probably stimulate the endogenous opioid system.

Hypnosis, which is not a placebo, is useful for a limited period in a wide variety of chronic painful conditions, including cancer. It differs from placebo therapy because patients' ability to be hypnotized does not correlate with their response to placebos, and hypnosis-induced analgesia is not naloxone-reversible.

Cognitive therapy, behavior modification, operant conditioning, biofeedback, and other psychologic therapies have been recommended when the response to the usual treatments is insufficient or when the pain is far greater than warranted by the bodily injury. They have also been used in cases of abnormal behavior, opioid abuse, or when family members have begun to reinforce maladaptive activities.

MALIGNANT PAIN

Although cancer-related situations can be highly variable, physicians have available several guidelines. They should monitor patients' pain as regularly as they monitor pulse, blood pressure, and respirations. They should generally accept patients' accounts of their symptoms without reservation (Fig. 14–3). Patients should have access to nonpharmacologic therapy, such as relaxation techniques, hypnosis, and psychotherapy, as well as the full arsenal of medications. Physicians should prescribe the three categories of analgesics—nonopioid, opioid, and adjuvant—early or preemptively, frequently, and generously. If undertreatment in pain management represents a physician's hesitancy, it represents an error in malignant pain.

A three-step treatment plan based on the World Health Organization Guidelines provides relief to as many as 90% of patients:

- Treat with a nonopioid analgesic with or without adjuvant medications until the ceiling is reached.

- Add a long-acting, oral opioid analgesic with or without adjuvant medications.

- Combine opioid and nonopioid analgesics given by different routes with adjuvant medications.

The doses of opioids must be readily increased as tolerance develops. Although long-acting oral preparations are preferable, transdermal, PCA, or other parenteral administrations may be required for severe pain, continuous administration, or other reasons.

Often local treatment with radiotherapy or opioid injection is helpful and avoids systemic side effects. Occasionally surgical procedures, such as a cordotomy or peripheral nerve block, are helpful.

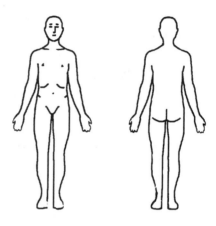

0 – 10 Numeric Pain Intensity Scale

0	1	2	3	4	5	6	7	8	9	10
No Pain					Moderate Pain					Worst Possible Pain

Visual Analog Scale

No Pain	Worst Possible Pain

FIGURE 14–3. Graphics are replacing verbal descriptions of the site and degree of pain. Patients describe their pain by circling the most intensely painful area on the sketch. Then they are asked either to circle the single number on the Numeric Pain Scale or mark the Visual Analog Scale at the point that describes the intensity of their pain: 0 = No Pain through 10 = The Worst Possible Pain. For children, for whom graphics are particularly useful, scales are based on the smiling face to crying face icons.

Variations of the basic scale measure maximum and minimum pain, response to treatment, insomnia, and functional impairment. (Adapted from Jacox A, Carr DB, Payne R, et al: Management of Cancer Pain: Adults Quick Reference Guide. No. 9. AHCPR Publication No. 94-0593. Rockville, MD: Agency for Healthcare Policy and Research, U.S. Department of Health and Human Services, Public Health Service.)

NONMALIGNANT PAIN SYNDROMES

Although agonizing pain is generally associated with malignancies, several non-cancerous conditions, such as postherpetic neuralgia, create comparable pain, suffering, and disability. Here also, physicians can apply the guidelines for management of malignant pain, except for freely dispensing opioids.

These severe nonmalignant conditions have several common features. They mostly stem from neuropathic pain, which is felt as a continual, dull, ache, worsened by superimposed, intermittent jabs of sharp (lancinating) pain. In these conditions, unlike simple painful conditions, such as degenerative arthritis, the pain is complicated by *allodynia* (pain produced by stimuli that ordinarily does not cause pain, such as cool air) and *hyperalgesia* or *hyperpathia* (an exaggerated painful response to mildly noxious stimuli, such as the point of a pin).

Patients and physicians should acknowledge frankly that most of these conditions are chronic and incurable, although not fatal. Their goals should be to psychologically accept persistent pain, reduce suffering, and restore ability to work and function socially. These goals, which are more limited than the traditional goal of a full cure and restoration of function, should be clearly stated, acceptable to the patient, and attainable within several months. Medications should usually consist of nonopioid analgesics, especially NSAIDs, and adjuvants.

Opioid Debate

Opioids are generally appropriate for a preplanned, limited course, but long-term opioid treatment remains controversial. Physicians who oppose prescribing opioids for chronic nonmalignant pain foresee several problems. Patients may demand opioids for conditions that usually do not warrant them or when simpler measures would probably suffice, often out of desire to achieve euphoria. Interest in continuing to obtain opioids might tempt patients to falsely report persistent symptoms, making it difficult to determine whether the basic illness was improving. Moreover, long-term treatment with opioids might produce cognitive, emotional, and behavioral changes far outweighing any potential benefits.

On the other hand, some physicians have advocated prescribing opioids for individuals who (1) have no alternative treatment for intractable, chronic, nonmalignant pain and (2) do not display abusive, destructive, drug-seeking behavior. They point out that opioids are highly effective, carry a very low morbidity and mortality rate, and, when used to control pain, are not addictive. Written, unequivocal drug schedules or "contracts" are said to prevent abuse. Advocates further assert that patients treated with an opioid for unequivocally severe pain do not experience either tolerance after pain control is reached or withdrawal symptoms when the medicine is discontinued.

Psychiatric Consultations

Physicians should be encouraged to refer patients for psychiatric consultation not only for evaluation and treatment of depression or anxiety but also for other psychologic disturbances and drug abuse. Physicians should obtain a psychiatric assessment early and as an integral part of the evaluation, not as a last resort or merely as a means of passing the patient on to a psychiatrist.

Whether acting individually or as part of a pain-management team, psychiatrists should evaluate patients (1) who have vegetative symptoms, regardless of the apparent connection to the pain; (2) whose pain or disability is refractory to several courses of medical treatment; (3) for whom excessive medications are required; (4) for psychopharmacology consultation; (5) for whom inpatient treatment or surgical procedures have been unsuccessful; or (6) who may have psychopathology that sabotages their treatment.

When possible, psychiatrists should examine the physical location of patients' pain. The touching might have a therapeutic benefit, albeit a primitive one. Also, in evaluating any functional disability brought on by the pain, psychiatrists should at least watch the patient sit, walk, and, if possible, use the affected part of the body.

With the possible exception of prescribing inadequate amounts of opioids, physicians tend to overmedicate patients. Where possible, they should consider supplementing or replacing medications with nonpharmacologic modalities, such as psychotherapy, hypnosis, cognitive-behavior techniques, and physical therapy.

Postmastectomy Axillary Pain

During a mastectomy, surgeons explore the axilla and remove lymph nodes. Often, they sever the cutaneous branch of the first thoracic nerve root, *the intercostobrachial nerve*. Several weeks later, some women develop searing axillary pain that extends to the inner aspect of the upper arm, well beyond the incision. Like many painful disorders, postmastectomy pain is worse at night. Because shoulder movement provokes the pain, this condition may lead to a "frozen shoulder." Common incision pain, which is only mildly to moderately intense, has an itching quality, and is confined to the scar, is different.

Assuming that the cause of postmastectomy pain is not tumor infiltration of the brachial plexus, infection in the incision, or radiation fibrosis, patients may benefit from nonopioid analgesics and TCAs. Massaging the painful skin with a damp cloth after applying a vapor-coolant, such as ethyl chloride spray, may also reduce the pain. Patients should exercise to increase shoulder mobility and upper arm strength. If conservative measures are ineffective, sometimes blocks administered to the sympathetic ganglion are helpful.

Even though postmastectomy pain carries little prognostic significance, it intensifies the surgery's psychologic impact. Moreover, it tempts physicians and psychologically oriented nonphysicians to conclude that postmastectomy pain originates in emotional factors.

Postherpetic Neuralgia

Acute *Herpes zoster* infection causes a vesicular skin eruption, *shingles,* usually in the distribution of one or two nerve dermatomes. Although any dermatome may be affected, the thoracic dermatomes and then the first branch of the trigeminal nerve, which includes the cornea, are most commonly involved. Reactivated varicella virus that has lain dormant in dorsal (sensory) nerve root ganglia causes the infection. *Herpes zoster* is common in individuals older than 65, even those in good health, and in those with immunosuppressive illnesses, such as lymphoproliferative disorders and acquired immune deficiency syndrome (AIDS).

The acute infection causes moderate severe burning and unrelenting pain that sometimes precede the vesicles by several days. In most cases, the pain and skin lesions recede within several weeks. During this period, the severe pain justifies the use of opioids. Antiviral agents, such as acyclovir (Zovirax) and famciclovir (Famvir), may speed healing of vesicles, shorten duration of the pain, and prevent spread of infection into the eye.

As excruciating as the pain of the initial infection may have been, patients are at risk for developing a more painful secondary phase, *postherpetic neuralgia*, typically 3 to 6 months after the initial infection. In an age-related risk pattern, few individuals younger than 50 years develop postherpetic neuralgia, but 50% of those older than 60 years and 75% of those older than 70 years develop it.

Patients with postherpetic neuralgia are left with a band of numb, scarred skin and, if a major motor nerve has been involved, muscle weakness and atrophy. The pain, which can last for months, tends to be a continual dull painful disturbance with superimposed lancinating pains. It wells up to cause anorexia, insomnia, and mood changes.

Postherpetic neuralgia is unequivocally an indication for opioids supplemented by TCAs. SSRIs are much less helpful. As in other chronic pain syndromes, gabapentin is helpful. However, other AEDs provide only limited benefit.

Local anesthesia can complement traditional analgesics. Cocaine injections, to which Sigmund Freud became addicted, provide the best-known historic example. Now, long-acting gels of lidocaine or NSAID provide some local anesthesia. Another preparation is a cream containing capsaicin (Zostrix), which depletes substance P in the spinal cord (see Fig. 14–1).

Complex Regional Pain Syndrome

A newly coined term, complex regional pain syndrome, encompasses *reflex sympathetic dystrophy (RSD)*, *causalgia*, and *sympathetically maintained pain (SMP)*. Their common factors are pain disproportionately greater than the injury, soft tissue changes, and autonomic dysfunction. These disorders typically follow seemingly minor compressive or traction injuries to a limb that do not necessarily involve overt nerve damage. Common immediate causes are gunshot wounds, wrist fractures, myocardial infarctions, and peripheral vascular disease.

Complex regional pain syndrome is characterized by relentless burning pain superimposed on irritating numbness developing several months after an injury. Touching or moving an affected limb produces greater pain. Patients tend to be preoccupied with the affected limb, which they protect with extravagant methods. For example, they assiduously shield an afflicted hand by wearing a sling and glove or a foot by using crutches. The combination of the injury, sensitivity, and protective maneuvers often incapacitate the affected limb.

In addition, complex regional pain syndrome may also include "trophic" or "sudomotor" soft tissue changes. The skin becomes smooth, shiny, pale, and scaly. Fingernails remain uncut and grow long and brittle. Although the skin may sweat excessively *(hyperhidrosis)*, it is usually cool, dry, and devoid of sweat. Severe cases can include muscle wasting (dystrophy), which has given rise to the term RSD. Rare cases involve tremors, dystonia, and other involuntary movement disorders.

In RSD, which remains the most common entity in this group, the pain and other sensory disturbances usually extend beyond the injury site. Sometimes the symptoms extend *far* beyond the injury. For example, after several months of left arm pain, a patient may describe similar symptoms in the left leg and then the right leg.

Causalgia is similar to RSD but usually follows an obvious injury of a limb's large peripheral nerve. Its criteria include a demonstrable peripheral nerve injury. The most common cause of causalgia is a partial transection of a nerve by a high velocity bullet.

Treatment for complex regional pain syndrome relies on adjuvant medications, physical therapy, and blockade of regional sympathetic ganglia. For example, patients with causalgia of the hand may benefit from blocking the stellate ganglion with an anesthetic agent. Alternatively, occasional dramatic pain relief can be produced by intravenous infusions of bretylium or guanethidine to block the region's α- and β-adrenergic sympathetic ganglion receptors. Response to sympathetic blocks, although brief, has diagnostic and therapeutic value.

Phantom Limb Pain

Phantom limb pain occurs at the site of an amputated limb. For example, a man may have had his leg severed at the thigh in an automobile accident and weeks later may still feel pain as though it were centered in his ankle. The pain is often accompanied by other noticeable but nonpainful sensations. For example, a patient with an amputation will often feel that the limb is an integral part of the body and may sense purposeful movements in an absent hand, finger, or toe. These sensations probably originate from a combination of sensory deprivation and cortical "reorganization," in which the cortical area that originally supplied the amputated region connects with adjacent regions. Whatever their origin, patients' sensations or misperceptions can reach the level of somatic hallucinations. They also resemble the visual hallucinations described by recently blinded people, which also stem, in part, from sensory deprivation (see Anton's syndrome, Chapter 12).

Phantom limb pain differs from pain at the site of a surgical incision, *stump pain*, which is usually attributed to scar tissue and nerve damage (neuromas). Phantom and stump pain, of course, may occur together.

The clinical problem of phantom pain should not be restricted to limb injuries. Virtually the same disorder might follow amputation of a breast, ear, or other body part. Physicians can apply the same general guidelines to these injuries.

Even in its most typical settings, phantom limb pain varies in quality, severity, and accompanying psychologic symptoms. It usually begins soon after a traumatic amputation of a limb and has a self-limited duration of several weeks. The pain is most likely to develop if a limb were chronically painful before the amputation (as with osteomyelitis) or if any amputation were suddenly traumatic. Because most cases result from war wounds, victims are usually young or middle-aged veterans. In addition to pain, many have sustained extensive injuries, including facial disfigurements, loss of several limbs, and castration.

Chronic pain from phantom limbs, brachial plexus avulsion, and thalamic infarctions (see below) is often attributed to the loss of sensory input and classified as *deafferentation pain*. One theory is that the pain does not result from irritation of nociceptors but from absence of normal sensation being converted into painful sensations.

Medical treatment alone is insufficient. Carbamazepine, especially for shooting pains, and conventional analgesics are inconsistently beneficial. TENS and acupuncture have been effective only in isolated cases. TCAs should be tried freely because of the high incidence of depression. Some physicians have claimed benefit from muscle relaxation and, through hypnosis, inducing the sensation that the phantom limb is shrinking to the point that it disappears. In most cases, psychotherapy and psychopharmacology are essential.

Thalamic Pain

Thalamic infarctions or other injuries, which themselves are usually painless, initially cause contralateral hemianesthesia. Depending on which nearby structures are damaged, the hemianesthesia may be accompanied by hemiparesis, hemiataxia, or a homonymous hemianopsia.

Subsequently, patients sometimes develop a painful condition, the *Déjérine-Roussy syndrome*, is characterized by spontaneous painful sensations on the hemianesthetic side of the body. The pain is typically perceived most strongly in the face and hand. In trying to ward off the pain, patients wear hats, long sleeves, and gloves. As in these other conditions, allodynia and hyperpathia complicate the picture.

A similar painful disturbance, *central pain*, follows other CNS injuries, such as spinal cord gun shot wounds, multiple sclerosis, and tabes dorsalis. Each of them typically causes lancinating pains, allodynia, and hyperpathia superimposed on paraparesis. Their common, underlying pathology is interruption of the spinothalamic tract and possibly other sensory systems.

Antiepileptics and analgesics fail to provide sustained relief in most cases. Even opioids are rarely satisfactory. Physical therapy and supportive psychotherapy can provide temporary relief. Fortunately, the pain generally subsides after 6 to 12 months.

REFERENCES

Ashburn MA, Staats PS: Management of chronic pain. Lancet *353:* 1865–1869, 1999

Borsook D, LeBel AA, McPeek B (eds): The Massachusetts General Hospital Handbook of Pain Management. Boston. Little, Brown and Company. 1996

Dotson RM: Causalgia—reflex sympathetic dystrophy—sympathetically maintained pain: Myth and reality. Muscle Nerve *16:* 1049–1055, 1993

Jacox A, Carr DB, Payne R, et al: Management of Cancer Pain: Adults Quick Reference Guide. No 9. AHCPR Publication No. 94-0593. Rockville, MD: Agency for Health Care Policy and Research, U.S. Department of Health and Human Services, Public Health Service

Kost RG, Straus SE: Postherpetic neuralgia—pathogenesis, treatment, and prevention. N Engl J Med *335:* 32–42, 1996

Loeser JD, Melzack R: Pain: An overview. Lancet *353:* 1607–1609, 1999

Melzack R: Phantom limbs. Sci Am *266:* 120–126, 1992

Meyler WJ, de Jongste MJ, Rolf CA: Clinical evaluation of pain treatment with electrostimulation: A study on TENS in patients with different pain syndromes. Clin J Pain *10:* 22–27, 1994

Nasreddine ZS, Saver JL: Pain after thalamic stroke: Right diencephalic predominance and clinical features in 180 patients. Neurology *48:* 1196–1199, 1997

Nurmikko T: Clinical features and pathophysiologic mechanisms of postherpetic neuralgia. Neurology *45* (Suppl 8): S54–S55, 1995

Portenoy RK, Kanner RM (eds): Pain Management: Theory and Practice. Philadelphia. F.A. Davis Co, 1996

Portenoy RK, Lesage P: Management of cancer pain. Lancet *353:* 1695–1700, 1999

Rowbotham MC (ed): Chronic pain mechanisms and management. Neurology *12* (Suppl 9): S1–S36, 1995

Rowbotham MC: Complex regional pain syndrome type I (reflex sympathetic dystrophy): More than a myth. Neurology *51:* 4–5, 1998

Schwartzman RJ: Reflex sympathetic dystrophy and causalgia. Neurol Clin *10:* 953–973, 1993

Stannard CF: Phantom limb pain. Br J Hosp Med *50:* 583–587, 1993

Turner JA, Deyo RA, Loeser JD, et al: The importance of placebo effects in pain treatment and research. JAMA *20:* 1609–1614, 1994

Watson CPN, Vernich L, Chipman M, et al: Nortriptyline versus amitriptyline in postherpetic neuralgia. Neurology *51:* 1166–1171, 1998

Woolf CJ, Mannion RJ: Neuropathic pain: Aetiology, symptoms, mechanisms, and management. Lancet *353:* 1959–1964, 1999

QUESTIONS and ANSWERS: CHAPTER 14

1–7. Match the substance (1–7) with its effect on the pain pathways (a–e).

1. Morphine

2. Endogenous opioids

3. Serotonin

4. Substance P

5. Enkephalin

6. Beta-endorphin

7. Nonsteroidal anti-inflammatory agents (NSAIDs)

a. Reduces tissue inflammation
b. Interferes with prostaglandin synthesis
c. Provides analgesia by acting within the CNS
d. Acts as a neurotransmitter of pain in the spinal cord
e. Is liberated in a spinal cord descending analgesic tract

ANSWERS: 1-c, 2-c, 3-c and e, 4-d, 5-c, 6-c, 7-a and b

8. Which property of morphine is *not* shared with endogenous opioids?

a. Tolerance
b. Effectiveness in deep brainstem structures and spinal cord
c. Ability to cause mood changes, as well as analgesia
d. Reversibility with naloxone
e. Commercial availability
f. Respiratory depression

ANSWER: e

9–17. What is the composition (a–h) of these substances (9–17)?

9. Leu-enkephalin

10. ACTH

11. Morphine

12. β-endorphin

13. Heroin

14. β-lipotropin

15. Met-enkephalin

16. Serotonin

17. Substance P

a. 11-amino-acid polypeptide
b. 5-amino-acid polypeptide
c. Diacetyl morphine
d. Greater than 30,000 amino acid polypeptide
e. An indole
f. An alkaloid of opium
g. 91-amino-acid polypeptide
h. 31-amino-acid polypeptide

ANSWERS: 9-b, 10-d, 11-f, 12-h, 13-c f, 14-g, 15-b, 16-e, 17-a

18. Which two of these fibers carry pain sensation?

a. A delta
b. C
c. A-beta
d. B-delta

ANSWER: a, b. Pain perception is transmitted by certain nerve fibers (*A-delta* and *C fibers*) rather than by all peripheral nervous system fibers. Thus, many patients have pain without disruption of other sensory modalities.

19. In which spinal cord tract does most pain sensation ascend?

a. Fasciculus gracilis
b. Fasciculus cuneatus
c. Lateral corticospinal tract
d. Lateral spinothalamic tract

ANSWER: d

20. In which tract do serotonin-based, analgesic fibers descend within the spinal cord?

a. Lateral spinothalamic tract
b. Dorsolateral funiculus
c. Fasciculus gracilis
d. Dentatorubral tract

ANSWER: b

21. Which two forms of analgesia are not naloxone-reversible?

a. Acupuncture
b. Opioid administration
c. Transcutaneous electrical stimulation (TENS)
d. Aspirin
e. Hypnosis
f. Placebo
g. Stimulation of periventricular gray matter
h. Intrathecal morphine injections

ANSWER: d, e

22. Why would the addition of aspirin or a NSAID increase the effectiveness of opioids?

a. Aspirin and NSAIDs are also opioids.
b. They actually do not increase analgesia.
c. They stimulate endogenous opioid release.
d. They interfere with prostaglandin synthesis.
e. They inhibit serotonin reuptake.

ANSWER: d

23. Regarding the treatment of chronic pain, which one of the following statements is incorrect?

a. Tricyclic antidepressants treat depression, which often coexists with chronic pain.
b. Tricyclic antidepressants help restore restful sleep patterns.
c. Tricyclic antidepressants increase serotonin levels.
d. Tricyclic antidepressants are less effective than serotonin reuptake inhibitors (SSRIs).
e. Tricyclic antidepressants block re-uptake of norepinephrine.

ANSWER: d. Blocking re-uptake of norepinephrine and increasing serotonin levels are both effective, but in many conditions, such as diabetic neuropathy, enhancing norepinephrine activity is more analgesic. However, tricyclic antidepressants' effects on the autonomic nervous system limit their usefulness. Although conventional SSRIs have been disappointing, mixed norepinephrine and serotonin re-uptake inhibitors show promise.

24. Which is not a potential complication of mixed agonist-antagonist opioids, such as pentazocine (Talwin)?

a. Normeperidine accumulation
b. Addiction
c. Delirium
d. Respiratory depression
e. They can precipitate withdrawal in patients using meperidine (Demerol).
f. Pentazocine can cause skin and subcutaneous scarring (sclerosis).
g. All of the above

ANSWER: a

25. What are the potential complications of meperidine (Demerol) use?

a. Marked undertreatment when a dose is switched from intramuscular to oral routes
b. Normeperidine toxicity
c. Overdose when the same dose is given parenterally as orally
d. Stupor
e. Seizures
f. Tremulousness
g. All of the above

ANSWER: g

26. Which one of the following features is *not* a characteristic of complex regional pain syndrome?

a. The sympathetic nervous system is involved.
b. The skin usually becomes shiny and often scaly.
c. The pain is usually relieved with blockade of the sympathetic ganglia.
d. The trunk and abdomen are typically included.
e. The pain spreads beyond the injured nerve.

ANSWER: d. "Complex regional pain syndrome" incorporates "reflex sympathetic dystrophy" and "causalgia."

27. A 39-year-old headache patient, who had had migraines since childhood, has been taking several tablets of an aspirin-butalbital-caffeine compound daily for at least 10 years. When the patient attempts to stop the medication, unbearable, generalized, dull headaches develop. What is the best descriptive term for this phenomenon?

a. Chronic migraine headache
b. Rebound headache
c. Status migrainosus
d. Addiction

ANSWER: b. Headaches following withdrawal of analgesics, especially if they are combined with vasoconstrictive medications, represent a major problem in headache management. Such "rebound headaches" are a form of withdrawal (see Chapter 9).

28. Which one of the following is *not* a complication of infarction of the thalamus and its surrounding structures?

a. Hemianesthesia
b. Allodynia
c. Patients protecting involved regions, such as their face and arm
d. Abnormal sweating
e. Hyperpathia

ANSWER: d

29. Which one of the following statements is false regarding the periaqueductal gray matter?

a. Stimulation of the periaqueductal gray matter produces analgesia.
b. Thiamine deprivation causes hemorrhage into the periaqueductal gray matter.
c. The periaqueductal gray matter surrounds the aqueduct of Sylvius.
d. The aqueduct of Sylvius is the conduit for CSF between the lateral and third ventricles.
e. The aqueduct of Sylvius is the conduit for CSF between the third and fourth ventricles.

ANSWER: d

30. Which one of the following statements is true regarding enkephalins?

a. They are tricyclic.
b. They are secondary messengers.
c. Naloxone inhibits enkephalins.
d. They are part of the serotonin system.

ANSWER: c. The enkephalins are peptide neurotransmitters that have a powerful, inhibitory effect on spinal cord interneurons. Their effects mimic morphine's because they are part of the opioid system.

31. Which one of the following statements is false regarding serotonin's role in pain and analgesia?

a. It often reduces pain before affecting mood.
b. Descending, serotonin-based spinal cord tracts induce analgesia.
c. In its analgesic role, serotonin is an inhibitory neurotransmitter.
d. Serotonin is an endogenous opioid.

ANSWER: d

32. Which statement most closely describes the gate control theory?

a. Descending corticospinal tract pathways inhibit pain.
b. The periaqueductal gray matter blocks pain transmission to the frontal lobes and limbic system.

c. Behavioral modification reduces pain-induced suffering.
d. Stimulation of large-diameter, heavily myelinated fibers inhibit pain transmission by small, sparsely myelinated fibers.

ANSWER: d

33. Which three are characteristics of NSAIDs?

a. They tend to cause gastrointestinal bleeding.
b. Additional medication produces greater analgesia, that is, they have no "ceiling."
c. Patients develop a tolerance to the analgesia.
d. They can be as effective as some opioids.
e. They can be combined with opioids to produce additional analgesia.
f. They cause opioid-like psychologic side effects.

ANSWER: a, d, e

34. For a given dose, which route of administration of an opioid provides the lowest blood concentrations?

a. Intramuscular
b. Oral, normal release
c. Intravenous

ANSWER: b. About 50% of orally administered opioid is metabolized on its first pass through the liver. Parenteral and transcutaneous administration is generally more effective than oral administration.

35. Which one of the following is not an advantage of patient-controlled analgesia (PCA) over analgesia administered on a "by the clock" or an "as needed" basis?

a. Lower cost
b. Steady levels of analgesia that avoid undertreatment and overtreatment
c. Better sleep schedules
d. Earlier hospital discharge

ANSWER: a. Despite the expense of training, close monitoring, and equipment, PCA has been a widely accepted and successful innovation in the management of postoperative and chronic malignant pain. It has also reduced potential friction among patients, families, physicians, and nurses. However, unless patients have the dexterity and cognitive capacity to adjust the system, PCA may be ineffective or dangerous. As with conventional administration, PCA opioid doses for patients with pulmonary disease should be carefully calculated.

36. Where do pain-carrying peripheral nerves synapse with the lateral spinothalamic tract?

a. Dorsal columns
b. Substantia gelatinosa
c. Limbic system
d. Thalamus

ANSWER: b. These peripheral nerves synapse in the substantia gelatinosa with the lateral spinothalamic tract, which ascends a short distance, crosses, and ascends to synapse in the thalamus.

37. Which two of the following painful conditions are considered examples of *deafferentation* pain?

a. Brachial plexus avulsion
b. Insect stings
c. Trigeminal neuralgia
d. Carcinoma metastatic to bones
e. Thalamic infarction
f. Migraine

ANSWER: a, e. When the brain is deprived of normal sensory input, pain is said to result from *deafferentation*. When nerves are directly injured, such as in trigeminal neuralgia, the pain is called *neuropathic*.

38. When a passing automobile catches his shirtsleeve, a 40-year-old man is dragged by his arm. The shoulder is dislocated. After it seems to heal, the arm develops an intense burning sensation that increases on movement or touching. The skin of the hand becomes smooth and dry. He cannot cut his fingernails because the pain is too intense. Which of the following three statements are true concerning his condition?

a. The disorder is maintained, at least in part, by the sympathetic nervous system.
b. The skin changes are an integral part of the condition.
c. TENS will be effective in most such cases.
d. Sympathetic blockage will provide partial, temporary relief in many cases.
e. Shoulder dislocations are painful injuries, but they do not cause nerve injury.

ANSWER: a, b, d. He has developed the reflex sympathetic dystrophy (RSD) variety of complex regional pain syndrome, which probably stems from autonomic nervous system as well as peripheral nerve injury. Shoulder dislocations are often part of traction injuries that often damage the nearby brachial plexus.

39. An 80-year-old man sustains an infarction that initially results in the loss of almost all sensation on the left face, trunk, and limbs. Several weeks later, the sensory loss is somewhat less pronounced, but he begins to develop a continual burning pain in the left face and arm. Also, the slightest stimulation, including people brushing against his hand or its being examined, causes him to have intolerable pain. He carefully shields the hand and arm under a glove and covers his arm with a blanket. What is the name of this condition?

a. Trigeminal neuralgia
b. Thalamic pain
c. Temporal arteritis
d. Postinfarction neoplasm
e. Psychogenic pain

ANSWER: b. The sensory loss indicates that he had sustained a thalamic infarction. The subsequent pain, the thalamic pain syndrome, is a frequently occurring, late complication. His extraordinary sensitivity—converting benign, nonpainful stimulation into unbearable pain (allodynia)—gives him the aura of a psychogenic disturbance, but this aspect of the problem is a common feature of neuropathic or other central pain.

40. Which of the following descriptions of withdrawal is false?

a. Withdrawal is roughly equivalent to dependence.
b. Abruptly stopping regular use of caffeine, tobacco, or alcohol causes withdrawal symptoms.
c. Withdrawal is equivalent to requiring additional doses of a substance.
d. Abruptly stopping treatment with insulin and some other medications causes withdrawal symptoms.
e. The most common symptom of stopping opioids is a flulike syndrome and anxiety.

ANSWER: c. Requiring additional doses of a substance is tolerance.

41. Match the term with the closest description:

a. Allodynia
b. Deafferentation pain
c. Physical dependence
d. Hyperalgesia
e. Hyperpathia

1. Testing for a Babinski sign provokes severe pain with crying
2. Spontaneous pain seeming to originate from denervated areas, as would follow avulsion of a limb
3. Patients' need for opioids increasing with progression of the disease
4. Patients' developing flulike symptoms with discontinuation of opioids
5. Nonpainful stimuli, such as a touch with a feather, provoking a pain

ANSWERS: a-5, b-2, c-4, d-1, e-1

15

Multiple Sclerosis Episodes

Multiple sclerosis (MS) is the most common disabling neurologic illness of North American and European young adults. Because it often starts with subtle and evanescent disturbances, MS may initially be misdiagnosed as a psychogenic disorder. Once MS progresses to its defining criteria of *multiple episodes of multiple neurologic deficits*, cognitive impairment and mood disorders often accompany physical disabilities. Despite highly sophisticated tests, the diagnosis of MS and its complications still rests on clinical grounds.

ETIOLOGY

MS is a chronic, usually recurring illness of unknown etiology that occurs when 1 mm to 3 cm patches of "white matter," the myelin sheaths of central nervous system (CNS) axons, become episodically inflamed, then stripped of myelin (demyelinated), and eventually sclerotic. Demyelinated patches, *plaques*, are scattered throughout the optic nerves, brain, and spinal cord. Thus, MS is called "disseminated sclerosis" in the United Kingdom.

Demyelinated patches produce neurologic deficits because axons, deprived of their myelin insulation, cannot properly transmit nerve impulses. These deficits partially resolve as the inflammation spontaneously subsides or is suppressed by anti-inflammatory medications, such as steroids. However, with repeated attacks more plaques develop and permanent neurologic deficits accumulate.

Although demyelination is the hallmark of MS, recent evidence indicates that the pathology includes transected axons. Moreover, it indicates that the permanent deficits are attributable to axonal degeneration.

The illness' mean age of onset is 33 years, with the vast majority of cases developing between 15 and 50 years. Some patients suffer their first or a subsequent MS attack after infection, childbirth, head or spine trauma, intervertebral disk surgery, electrical injury, or psychologic stress. However, studies have shown that these factors are neither the cause of MS nor responsible for any exacerbations.

The specific cause of MS still remains unknown, but studies indicate that it is probably a complex interaction of genetic susceptibility with environmental factors. Multiple sclerosis occurs 1.5 times more frequently in women than in men and 20 to 40 times more frequently in first-degree relatives of MS patients than in the general population. Although the genetic factors confer susceptibility, they cannot represent the entire explanation. For example, at most, only 30% of monozygotic twins and 5% of dizygotic twins are concordant for MS, and each twin in the affected pairs tends to display a different phenotype. Several different chromosomes have been implicated, but none are necessary or sufficient.

Epidemiologic findings have suggested an important environmental factor. The incidence of MS is greatest in patients who have lived, at least through age 15 years, in cool northern latitudes (above the 37th parallel) in the United States and Europe. Likewise, the incidence in Australia is greater in the cool, southern region. The incidence of MS is higher in Boston than New Orleans. It is extremely low in Central Africa, Asia, and Latin America. In Israel, the incidence is higher in those who emigrated from Northern Europe as adults than as children. Because spouses are not particularly vulnerable, environmental factors that adults encounter are unlikely to be the cause.

CLINICAL MANIFESTATIONS

Course

The initial episode of MS may range from a single trivial impairment lasting several days to a group of debilitating deficits that remain for several weeks and do not fully recede. Subsequent episodes vary considerably in their manifestations, severity, and number. For most MS patients, 2 to 3 years elapse before a recurrence (exacerbation) develops. In exacerbations, the initial symptoms, accompanied by additional ones, generally recur.

The overall course of MS generally consists of multiple discrete attacks, a steady deterioration, or several attacks followed by steady deterioration. Almost all MS patients follow one of four reasonably distinct courses called *disease categories* (Fig. 15–1, top). The categories do not take into account the results of magnetic resonance imaging (MRI) and other testing. *Relapsing-remitting MS*, which includes the majority of MS cases in the initial years, is characterized by discrete attacks followed by partial or complete recovery. Although deficits may accumulate from each attack, patients are stable between them. Most patients in the relapsing-remitting category eventually change to a *secondary progressive* category, which consists of further, steady progression.

Primary progressive MS, characterized by a steady deterioration from the illness' onset, accounts for only about 10% of cases. Unlike the other disease categories, primary progressive MS first develops in individuals who are in their fifth or sixth decade, rather than their third or fourth. Also, it primarily or exclusively affects the spinal cord. *Progressive-relapsing MS*, the most rarely occurring category, consists of a steady deterioration with superimposed attacks.

In addition to being descriptive, the disease categories indicate a patient's prognosis and probable response to the new immunomodulating treatments. Of the various categories, relapsing-remitting MS is the most amenable to treatment; progressive MS, the least (see below).

Frequent Symptoms

Although numerous symptoms may occur during the illness, the most frequent result from plaques in the white matter tracts of the spinal cord, brainstem, and optic nerves (Fig. 15–1, bottom). Many symptoms tend to arise together because they all stem from involvement of a particular area of the CNS.

Cerebellar Symptoms and Signs. MS patients typically develop ataxia and other signs of cerebellar injury. Their gait is typically ataxic (see Fig. 2–13); however, if the cerebellar involvement is minimal, patients' only impairment may be in walking heel-to-toe *(tandem gait)*. Cerebellar involvement also typically causes *scanning speech,* a variety of dysarthria analogous to a "speech ataxia," characterized by irregular cadence and uneven emphasis on words. For example, when asked to repeat a pair of short syllables, such as "ba . . . ga . . . ba . . . ga . . . ," the patient might place unequal stress on different syllables, blur them together, or pause excessively. Other

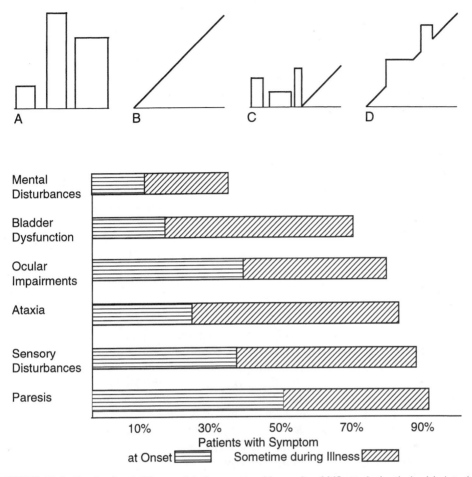

FIGURE 15–1. *Top,* Graphs of different clinical courses—with severity of MS attacks (vertical axis) plotted against time (horizontal axis)—reveals four patterns or disease categories: **A**, Relapsing-remitting; **B**, primary progressive; **C**, secondary progressive; **D**, progressive-relapsing. *Bottom,* This chart of initial and cumulative manifestations of MS indicates that mental disturbances are rarely present at the onset.

manifestations of MS cerebellar involvement include intention tremor (see Fig. 2–11), dysdiadochokinesia, and an irregular, conspicuous, head tremor *(titubation).*

Sensory Symptoms. Sensory disturbances are a frequent and prominent, although usually nonspecific, symptom of MS. Patients often describe only hypalgesia or paresthesias that are sometimes painful in scattered areas of their limbs or trunk or below a particular spinal cord level (see Fig. 2–15). They typically lose ability to appreciate vibration and position sensations more than other sensations.

One specific sensory symptom is trigeminal neuralgia developing in young adults. In them, it results from demyelination of the trigeminal nerve's brainstem sensory tract. It responds to antiepileptic drug (AEDs). (Trigeminal neuralgia in older adults usually results from an aberrant blood vessel pressing on the trigeminal nerve as it exits from the cerebellopontine angle. Their variety of trigeminal neuralgia, which is more common than MS-induced neuralgia in young adults, responds to trigeminal nerve decompression surgery if AEDs are unsatisfactory [see Chapter 9].)

Aside from this pattern, patients with only sensory disturbances are liable to be misdiagnosed as expressing a psychogenic condition. This misinterpretation usually results because their sensory symptoms often overshadow their objective findings, which may be subtle, and usually do not conform to commonplace neurologic patterns.

"Eye Signs." Ocular impairments, often early MS manifestations, include impaired visual acuity and disordered ocular motility. Visual acuity impairment results from inflammatory attacks of the retrobulbar portion of the optic nerve, *retrobulbar (optic) neuritis* (see Fig. 12–6), rather than plaques developing in the occipital cortex. Optic neuritis causes a characteristic, irregular area of visual loss in one eye, a *scotoma*, that includes the center of vision, a *cecocentral scotoma* (Fig. 15–2). It also leads to *color desaturation*, which is a symptom in which colors, especially red, are less intense than normal.

The affected eye is painful. Moreover, the pain increases when patients look from side to side, probably because the movement puts traction on the inflamed optic nerve.

Unless the optic disk is swollen, which is difficult to detect, ophthalmoscopic examination typically reveals no abnormality. This discrepancy between visual loss and normal ophthalmoscopy has given rise to the saying "The patient sees nothing and the physician sees nothing." As an optic neuritis attack subsides, most, if not all, vision returns and the pain disappears. However, with repeated attacks, progressive visual loss ensues and the disk becomes atrophic.

Statistics vary on the relationship of optic neuritis to MS, mostly because of problems making a definite diagnosis of each condition. Also, some studies include asymptomatic, as well as symptomatic, patients. Roughly 25% of MS patients have had overt optic neuritis as their initial symptom. About 80% have it at some time during their illness. On the other hand, only about 30% of young adults who develop optic neuritis as an isolated condition will develop MS during the next 5 years. A single attack of optic neuritis, devoid of other neurologic symptoms, is therefore not diagnostic of MS; however, finding three or more MRI lesions greatly increases the likelihood of a patient subsequently developing MS.

Multiple sclerosis also causes ocular motility disturbances: *nystagmus* and the characteristic *internuclear ophthalmoplegia (INO)*, which is also called the *medial longitudinal fasciculus (MLF) syndrome*. Nystagmus results from either brainstem or cerebellar MS involvement. Although MS-induced nystagmus is clinically indistinguishable from nystagmus induced by other conditions (see Chapter 12), it frequently occurs in combination with dysarthria and tremor (Charcot's triad).

The INO produces diplopia on lateral gaze because of paresis of the adducting eye. In this syndrome, demyelination or other MLF damage interrupts nerve impulse transmission from the pontine conjugate gaze centers to the oculomotor nuclei (Figs. 15–3 and 15–4). This disorder is so characteristic that one of the most closely held rules in clinical neurology is that unilateral or bilateral INO, when found in conjunction with other signs of CNS injury, is virtually diagnostic of MS. Neurologists must concede, however, that INO may also result from systemic lupus erythematosus (SLE or lupus), small basilar artery strokes, and botulism. In addition, myasthenia gravis can produce an ocular muscle weakness that mimics an INO. From a physiologic viewpoint, INO is analogous to disconnection syndromes, such as conduction

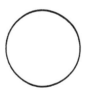 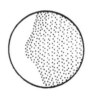

FIGURE 15–2. Optic (retrobulbar) neuritis causes impaired vision in a large, irregular area *(scotoma)* in the affected eye (see Fig. 12–6). It also causes pain, especially when the eye moves. The optic nerve is susceptible because, unlike almost all other cranial nerves, a CNS myelin covering surrounds it.

MEDIAL LONGITUDINAL
FASCICULUS (MLF)

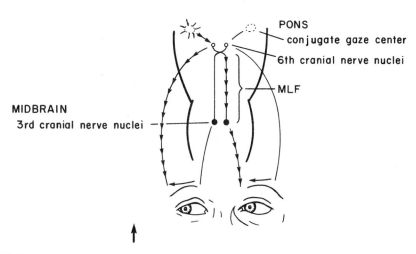

FIGURE 15–3. When looking laterally, the pontine conjugate gaze center stimulates the adjacent abducens (sixth) nerve nucleus and, through the *medial longitudinal fasciculus (MLF),* the contralateral oculomotor (third) nerve nucleus. Thus, when looking to the right, the right abducens and the left oculomotor nuclei are both stimulated (see Fig. 12–12). The MLF is therefore a crucial link in the complementary innervation of the third and sixth cranial nerve nuclei, which is required for lateral conjugate gaze.

INTERNUCLEAR
OPHTHALMOPLEGIA

FIGURE 15–4. In *internuclear ophthalmoplegia (INO),* also called the *MLF syndrome,* an interruption of the MLF prevents impulses from reaching the oculomotor (third) nuclei. Because the nuclei themselves are intact, the pupils and eyelids are normal in both eyes. However, when looking to the right, because the oculomotor nuclei are not stimulated, the left eye fails to adduct. The right eye abducts, but nystagmus develops. With bilateral INO, which is characteristic of MS, neither eye adducts and the abducting eye has nystagmus.

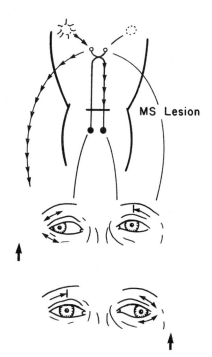

aphasia, in which communicating links are severed but each neurologic center is intact (see Chapter 8).

Spinal Cord Symptoms and Signs.   Patients with spinal cord involvement, which may be the illness' primary or exclusive site, as in primary progressive MS, have obvious paraparesis with hyperactive DTRs and Babinski signs (see Fig. 2–17*D*). They usually have three troublesome, common symptoms ("the 3 Is")—incontinence, impotence, and impairment of gait. In addition, spinal cord involvement almost invariably produces spasticity, which is a major impediment. Spasticity causes further gait impairment, painful leg spasms, and, in part, the bladder and sexual disturbances. Patients with cervical spinal cord involvement often describe a characteristic electrical sensation elicited by neck flexion that extends from the neck down the spine *(Lhermitte's sign)*.

Spinal cord involvement typically leads to *spastic urinary incontinence* from a combination of spasticity, paresis, and incoordination *(dyssynergia)* of the bladder sphincter muscles (Fig. 15–5). MS patients initially have incontinence during sleep and sexual intercourse. Even at its onset, the incontinence is closely associated with sexual impairment (see Chapter 16). As the disease progresses, patients develop intermittent urinary retention and then complete loss of control. Many patients must undergo intermittent or continuous catheterization.

Sexual impairment, with or without bladder dysfunction, plagues about 85% of MS patients (see Chapter 16). About 40% of women with MS do not engage in sexual intercourse. Men often have premature or retrograde ejaculation, as well as urinary incontinence, before erectile dysfunction develops. With spinal cord damage severe enough to cause paraplegia, men have lowered and abnormal sperm production.

Other Important Symptoms.   An inexplicable generalized *fatigue* affects about 50% of MS patients, including those with no paresis. This persistent sense of tiredness, which is entirely subjective, does not correlate with patients' physical disability, age, or mood. It is not a manifestation of depression. In fact, MS-induced fatigue, which can reach a state of exhaustion, represents a physiologic cause of chronic fatigue syndrome (see Chapter 6). Amantadine may reduce MS-induced fatigue.

Some symptoms occur rarely, if at all. Because the cerebral cortical "gray matter," which has no myelin, is relatively spared, MS patients rarely develop signs of cerebral

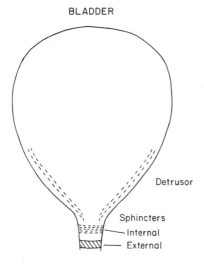

BLADDER

Detrusor

Sphincters
— Internal
— External

FIGURE 15–5. The urinary outflow of the bladder has two sphincters: an internal sphincter is controlled by the autonomic nervous system (ANS), and an external sphincter is under voluntary control. Normal urinary bladder emptying (urination) occurs when the detrusor (wall) muscle contracts and *both* sphincter muscles relax. Purposefully urinating requires the simultaneous voluntary action (to relax the external sphincter) and reflex parasympathetic (ANS) activity (to contract the detrusor and relax the internal sphincter). Urinary retention occurs with either anticholinergic medications or excessive sympathetic activity because both inhibit detrusor contraction and internal sphincter muscle relaxation. Urinary retention also occurs with spinal cord injury because the external sphincter is spastic, paretic, and unable to relax (dyssynergia).

cortical dysfunction, such as seizures or aphasia. Similarly, because the basal ganglia are also devoid of myelin, involuntary movement disorders (see Chapter 18) are virtually never manifestations of MS.

Pregnancy

Women with MS remain fertile. If they conceive, they do not have an increased rate of miscarriages, obstetric complications, or fetal malformations. Their pregnancies do not worsen the long-term course of MS. The rate of either first MS attacks or exacerbations is actually reduced throughout pregnancy. In fact, during the third trimester, the exacerbation rate falls to 70% of its baseline. If MS exacerbations do occur, they do not affect the pregnancy. MS patients require cesarean sections for only the usual indications. Epidural anesthesia has no effect on the course of MS.

On the other hand, during their first 3 postpartum months, mothers with MS have an increased rate of exacerbations that might interfere with the mother's care of her infant. After that period, the rate returns to its baseline. Although the pregnancy has little or no effect on the mother or child, the mother passes to her child an increased genetic-based susceptibility to the illness.

DEPRESSION AND COGNITIVE IMPAIRMENT IN MS

Depression

Depressive symptoms that do not reach the point of depressive illness are common in MS patients. They are most often attributable to a nonspecific psychologic response to a chronic, serious illness. These symptoms correlate with MS-induced physical impairments, loss of bodily function, inability to work, and lack of social support.

Major depressive illness (depression) occurs in about 50% of MS patients during their lifetime. It develops more frequently in patients with MS than in patients with other chronic illnesses (who have a 13% incidence), even if those illnesses produce comparable physical impairments.

Depression is especially frequent during certain periods of MS: at the onset of the illness, during exacerbations, late in the course of the illness, and when cognitive impairment develops. Unlike major depressive illness that occurs in families without MS, genetic influence in MS-induced depression is negligible. For example, the rate of depression in first-degree relatives of depressed MS patients is considerably lower than the rate of depression in first-degree relatives of depressed individuals who do not have MS.

Yet, the suicide rate of patients in MS clinics is 7.5 times greater than that of a comparably aged group. Moreover, of deaths among MS patients that are not due to the disease, about 30% have been attributed to suicide. Compared to all MS patients, those who have attempted suicide have been relatively young, less disabled, and symptomatic for fewer years.

In the debate about assisted suicide, MS will undoubtedly become a battleground. Many MS patients will probably seek an assisted suicide that will be resisted with more than the usual arguments. Unlike terminal cancer patients, for whom the concept is most understandable, MS patients are generally young, have a life expectancy of many years, and have little or no physical pain. More important, their thinking may be distorted by depression and impaired cognitive capacity.

Although bipolar affective disorder occurs at a higher rate in MS patients than in the general population, mania occurs rarely in MS patients. Instead, episodes that appear as mania may result from steroid treatment of MS (see below).

In view of the consequences of MS, the apparent elevation of mood in some patients, MS-induced "euphoria," has been a striking paradox. Certainly, some euphoric patients are masking depression or protecting themselves with denial. Others simply feel relieved as an MS attack subsides.

On the other hand, euphoria, along with other symptoms of emotional lability, is usually a manifestation of extensive cerebral involvement. These symptoms may actually represent an example of pseudobulbar palsy (see Chapter 4). Individually or together, they are associated with physical deterioration, chronicity of the illness, and subtle, if not overt, intellectual impairment. In addition, steroid treatment may induce euphoria with or without emotional or cognitive disturbances.

Cognitive Impairment

Cognitive function in MS patients may be difficult to assess because their slow and inarticulate speech, fatigue, and visual impairments impair mental status assessment. Allowing for such impediments, almost all MS patients initially have normal cognitive function based on their satisfactorily completing their day-to-day functions, routine mental status examination, and the Mini-Mental State Examination (MMSE) (see Fig. 7–2). Still, complex neuropsychologic tests, such as the Wechsler Adult Intelligence Scale (WAIS), Selective Reminding Test, and Halstead Category Test, might reveal clinically silent deficits.

Declining cognitive function in MS initially impairs concentration and memory. It eventually deteriorates to the level of dementia, which typically appears only late in the course of MS. Superimposed on physical impairments, MS-induced cognitive impairment, no matter how mild, can hamper activities of daily living, prevent full compliance with medical regimens, and strain interpersonal relationships. Moreover, it can precipitate thought or mood disorders.

MS-induced dementia correlates, in general, with physical disability, duration of the illness, and certain changes in the brain: enlarged cerebral ventricles, corpus callosum atrophy, periventricular white matter demyelination, total lesion area or volume (the *lesion load*) determined by MRI, and cerebral hypometabolism determined by positron emission tomography (PET). Of all these factors, cognitive impairment correlates most closely with the lesion load in the periventricular region.

Nevertheless, some MS patients who are severely disabled—even quadriplegic with incomprehensible speech, and incontinence—retain normal or near normal cognitive function. Clinicians should be aware that cursory evaluation might incorrectly indicate that MS patients have cognitive deficits comparable to their physical deficits. In other words, MS stands as another disease that can cause devastating physical impairments but may not impair cognitive function. Other diseases capable of producing this discrepancy include athetotic cerebral palsy, torsion dystonia, amyotrophic lateral sclerosis (ALS), and poliomyelitis.

Cognitive impairment in MS differs from that in Alzheimer's disease in several respects. If one accepts the classification, MS would produce a subcortical dementia, but Alzheimer's would produce a cortical dementia (see Chapter 7). MS-induced cognitive impairment results from CNS demyelination rather than from cerebral cortex gray matter degeneration. Another distinguishing feature is that in MS, clinically apparent cognitive impairment typically develops long after incapacitating physical impairments, relatively late in the illness. In Alzheimer's disease intellectual impairment occurs first and becomes profound long before onset of physical impairments. By contrast, in multi-infarct (vascular) dementia, where both gray and white matter are simultaneously affected, intellectual and physical deficits develop together.

Although the thought disorder in MS occasionally mimics psychosis, the incidence of psychosis in MS patients is remarkably lower than in other neurologic illnesses, including Alzheimer's disease, head trauma, and epilepsy, even partial complex epilepsy. In MS, psychosis undoubtedly originates partly from cognitive impairment and sensory deprivation. Other contributing factors may be steroid therapy (see below) or systemic infections causing delirium. On a practical level, psychiatrists should at least initially assume that psychosis in MS patients is a manifestation of cerebral demyelination, medications, or a concomitant physical illness rather than of psychologic stress, depression, or a latent, preexisting mental disorder. Except in scattered reports in the literature, MS virtually never presents with depression, cognitive impairment, or psychosis.

LABORATORY TESTS

No particular test is diagnostic of MS. In fact, when patients' symptoms are vague, few objective signs are present, only a single episode has occurred, or only a single CNS area is affected, several tests must be performed to diagnose MS and exclude other illnesses. In diagnosing MS, all currently available tests still produce both occasional false-negative and false-positive results.

Cerebrospinal Fluid

Routine cerebrospinal fluid (CSF) analysis during an MS attack will usually reveal that the protein concentration is either normal (40 mg/100 ml) or only slightly elevated, but the gamma globulin portion is elevated (9% or greater), which is a nonspecific finding. MS is more closely associated with an increased rate of synthesis of *CSF IgG*; the presence of CSF *oligoclonal bands,* which constitute a discrete IgG antibody; and the presence of CSF *myelin basic protein,* which probably represents a myelin breakdown product. However, these abnormalities may be found in other chronic inflammatory CNS illnesses, such as chronic meningitis, sarcoidosis, neurosyphilis, and Lyme disease.

Evoked Responses

Although routine electroencephalograms (EEGs) do not help in the diagnosis, related electrophysiologic testing, *evoked response* or *evoked potential tests,* can reveal characteristic interruptions in the visual, auditory, or sensory pathways. Evoked potential testing is based on repetitive stimulation of these pathways, which are heavily myelinated, and then detecting the responses with scalp electrodes similar to those used for EEGs. Normal responses are so small that they are lost in the normal cerebral electrical patterns and background noise but, in evoked testing, hundreds of responses are computer-averaged. After canceling out normal electrical activities, computer averaging displays an otherwise undetectable composite wave pattern. With injury to the pathways, the evoked response shows an increased interval *(latency)* between the stimulus and the composite response or a distortion in the wave form.

Evoked response tests are particularly useful in demonstrating lesions that are not detectable on neurologic examination. For example, if a patient has deficits referable only to the spinal cord but evoked response tests reveal a subclinical optic nerve injury, the physician would know that at least two CNS areas were injured.

Visual evoked responses (VERs) reveal visual pathway lesions. VERs are performed by having the patient stare at a rapidly flashing pattern on a television screen and averaging responses detected over the occipital cortex. Abnormalities are found with optic neuritis from MS or any other cause. They are also found with other optic nerve lesions, such as optic nerve gliomas (see Chapter 19) and congenital injuries (see Chapter 13). Because VERs can indicate the site of an interruption in the visual pathway, they are helpful in distinguishing ocular from cortical blindness. When the test is entirely normal, VERs are helpful in identifying psychogenic visual loss (see Chapter 12).

Brainstem auditory evoked responses (BAERs) reveal auditory pathway lesions. By measuring responses to a series of clicks in each ear, BAERs help indicate MS brainstem involvement. They are also useful in a variety of diagnostic tasks related to hearing: characterizing hearing impairments, diagnosing acoustic neuromas, and evaluating hearing in people unable to cooperate, such as infants and those with autism.

Somatosensory evoked responses reveal lesions in the sensory system from the limbs to the cerebral cortex. This test involves stimulating the limbs and detecting the resulting cerebral potentials. MS or other spinal cord injury causes abnormal latencies.

Imaging Studies

Computed tomography (CT) can occasionally reveal areas of demyelination. However, it is so insensitive that it is not useful for routine diagnosis of MS.

MRI—unequivocally the most valuable test—can readily reveal numerous or widely distributed demyelinated areas indicative of MS plaques in the brain (Figs. 15–6 and 20–17). It can detect demyelinated areas in both the cerebral and cerebellar white matter and in structures that are small or encased in bone, such as the optic nerves and spinal cord (Fig. 15–7). It can show asymptomatic as well as symptomatic plaques and thus indicate when a neurologic disease is disseminated. T1 gadolinium enhanced images show active lesions, but T2 proton density weighted images show new and old lesions.

The MRI indicates MS when it shows at least three white matter lesions; lesions in heavily myelinated areas, especially in the periventricular region and corpus callo-

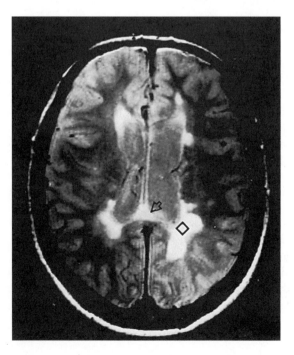

FIGURE 15–6. This MRI cuts through the cerebrum of an MS patient. Plaques, identifiable by their increased signal intensity, are multiple, irregular, white, and located in the deeply situated myelin. They are characteristically concentrated in the periventricular region and other heavily myelinated regions, such as the corpus callosum. In this MRI, of several periventricular plaques, one is marked *(diamond)* and another is located in the posterior limb of the corpus callosum *(arrow)* (see Figs. 8–4, 8–8, 20–17).

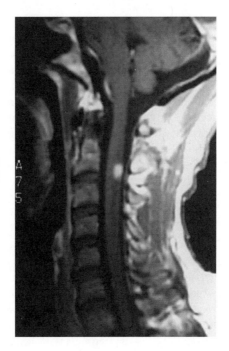

FIGURE 15–7. This MRI of an MS patient reveals a plaque—the hyperintense lesion—in the high cervical spinal cord.

sum; and, in gadolinium enhanced studies, open rings. Overall, MRI shows lesions in 90% of patients with clinically definite MS.

In MS patients, the lesion load closely correlates with physical and, more so, cognitive impairment. The lesion load is more reliable than the location of individual lesions in predicting cognitive impairment. Also, the appearance of new lesions in successive MRIs in established MS cases is generally accepted as a reliable marker of active disease or exacerbations. In fact, the development of new MRI lesions is a more sensitive indicator of disease activity than the clinical examination.

In established cases, the MRI shows, as previously mentioned, various structural changes: enlarged cerebral ventricles, corpus callosum atrophy, and periventricular white matter demyelination.

The MRI might lead to false-positive interpretations if it shows only one or two hyperintense lesions or many small, scattered, hyperintense lesions ("unidentified bright objects" [*UBOs*]). These potentially misleading hyperintensities, which are found predominantly in individuals older than 50 years, probably result from cerebrovascular disease, healed infection, or normal variations.

Although the MRI can readily reveal areas of demyelination, diseases other than MS, such as the leukodystrophies (see below), can cause a similar pattern. However, these other diseases usually do not cause the multiple, relatively large, dispersed plaques.

"Definite MS"

The characteristic courses, symptoms, signs, and results of MRI and other testing provide approximately 90% accuracy in diagnosing MS. In view of the small but persistent error rate, absence of a definitive clinical sign or laboratory test, and need for stringent research criteria, neurologists distinguish between *clinically definite MS* and *clinically probable MS*—each with a *laboratory-supported* version. Their criteria for clinically definite MS include a relapsing-remitting or progressive course, two or more distinct signs of CNS injury, and onset between ages 10 and 50 years. Clinically probable MS is based on either a single attack or area of involvement. The clinical diagnoses can be given "laboratory support" by the presence of multiple MRI hyperintensities, abnormal evoked responses, CSF oligoclonal bands, and increased CSF IgG.

Several clinical problems have caused most of the diagnostic errors. Warning signs that the diagnosis may *not* be MS include a progressive neurologic deterioration rather than a relapsing-remitting course; neurologic deficits confined to a single CNS region; absence of eye findings or urinary incontinence; normal CSF results; and a normal MRI. Erroneous diagnoses of MS were made most often in patients with conversion disorder and other psychiatric conditions, complicated migraines, and strokes. In addition, although they occur less frequently, many other conditions mimic MS (see below).

THERAPY

For attacks of MS or optic neuritis, with or without other signs of MS, neurologists generally administer high doses of intravenous steroids, such as methylprednisolone, which shorten attacks and may reduce residual deficits. Steroid treatment may lead to steroid psychosis (see below), as well as other potential complications. However, it almost never produces opportunistic infections, such as tuberculosis or cryptococcal meningitis—as happens with long-term steroid treatment of lupus or renal transplantation rejection.

With the introduction of immunomodulators, neurologists now have the expectation of reducing the frequency, severity, and residue of exacerbations and of prolonging the patient's ability to function. However, these medicines still cannot arrest MS, much less cure it.

This new and different approach to MS treatment requires that patients inject themselves with recombinant beta-interferon preparations (Betaseron and Avonex) or a preparation of four amino acids similar to myelin basic protein (glatiramer [Copaxone]). Immunomodulator treatment is indicated for those who have relapsing-remitting MS and have remained ambulatory. Patients are usually able to tolerate the medicines' side effects, which include fatigue, depression, and flulike symptoms after the injections. These medicines are also expensive (see Appendix 2). This treatment, compared to the natural history of MS, not only reduces the illness' symptoms, signs, and disability but also the lesion load.

For patients with progressive disease and for those who do not respond to these immunomodulators, neurologists administer other immunosuppressors. However, popular "treatments," such as snake and bee venom, vitamins in megadoses, and electric stimulation—generally born out of naturally occurring spontaneous remissions, folklore, or desperation—have been ineffective when scientifically tested.

In addition, neurologists administer symptomatic treatments. For example, depending on the nature of a patient's bladder dysfunction, medications that are cholinergic, such as bethanechol (Urecholine) or anticholinergic, such as imipramine (Tofranil), might be helpful; however, patients with advanced disease often require self-catheterization or sphincter bypass. Men with MS-induced erectile dysfunction may be helped by sildenafil (Viagra) pills or vasodilators injected directly into the penis (see Chapter 16). Although paresis cannot be improved, the accompanying spasticity, which is just as much of an impediment, usually responds to baclofen, diazepam, muscle relaxants, or injections of botulinum toxin (see Chapter 18). Also, formal exercise programs reduce disability and promote social contacts. MS-induced chronic fatigue, unlike idiopathic chronic fatigue, may respond to pemoline (Cylert), amantadine (Symmetrel), or modafinil (Provigil) (see Chapters 17 and 18).

Psychopharmacology can elevate or modulate MS patients' mood, reduce their discomfort associated with immobility, and help restore restful sleep. Depressed patients generally respond to both tricyclics and selective serotonin reuptake inhibitors (SSRIs); however, antidepressants with anticholinergic side effects should be used cautiously because they are particularly liable to cause urinary retention. In addition, SSRIs may increase spasticity.

Antidepressants' effective doses in depression associated with MS are generally lower than in depression not associated with neurologic disease. Electroconvulsive therapy (ECT) is also usually effective, and it can be administered with only the usual precautions (i.e., MS cerebral lesions are not a counterindication to ECT). Whichever treatment is chosen, in order to be maximally effective it might need to be administered along with psychotherapy, social services, occupational counseling, or physical therapy.

STEROID PSYCHOSIS

Steroid treatment of MS—as with steroid treatment of lupus, organ transplant rejection, and acute asthma—can induce anxiety, euphoria, mania, depressive symptoms, or psychosis. Likewise, conditions that generate excessive production of steroids, such as Cushing's syndrome, can produce similar symptoms. Even athletes who may surreptitiously use steroids for bodybuilding and energy can develop personality and behavioral changes. When steroid treatment causes a psychosis that includes prominent hallucinations or delusions, the mental disorder meets the *Diagnostic and Statistical Manual of Mental Disorders-IV (DSM-IV)* criteria for a *Substance-Induced Psychotic Disorder*, which is commonly known as a "steroid psychosis."

Even without excessive doses, steroids often produce a ravenous appetite, insomnia, and tremor. The steroid-induced tremor is fine and rapid, which gives it the appearance of anxiety-induced and essential tremors (see Chapter 18).

Glucocorticoid steroids, such as prednisone, are more apt than mineralocorticoid steroids, such as dexamethasone, to induce a steroid psychosis. The incidence of steroid psychosis, which usually begins 1 to 4 days after starting treatment, increases from 4% of patients receiving less than 40 mg of prednisone daily to 20% of patients receiving more than 80 mg daily. When steroid treatment is discontinued, symptoms generally recede. If the euphoria persists and reaches the point of mania, mood-modulating medications, such as valproate, may be required.

Psychosis in a patient with lupus or other systemic inflammatory disease receiving high-dose steroids poses a clinical dilemma. Because these diseases can directly affect the brain, abruptly decreasing the steroids might intensify their cerebral involvement. In addition, at a time when the body is under stress and consequently requires increased steroids, suddenly stopping them may precipitate adrenal insufficiency. Thus, as a general rule, in patients with a systemic inflammatory disease, until the evaluation is completed, steroids should be maintained or increased. On the other hand, in MS patients, because the benefit of steroids is marginal and they are certainly not life-saving, steroids should be discontinued as soon as possible. In the interim, antipsychotic medicines or, according to a few reports, lithium should be used to treat psychotic disturbances. Antidepressants should be avoided because they may exacerbate steroid-induced psychosis.

CONDITIONS THAT MIMIC MS

Many other physically incapacitating conditions frequently develop in young people. Several of them can reasonably be confused with MS because of its innumerable clinical manifestations. As previously mentioned, many individuals initially thought to have MS were eventually diagnosed as having conversion disorder and other psychiatric conditions, complicated migraines, or strokes.

The confusion between MS and psychogenic disturbances is understandable. Depending on the mental disorder, patients might have clumsiness, sexual impairments, nonspecific sensory loss, fatigue, or even several weeks of paraparesis or blindness. Indeed, some young paraplegic patients described in the original psychoanalytic literature who improved after a course of psychoanalysis may actually have had the spontaneous resolution of an MS episode.

Today, most conditions that mimic MS develop in young adults and cause PNS or CNS demyelination. In addition, illnesses that damage the CNS without primarily attacking myelin can mimic MS.

Non–MS Demyelinating Diseases

Guillain-Barré Syndrome.   Even though it is a demyelinating disease of the peripheral nervous system (PNS) rather than of the CNS, Guillain-Barré syndrome may resemble MS because it generally strikes young and middle-aged adults and causes paraparesis or quadriparesis (see Chapter 5). In contrast to MS, it is characterized by a single monophasic attack, lasting several weeks to several months, of symmetric, flaccid, areflexic paresis. In addition, although Guillain-Barré syndrome may be physically devastating, it does not cause cognitive impairment, depression, or psychosis unless medical complications have supervened.

Leukodystrophies.   Destruction of CNS white matter, alone or in combination with PNS myelin, is the hallmark of a rare group of genetically transmitted illnesses, the leukodystrophies. As with MS, the leukodystrophies cause optic nerve, cerebellum, and spinal cord myelin degeneration that leads to progressively severe visual impairment, ataxia, and spastic paraparesis. However, in contrast to MS, the leukodystrophies are entirely genetically determined. They usually first manifest in infants or children but occasionally not until the victims are teenagers or young adults, at which times they may present with behavioral problems, emotional changes, and cognitive impairment. During the next several years, they rapidly progress to psychosis and dementia. In contrast to the common relapsing-remitting variety of MS, the leukodystrophies cause unremitting physical and mental deterioration.

Two well-known leukodystrophies are *adrenoleukodystrophy (ALD)* and *metachromatic leukodystrophy (MLD*; see Chapter 5). ALD, which is transmitted as a sex-linked trait, typically first produces neurologic symptoms and adrenal insufficiency in boys between 5 and 15 years old. However, sometimes symptoms emerge only when the men carrying the defective gene reach 20 to 30 years. When ALD develops in this older group, CNS demyelination induced by it typically first causes mania and gait impairment and eventually dementia. In addition to the demyelination, which often has an inflammatory component, ALD causes peripheral neuropathy.

The biochemical defect in ALD results in accumulation of unbranched saturated very long chain fatty acids (VLCFAs). It stems from an oxidation enzyme defect in *peroxisomes,* which are intracellular organelles. The widely publicized treatment—developed by two self-trained biochemists who were parents of a victim—with Lorenzo's oil reduced VLCFA concentrations but failed to alter the disease's course. Similarly, treatment by adrenal hormone replacement does not arrest the demyelination. Some research has indicated that bone marrow transplants, before symptoms develop, may prevent both brain and adrenal damage.

Infections.   Certain infectious agents produce demyelination not by an actual infection (invasion) of the CNS but by provoking an antibody response that disrupts the myelin. For example, *postinfectious* and *postimmunization encephalomyelitis,* which occur 1 to 4 weeks after an infection or immunization, consist of an attack on the cerebral and spinal cord myelin that is often extensive and permanent. (Postimmunization encephalomyelitis, although rare and unpredictable, carries a major liability risk for pharmaceutical firms.)

Progressive multifocal leukoencephalopathy (PML), a true infection, leads to CNS demyelination. PML is a late complication of acquired immune deficiency syndrome (AIDS) and several other illnesses characterized by immunologic impairment. Like MS, PML leads to patchy areas of demyelination throughout the CNS.

Several other CNS infections, even though they do not primarily attack CNS myelin, can mimic MS. In particular, an infection with the retrovirus *HTLV-1* causes a *myelitis* (infection of the spinal cord) that closely resembles MS restricted to the spinal cord. This virus is related to *human immunodeficiency virus (HIV)*. It was initially labeled *HTLV-3* and is endemic in the Caribbean islands, where MS is uncommon. HTLV-1 myelitis often causes a slowly evolving, painless, spastic paraparesis in Caribbean residents.

Toxins.   Numerous toxins preferentially attack CNS myelin. *Marchiafava-Bignami syndrome,* which is probably caused by a substance in homemade Italian red wine, consists of degeneration of the heavily myelinated corpus callosum. Thus, theoretically at least, the Marchiafava-Bignami syndrome can cause split brain syndrome (see Chapters 7 and 8).

Chronic toluene exposure, whether from poor industrial ventilation or recreational volatile substance abuse, damages cerebral myelin. Although it rarely produces objective physical abnormalities, toluene reportedly often impairs cognitive ability and causes personality changes (see Chapter 5). Sometimes the MRI will show dramatic demyelination.

A small group of lawyers and physicians, but not neurologists, have claimed that silicone breast implants cause MS, "multiple sclerosis-like symptoms," chronic fatigue syndrome, cognitive impairment, chronic inflammatory demyelinating polyneuropathy, and other neurologic disorders. However, after several major national studies, a wide spectrum of physicians and scientists, individually and in groups, concluded that silicone breast implants do not cause any neurologic disease. Women who have received silicone breast implants and described neurologic disorders had no consistent pattern of symptoms, virtually no objective signs, and no significant laboratory abnormalities—except in the normal number of women who would be expected to have contracted various neurologic illness before or after the surgery. Women with unruptured implants reported the same incidence of postoperative neurologic problems as women with ruptured implants. Women in Sweden and Denmark who had the implants reported essentially the same incidence of neurologic symptoms as those who underwent breast reduction. In other settings, such as its use as cardiac pacemaker coverings, silicone has not been associated with neurologic disease. In individual cases, physicians have established more plausible alternative diagnoses: most often, depression and anxiety, carpal tunnel syndrome, neuropathies, and preexisting MS.

Lupus

Other vascular inflammatory diseases, such as lupus, may produce multiple CNS abnormalities in young adults. At its onset, lupus affects the CNS in only about 5%

of cases, but it eventually produces neurologic complications in approximately 75%. The most frequently occurring pattern consists of seizures and cerebral infarctions, including those that cause mental aberrations, chorea, and the MLF syndrome—the "three Ss: seizures, strokes, and psychosis." Of these various CNS complications, the most life-threatening is seizures.

MRIs might show the cerebral infarctions that characterize lupus cerebritis but only in its late stage. In contrast, single photon emission tonography (SPECT) can detect lupus cerebritis in its early stage. In addition, SPECT can distinguish lupus cerebritis from steroid psychosis.

Lupus causes neuropathy, mononeuropathy multiplex, and other PNS abnormalities, alone or in conjunction with cerebritis. Both the CNS and PNS neurologic complications have been attributed to immune complexes producing an arteritis, but many complications are manifestations of cardiac valvular disease, a tendency to develop thromboses, opportunistic infections, hypertension, renal failure, or possibly the elaboration of false neurotransmitters.

Other inflammatory illnesses, such as Sjögren's syndrome and sarcoidosis, may cause cognitive impairment, facial nerve injury, and neuropathy. As with lupus, these illnesses can almost always be diagnosed by their systemic symptoms and various laboratory tests.

Spinal Cord Disorders

Insidiously developing, painless paraparesis is a relatively common, important clinical problem. Numerous unrelated diseases that affect the spinal cord can be responsible: combined system disease (B_{12} deficiency), cervical spine degeneration, ALS, HTLV-1 infection, and spinal meningiomas, as well as MS. To diagnose spinal cord disorders, neurologists often require an MRI of the spinal cord, serum B_{12} level determinations, electromyographic studies, and various blood and CSF tests.

REFERENCES

Multiple Sclerosis

Abramowicz M (ed): Interferon beta-1A for multiple sclerosis. Med Lett *38:* 63–64, 1996
Confavreux C, Hutchinson M, Hours MM, et al: Rate of pregnancy-related relapse in multiple sclerosis. N Engl J Med *339:* 285–291, 1998
Diaz-Olavarrieta C, Cummings JL, Velazquez J, et al: Neuropsychiatric manifestations of multiple sclerosis. J Neuropsychiatry Clin Neurosci *11:* 51–57, 1999
Feinstein A, Feinstein K, Gray T, et al: Prevalence and neurobehavioral correlates of pathologic laughing and crying in multiple sclerosis. Arch Neurol *54:* 1116–1121, 1997
Hohol MJ, Guttmann CRG, Orav J, et al: Serial neuropsychological assessment and magnetic resonance imaging analysis in multiple sclerosis. Arch Neurol *54:* 1018–1025, 1997
The IFNB Multiple Sclerosis Study Group: Interferon beta-1b in the treatment of multiple sclerosis: Final outcome of the randomized trial. Neurology *45:* 1277–1285, 1995
Kurtzke JF, Page WF: Epidemiology of multiple sclerosis in US veterans. Neurology *48:* 204–213, 1997
Lublin FD, Reingold SC: Defining the clinical course of multiple sclerosis. Neurology *46:* 907–911, 1996
McFarland HF: Editorial: Twins studies and multiple sclerosis. Ann Neurol *32:* 722–723, 1992
Minden SL, Schiffler RB: Affective disorders in multiple sclerosis. Arch Neurol *47:* 98–104, 1990
Mumford CJ, Wood NW, Kellar-Wood H, et al: The British Isles survey of multiple sclerosis in twins. Neurology *44:* 11–15, 1994
Optic Neuritis Study Group: The 5-year risk of MS after optic neuritis. Neurology *49:* 1404–1413, 1997
Poser CM, Roman GC, Vernant JC: Multiple sclerosis or HTLV-1 myelitis? Neurology *40:* 1020–1022, 1990
Rao SM, Leo GJ, Bernardin L, et al: Cognitive dysfunction in multiple sclerosis. Neurology *41:* 685–691, 1991
Rovaris M, Filippi M, Falautano M, et al: Relation between MR abnormalities and patterns of cognitive impairment in multiple sclerosis. Neurology *50:* 1601–1608, 1998
Rudick RA, Cohen JA, Weinstock-Guttman B, et al: Management of multiple sclerosis. N Engl J Med *337:* 1604–1611, 1997

Sadovnick AD, Remick RA, Allen J, et al: Depression and multiple sclerosis. Neurology 46: 628–632, 1996

Scott TF, Allen D, Price TRP: Characterization of major depression symptoms in multiple sclerosis patients. J Neuropsychiatry Clin Neurosci 8: 318–323, 1996

Stenager EN, Stenager E: Suicide and patients with neurologic diseases. Arch Neurol 49: 1296–1303, 1992

Swirsky-Sacchetti T, Mitchell DR, Seward J, et al: Neuropsychological and structural brain lesions in multiple sclerosis. Neurology 42: 1291–1295, 1992

Therapeutics and Technology Assessment Subcommittee of the American Academy of Neurology: The relationship of MS to physical trauma and psychologic stress. Neurology 52: 1737–1745, 1999

Tselis A, Lisak RP: Multiple Sclerosis: Therapeutic update. Arch Neurol 56: 277–280, 1997

Trapp BD, Peterson J, Ransohoff RM, et al: Axonal transection in the lesions of multiple sclerosis. N Engl J Med 338: 278–285, 1998

Vercoulen JHMM, Hommes OR, Swanink CMA, et al: The measurement of fatigue in patients with multiple sclerosis: a multidimensional comparison with patients with chronic fatigue syndrome and healthy subjects. Arch Neurol 53: 642–649, 1996

Other Illnesses

Angell M: Shattuck Lecture—Evaluating the health risks of breast implants: The interplay of medical science, the law, and public opinion. N Engl J Med 334: 1513–1518, 1996

Ferguson JH: Silicone breast implants and neurologic disorders: Report of the Practice Committee of the American Academy of Neurology. Neurology 48: 1504–1507, 1997

Futrell N, Schultz LR, Millikan C: Central nervous system disease in patients with systemic lupus erythematosus. Neurology 42: 1649–1657, 1992

Hietaharju A, Yli-Kerttula U, Hakkinen V: Nervous system manifestations in Sjögren's syndrome. Acta Neurol Scand 81: 144–152, 1990

Rosebush PI, Garside S, Levinson AJ, et al: The neuropsychiatry of adult-onset adrenoleukodystrophy. J Neuropsychiatry Clin Neurosci 11: 315–327, 1999

Scott TF: Neurosarcoidosis: Progress and clinical aspects. Neurology 43: 8–12, 1993

Shapiro EG, Lockman LA, Knopman D, et al: Characteristics of the dementia in late-onset metachromatic leukodystrophy. Neurology 44: 662–665, 1994

Wolkowitz OM, Reus VI, Canick J, et al: Glucocorticoid medication, memory and steroid psychosis in medical illness. Ann NY Acad Sci 823: 81–96, 1997

QUESTIONS and ANSWERS: CHAPTER 15

1–4. Over four days, a 25-year-old salesman developed paraparesis. Then his left eye became painful and blind. The left pupil reacts slowly to light. His legs have hyperactive deep tendon reflexes (DTRs) and bilateral Babinski signs. His arms have normal strength, reflexes, and coordination. He does not have Lhermitte's sign.

1. Which of the following disorders is the most likely cause of his neurologic deficits?

a. Spinal cord tumor
b. Psychogenic disturbances
c. Multiple sclerosis (MS)
d. Postvaccinal or postinfectious encephalomyelitis
e. HTLV-1 myelitis

> **ANSWER:** c. The salesman may have developed MS affecting the optic nerve and spinal cord, but, in the absence of a second event or consistent MRI studies, the diagnosis cannot be confirmed. Yet, it remains the most likely ultimate diagnosis. It may be a demyelinating inflammatory reaction to an infection or vaccination, especially one against smallpox or rabies, but this is rare. Spinal cord tumors would create spastic paraparesis but, of course, not visual impairment. Psychogenic disturbances might lead to visual and motor symptoms and possibly feigned Babinski signs; however, people cannot mimic abnormal pupil reactions. HTLV-1 myelitis typically causes spastic paraparesis but does not affect vision or pupil reactions.

2. In regard to the patient described in Question 1, which regions of the CNS are most likely to be affected?

a. Right occipital lobe and thoracic spinal cord
b. Thoracic spinal cord and left optic nerve

   c. Sacral spinal cord and left optic nerve
   d. Left optic nerve and cervical spinal cord

> **ANSWER:** b. He has retrobulbar neuritis and thoracic myelitis. Unlike the other cranial nerves, the optic nerve (cranial nerve 2) is an outgrowth of the CNS. Only the optic nerve and a small portion of the acoustic nerve (cranial nerve 8) are covered by CNS myelin.

3. After three weeks, the patient in Question 1 became ambulatory and had recovered his vision. One year later, he returns with new symptoms: dysarthria, ataxia, nystagmus, and tremor of the arms. In which two CNS regions are the new lesions located?

   a. Cerebrum   c. Brainstem
   b. Cerebellum   d. Spinal cord

> **ANSWER:** b, c

4. At this visit, with which diagnosis is this patient's illness most consistent?

   a. Clinically definite MS   c. Clinically possible MS
   b. Clinically probable MS   d. None of the above

> **ANSWER:** a. Clinically definite MS. With the two attacks and their two locations, as well as the classic symptoms and signs, his diagnosis reaches the level of *clinically definite MS* instead of *clinically probable MS*. In practice, neurologists seek to support any clinical MS diagnosis with an MRI and often CSF analysis. If these studies are positive, then the clinical diagnosis is designated *laboratory-supported.* On the other hand, if testing fails to confirm the clinical diagnosis, the entire case must be reevaluated.

5. Of the various MRI abnormalities in MS, which one correlates most closely with cognitive impairment?

   a. Enlarged cerebral ventricles
   b. Corpus callosum atrophy
   c. Lesions seen with gadolinium enhancement
   d. Total lesion area or volume

> **ANSWER:** d. MS-associated cognitive impairment is most closely associated with total MRI lesion area or volume ("the lesion load"), particularly in the periventricular region. Gadolinium infusion during T1 sequences highlights active lesions.

6. Which three of the following substances produces optic neuritis?

   a. Tobacco   d. Methyl alcohol
   b. Oral contraceptives   e. Penicillin
   c. Ethyl alcohol   f. Heroin

> **ANSWER:** a, c, d

7. Which four of these illnesses are associated with optic neuritis?

   a. Rubella   e. Sarcoidosis
   b. Gonorrhea   f. Vasculitis
   c. MS   g. Syphilis
   d. AIDS   h. Lyme disease

> **ANSWER:** c, e, f, g. Although MS is not the only cause of optic neuritis, it has the closest association. After an episode of isolated optic neuritis, the overall risk is only about 30% of subsequently developing MS; however, if the MRI shows three or more cerebral lesions, MS is more than 50% likely to develop during the next five years.

8. Which four of the following conditions may lead to internuclear ophthalmoplegia (INO)?

   a. MS   d. Lupus
   b. Subdural hematoma   e. Thiamine deficiency
   c. Conversion reaction   f. Brainstem infarctions

> **ANSWER:** a, d, e, f. In other words, INO, like optic neuritis, is not pathognomonic of MS.

9–12. A 60-year-old man has difficulty walking and suffers from lower back pains that radiate to the trunk and legs. He walks with a broad-based gait and excessively lifts his knees. He has no dysmetria or intention tremor of his arms. Although strength in his legs is normal, his DTRs are absent. He has lost position sense (but not pain or touch sense) in the feet. He has small pupils that are unreactive to light.

9. Which one of the following is the most likely cause of his gait disturbance?

a. Cerebellar damage

b. Spinal cord compression

c. MS

d. Posterior column dysfunction

ANSWER: d. The gait disturbance is entirely explainable by the loss of proprioception in his legs causing him to have ataxia and a "steppage gait" (see Fig. 2–18). Neurologists might say that he has "sensory ataxia."

10. Although his pupils were small and unreactive to light, they constricted when he looked at a closely held (regarded) object. What is the pupillary disturbance called?

a. Argyll-Robertson pupils

b. Optic neuritis

c. INO

d. Miosis

ANSWER: a. He has small pupils with lack of light reaction but preserved accommodation. This pattern is called "Argyll-Robertson pupils." His neurologic signs indicate tabes dorsalis.

11. What laboratory finding would be most reliable in confirming a diagnosis of CNS syphilis?

a. A positive CSF MHA

b. Periventricular white matter changes on an MRI

c. A positive CSF VDRL

d. Detecting oligoclonal bands in the CSF

ANSWER: c. Keeping in mind that many serum and CSF test results are false-negative, the most reliable test for confirming CNS syphilis is a positive CSF VDRL. Determining a CSF MHA is an unreliable test. Periventricular white matter changes on the MRI indicate MS. CSF oligoclonal bands are found in a variety of CNS infectious or inflammatory illnesses.

12. Many features of internuclear ophthalmoplegia (INO) are shared by oculomotor cranial nerve palsy (CN III). Which of the following indicates that a patient has an INO rather than a CN III palsy?

a. In INO, there is no ptosis or dilation of the pupil.

b. In INO, the affected eye fails to adduct.

c. In INO, the adducting eye has nystagmus.

d. A CN III palsy is characterized by ptosis, miosis, and anhidrosis.

ANSWER: a. Ptosis or dilation of the pupil characterizes a CN III palsy. In both conditions, the affected eye cannot adduct. In INO, the abducting eye has nystagmus. Ptosis, miosis, and anhidrosis are features of the Horner's syndrome.

13. During which obstetrical period is MS most likely to become exacerbated?

a. First trimester

b. Second trimester

c. Third trimester

d. First 3 postpartum months

ANSWER: d. The first three postpartum months are associated with MS exacerbations. Pregnancy is associated with reduced attacks.

14. What is the effect of one or more pregnancies on the course of a woman's MS?

a. Her functional status deteriorates with each succeeding pregnancy.

b. Her functional status is better with each succeeding pregnancy.

c. There is little or no effect.

ANSWER: c. Contrary to previous thinking, pregnancy and delivery have little or no effect on the mother's MS.

15. Which other statement regarding pregnancy and MS is true?

a. MS causes a high rate of spontaneous abortions.
b. Obstetric complications are frequent.
c. Fetal malformations are common.
d. Cesarean sections are indicated in most deliveries.
e. Offspring have a greater risk than the general population of developing MS.

ANSWER: e. Children of MS patients have an increased incidence of the illness.

16. Which MS features are associated with cognitive impairment?

a. Physical impairments
b. Duration of the illness
c. Enlarged cerebral ventricles
d. Corpus callosum atrophy
e. Periventricular demyelination
f. Total lesion area
g. Cerebral hypometabolism

ANSWER: All

17. What is the approximate concordance rate of MS among monozygotic twins?

a. 25%
b. 50%
c. 75%
d. 100%
e. 200%

ANSWER: a. Most studies describe an MS concordance rate for monozygotic twins of 25% to 30% and for dizygotic twins of 5%. Moreover, the symptoms (phenotypes) of twins differ when both are affected. This data diminishes the importance of genetic factors in MS. If MS were determined by a genetic abnormality, when one monozygotic twin developed MS, the other twin would develop the illness (to give 100% concordance), and affected twin pairs would have similar symptoms (i.e., have the same phenotype).

18–24. Match the ocular motility disorder (18–24) with the most likely cause (a–g).

a. Wernicke's encephalopathy
b. Labyrinthitis
c. Psychogenic disorders
d. Myasthenia gravis
e. MS
f. Midbrain infarction
g. None of the above

18. Pupillary dilation, ptosis, and paresis of adduction

ANSWER: f (oculomotor nerve palsy)

19. Bilateral ptosis

ANSWER: d

20. Bilateral horizontal nystagmus

ANSWER: a, b, e

21. Bilateral horizontal nystagmus, unilateral paresis of abduction, and areflexic DTRs

ANSWER: a

22. Nystagmus in abducting eye and incomplete adduction of the other eye when looking horizontally

ANSWER: e (INO or the MLF syndrome)

23. Ptosis bilaterally, paresis of adduction of one eye, and normal pupils

ANSWER: d

24. Nystagmus in adducting eye and paresis of abduction of the other eye

ANSWER: g

25. A 58-year-old man with MS is brought to the emergency for urinary incontinence. He has a distended bladder, paraparesis, and sensory impairment in his lower trunk and legs. Although he is fully alert, he is very uncomfortable. Which should be the first step in alleviating his distress?

a. Administer cholinergic medications
b. Do an MRI of the spinal cord
c. Stop any anticholinergic medications
d. Administer analgesics that have no anticholinergic side effects
e. None of the above

ANSWER: e. He has overflow incontinence and needs to have a catheter inserted into his bladder to drain the urine. However, the drainage should be interrupted after removing each liter to avoid precipitating a hypotensive episode. Not all cases of bladder distention and overflow incontinence in MS are due to the illness. Instead, the cause may be prostatic hypertrophy, other obstructions, anticholinergic medications, or detrusor muscle weakness.

26. A 9-year-old boy has developed social difficulties and then academic difficulties. He has hyperactive DTRs, clumsiness, and an awkward gait. His older brother had similar symptoms and then died of adrenal failure before the correct diagnosis was made. The patient's MRI of the brain shows extensive demyelination. Which of the following statements is correct?

a. Lorenzo's oil will arrest the disease.
b. The illness is transmitted in an autosomal recessive pattern.
c. The illness results from defective mitochondria.
d. The disease is characterized by the accumulation of unbranched saturated very long chain fatty acids (VLCFAs).

ANSWER: d. The patient and his brother have adrenoleukodystrophy (ALD), which is a relatively common leukoencephalopathy. ALD is characterized by accumulation of VLCFAs because of defective peroxisomes. The illness is an X-linked disorder that usually presents in boys and runs a fulminant course over 5 years. Neither Lorenzo's oil nor adrenal replacement therapy will arrest the disease's neurologic consequences.

27. Which one of the following descriptions best characterizes MS-induced MRI changes?

a. Multiple, white areas scattered in the cerebrum
b. Conversion of the cerebral hemisphere white matter to gray
c. Loss of the myelin signal throughout the corpus callosum
d. Periventricular, high-intensity abnormalities
e. Periventricular, high-density abnormalities

ANSWER: d. MS is characterized by multiple, relatively large patches (plaques) in the cerebral periventricular white matter. Plaques are also often routinely detected in other areas of the cerebrum, especially the corpus callosum, and the cerebellum. With high-resolution MRI, plaques can even be visualized in the optic nerves and spinal cord. Plaques are visualized on an MRI as high-intensity abnormalities. However, scattered, small white matter hyperintense lesions—unidentified bright objects (UBOs)—are a nonspecific finding. High-density abnormalities generally refer to findings on a CT, which is based on lesions absorbing x-rays. In technical terms, MS plaques on MRIs show high intensity on T2 images and low intensity on T1 images.

28. Natives of which of the following cities have the highest MS incidence?

a. New Orleans
b. Boston
c. Philadelphia
d. Seattle

ANSWER: Boston. Higher latitudes are usually associated with a greater incidence of MS. Cities in Colorado, an exception in terms of latitude but not climate, have a higher incidence than most of the West Coast states.

29. Which of the following regions has the lowest MS incidence?

a. New England
b. Colorado
c. Scotland
d. Caribbean islands

ANSWER: Caribbean islands. The incidence of all the other regions is high.

30. Of the following Israeli groups, which would have the highest and lowest incidence of MS?

a. Native Israelis (Sabras)
b. European immigrants to Israel
c. Black African Israelis

ANSWER: Highest-European immigrants; lowest-Black Africans. The period when vulnerability is conveyed last from birth to about 16 years. In other words, adults emigrating from one region to another carry the incidence of their homeland.

31. In which conditions do visual evoked responses (VERs) typically show prolonged latencies or other abnormal pattern?

a. Asymptomatic optic neuritis
b. Retrobulbar neuritis
c. Most patients with long-standing MS
d. Patients with "blindness" from a conversion reaction
e. Optic nerve gliomas
f. Deafness

ANSWER: a, b, c, e. Almost any lesion in the visual pathway will slow the nerve action potential, which prolongs the latency and distorts the wave form.

32. In MS patients, which three findings are most often associated with urinary incontinence?

a. Leg spasticity
b. Ataxia
c. Spasticity of the external sphincter of the bladder
d. Sexual impairment
e. MLF syndrome

ANSWER: a, c, d. Urinary incontinence, sexual impairment, and spastic paraparesis all result from spinal cord involvement. In MS, the spinal cord is often the sole or primary site of involvement. Its pathways are quite sensitive.

33. Which symptoms typically develop only late or not at all in the course of MS?

a. Pseudobulbar palsy
b. INO
c. Optic neuritis
d. Bladder dysfunction

e. Psychosis
f. Depression
g. Sexual dysfunction
h. Dementia

ANSWER: a, e, h

34. Which of the following statements is not true for relapsing-remitting MS?

a. Of the major MS disease categories, relapsing-remitting is the most amenable to immunologic modulation.
b. As with other categories, the determination is based on the clinical course.
c. Relapsing-remitting disease usually evolves into secondary progressive disease.
d. The presence of additional MRI abnormalities in relapsing-remitting disease changes its designation to secondary progressive disease.
e. Progressive disease is the least amenable to immunologic modulation.

ANSWER: d. MRI results are not considered in determining the disease category.

35. Which five of the following conditions may lead to apparent euphoria in MS patients?

a. Pseudobulbar palsy
b. Steroid treatment
c. Cerebellar cortex demyelination
d. Cerebral demyelination
e. Depression
f. Remission of an acute attack
g. Partial complex seizures
h. Optic nerve demyelination

ANSWER: a, b, d, e, f

36. Fatigue in MS is often a prominent symptom. With which other symptom does it correlate?

a. Physical disability
b. Older age
c. Depression
d. Optic neuritis
e. Fibromyalgia
f. None of the above

> **ANSWER:** f. MS-induced fatigue, which is entirely subjective, does not correlate with patients' physical disability, older age, or mood. It is not related to depression. It may respond to pemoline or amantadine.

37. Which of the following cells produces CNS myelin?

a. Glia cells
b. Neurons
c. Schwann cells
d. Oligodendroglia
e. Lymphocytes

> **ANSWER:** d. Oligodendroglia produce CNS myelin. Schwann cells produce peripheral nervous system myelin.

38. In regard to the allegation that silicone breast implants cause MS, which of the following statements is true?

a. The incidence of symptoms is greater in women with ruptured than unruptured implants.
b. The incidence of symptoms is greater in women who have had breast implants than in women who have undergone breast reduction surgery.
c. Silicone-covered pacemakers produce similar neurologic problems.
d. Neurologic symptoms associated with silicone breast implants are consistent from patient to patient.
e. None of the above

> **ANSWER:** e. There is no credible evidence that silicone breast implants cause neurologic disease.

16

Neurologic Aspects
of Sexual Function

Whatever its underlying psychology, sexual function depends on two major neurologic pathways that are complex and delicate: (1) a highway between the brain and the genitals and (2) in essence, a short reflex loop between the genitals and spinal cord. Both involve the central nervous system (CNS), peripheral nervous system (PNS), and autonomic nervous system (ANS).

In the first pathway, the brain converts various cerebral stimuli, including sleep-related events, into sexually arousing neurologic impulses. These impulses travel down the spinal cord, which is also part of the CNS. Some impulses exit at its sacral region to be carried by the *pudendal nerve,* which is part of the PNS (Fig. 16–1). As if diverted to a parallel route, other impulses leave the spinal cord's low thoracic and upper lumbar areas (T11–L2) to join the *sympathetic* ANS. Still others leave the spinal cord's lower sacral segments (S2–S4) to join the *parasympathetic* ANS. Increased parasympathetic ANS activity reduces the tone of the genital arteries' wall muscles. Relaxed arteries dilate, which allows increased genital blood flow. In men, the increased parasympathetic-mediated blood flow inflates the penis and produces an erection. In women, it produces clitoral engorgement.

With continued stimulation, a complex series of predominantly sympathetic ANS-mediated events produce an orgasm. Afterward, a return to normal, relatively constricted arterial wall muscle tone reduces blood flow. Lack of vascular engorgement leads to detumescence.

The sympathetic and parasympathetic components of the ANS have different roles in sexual function and depend on different neurotransmitters—acetylcholine in the parasympathetic and monoamines in the sympathetic. However, they are complementary and vulnerable to similar injuries. An admittedly crude mnemonic describes the *p*arasympathetic and *s*ympathetic ANS roles in sexual response: "*p*oint and *s*hoot."

In the second pathway, which is simpler, erotic impulses from genital stimulation pass through the dorsal and then pudendal nerves to the spinal cord. Some impulses, in a *genital-spinal cord reflex,* synapse in the sacral region of the spinal cord and return, via the ANS, to the genitals. Other impulses ascend through the spinal cord to join other cerebral stimuli.

The mnemonic just cited also crystallizes another point. The current state of knowledge of sexual function rests on male physiology, evaluation, and treatment. This chapter's predominant references to male function do not reflect a bias, simply that the neurologic aspects of female sexual activity, for a variety of reasons, have received much less investigation.

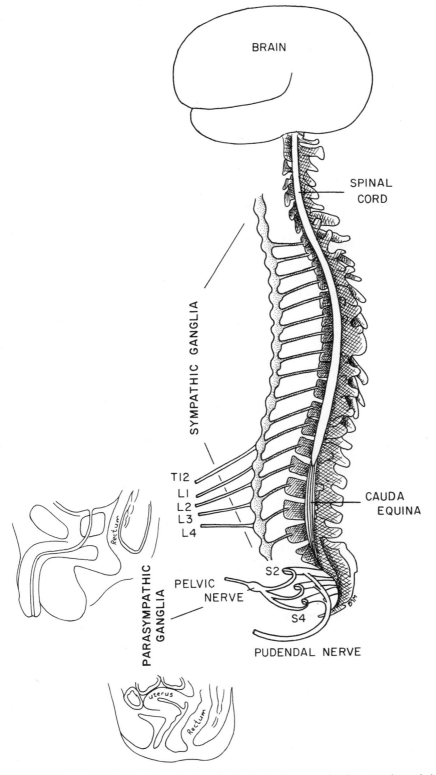

FIGURE 16–1. The sacral (S2–S4) spinal cord segments give rise to the nerves that innervate the genitals. In addition, the sympathetic and parasympathetic components of the autonomic nervous system (ANS) innervate the genitals. Branches of the pudendal nerve supply the genital muscles and skin. The ANS innervates the genitals, reproductive organs, bladder, sweat glands, and artery wall muscles.

TABLE 16–1. *Indications of Neurologic Sexual Impairment*

Continual erectile dysfunction
    Absence of morning erections
    No erection or orgasm during masturbation or sex with different partners
Related somatic complaints
    Sensory loss in genitals, pelvis, or legs
    Urinary incontinence
Certain neurologic conditions
    Spinal cord injury
    Diabetic neuropathy
    Multiple sclerosis
    Herniated intervertebral disk
    Use of medications

NEUROLOGIC IMPAIRMENT

Without accepting a strict distinction between neurologic and psychogenic sexual impairment, a neurologic origin is reliably indicated by certain elements of the patient's history (Table 16–1) and routine neurologic examination (Table 16–2). Either spinal cord or peripheral nerve injury might lead to a pattern of weakness and sensory loss below the waist or one confined to the genitals, anus, and buttocks—the "saddle area" (Fig. 16–2). Plantar and deep tendon reflex (DTR) testing will indicate which system is responsible: spinal cord injury causes hyperactive DTRs and Babinski signs, whereas peripheral nerve injury causes hypoactive DTRs and no Babinski signs. Both CNS and PNS impairment lead to loss of the relevant "superficial reflexes": scrotal, cremasteric, and anal (Fig. 16–3).

Signs of ANS impairment, which may be subtle, are equally important. A classic sign is *orthostatic hypotension*, which is usually defined as a fall of 10 mm Hg in blood pressure on standing. It is strong evidence of diabetic, medication-induced, or spontaneous ANS impairment. Another sign is *anhidrosis*, lack of sweating, in the groin and legs. It is usually found with hairless and sallow skin, and *urinary incontinence.* Finally, *retrograde ejaculation* can be detected if microscopic examination of urine obtained after orgasm reveals sperm.

Neurologic-induced sexual impairment is frequently accompanied by urinary and fecal incontinence because the bladder, bowel, and genitals share many elements of

TABLE 16–2. *Signs of Neurologic Sexual Impairment*

Signs of spinal cord injury
    Paraparesis or quadriparesis
    Leg spasticity
    Urinary incontinence
Signs of autonomic nervous system injury
    Orthostatic hypotension or lightheadedness
    Anhidrosis in groin and legs
    Urinary incontinence
    Retrograde ejaculation
Signs of peripheral nervous system injury
    Loss of sensation in the genitals, "saddle area," and legs
    Paresis and areflexia in legs
    Scrotal, cremasteric, and anal reflex loss*

*Also found with spinal cord injury.

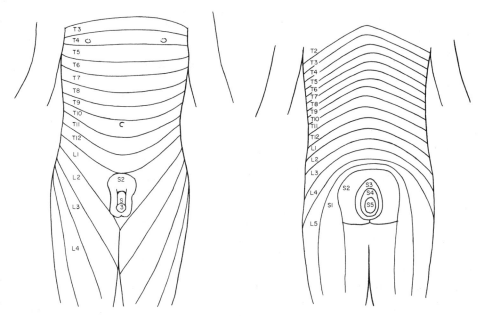

FIGURE 16–2. The sacral dermatomes (S2–S5) innervate the skin overlying the genitals and anus, but the lumbar dermatomes innervate the legs.

spinal cord, PNS, and ANS innervation. The anus, like the bladder, has two sphincters (see Fig. 15–5). The anus' internal sphincter, the more powerful one, is controlled by ANS activity. Sympathetic ANS activity constricts the sphincter, and increased parasympathetic ANS activity relaxes the sphincter. The anus' external sphincter, is under voluntary control through the pudendal nerves and other branches of the S3 and S4 peripheral nerve roots. Thus, to produce a bowel movement, individuals must

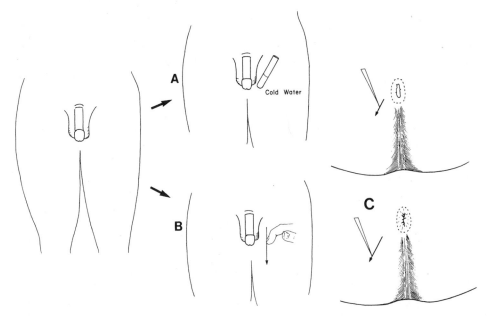

FIGURE 16–3. A, The *scrotal reflex:* Normally when a cold surface is applied to the scrotum, the testicle retracts and the skin surface contracts. B, The *cremasteric reflex:* Likewise, when the inner thigh is stroked, the testicle retracts and the skin surface contracts. C, The *anal reflex:* When the perianal skin is scratched, the anus tightens.

allow the external sphincter to relax, while the internal sphincter, which is under parasympathetic control, simultaneously relaxes.

As could be anticipated, excess sympathetic ANS activity, as in the "flight and fright" model, usually inhibits both urinating and defecating. Moreover, excess sympathetic ANS activity would usually impair sexual arousal and inhibit an erection before orgasm. In addition, excessive sympathetic activity, which might be a manifestation of anxiety, causes premature ejaculation.

Laboratory Tests

Men with suspected erectile dysfunction might choose to undergo a series of tests, but few tests are applicable to women with sexual dysfunction. Sleep-related studies can document the presence or absence of nocturnal erections. Electrical tests can assess the status of the genitals' nerve supply. Vascular tests can measure the blood flow of the penis. These tests may be expensive, painful, and inconclusive. As an alternative, if an affected man's clinical evaluation suggests certain neurologic disorders, he may reasonably elect to dispense with laboratory testing and proceed directly to medical treatment, which might be as simple a taking a pill, before attempting sexual intercourse (see below).

The traditional assumption had been that erectile dysfunction generally resulted from anxiety or another psychologic cause. Modern studies have shown, in view of the results of these laboratory tests and response to simple treatments, that the majority of men with erectile dysfunction—possibly 80%—have an underlying or coexisting neurologic or other physical abnormality. Comparable data about women are not available.

Sleep-Related Studies.   During their rapid eye movement (REM) periods of sleep, from infancy to old age, normal men have erections and other signs of ANS activity. The erections develop during dreams, regardless of their overt content. Thus, normal men have three to five erections lasting about 30 minutes each night. In a standard overnight clinic or hospital-based test, the *nocturnal penile tumescence (NPT) study*, devices monitor the man's erections and correlate them with REM periods during one to three nights. An alternative, "simple stamp" test consists of affixing a ring of postage stamps around the base of the penis at bedtime: a broken ring in the morning indicates that the man developed at least one erection.

When freed from social and psychologic influences during NPT studies, many men who had reported sexual impairment can be shown to have had erections. These men may have a psychogenic sexual dysfunction. In contrast, men who do not develop any erections during NPT studies may be suspected of having a neurologic basis or other "organic cause" of their sexual dysfunction. These men are usually asked to undergo further testing.

A failure to have erections during the NPT study, however, may have alternative explanations, such as profound depression, a sleep disorder, and testing-induced artifacts. In addition, some otherwise normal men inexplicably fail to develop erections during sleep.

Other Tests.   Physicians can assess the blood pressure and blood flow in the dorsal artery of the penis with a small blood pressure cuff, Doppler ultrasound examination, and other devices. These tests may be useful in assessing men with peripheral vascular disease, atherosclerosis, diabetes, or pelvic injuries. On the other hand, a simple, direct test of the patient's vascular status consists of an injection of a vasodilator into the penis (i.e., an intracorporal vasodilator injection). If the injection produces an erection, this result excludes vascular insufficiency as the cause of erectile dysfunction. In fact, injections could provide treatment.

Electrophysiologic studies, such as nerve conduction velocities and evoked potentials, could reveal that a polyneuropathy, pudendal nerve damage, or spinal cord injury is the cause of sexual dysfunction in women, as well as men. In addition, the conduction of the penile nerve can be measured. Electrophysiologic studies are performed most often in patients with diabetes, following prostate surgery, and when trauma or multiple sclerosis (MS) (see Chapter 15) might have injured the spinal cord.

Individuals with an endocrinologic basis of their sexual dysfunction usually have other signs of hormone imbalance. The screening tests usually determine their blood glucose prolactin, testosterone, estrogen, and gonadotropic hormone concentrations. An elevated serum prolactin concentration indicates a pituitary adenoma or tumor. Other tests might reveal hypogonadism, hypothyroidism, diabetes, or a disruption of the hypothalamic-pituitary-gonadal axis.

Medical Treatment of Erectile Dysfunction

Several medications can produce erections adequate for sexual intercourse in spite of neurologic injury or vascular insufficiency. They can also restore erections in men thought to have psychogenic erectile dysfunction.

Yohimbine (Aphrodyne, Yocon, Yohimex), an alpha-2 adrenergic receptor antagonist (see Chapter 21), has been widely prescribed, even though its benefits have never been substantiated in either men or women. It may slightly increase sympathetic vasomotor activity and act as a mild psychologic stimulant that produces an aphrodisiac sensation. However, it may act mostly as a placebo and usually does not promote sexual function. It often causes anxiety.

Testosterone injections have also been popular but have been mostly ineffective. Although they may increase muscle mass, especially in body builders, and provide psychologic stimulation, testosterone injections have no effect on sexual function, unless a man has hypogonadism. In high doses for long periods, they may induce prostate cancer.

In contrast, intracorporal injections of vasoactive medicines have been invasive but helpful. This treatment can induce erections in men with spinal cord damage from trauma or MS, or peripheral nerve damage from prostate surgery, diabetic neuropathy, or vascular disease. The most effective medicines have been a smooth muscle relaxant, papaverine; an alpha-adrenergic blocker, phentolamine (Regitine); and, the most popular, a synthetic prostaglandin E1, alprostadil (Prostin or Caverject). For example, a man with erectile dysfunction can inject these medicines into the base of his corpus cavernosum (the erectile tissue). The pain from the injection, especially with its automated device, is minimal. Alternatively, he can insert a short, thin alprostadil suppository into his urethra, which is initially uncomfortable. These medications promote blood flow into the penis while retarding its outflow. The penis, then congested with blood, widens and elongates. After an orgasm, the erection usually subsides spontaneously during the following one to three hours.

However, in one of the complications of this treatment, persistent erections (priapism) can last for more than eight hours and be uncomfortable and embarrassing. These erections can be aborted with epinephrine injections, which is an α-adrenergic receptor agonist that acts as a vasoconstrictor (see Table 21–2). Patients with spinal cord injury are susceptible to another potential complication of intracorporal vasodilator injections: they tend to have overreaction to the treatment probably because of denervation hypersensitivity.

The new treatment, sildenafil (Viagra) revolutionized the treatment of erectile dysfunction at the same time that it brought to light that approximately 30 million

American men have the problem. Sildenafil greatly assists men with erectile dysfunction from diabetes, multiple sclerosis, spinal cord injury, and nerve damage from prostate surgery. It also helps men with erectile dysfunction associated with decreased libido, depression, and other psychiatric disturbances. Sildenafil partially or completely reverses sexual dysfunction caused by selective serotonin reuptake inhibitors (SSRIs) in both sexes. Otherwise, studies regarding its usefulness in women have not as yet been published.

Sildenafil has a well-established, rational mechanism of action. Under normal circumstances, psychologic or tactile sexual stimulation provokes parasympathetic neurons to produce and release the neurotransmitter nitric oxide (NO) in the penis. NO, in turn, promotes the production of cyclic guanylate cyclase monophosphate (cGMP). The cGMP dilates the vascular system and creates the erection. Sooner or later, an enzyme, cGMP-phosphodiesterase, metabolizes cGMP and the erection subsides. Sildenafil inhibits this enzyme and thus slows the metabolism of cGMP. The increased cGMP concentrations enhance the strength and duration of erections.

The alternatives to medical treatment are rarely satisfactory. Delicate and tedious arterial reconstructive procedures are often performed; however, except in men with localized vascular injuries, the results are disappointing. Surgically implanted devices, such as rigid or semirigid rods or a balloonlike apparatus, can mimic an erection. Unfortunately, they are costly and prone to mechanical failures, infections, or aesthetic difficulties.

ASSOCIATED NEUROLOGIC ILLNESSES

Although most patients with certain neurologic illness have predictable sexual impairments, those with other illnesses, even when incapacitated in many ways, have no sexual impairment. Some textbooks, while technically correct, list dozens of illnesses that can impair sexual function; however, only a few are responsible for the majority of cases.

Spinal Cord Injury

Every year hundreds of teenagers and young adults sustain spinal cord injuries from automobile, diving, horseback riding, and trampoline accidents; knife or bullet wounds; and MS. The spinal cord is also subject to congenital injuries, such as the myelomeningocele (see Chapter 13). Depending on the level of the spinal cord injury and whether the cord is partially or completely transected, patients have an easily recognizable triad of symptoms:

- Paraparesis or quadriparesis with spasticity, hyperactive reflexes, and Babinski signs
- Sensory loss up to a certain spinal level (Fig. 16–2)
- Bladder, bowel, and sexual difficulties

In addition, when the upper cervical cord is damaged, the respiratory center is impaired and the sympathetic nervous system is released from CNS control. Although cerebral sexual pathways remain intact, spinal cord injury is typically associated with anxiety, depressive symptoms, and diminished libido.

Cervical and Thoracic Spinal Cord Injury.   When the cervical spinal cord is severed, quadriparesis develops. When the thoracic portion is severed, paraparesis develops. In both of these injuries, ascending sensory impulses are interrupted, and patients cannot sense genital stimulation. Nevertheless, because the genital-spinal cord reflex remains intact, patients retain the capacity for reflex genital arousal. They can achieve an orgasm even though they are unable to appreciate the sensations.

With these injuries, men's erections are usually too weak for intercourse. If orgasms occur, they may produce an excessive, almost violent ANS response. This *autonomic hyperreflexia* causes hypertension, bradycardia, nausea, and lightheadedness. It can even, rarely, lead to an intracerebral hemorrhage.

Most spinal cord injury patients develop urinary incontinence and constipation that require catheters and enemas. Infections of the urinary tract and decubitus ulcers are constant threats. Men lose fertility because of inadequate and abnormal sperm production. In contrast, women continue to ovulate, menstruate, and retain their capacity to conceive and bear children.

With incomplete spinal cord injuries, as typically occurs in MS and many non-penetrating injuries, neurologic deficits are less pronounced. Still, because of the delicate nature of the neurologic pathways, problems with genital arousal and anorgasmia plague most individuals with incomplete spinal cord injury.

Lumbosacral Spinal Cord Injury.   As with thoracic spinal cord transection, patients with lumbosacral spinal cord injury have paraparesis and incontinence. In addition, because both the genital-spinal cord reflex and descending tracts are interrupted, neither genital nor cerebral stimulation produces arousal or orgasm. Nevertheless, the ANS, which travels in a parallel pathway, may remain undamaged and can continue to innervate the genitals. It preserves fertility in men as well as women. Also in contrast to higher spinal cord injuries, sensation of the breasts and their erotic capacity is preserved—and possibly enhanced—because upper chest sensation is unaffected.

Poliomyelitis and Other Exceptions

Several neurologic illnesses that spare sexual function can be so devastating that the untrained physician might assume that victims are "impotent." Two relatively common motor neuron diseases, poliomyelitis (polio) and amyotrophic lateral sclerosis (ALS), devastate the voluntary motor system. Survivors of polio were often confined to wheelchairs and braces. ALS is a progressively incapacitating illness that is usually fatal in 6 months to 2 years. Nevertheless, these illnesses spare the victim's intellect, sensation, involuntary muscle strength, and ANS. Thus, motor neuron disease patients have normal sexual capacity, genital sensation, bladder and bowel control, fertility, and libido.

Similarly, most extrapyramidal illnesses (see Chapter 18), despite causing difficulties with mobility, also do not impair sexual desire, sexual function, or fertility. For example, Parkinson's disease patients have an intact sexual drive that may be acted upon once dopa-repleting medications are introduced. Moreover, illness-induced impairment of inhibition, as in frontal lobe trauma and Alzheimer's disease, can lead to sexual aggressiveness.

Diabetes Mellitus

Sexual dysfunction, especially retrograde ejaculation and erectile dysfunction, eventually affects almost 50% of diabetic men. It is the first sign of diabetes in about 5% of patients. Diabetic sexual impairment results not only from ANS and PNS injury but also from atherosclerosis of the genital arteries (see below). In addition, urinary incontinence often accompanies sexual dysfunction because the bladder and genitals have a common ANS innervation. The bladder of affected patients is typically large, flaccid, and poorly controlled (Fig. 16–4). Moreover, patients with diabetes-induced sexual dysfunction typically have other manifestations of ANS impairment, such as anhidrosis and orthostatic hypotension. However, they do not necessarily have other complications of diabetes, such as retinopathy, nephropathy, or peripheral vascular disease. Although many diabetic men with erectile dysfunction have low testosterone concentrations, testosterone therapy generally has only a placebo effect.

The few available descriptions of sexual impairment in diabetic women conflict. Some authors found that 35% of diabetic women had anorgasmia and that sexual impairment was related to neuropathy; however, others found that diabetic women were no more prone than nondiabetic ones to sexual impairment and that diabetic women, even with profound neuropathy, had full sexual function. Vaginal infections are undoubtedly more common in diabetic women. In addition, although diabetic

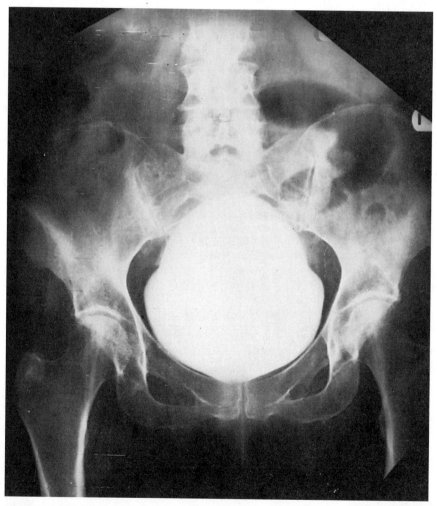

FIGURE 16–4. A patient had diabetes mellitus complicated by impotence and urinary incontinence, which are both typically associated with a large, flaccid bladder. An intravenous pyelogram (IVP) revealed a distended bladder (the large white area). In many conditions, such as diabetes and multiple sclerosis, urinary incontinence and sexual dysfunction develop together. Current tests, such as sonography and CT, show the same information and do not subject patients to infusions of a contrast solution.

women remain fertile, pregnancies are more often complicated by miscarriages and fetal malformations.

Multiple Sclerosis

Sexual impairment can be the most bothersome or even the sole symptom of multiple sclerosis (MS) (see Chapter 15). In typical cases, MS causes premature ejaculation, erectile dysfunction, retrograde ejaculation, and anorgasmia. Early stage MS patients might have few persistent neurologic deficits, but when episodes develop repeatedly, the incidence of sexual impairment, urinary incontinence, and extrasexual deficits all rise dramatically. With advanced MS, women have decreased sexual desire in conjunction with sensory impairments and decreased vaginal lubrication. In 90% of cases, sexual impairments are associated with urinary bladder dysfunction.

Fertility is preserved. Pregnancies do not affect the overall course of MS. Similarly, MS does not complicate the pregnancy or lead to fetal malformations. When women are pregnant, they have a reduced rate of MS exacerbations. However, during the first three postpartum months, the rate of exacerbations increases. Male fertility is impaired by decreased sperm production.

Medication-Induced Impairment

Although over 100 medications have been implicated, only a few categories consistently impair sexual function. The most common offenders are antihypertensive medications, including clonidine (Catapres), thiazide diuretics, and beta-blockers (e.g., propranolol). Fortunately, the newer antihypertensive medications—angiotensin-converting enzyme (ACE) inhibitors and the calcium-channel blockers—cause little or no sexual impairment.

Typical antipsychotic medications cause erectile dysfunction and other sexual impairments. Their side effects are consistent with observations that decreased dopamine leads to sexual dysfunction, but increased dopamine stimulates it. In contrast, clozapine and quetiapine carry a low risk of sexual impairment.

Anticholinergic medications, often given to counteract antipsychotic medication-induced parkinsonism, cause sexual impairment, as well as other bothersome symptoms: cognitive impairments, dry mouth, orthostatic hypotension, accommodation paresis (see Fig. 12–4), and urinary hesitancy (see Fig. 15–5). Clozapine (Clozaril) and trazodone (Desyrel) cause priapism.

Almost all antidepressants—tricyclics, heterocyclics, monoamine oxidase inhibitors, and SSRIs—lead to sexual dysfunction. Medication-induced sexual dysfunction is primarily dose-related. It also correlates with medications' suppression of dopamine activity, as well as their increase in serotonin activity, stimulation of prolactin release, and inhibition of nitric oxide (NO) synthetase. SSRIs are more likely than tricyclic antidepressants to delay or prevent orgasm. They also interfere with erectile function and vaginal lubrication. For any particular SSRI, the rate of adverse sexual side effects greatly varies among different studies. Bupropion (Wellbutrin), which is a relatively strong dopamine reuptake inhibitor, has infrequent sexual side effects.

When SSRIs cause sexual side effects, several options are available. Because the side effects may recede with continued use, the physician can continue to prescribe the SSRI at the same dose for four to six weeks, reduce the dose, prescribe sildenafil as a presex antidote, substitute an SSRI that may be more tolerable, such as nefazodone (Serzone), or substitute an agent from a different class, such as bupropion.

Physicians may capitalize on certain psychotropic medications' delaying orgasm so that they may counter premature ejaculation. For example, clomipramine (Anafranil), sertraline (Zoloft), and trazodone, at least in men, prolong arousal and delay orgasm.

LIBIDO EFFECTS

From a neurologic viewpoint, the *limbic system* is the source of libido (Fig. 16–5). When the limbic system is damaged, usually through injury of the frontal or temporal lobe, hypothalamus, or the entire brain, libido is usually reduced. However, sometimes it is heightened.

The Klüver-Bucy Syndrome

The closest example of a pure limbic system injury is the *Klüver-Bucy syndrome.* This disorder, which is famous and quite dramatic, was first introduced by a laboratory experiment produced in rhesus monkeys. Neurosurgeons performed bilateral anterior temporal lobectomies, which included removal of both amygdalae. Postoperatively, the monkeys displayed increased heterosexual and homosexual activity, aggression, and other behavioral changes. Their increased sexuality was accompanied by continual tactile activity and placing inedible objects in their mouth, which is called "psychic blindness" or *oral exploration* (similar to visual agnosia, see Chapter 12).

A modified form of this syndrome, the *human Klüver-Bucy syndrome,* occasionally develops in both children and adults. As with the monkeys, this syndrome has re-

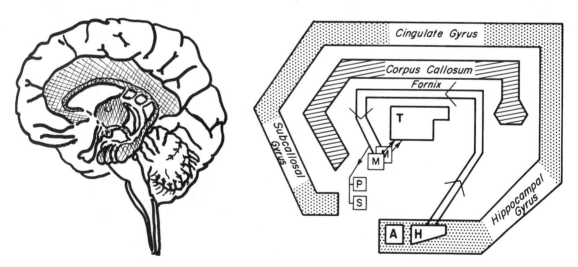

FIGURE 16–5. *Left,* The *limbic system* (shaded) is a circuit deep in the brain that connects with the overlying cerebral cortex. *Right,* This schematic portrayal of the *limbic system* shows its main features:

Hippocampus (H) with the adjacent amygdala (A)
  ↓
Fornix
  ↓
Mamillary bodies (M) that send off a mamillothalamic tract
  ↓
Anterior nucleus of the thalamus (T)
  ↓
Cingulate gyrus that connects to the overlying cerebral cortex and back to the hippocampus ↑

sulted from bilateral temporal lobe damage; however, the causes in humans have been Herpes simplex encephalitis, Pick's disease and other forms of frontotemporal dementia, infarctions of both posterior cerebral arteries, head trauma, and Alzheimer's disease. People with the Klüver-Bucy syndrome, like the experimental monkeys, tend to eat excessively and show oral exploration. Instead of excessive eating, they sometimes smoke or drink in excess or compulsively.

In other respects, the human syndrome differs considerably from the animal model. Despite their oral tendencies, the patients rarely become obese. Only about one-half of Klüver-Bucy syndrome patients show any increase in heterosexual activity or masturbation. Most of them only make suggestive gestures. Whatever their sexual proclivities, patients are more handicapped by other manifestations of temporal lobe injury, such as memory impairment (amnesia), aphasia, and dementia. In particular, children who develop the Klüver-Bucy syndrome, which usually results from hypoxic cerebral damage, are most impaired by the amnesia.

Other Conditions

Certain medications that act as stimulants, including hallucinogens, amyl nitrate, and L-dopa preparations, can increase sexual interest or increase sexual activity. Of course, numerous substances are purported to have aphrodisiac qualities, but their effect is minimal or nil, and many may be dangerous. (Sildenafil, despite its ability to enhance sexuality, is not an aphrodisiac because it requires stimulation to be effective and does not affect the libido.)

A different mechanism can produce the same effect: damage to cerebral centers that ordinarily inhibit sexual activity can increase sexual interest or unleash suppressed sexual impulses. For example, Alzheimer's disease and Parkinson's disease patients occasionally increase their sexual activity from a loss of cerebral inhibition. These patients usually have other inhibited behavior and at least moderate cognitive impairment.

Otherwise, most neurologic damage decreases the libido. Lesions of the pituitary, hypothalamus, and diencephalon have been associated with hypersexuality; however, usually these injuries cause hyposexuality. For example, the Wernicke-Korsakoff syndrome and transient global amnesia, conditions in which limbic system structures are injured, are characterized by amnesia, not libido changes. Lesions in this region also lead to appetite changes in either direction accompanying alterations in libido. For example, in Sheehan's syndrome (see Chapter 19), women lose weight and have other physical and mental signs of hypothalamic-pituitary insufficiency, but with hypothalamic tumors, patients typically have ravenous appetites.

Partial complex epilepsy, which originates in temporal lobe dysfunction in most cases, is sometimes associated with simple actions that appear to be sexual to some degree. During seizures, patients may seem to engage in rudimentary masturbation or even partially undress; however, they do not engage in any franker sexual activity. During interictal periods, these patients are prone to hyposexuality (see Chapter 10).

The libido is also indirectly vulnerable to neurologic impairments that lessen sexual satisfaction. For example, some men with MS or diabetes who have chronic erectile dysfunction often suppress their sexual desires, as through a "negative feedback loop." On the other hand, sexual desire was found to be similar in women with and without physically disabilities.

Although the libido resists mild fatigue, hunger, and fear, it is almost always dampened by pain. In addition, patients with chronic pain may have an associated depression or use potent analgesics that produce sexual dysfunction.

REFERENCES

Abramowicz M (ed): Yohimbine for male sexual dysfunction. Med Lett *36*: 115–116, 1994

Berman JR, Berman L, Goldstein I: Female sexual dysfunction: incidence, pathophysiology, evaluation, and treatment options. Urology *54*: 385–391, 1999

Goldstein I, Lue TF, Padma-Nathan H, et al: Oral sildenafil in the treatment of erectile dysfunction. N Engl J Med *338*: 1397–1404, 1998

Harrison J, Glass CA, Owens RG, et al: Factors associated with sexual functioning in women following spinal cord injury. Paraplegia *33*: 687–692, 1995

Hulter BM, Lundberg PO: Sexual function in women with advanced multiple sclerosis. J Neurol Neurosurg Psychiatry *59*: 83–86, 1995

Kim SC, Seo KK: Efficacy and safety of fluoxetine, sertraline, and clomipramine in patients with premature ejaculation: A double-blind, placebo controlled study. J Urol *159*: 425–427, 1998

Lilly R, Cummings JL, Benson DF, et al: The human Klüver-Bucy syndrome. Neurology *33*: 1141–1145, 1983

Madoff RD, Williams JG, Caushaj PF: Fecal incontinence. N Engl J Med *326*: 1002–1007, 1992

Nosek MA, Rintala DH, Young ME, et al: Sexual functioning among women with physical disabilities. Arch Phys Med Rehabil *77*: 107–115, 1996

Padma-Nathan H, Hellstrom WJG, Kaiser FE, et al: Treatment of men with erectile dysfunction with transurethral alprostadil. N Engl J Med *336*: 1–7, 1997

Piletz JE, Segraves KB, Feng YZ, et al: Plasma MHPG response to yohimbine in women with hypoactive sexual desire. J Sex Marital Ther *24*: 43–54, 1998

Report of the Therapeutics and Technology Assessment Subcommittee of the American Academy of Neurology: Assessment: Neurologic evaluation of male sexual dysfunction. Neurology *45*: 2287–2292, 1995

Rosen RC, Lane RM, Menza M: Effects of SSRIs on sexual function: A critical review. J Clin Psychopharmacology *19*: 67–85, 1999

Salloway S, Malloy P, Cummings JL (eds): The Neuropsychiatry of Limbic and Subcortical Disorders. Washington, American Psychiatric Press, 1997

Tonsgard JH, Harwicke N, Levine SC: Klüver-Bucy syndrome in children. Pediatr Neurol *3*: 162–165, 1987

QUESTIONS and ANSWERS: CHAPTER 16

1. A 40-year-old man complains of long-standing erectile dysfunction. He has severe low back pain, mild hypertension, and borderline diabetes. Which condition should be considered as possible causes of his sexual dysfunction?

a. Herniated lumbar intervertebral disk
b. Antihypertensive medications
c. Diabetic neuropathy
d. Psychogenic factors
e. Narcotic analgesics
f. All of the above

ANSWER: f. This man might have sexual impairment because of the various medical or psychogenic disorders.

2. A 24-year-old man who complains of premature ejaculation also had episodes of unsteady gait, diplopia, and paraparesis. Which of the following might a neurologic examination reveal?

a. Internuclear ophthalmoplegia
b. Absent abdominal reflexes
c. Ataxia of gait
d. Babinski signs
e. Hyperactive deep tendon reflexes (DTRs)
f. All of the above

ANSWER: f. The patient is likely to have multiple sclerosis (MS) with cerebellar, brainstem, and spinal cord involvement. Between episodes, when the patient is likely to have residual neurologic signs (a–e), including sexual dysfunction. Premature ejaculation and erectile dysfunction are often manifestations—and possibly the only ones—of quiescent MS that has affected the spinal cord. MS is only one of numerous potential disorders of the spinal cord that can disrupt its intricate, delicate pathways.

3. Which one of the following conditions might cause retrograde ejaculation?

a. Ovarian dysfunction
b. Diabetic autonomic neuropathy
c. Psychogenic influence
d. Yohimbine
e. Sexual inexperience
f. All of the above

ANSWER: b. In retrograde ejaculation, semen is propelled by involuntary mechanisms into the bladder instead of the urethra. It is always the result of neurologic, muscular, or other organic impairment—particularly autonomic nervous system dysfunction.

4. In which illnesses might a physician assume that sexual dysfunction has a neurologic basis?

a. XYY syndrome
b. Mild mental retardation
c. Parkinson's disease
d. Poliomyelitis
e. Amyotrophic lateral sclerosis
f. None of the above

ANSWER: f. Although each of these illnesses may cause weakness, the patient's sexual drive, genital sensation, and orgasmic reactions are all preserved.

5. In which three illnesses is medication-induced sexual dysfunction likely to be encountered?

a. Psychosis
b. Migraine headache
c. Hypertension
d. Low back pain
e. Duodenal ulcer
f. Glaucoma

ANSWER: a, c, e. Medications that cause sexual impairments are usually antihypertensive medications and those with systemic anticholinergic properties, including neuroleptics and ulcer therapies.

6. During sleep, when do erections and emissions occur?

a. NREM stages 1 and 2
b. NREM stages 3 and 4
c. REM
d. All of the above

ANSWER: c. Erections and emissions occur during REM sleep. Erections are also characteristically present on awakening.

7. In which situation is fertility lost?

a. Women with cervical spinal cord transection
b. Men with cervical spinal cord transection
c. Men with diabetes mellitus and neuropathy
d. Women with diabetes mellitus and neuropathy

ANSWER: b. Men with upper spinal cord injury have reduced concentration and abnormalities of their sperm. Women are able to conceive and bear children despite spinal cord injury. Both men and women with diabetes remain fertile.

8. A 43-year-old man describes several days of erectile dysfunction each time he completes a bicycle ride of several hours. A less severe impairment follows his practicing on a stationary bicycle. He has no diabetes and takes no medications. Which is the most likely cause of his sexual difficulty?

a. Compression of the pudendal nerve
b. Excessive sympathetic autonomic nervous system
c. A muscle disorder
d. Excessive parasympathetic autonomic nervous system
e. Psychologic factors

ANSWER: a. He has a classic case of compression of the pudendal nerve between the seat and his symphysis pubis when he rides his bicycle. Sometimes bicycle riders compress the vessels, which can also cause erectile dysfunction. Such nerve or vessel compression is a relatively common cause of sexual dysfunction.

9. In which two conditions would cremasteric reflexes be lost?

a. Diabetic autonomic neuropathy
b. Anxiety
c. Sacral spinal cord injury
d. Frontal meningiomas

ANSWER: a, c. Cremasteric reflexes, which are "superficial reflexes" rather than DTRs, require that the pudendal nerves, autonomic nervous system, and spinal cord be intact.

10. One month after falling down a flight of stairs, a 35-year-old man complains of low back pain and erectile dysfunction. Examination reveals loss of pinprick sensation from the waist down to the toes but intact position, vibratory, and warm-cold sensation. Deep tendon and cremasteric reflexes are intact, and plantar reflexes are flexion. Which is the most likely cause of the erectile dysfunction?

a. Spinal cord injury
b. Autonomic nervous system dysfunction
c. Peripheral neuropathy
d. Multiple sclerosis
e. Alcoholism
f. None of the above

ANSWER: f. The lack of objective neurologic deficit indicates that no neurologic injury has occurred. In fact, a structural lesion cannot cause the dissociation of pinprick and warm-cold sensation because both sensations travel in the same nerve pathways. Alcoholism may blunt the libido and cause a neuropathy. In alcoholic peripheral neuropathy, DTRs and sensation are lost.

11. In monkeys, which is not a component of the Klüver-Bucy syndrome?

a. Psychic blindness
b. Apathy
c. Frontal lobectomy
d. Loss of amygdalae
e. Increased homosexual, heterosexual, and autosexual activity

ANSWER: c. After temporal lobectomy including removal of the amygdalae, monkeys have oral exploratory behavior. They are said to have visual agnosia because they do not identify objects by their appearance even though their vision is intact. The monkeys characteristically lose extreme emotion. Sometimes appearing fearless, they are actually apathetic. Most striking, they have increased and indiscriminate sexual activity.

12. In humans who have had bilateral temporal lobe damage, which two of the following conditions are almost always found?

a. Memory impairment
b. Placing food and inedible objects in their mouths
c. Hypersexuality
d. Rage attacks
e. Obesity

ANSWER: a, b. The human variety of the Klüver-Bucy syndrome is characterized by impaired memory, a tendency to eat excessively, and, like monkeys, placing inedible objects in their mouths. Contrary to expectations, these people have little increased sexual appetite or violent outbursts. Even though they eat excessively and put inanimate objects into their mouth, they are usually not obese.

13. Which one of these conditions does not usually damage the limbic system in humans?

a. *Herpes simplex*
b. Alcoholism
c. TIAs of the posterior cerebral arteries
d. *Herpes zoster*
e. Frontotemporal dementia

ANSWER: d. Because the amygdala and hippocampus are situated in the temporal lobes, these limbic system structures are vulnerable to conditions that damage the temporal lobe. *Herpes simplex* virus, which has a predilection for the frontal and temporal lobes, is a frequent cause of encephalitis characterized by memory impairment and partial complex seizures. Although *herpes zoster* often causes painful neuralgia in the trigeminal nerve distribution, it usually does not infect the CNS. Posterior cerebral TIAs cause ischemia of the temporal lobes. These TIAs induce episodes of confusion and memory impairment that are called "transient global amnesia." Chronic alcohol abuse can cause the Wernicke-Korsakoff syndrome, which is associated with hemorrhage into the mamillary bodies and other parts of the limbic system. Frontotemporal dementia, which includes Pick's disease, causes early and severe atrophy of the frontal and temporal lobes.

14. Which two of the following are not consequences of a pituitary microadenoma?

a. Headaches
b. Hyperprolactinemia
c. Optic atrophy
d. Homonymous superior quadrantanopia
e. Infertility
f. Irregular menses

ANSWER: c, d. Optic atrophy and homonymous superior quadrantanopia are manifestations of large (macroscopic) pituitary adenomas. Microadenomas can cause headaches, hyperprolactinemia, and infertility.

15. In normal males, which of the following is not associated with REM-induced erections?

a. Dreams with or without overt sexual content
b. Most dreams with even frightful or anxiety-producing content
c. Increased pulse and blood pressure
d. Increased testosterone level
e. An EEG that appears, aside from eye movement artifact, as though the patient were awake

ANSWER: d. In REM sleep, individuals have increased ANS activity and an EEG that has ocular movement artifact superimposed on an "awake" background pattern.

16. In the treatment of men with erectile dysfunction, an intracorporal injection of which substance will abort a medication-induced erection?

a. Epinephrine
b. Phentolamine
c. Papaverine
d. Prostaglandins

ANSWER: a. In men who have erectile dysfunction because of multiple sclerosis, diabetes, spinal cord injury, or many other illnesses, injections into the dorsum of the penis (intracorporal injections) of phentolamine (Regitine), papaverine, or prostaglandins, which are vasodilators, will produce an erection. The injections are so effective that they may be appropriate in some men with psychogenic erectile dysfunction. However, they must be used with caution in men with vascular disease or spinal cord injury. They can be complicated by priapism, which can be terminated by an injection of epinephrine, which is a vasoconstrictor.

17. What is the origin of the sympathetic autonomic nervous system supply of the sexual organs?

a. Lower cranial nerves
b. Cervical and upper thoracic spinal cord
c. Lower thoracic and upper lumbar spinal cord
d. Sacral spinal cord

ANSWER: c

18. What is the origin of the parasympathetic autonomic nervous system supply of the sexual organs?

a. Lower cranial nerves
b. Cervical and upper thoracic spinal cord
c. Lower thoracic and upper lumbar spinal cord
d. Sacral spinal cord

ANSWER: d

19. What is the effect of hyperprolactinemia?

a. Increased libido
b. Decreased libido
c. Priapism
d. Erectile dysfunction

ANSWER: b

20. What is the mechanism of action of sildenafil (Viagra)?

a. It provokes the release of nitric oxide (NO).
b. It promotes the production of cyclic guanylate cyclase monophosphate (cGMP).

c. It enhances cGMP-phosphodiesterase, which metabolizes cGMP.
d. By inhibiting cGMP-phosphodiesterase, it increases or prolongs cGMP activity.

ANSWER: d. Sildenafil (Viagra) inhibits the enzyme cGMP-phosphodiesterase. Increased or prolonged cGMP activity promotes genital blood flow.

21. Which president survived poliomyelitis (polio)?

a. J. Carter
b. T. Roosevelt
c. F.D. Roosevelt
d. J.F. Kennedy

ANSWER: c. As a young man, FDR contracted polio. When president, he required heavy braces for his legs and eventually was confined to a wheelchair. Polio is an example of a neurologic illness that causes marked disability but spares intellectual and sexual abilities.

22. Which of the following sequences is the generally described path of the limbic system?

a. Fornix, mamillothalamic tract, amygdala, anterior nucleus of the thalamus, cingulate gyrus
b. Cingulate gyrus, mamillary bodies, mamillothalamic tract, anterior nucleus of the thalamus, hippocampus and adjacent amygdala
c. Hippocampus and adjacent amygdala, fornix mamillary bodies, mamillothalamic tract, anterior nucleus of the thalamus, cingulate gyrus
d. Hippocampus and adjacent amygdala, mamillothalamic tract, fornix, hippocampus and adjacent amygdala, mamillary bodies, anterior nucleus of the thalamus, cingulate gyrus

ANSWER: c

23. During sexual function, which of the following acts as the neurotransmitter for *sympathetic* nervous system activity?

a. Acetylcholine
b. Monoamines
c. Serotonin
d. Nitric oxide

ANSWER: b. Monoamines, such as norepinephrine, are the neurotransmitters in the sympathetic system.

24. During sexual function, which of the following act as the neurotransmitter for *parasympathetic* nervous system activity?

a. Acetylcholine
b. Monoamines
c. Serotonin
d. Dopamine

ANSWER: a. Acetylcholine is the neurotransmitter in the parasympathetic system. The actual genital engorgement may be initiated by nitric oxide (NO).

25. A 45-year-old diabetic man who is being evaluated for erectile dysfunction fails to have erections during a NPT study. Which of the following is the least likely explanation?

a. Profound depression
b. A sleep disorder
c. Use of medications or alcohol
d. Anxiety

ANSWER: d. Men with anxiety-induced or other psychologic erectile dysfunction, as well as normal men, typically develop erections during REM sleep, which can be documented during NPT studies. An absence of erections, however, does not necessarily mean that men have a serious neurologic or vascular disease. Erectile dysfunction during NPT studies can also be due to profound depression, a sleep disorder (especially ones that abolish REM sleep), and long-term use of certain medications or alcohol.

26. Which autonomic nervous system activity produces an erection?

a. Increased parasympathetic tone
b. Decreased parasympathetic tone
c. Increased sympathetic tone
d. Decreased sympathetic tone

ANSWER: a

27. Which autonomic nervous system activity produces ejaculation?

a. Increased parasympathetic tone

b. Decreased parasympathetic tone

c. Increased sympathetic tone

d. Decreased sympathetic tone

> *ANSWER:* c. Under normal circumstances, a switch from predominately parasympathetic to sympathetic tone advances the sexual response from arousal to orgasm. In highly anxious individuals, excessive sympathetic activity may suppress an erection or, if one occurs, precipitate a premature ejaculation.

17

Sleep Disorders

Sleep and its stages are defined by physiologic information that is almost entirely derived from a monitoring system, the *polysomnogram (PSG)*. In sleeping individuals, the PSG simultaneously records (a) cerebral activity through several electroencephalogram (EEG) channels; (b) ocular movement through an electro-oculogram (EOG); (c) chin, limb, or other muscle movement and tone through an electromyogram (EMG); and (d) oxygen saturation and other vital signs.

The discipline of sleep studies rests on the distinction between two phases of sleep detected by the PSG. In one phase, *rapid eye movement (REM) sleep*, dreaming and flaccid limb paralysis accompany eye movements that are rapid, conjugate, and predominantly horizontal. The other phase, *nonrapid eye movement (NREM) sleep*, consists of relatively long stretches of essentially dreamless sleep and, approximately every 15 minutes, repositioning movements of the body (Table 17–1).

NORMAL SLEEP

REM Sleep

Because most people awakened during a REM period report that they were having a dream, REM sleep has become synonymous with dreaming. Dreams during REM sleep are intellectually complex, at least on a superficial level, and rich in visual imagery. The vigorous eye movements are attributed to people watching or feeling themselves participating in a dream.

Except for the eye movements and normal breathing, people in REM sleep are immobile and their muscles are paretic, areflexic, and flaccid. EMGs recorded from chin and limb muscles, which is standard placement, show no electric activity (Fig. 17–1). The paralysis is fortuitous because it normally prevents people from acting on their dreams.

In marked contrast to the extensive muscle paralysis, the autonomic nervous system activity (ANS) becomes highly active. REM sleep produces increased pulse, elevated blood pressure, raised intracranial pressure, increased cerebral blood flow, greater muscle metabolism, and, in men, erections. As though defying psychoanalytic interpretation, erections develop regardless of the content of boys' and men's dreams. ANS activity during REM sleep is so intense that REM sleep has been labeled "activated" or "paradoxical sleep." In fact, REM-induced ANS activity has been implicated in the increased incidence of myocardial infarctions and ischemic strokes that develop between 6:00 AM and 11:00 AM.

The EEG is also surprisingly active during REM sleep. Aside from eye-movement artifact, the REM-induced EEG is similar to EEGs in wakefulness. Overall, REM sleep with its bodily activities and EEG, although not the EMG, is more similar to wakefulness than to NREM sleep.

Nuclei in the pons generate several physical elements of REM sleep. The pontine vestibular nuclei generate the rapid eye movements. At the same time, a region im-

TABLE 17–1. *Normal Sleep*

Stage	Bodily Movements	Ocular Movements	EMG	EEG
NREM				
1 Light	Persistent face and limb tone with repositioning every 15–20 minutes	Slow, rolling	Continual activity	Loss of alpha (8–12 Hz) activity
2 Intermediate	Same	Slow, rolling	Further reduction	Sleep spindles and K complexes
3 Slow-wave, deep, delta	Same	Slow, rolling	Further reduction	Increased proportion of slow-wave (1–3 Hz) activity
4 Slow-wave, deep, delta	Same	Slow, rolling	Further reduction	Greatest proportion of slow-wave activity
REM Activated, paradoxical	Flaccid, areflexic paresis, except for brief face and limb movements	Rapid, conjugate	Silent	Low-voltage fast with ocular movement artifacts

mediate adjacent to the pons' locus ceruleus completely suppresses muscle tone (see Chapter 21). In other words, an active process, rather than simply reduction of normal muscle tone, produces the flaccid paresis during REM sleep.

On a biochemical level, REM sleep is associated with increased acetylcholine (cholinergic) activity. Thus, cholinergic agonists, such as arecoline, physostigmine, and nicotine, induce or enhance REM activity. In contrast, anticholinergic medications, including antidepressants with anticholinergic activity, suppress it. REM sleep is associated with decreased activity of dopamine, norepinephrine, and epinephrine (adrenergic systems).

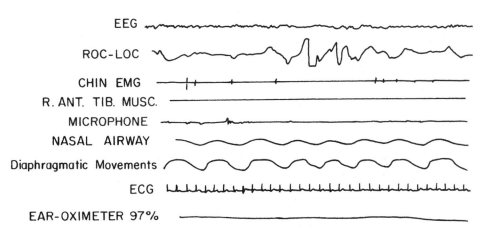

FIGURE 17–1. Polysomnography (PSG) of REM sleep displays nine channels, which each monitor a physiologic function. Depending on the clinical problem, even more could have been added. The EEG has low-voltage, fast activity that is similar to the EEG activity of individuals when they are awake. The electro-oculogram (EOG) channel—ROC-LOC—reflects several rapid eye movements (REM) by large-scale, quick fluctuations. Electromyograms (EMGs) of the chin and right anterior tibialis muscles show virtually no activity, which indicates an absence of muscle movement and tone (flaccid paresis). The microphone detects a little noise, which is probably a snore. The regular, undulating airway and diaphragm recordings indicate normal breathing and air movement.

NREM Sleep

NREM sleep, in contrast to REM sleep, is divided into four stages that are distinguished by progressively greater depths of unconsciousness and slower, higher-voltage EEG patterns. In early NREM sleep, the eyes roll slowly and thinking is brief, rudimentary, and readily forgotten. Unlike people's ability to recall dreams from REM sleep, the NREM period is characterized by amnesia for whatever thought processes take place during it. In NREM sleep, bodily repositioning movements are conspicuous. Relatively normal muscle tone persists, and DTRs can be elicited. EMG activity is detectable in the chin and limb muscles (Fig. 17–2).

People in NREM sleep, unlike those in REM sleep, have a generalized decrease in ANS function accompanied by hypotension and bradycardia. Similarly, cerebral blood flow and oxygen metabolism fall to about 75% of the awake state, which is the level produced by light anesthesia.

Nevertheless, important hypothalamic-pituitary (neuroendocrine) activity ensues. The daily secretion of growth hormone occurs almost entirely during NREM sleep, about 30 to 60 minutes after sleep begins. Likewise, serum prolactin concentration is highest soon after sleep begins. In contrast, cortisol is secreted in 5 to 7 discrete late nighttime episodes, which accumulate to yield the day's highest cortisol concentration at about 8:00 AM.

Overall, the third and fourth stages of NREM sleep, which are called *slow-wave*, *delta*, or *deep NREM* sleep, provide most of the physical recuperation derived from a night's sleep. As if the immediate role of sleep were to revitalize the body, slow-wave sleep occurs predominantly in the early night. After "squeezing in" slow-wave sleep at the beginning of the night, the remaining sleep becomes lighter and more dream-filled.

NREM sleep is associated with increased serotonin and noradrenergic activity. The activity of these neurotransmitters may be more influential in terminating REM sleep than initiating NREM sleep.

Patterns

After retiring, people usually fall asleep within 10 to 20 minutes. The interval, sleep *latency*, is inversely related to sleepiness: the shorter the interval, the greater the sleepiness. During daytime, sleep latency is actually shortest at 4:00 PM but is potentially altered by numerous psychologic and physical factors. In general, adolescents, who never seem to want to sleep, have the longest sleep latency. Latencies are rela-

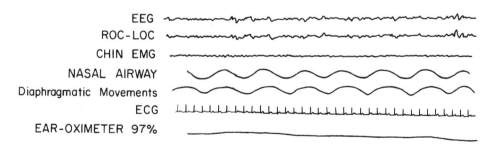

FIGURE 17–2. PSG of stage I NREM sleep reveals slow EEG activity. Stages 3 and 4 NREM sleep (slow-wave sleep) would show higher-voltage, slower EEG activity. The ROC-LOC channel shows virtually no ocular movement (i.e., no REM activity). Continual, low-voltage EMG activity in the chin muscles reflects persistent muscle tone.

TABLE 17–2. *Sleep Latency Changes in Sleep Disorders*

Shortened sleep latency*
  Alcohol- and drug-induced sleep
  Narcolepsy
  Sleep apnea
  Sleep deprivation
Prolonged sleep latency
  Delayed sleep phase syndrome
  Inadequate sleep hygiene
  Psychiatric disorders
      Acute schizophrenia
      Major depression
      Mania
  Restless leg syndrome

*Normal sleep latency is 10 to 20 minutes.

tively short in elderly people, college students, and individuals with specific sleep disorders (Table 17–2).

Once asleep, normal individuals enter NREM sleep and pass in succession through its four stages. After 90 minutes to 120 minutes of NREM sleep, they enter the initial REM period. The interval from falling asleep to the first REM period is called *REM latency*. Determining the REM latency can be helpful in diagnosing many sleep disorders, especially narcolepsy (Table 17–3).

Bedtime   Sleep   First REM period

◄──────────────────► ◄──────────────────►

Sleep latency (10–20 min)   REM latency (90–120 min)

The NREM-REM cycle repeats itself throughout the night with a periodicity of approximately 90 minutes. REM periods occur 4 or 5 times nightly and are progressively longer and more frequent (Fig. 17–3). In later sleep, when the tendency toward REM sleep is the greatest, the body's temperature falls to the day's lowest point (the nadir). The final REM period can merge with awakening. Consequently, surrounding morning household activities may influence a person's final dream. In addition, on awakening, men usually have erections.

Without external clues, an "internal biological clock," which is centered in the *suprachiasmatic nucleus* of the hypothalamus, would set individuals' daily *(circadian)* cycles at 24.5 to 25 hours (Fig. 17–4). When individuals are forced to rely exclusively on their internal biologic clocks, such as if they participate in experiments that isolate them in caves, they gradually lengthen their cycle to almost 25 hours and go to sleep later each day.

TABLE 17–3. *Causes of Shortened or Sleep-Onset REM Latency**

Depression
Narcolepsy
Sleep apnea
Sleep deprivation†
Withdrawal from alcohol, hypnotics, tricyclic antidepressants

*Normal REM latency is about 90 to 120 minutes.
†As part of REM rebound.

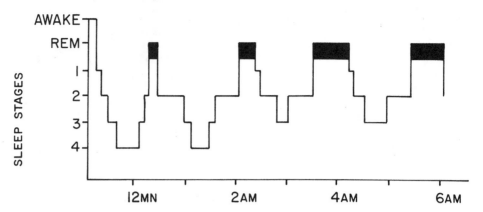

FIGURE 17–3. In the conventional representation of a normal night's sleep pattern—its sleep *architecture*—the first REM period starts about 90 minutes after sleep begins and has a duration of approximately 10 minutes. Later in the night, REM periods recur more frequently and have longer duration. NREM sleep progresses through regular, progressively lighter stages.

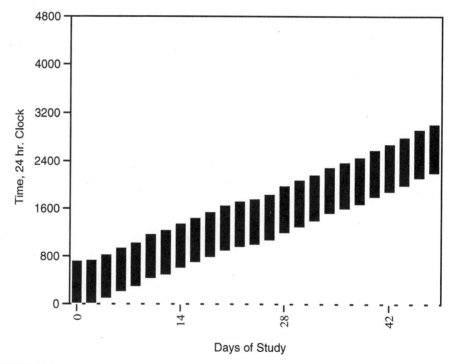

FIGURE 17–4. In experiments, healthy, young adults are allowed to *free run:* sleep and arise at will in rooms sequestered from time cues, such as clocks, daylight, daytime sounds, delivery of meals on a fixed schedule. Individuals in this situation typically go to sleep later each day (delay their sleep phase) and extend their sleep-wake (circadian) cycle to 24.5 to 25 hours. As shown in this sleep graph, a typical circadian duration extends to almost 24.5 hours.

The average adult has a total sleep time of 7.5 to 8 hours, with a range of 4 to 10 hours. Although an individual's total sleep requirement seems to be genetically based, the actual total sleep time is determined predominantly by the environment's light-dark timing and immediate social and occupational conventions.

Melatonin. The environment's light-dark cycles regulate the sleep-wake cycle in part through their effect on the pineal gland's synthesis and release of melatonin (*N*-acetyl-5-methoxytryptamine). Melatonin possibly regulates the suprachiasmatic nucleus of the hypothalamus through melatonin receptors on its surface.

The pineal gland synthesizes melatonin, which is an indolamine, through the following pathway:

Tryptophan → Serotonin → *N*-acetyl-serotonin → Melatonin.

Darkness promotes melatonin synthesis and its release into the plasma. Thus, high melatonin concentrations are found at night. Either natural or artificial light suppresses melatonin synthesis and release. Because of its relationship to light, melatonin may play a role in seasonal affective disorder.

Medications that increase melatonin concentration include noradrenergic and selective serotonin reuptake inhibitors (SSRIs) and neuroleptics. Factors that decrease melatonin concentration include benzodiazepines, monoamine depleting medications, and tryptophan deficiency.

Melatonin, as a medication, increases sleepiness and may be useful in treating conditions characterized by insomnia (see below). It may be particularly useful for blind individuals who would benefit from medications that, in at least a small way, re-created physiologic changes induced by light and dark.

Sleep Deprivation. In the conventional 24-hour-a-day world, important changes can be observed after sleep deprivation. Adults who have worked all night and children who skip a customary afternoon nap, for example, have predictable sleep pattern alterations: a short sleep latency, increased sleep time, and more slow-wave sleep.

In addition, they have a characteristic *REM rebound*, which has several components: the first REM period occurs soon or immediately after falling asleep *(sleep onset REM)*; subsequent REM periods are longer than normal; and REM sleep occupies a greater proportion of sleep time. Also, sleep-deprived individuals often have sleep paralysis on awakening. In other words, after missing sleep, people usually fall asleep almost immediately, soon start to dream, then recoup their dreamtime, and sleep late the next morning. As could be anticipated, REM rebound also occurs after withdrawal from REM-suppressing substances, such as alcohol, hypnotics, cocaine and amphetamine, and tricyclic antidepressants (Table 17–3).

Effects of Age

The first REM-NREM cycles can be detected in the 20-week fetus. Neonates sleep 16 to 20 hours a day, with about 50% of that time spent in REM sleep. As individuals mature, they spend less total time sleeping and proportionately less in dreaming. Young children spend 10 to 12 hours sleeping during the night and in afternoon naps, with about 30% in REM sleep. By age 6 years, however, they give up their afternoon nap to consolidate their sleep into the night.

Adolescents and teenagers allow themselves less time for sleep, despite their great need for sleep. In addition, they have erratic sleep patterns that are strongly influenced by social "cues."

Adults average 6 to 8 hours of total sleep time with 20% to 28% in REM sleep. Adults who are accustomed to relatively little sleep increase the proportion of slow-wave NREM sleep. In other words, the *quantity* of their slow-wave NREM sleep tends to be preserved at the expense of their REM and lighter stages of NREM sleep.

The elderly sleep somewhat less than young adults. Their nighttime sleep is shorter and fragmented by multiple brief awakenings, especially in the early morning. They recoup their sleep during daytime naps not only after meals, in the late afternoon, and other periods of normal sleepiness but also irresistibly at any time, including during social activities. In what is termed *phase*-advanced sleep, they go to sleep in the earlier evening and awaken earlier in the early morning than they did as younger adults. Thus, early morning awakening—as an isolated symptom—in an elderly person does not necessarily represent depression.

Another aspect of sleep in the elderly is decreased total REM time. Moreover, REM periods, instead of being longer and more frequent in the later night, do not change in duration or frequency. During REM sleep, often because of their use of hypnotics and certain medications, such as L-dopa, the elderly have relatively frequent nightmares. NREM sleep, especially its slow-wave phase, also diminishes in the elderly. In fact, slow-wave sleep shows the greatest loss as a percent of total sleep time. It almost entirely disappears in people older than 75 years. Unlike in younger adults, reductions in the sleep of elderly individuals are taken at the expense of slow-wave NREM sleep.

In addition to these normal variations, people older than 55 years are prone to certain sleep disorders, including various leg movement disorders, REM behavior disorder, and sleep apnea syndrome (see below). Also, they are subject to sleep disturbances induced by medications, medical disorders, especially cardiovascular disturbances, pain, depression, dementia, and other neurologic illnesses.

SLEEP DISORDERS

Neurologists, as well as the academic "sleep community," follow the *International Classification of Sleep Disorders* manual, which is, for the most part, consistent with the *Diagnostic and Statistical Manual-IV (DSM-IV)*. Both are based on the three major categories of sleep disorders (Table 17–4):

- Dyssomnias
- Parasomnias
- Medical/Psychiatric Disorders

DYSSOMNIAS

The dyssomnias are sleep disorders that either impair initiating or maintaining sleep (falling asleep or staying asleep) or cause *excessive daytime sleepiness (EDS)*. This category is divided into *Intrinsic, Extrinsic*, and *Circadian Disorders*.

Intrinsic Sleep Disorders

Intrinsic Sleep Disorders are important, discrete, and well-established neurophysiologic disturbances. Patients typically come to medical attention because of EDS.

Narcolepsy.   Narcolepsy, the most dramatic of the Intrinsic Disorders, starts in 90% of patients between their adolescence and 25th year, with men and women

TABLE 17–4. *Classifications of Sleep Disorders**

American Sleep Disorders Association	*DSM-IV*
1. Dyssomnias	1. Primary Sleep Disorders
A. Intrinsic	A. Dyssomnias
Insomnia	Primary Insomnia
Psychophysiological	
Idiopathic	
Narcolepsy	Narcolepsy
Sleep Apnea Syndrome	Breathing-Related Sleep Disorder
Periodic Limb Movements	
Restless Legs Syndrome	
Hypersomnias	Primary Hypersomnia
B. Extrinsic	
Inadequate Sleep Hygiene	
Environmental Sleep Disorder	
Hypnotic, Stimulant, Alcohol, and Toxin	
Dependency	
C. Circadian	Circadian Rhythm Sleep Disorder
Time Zone Change (Jet Lag)	
Shift Work	
Delayed Sleep Phase	
2. Parasomnias	B. Parasomnias
A. Arousal Disorders	
Confusional Arousals	
Sleep Terrors	Sleep Terror Disorder
Sleepwalking	Sleepwalking Disorder
B. Sleep-Wake Transition Disorders	
Rhythmic Movement Disorder	
Sleep Talking	
C. Parasomnias usually associated with REM Sleep	
Nightmares	Nightmares
REM Sleep Behavior Disorder	
D. Other Parasomnias	
Bruxism	
Enuresis	
3. Medical/Psychiatric Disorders	2. Sleep Disorders Related to Another Mental
A. Psychiatric	Disorder
Psychoses	A. Insomnia (Axis I or Axis II)
Depression	B. Hypersomnia (Axis I or Axis II)
Alcoholism	
B. Neurologic	3. Sleep Disorder Related to a General Medical
Dementia	Condition[†]
Parkinson's disease	
Fatal Familial Insomnia	4. Substance-Induced Sleep Disorder[‡]
Epilepsy	
Headaches	
C. Other	

*Major categories and examples in the classification by the American Sleep Disorders Association, 1991, compared to the counterparts of the major categories in the *DSM-IV.*

[†]Including neurologic conditions.

[‡]Including medication-induced disorders.

equally affected. Its salient feature is EDS that takes the form of brief, irresistible sleep episodes (attacks) that initially mimic normal daytime naps. Narcoleptic sleep attacks usually occur when patients are bored, comfortable, and engaged in monotonous activities. Each attack usually lasts less than 15 minutes and can be easily interrupted by noise or movement. As narcolepsy progresses, the attacks evolve into episodes that clearly differ from naps. Narcolepsy attacks have a relatively abrupt onset and take place when patients are standing, having a lively interchange, or engaged in activities that require constant attention, including driving. Multiple attacks occur daily. Moreover, the episodes cause momentary amnesia, confusion, and autonomic behavior.

In children, the EDS from narcolepsy, sleep apnea, and other disorders leads to somewhat different symptoms than in adults with the same disorders. Instead of being merely sleepy, children typically respond with inattention and often "paradoxical hyperactivity" (increased, usually purposeless, activity). These children also display behavioral, cognitive, and scholastic problems that can resemble symptoms of Attention Deficit Hyperactivity Disorder.

Narcolepsy's other cardinal symptoms, which develop after the sleep attacks, are manifestations of disordered REM sleep: *cataplexy, sleep paralysis,* and *sleep hallucinations.* Combined with the sleep attacks, these symptoms form the *narcoleptic tetrad.* However, the more common condition is restricted to a *narcolepsy-cataplexy syndrome.*

Cataplexy consists of episodes, typically lasting 30 seconds or less, of sudden weakness precipitated by emotional situations. Unless patients have a simultaneous sleep attack, they remain alert. The three most common situations that lead to cataplexy are hearing or telling a joke, laughing, or developing anger. Other situations that provoke cataplexy include being surprised, being frightened, or having sex.

The episodes begin about 4 years after the onset of narcolepsy. Eventually, by definition, all true narcolepsy patients develop cataplexy. In other words, cataplexy is a requirement for the diagnosis of narcolepsy.

Cataplexy typically occurs 1 to 4 times daily. The weakness tends to be symmetric and proximal. For example, the neck, trunk, hips, knees, and shoulders are affected first. Sometimes the eyelids, jaw, or face are affected alone or in combination with the trunk and limbs. In manifestations that could easily be dismissed, cataplexy induces only a brief period of a patient's jaw dropping open or head nodding. In only its most sensational and rare form, patients' entire body musculature becomes limp and they collapse to the floor. Whether a group of muscles or the entire musculature is weakened, affected muscles become flaccid and areflexic. Nevertheless, as in normal REM sleep, patients breathe normally and retain complete ocular movement.

Sleep paralysis and sleep hallucinations—other components of the tetrad—affect only about 10% of patients. They develop several years after the onset of narcolepsy, and can occur independently. In other words, only 10% of narcolepsy patients have the full narcoleptic tetrad. These symptoms may be present on awakening (hypnopompic) or while falling asleep (hypnagogic). In sleep paralysis, patients are unable to move for several seconds on awakening or when falling asleep, but they can breathe and move their eyes. Although sleep paralysis is a hallmark of narcolepsy, it is not peculiar to narcolepsy. Sleep paralysis routinely occurs in individuals who have been sleep deprived, such as adolescents and house officers.

While having hypnopompic or hypnagogic hallucinations, patients essentially experience vivid twilight dreams that qualify as an organic cause of visual hallucinations (see Chapters 9 and 12). As with the other features of narcolepsy, these hallucinations represent REM sleep intruding into people's wakefulness (Fig. 17–5).

In addition to the narcolepsy tetrad, nighttime is restless and interrupted by multiple, brief, spontaneous awakenings. Thus, narcolepsy patients' EDS partly reflects their inadequate nighttime sleep.

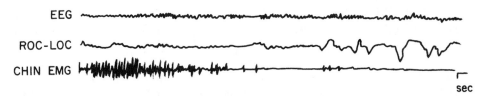

EEG

ROC-LOC

CHIN EMG

sec

FIGURE 17–5. A narcoleptic attack begins when the EEG channel shows low-voltage fast activity that is characteristic of REM sleep. The loss of chin EMG activity indicates that muscles are flaccid. After several seconds, rapid ocular movements begin. The multiple sleep latency test (MSLT) would show similar, characteristic sleep-onset REM periods (SOREMPs). However, one SOREMP does not constitute a diagnosis of narcolepsy.

A standard test for narcolepsy is the *multiple sleep latency test (MSLT)*. Using PSG recording techniques, the MSLT determines both sleep latency and REM latency during 4 or 5 "nap opportunities" presented at 2-hour intervals during daytime. Compared to the normal adult sleep latency of 10 to 20 minutes, narcoleptic patients have a sleep latency of 5 minutes or less. Another abnormality of REM sleep in narcolepsy is that it characteristically starts immediately or within 10 minutes of falling asleep, rather than following the normal, preliminary 90 minutes of NREM stages. These short narcolepsy REM latencies fall into the category of *sleep onset REM periods (SOREMPs)*. More than 70% of narcoleptic patients have 2 or more SOREMPs during their MSLT.

A complementary test measures daytime sleepiness by assessing an individual's ability to remain awake. In the *Repeated Test of Sustained Wakefulness (RTSW)*, individuals are monitored as they attempt to remain awake in a quiet, dark room throughout the daytime. Individuals who tend to fall asleep have EDS, but such a determination is nonspecific.

Narcolepsy undoubtedly results, in part, from a genetic predisposition. Almost 90% of narcolepsy-cataplexy patients have a certain major histocompatibility complex designated human leukocyte antigen (HLA) DQB1, which is located on chromosome 6. This association is the closest known link between any illness and an HLA antigen. On the other hand, genetic studies have also shown that the antigen is neither sufficient nor necessary for narcolepsy-cataplexy. About 25% of the general population have the same antigen, but less than 1% of them has narcolepsy. In fact, only about 1% of narcolepsy patients has an affected first-degree relative. Moreover, only about 25% of monozygotic twins are concordant for the illness. An unidentified factor most likely triggers the illness in individuals who are susceptible because they carry the antigen.

Some cases of narcolepsy without the other elements of the tetrad have followed head trauma, multiple sclerosis, or tumors in the diencephalon. It also occurs in ponies and dogs that have been bred in research colonies.

The primary goal in treatment of narcolepsy is for the patient to remain awake at critical times, particularly when driving, attending school, and working. Methylphenidate (Ritalin) and amphetamines, which enhance dopamine, reduce EDS and the naps. A new nonamphetamine medication, modafinil (Provigil), which probably acts as an α-1 adrenergic agonist, promotes wakefulness without causing excitation or nighttime insomnia. Moreover, unlike stopping amphetamines and other stimulants, stopping modafinil does not lead to a rebound in sleep. On the other hand, despite their help in keeping patients awake, these medications have little effect on cataplexy.

Cataplexy, which is treated differently than sleepiness, often responds to chlorimipramine, imipramine, protriptyline, and possibly SSRIs. These medications probably lessen cataplexy by inhibition of adrenergic reuptake. Benzodiazepines, such as triazolam (Halcion), help assure nighttime sleep.

Patients should arrange regular, strategically placed daytime naps ("nap therapy"). The naps should be brief because short naps are just as restful as long ones. Patients should maintain regular bedtimes.

Sleep Apnea.   Sleep apnea, one of the most common causes of EDS, is characterized by multiple, 10-second to 2-minute interruptions in breathing (apnea) during sleep. Each hour, five or more episodes of apnea produce partial awakenings ("micro-arousals"), as though the brain were interrupting sleep in order to breathe. Patients are usually unaware of the awakenings because they are so brief and incomplete. Nevertheless, the awakenings lead to restless sleep and then EDS.

Another characteristic of sleep apnea is that, as breathing resumes at the end of an apneic episode, patients have loud, irregular snoring that is part of a resuscitative mechanism. In practice, loud nighttime snoring in individuals with irresistible napping is virtually diagnostic of sleep apnea.

During the day, because of their EDS, sleep apnea patients succumb to relatively long but unrefreshing naps. Between attacks, patients are often physically fatigued, as well as lethargic. Whether patients have EDS from sleep apnea, narcolepsy, or another condition, they have a markedly increased rate of traffic accidents.

Sleep apnea includes an *obstructive* and *central* variety. Obstructive sleep apnea is usually caused by mechanical obstructions, such as thickened soft tissues of the pharynx, congenital cranial deformities, hypertrophied tonsils or adenoids, trauma, and other pharyngeal abnormalities. In addition, neuromuscular disorders, such as bulbar poliomyelitis, can also produce weakness of the pharynx.

The central variety, which is rare, results from reduced or inconsistent central nervous system (CNS) ventilatory effort. Patients who have sustained lateral medullary infarctions (see Fig. 2–10), bulbar poliomyelitis, and other injuries to the medulla, which is the site of the respiratory drive, are prone to develop central sleep apnea.

Both varieties can produce arterial blood oxygen desaturation (hypoxia) with oxygen saturation as low as 40%, cardiac arrhythmias, and pulmonary and systemic hypertension. Thus, sleep apnea is a risk factor for stroke. Directly or indirectly, sleep apnea causes morning headache and confusion. It also may cause persistent intellectual impairment and depression.

Patients are typically but not exclusively men who are middle-aged, hypertensive, and overweight. In addition, sleep apnea may affect older children, adolescents, and young adults. Even young children, who have enlarged tonsils and adenoids, may have sleep apnea. Unlike adults, children with sleep apnea usually have normal weight.

The diagnosis of sleep apnea can be confirmed by a PSG that shows periods of apnea, arousals, and hypoxia. In the obstructive variety, airflow is absent despite chest and diaphragm respiratory movements and episodic snoring is prominent (Fig. 17–6). Because of sleep deprivation, sleep latency is short, REM latency is short, and SOREMPs appear. During the night, episodes of sleep apnea occur in either phase of sleep, but they are more pronounced in REM sleep.

The initial management of this condition, in almost all cases, is to lose weight, stop smoking, and stop using hypnotics and alcohol. If those strategies do not alleviate the problem, physicians prescribe ventilation by nasal continuous positive airway pressure (CPAP). Although the device is cumbersome, CPAP remains the best specific treatment. Alternative devices that might secure a patent airway include a tongue-retainer, mandibular advancement prosthesis, or a small nasopharyngeal tube. In the past, tracheostomies were performed to bypass the pharynx, but now surgeons perform other procedures, such as jaw reconstruction or, in children, tonsillectomy. The uvulopalatopharyngoplasty (UPPP)—a laser-assisted plastic proce-

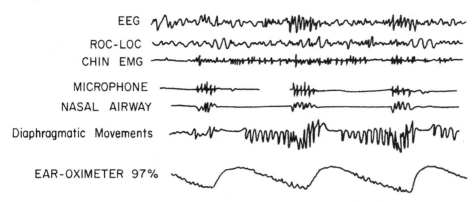

FIGURE 17–6. In sleep apnea, the PSG shows that, during a period of NREM sleep, the oxygen saturation falls. Hypoxia triggers a partial arousal, which is indicated by faster EEG activity. Diaphragmatic movements reach a crescendo and loud snoring begins. After strenuous diaphragm movements, air moves through the nasal airway and oxygen saturation improves.

dure—was also popular, but the results have been disappointing and the procedure may be complicated by a voice change. Fluoxetine, protriptyline, or medroxyprogesterone may be useful for central sleep apnea.

Periodic Limb Movement Disorder. *Periodic limb movement disorder*, also called *nocturnal myoclonus* or, when confined to the legs, *periodic leg movements*, consists of regular (periodic), episodic movements of the legs or, less often, arms during sleep. The movements consist most often of stereotyped, brief (0.5 to 5.0 second), dorsiflexion movements of the feet. They take place at 20- to 40-second intervals, for periods of 10 minutes to several hours primarily during NREM sleep (Fig. 17–7). Because periodic limb movements—like apneas—continually arouse patients, the disorder leads to EDS.

During periodic limb movements, EMG leads show regular muscle contractions that lead to arousals. The disorder usually develops in individuals older than 55 years. It can occur in association with sleep apnea, restless leg syndrome, and other sleep disorders, use of antidepressants, withdrawal from various medications, or medical illnesses, such as uremia. Treatment with benzodiazepines or dopamine agonists may be helpful.

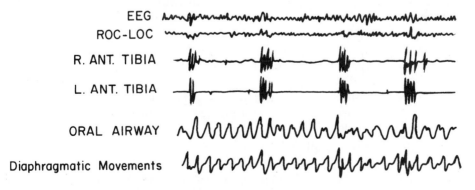

FIGURE 17–7. Periodic limb movements, a variety of nocturnal myoclonus, are represented by approximately 30-second intervals of synchronous anterior tibialis EMG activity. The muscle contractions dorsiflex the patient's ankles.

Restless Leg Syndrome. *Restless leg syndrome* consists of random, irregular movements of the feet and legs during the evening and early portion of sleep but also to a lesser extent during wakefulness. In addition to patients' irregular movements, about 80% of them have periodic leg movements. The nocturnal movements delay the onset of sleep (prolong sleep latency) and later interrupt it.

A distinctive aspect of this disorder is that unpleasant sensations (dysesthesias or painful paresthesias), such as burning and aching, situated deeply in the feet and legs seem to initiate the movements. As if to satisfy an urge, patients walk, pace, or, in bed, make bicycle movements or shuffle. These actions only temporarily alleviate the sensations and stop the involuntary movements. The combination of the involuntary movements and the attempts to relieve the unpleasant sensations cause insomnia and EDS in both the patient and bed partner.

Restless leg syndrome is usually a manifestation of a polyneuropathy or other underlying condition. Diabetic and uremic polyneuropathies, in which paresthesias are prominent symptoms, routinely lead to restless leg syndrome (see Chapter 5). Other common causes, not associated with polyneuropathy, include pregnancy and iron deficiency.

About one-third of patients have no known underlying condition. The majority of them, who are said to have primary restless leg syndrome, have a family history of the disorder. Preliminary information indicates that primary restless leg syndrome is transmitted as an autosomal dominant trait.

Restless leg syndrome is one of several conditions characterized by prominent involuntary leg movements. In contrast to restless leg movements, periodic limb movements occur at regular intervals, are confined to sleep, and are not associated with sensory symptoms. Akathisia (see Chapter 18) results from a CNS drive rather than peripheral sensations. In addition, akathisia is not associated with leg movements when the patient is in bed. It is also not associated with sleep disturbances.

Another condition characterized by involuntary nocturnal leg movements is the familiar, benign leg thrusts that seem to protect against falling when people "fall" asleep. These movements, *sleep starts* or *hypnic* or *hypnagogic jerks,* occur in the twilight of sleep. In view of their time of onset, they are classified as a sleep-wake transition disorder parasomnia.

Although the rationale remains unclear, dopamine precursors and dopamine agonists (see Chapter 18) have the greatest efficacy with the fewest risks in suppressing the movements and promoting restful sleep. Opioids, including codeine, are also effective but risky. Tricyclic antidepressants that reduce dysesthesias and promote sleep may be helpful for patients with polyneuropathy-induced restless leg syndrome.

Hypersomnias. The Kleine-Levin syndrome, *periodic hypersomnia,* is a rare sleep disorder in which patients, who are predominantly adolescent males, have lengthy but otherwise normal sleep. Their sleep lasts for periods of several days to two weeks, 3 or 4 times yearly. Patients awaken during these periods to eat great quantities of food and display unusual behavior, typically hypersexuality and irritability. During this time, they are withdrawn and apathetic. No laboratory abnormality proves that the disorder is clearly "organic."

Encephalitis, brain tumors, hypothalamic injuries, and head trauma (see postconcussive syndrome, Chapter 22) cause EDS. Nevertheless, patients typically sleep poorly at night and have other signs of cerebral dysfunction, such as personality changes and intellectual impairment.

Extrinsic Sleep Disorders

Extrinsic sleep disorders result from personal, social, or drug and alcohol-related factors interfering with a presumably normal brain. Removing such factors should restore a normal sleep-wake schedule in affected individuals.

Inadequate or Poor Sleep Hygiene includes use of caffeine, alcohol, and certain medications at night; performing exercise, mental challenging, or anxiety-provoking activities before bed; and engaging in other activities counterproductive to sleep. Related conditions, such as an environmental sleep disorder, also result from outside interference. In most of these conditions, the PSG shows prolonged sleep latency, which is the physiologic counterpart of tossing and turning in bed, frequent arousals, and advanced (early morning) awakening.

Hypnotic, Stimulant, Alcohol, or other Toxin Dependency is a major cause of insomnia, as well as EDS. These disorders are defined by the use of various substances for their hypnotic effect, but, cutting a fine line, they exclude frank addiction, such as alcoholism. The PSG, in general, shows a short sleep latency, disrupted sleep, and fragmented or suppressed REM phases. In common terms, people who take bedtime drinks ("nightcaps") soon fall deeply asleep, but the sleep is disrupted and normal dreaming is reduced or fragmented.

Sleep impairment may also be caused by medicines that have unappreciated stimulant effects, such as steroids, aminophylline, or pseudoephedrine (Actifed). The most common stimulant is caffeine. Coffee has 60 to 175 mg of caffeine per cup; tea, 25 to 100 mg; cola drinks, 25 to 60 mg; weight-loss drugs, 100 to 200 mg; and headache medicines, 130 mg in 2 aspirin-caffeine compound tablets. Many Americans easily and often inadvertently ingest so much caffeine (250 to 500 mg per day) that they develop *caffeinism:* insomnia, agitation, tremulousness, palpitations, gastric distress, and diuresis.

When medications that suppress sleep are withdrawn, people naturally have insomnia, greater EDS because of less nighttime sleep, and psychological agitation. When finally able to fall asleep, they typically have REM rebound—as though their previously suppressed REM sleep were trying to catch up. In addition, abrupt withdrawal from alcohol or barbiturates, especially short-acting ones, may lead to generalized, tonic-clonic seizures and delirium tremens (DTs).

Circadian Rhythm Disorders

Both neurophysiologic and external factors can alter the sleep-wake schedule to produce *circadian rhythm disorders.* In the best known example, *Time Zone Change (Jet Lag) Syndrome,* people who rapidly traverse at least two time zones develop insomnia and EDS accompanied by changes in digestion and other autonomic behavior. Many travelers feel as though their mind and body have remained on the schedule of their city of origin.

Going east to west is easier than west to east because travelers can more easily postpone (delay) their night's sleep than fall asleep earlier (advance it). When going in either direction, travelers can facilitate the transition by shifting their sleep-wake schedule to their destination city's day-night schedule by initiating it *before* the trip or assuming it immediately on arrival. Travelers also can further facilitate the adjustment by exposing themselves to daylight once they have reached their destination. (Light is more powerful than noise in entraining people to a new sleep-wake schedule.) On long west-to-east flights, which are the most taxing, travelers can take a hypnotic to advance their sleep schedule so that it will conform to the new time zone.

A related cause of insomnia and EDS is *Shift Work Sleep Disorder*. A well-known example is the worker who begins work on a night shift suffering daytime fatigue and inattention and then an inability to fall asleep. Although most workers can make the transition after several days, some may be unsuccessful because their internal schedule is too ingrained or they continue to follow their old schedule on weekends or holidays.

In contrast to the previous disorders that result from outside scheduling, the *Delayed Sleep Phase Syndrome* results—in technical terms—from an intrinsic, neurophysiologic delay in falling asleep (prolonged sleep latency) followed by a sleep of normal quality and duration. Most commonly, the delayed sleep phase syndrome first develops in adolescents during long vacations when they remain active until the early morning. The late hour of sleep postpones the time that they awaken. Although the delay may seem benign, these adolescents and other affected individuals find that either they do not attend to school or work because of their unconventional schedule or they are perpetually tired because of inadequate sleep. Their sleep-wake schedule and the resultant disruptions seem intractable to the usual sleep-altering interventions, such as hypnotics and going to bed earlier.

In a physiologic, nonpharmacologic, and usually successful treatment of the Delayed Sleep Phase Syndrome, *chronotherapy*, affected individuals delay their sleep time by 30 to 60 minutes successively each night. They postpone (delay) their sleep onset time—with activities, coffee and other stimulants, and light—by *almost* 24 hours. They eventually fall asleep at a conventional time, such as 11 PM, and, with effort, maintain that schedule (Fig. 17–8).

PARASOMNIAS

Behavioral or physiological aberrations, the *parasomnias*, originate in neurophysiologic dysfunction and intrude into otherwise normal sleep. Parasomnias are usually associated with full or partial arousal, the sleep-wake interface, and slow-wave NREM sleep. Aside from these interruptions, patients usually have normal restful sleep. In particular, their REM latency is normal (Tables 17–2 and 17–3), and they usually do not have EDS.

Arousal Disorders

A subgroup of parasomnias, which are provoked by arousals during slow-wave sleep, occur overwhelmingly during the first 2 hours of sleep when this phase predominates. They are not manifestations of dreams or REM sleep disturbances.

Confusional Arousals consist of disorientation and amnesia when the individual is roused from slow-wave sleep. It develops in physicians "on call" who are awakened for medical decisions but remain confused. In the morning, they are unable to recall conversations in which they engaged.

Sleepwalking.   Sleepwalking (somnambulism) usually consists just of sitting or standing but can include activities that are more complex. During a typical episode, children walk slowly, with their eyes open, along familiar pathways. Although sleepwalking children seem to be partially awake, they cannot be aroused fully. When questioned, they are confused, inappropriate, and amnestic.

Sleepwalking and sleep terrors (see below) usually develop in early childhood, affect boys more often than girls, and cease before puberty. Studies of twins indicate that sleepwalking has, in part, a genetic basis. Treatment of an episode is not feasible because of its brevity, but when episodes occur several times a week, a trial of prophylactic benzodiazepine or imipramine may be worthwhile.

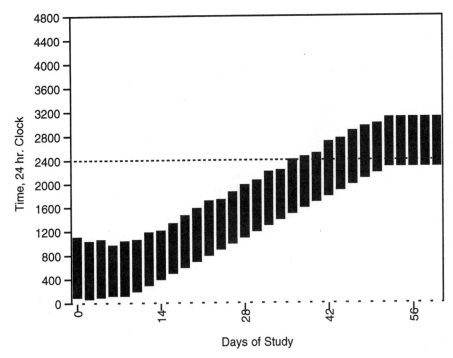

FIGURE 17–8. A 17-year-old high-school student has been unable to fall asleep before 1:00 AM or to arise before 9:00 AM. He has been unable to attend school on a regular basis and tends to associate with unsupervised friends who have no curfews. Brought into a sleep laboratory, his sleep graph demonstrates a delayed sleep phase during the first week of study. Then each succeeding night, he is "encouraged" to remain awake for an additional 30 minutes. By the end of 6 weeks, he has postponed (delayed) his sleep time to 2300 hours (11:00 PM) and he is awakened at 8:00 AM. For the next week, the 11:00 PM to 8:00 AM is reinforced. The young man stays on this schedule for many months. If this strategy, chronotherapy, is successful, it does not require hypnotics, stimulants or other medication, a sleep laboratory, or trained personnel.

Children are liable to have more than one variety of parasomnia and display complex behaviors during each of them. Parasomnias might be confused with a partial complex seizure (see Chapter 10), but such seizures tend to be stereotyped, undergo secondary generalization, and be followed by (postictal) confusion. A PSG during an episode would be diagnostic of a seizure.

Parasomnias are not associated with psychiatric disturbances in children. In adults, however, parasomnias have been associated with psychiatric disturbances, including violence, and CNS pathology.

Sleep Terrors. Completely different from nightmares (see below), sleep terrors in children consist of episodes in which they suddenly, after a partial or full awakening, behave as though they were in great danger. The children stare, moan, and sometimes speak a few words with their eyes fully open and their pupils dilated. They characteristically sweat, hyperventilate, and have tachycardia. They resist their parents' attempts to wake them up, put them back to sleep, or comfort them. They often leave their parents' arms to walk aimlessly. The episode lasts for several minutes and ends abruptly with a return to deep sleep. Despite the episode's vivid and awesome features, children do not recall it in the morning.

Sleep terrors usually develop several hours after bedtime and especially after sleep deprivation. PSG studies show that they arise in slow-wave rather than REM sleep. Noises or other disruptions during slow-wave sleep can arouse children and precipitate the episodes. Unlike dreams, sleep terrors are unrelated to frightening events of the day and no REM activity is detectable during the episode. In addition, sleep terrors usually take place only a few times a month.

Night terrors and other parasomnias frequently develop or become more common when children give up their afternoon nap. Children are susceptible when reaching this milestone because they are "overtired" when they fall asleep and quickly lapse into slow-wave sleep, from which most parasomnias originate.

Sleep terrors can be prevented in some children by enforcing an afternoon nap and avoiding sleep disruptions, such as loud noises. Similarly, predisposed children should be limited to a few sips of water at bedtime to avoid awakening to urinate. A course of medication may be used as a last resort. Studies have suggested imipramine, benzodiazepines, and paroxetine; however, they have been unable to specify the duration of treatment, likelihood of tolerance developing, or length of posttreatment effectiveness.

Sleep-Wake Transition Disorders

As people fall asleep and progress through the various sleep stages, they are subject to certain parasomnias at each stage or during transitions. In one disorder, *Rhythmic Movement Disorder*, infants, children, and occasionally adults have rhythmic, repetitive, stereotyped movements of their head, trunk, or entire body while lying in bed during the initial stages of falling asleep and during daytime naps. The movements usually begin in infancy and disappear by age 5 years. They usually consist of slow *head-banging* on the pillow. However, they can persist into the teenage years and be a relatively violent rocking from side to side.

Another sleep-wake transition disorder is *Sleep Talking*. The common phenomenon of people "talking" in their sleep is an overstatement because they merely utter a few words that are difficult to comprehend. This parasomnia affects adults and children and occurs in all sleep stages. It is benign and usually independent of dreams but can be associated with sleepwalking and REM sleep behavior disorder (see below).

Parasomnias with REM Sleep

Nightmares.   In contrast to sleep terrors, *nightmares* are essentially dreams that have a frightening content (i.e., "bad dreams"). They contain complex imagery that the dreamer is often able to recall when awakened during the nightmare or on arising in the morning. Nightmares are usually unaccompanied by any bodily movement except for crying, or autonomic response other than mild tachycardia. Typically, a nightmare ends by itself, but awakening the dreamer can interrupt it. After becoming fully awake, the dreamer has a slow, difficult return to sleep.

Although nightmares are commonly assumed to be a childhood sleep disorder, they also occur in adults. In them, as in children, nightmares occur during REM periods and particularly when REM activity is increased. Thus, adults tend to have nightmares following sleep deprivation, during alcohol withdrawal, when using or discontinuing medications, and when suffering from Posttraumatic Stress Disorder (PSD). Evaluation of frequent nightmares in adults requires exploring not only the circumstances and content of the dreams but also the use of medications, alcohol, and drugs.

REM Sleep Behavior Disorder.   During normal REM sleep, even during nightmares, the bodily musculature is motionless, flaccid, and areflexic. This normal immobility, among other purposes, protects people from participating in their dreams. In comparison, the *REM Sleep Behavior Disorder* restores individuals' ability to move and their normal muscle tone during dreams. Affected individuals thrash, hit, and make running movements during their REM sleep.

Their violent motor activity seems to result from "acting out" their dreams. When awakened from an episode, they typically either recall a dream or explain that they were only defending themselves against attack. They deny deliberately aggressive behavior. Individuals with REM sleep behavior disorder, who are usually men older than 65 years, are potentially injurious to themselves and their bed partner.

REM sleep behavior disorder is associated with lacunar cerebral infarctions, diffuse Lewy body disease, Parkinson's disease, and other neurologic illnesses that cause dementia. It is also associated with increased REM activity, especially the REM rebound that follows medication withdrawal. Clonazepam taken at night reduces or eliminates the problem but at the necessary doses causes daytime sleepiness. SSRIs and tricyclic antidepressants, even though they suppress REM sleep, are ineffective or can exacerbate the problem.

Other Parasomnias

Bruxism.   Sleep-related, stereotyped, forceful teeth grinding or clenching, *bruxism*, is a parasomnia. Bruxism makes a loud, disconcerting sound and leads to wearing away of teeth, headaches, and temporomandibular joint dysfunction. Although bruxism occurs in all sleep stages, it occurs mainly in the transition from wakefulness to sleep and during light sleep. It is also associated with dementia, mental retardation, and Parkinson's disease. Individuals with these disorders often have bruxism while awake, as well as when asleep. Nighttime dental devices are helpful.

Enuresis.   Bed-wetting (enuresis) is considered a parasomnia in children older than 5 years and in all adults. Like bruxism, it is not restricted to a particular sleep stage or transition. Enuresis occurs mostly in slow-wave sleep during the first third of the night. Boys are affected more than girls. Imipramine may be helpful for children and some adults. Behavior modification therapy devices, such the "bell and pad," can suppress enuresis. Alternatively, single injections or nasal sprays of desmopressin (DDAVP), which is a synthetic form of the antidiuretic hormone (ADH) vasopressin, promotes enough water retention to stop enuresis for one night. DDAVP is indicated for refractory situations or when enuresis would be especially embarrassing (such as during a "sleep-over"). However, excessive use can lead to excessive water retention with water intoxication.

In adults, enuresis can result not only from a parasomnia but also from a variety of neurologic and urologic conditions. For example, it can result from degenerative cerebral disease and thus can be associated with dementia. In addition, a single episode can be the residue of a seizure. Chronic enuresis can result from spinal cord damage, as with multiple sclerosis; cauda equina injuries, as with meningomyeloceles; and ANS damage, as with diabetes.

MEDICAL/PSYCHIATRIC DISORDERS

Mental Disorders

Schizophrenia, schizophreniform disorder, and other functional psychoses are associated with both insomnia and EDS. However, probably because of the diverse nature of these disorders, fluctuations in their activity and severity, and patients' exposure to antipsychotic medications, PSG results are variable, often overlap with normal values, and are too inconsistent to serve as a biological marker.

Only generalizations are possible in *acute schizophrenia*. The PSG usually shows a decreased total sleep time, increased sleep latency, and frequent, long awakenings that reflect restlessness ("decreased sleep efficiency"). It also shows normal or slightly reduced REM sleep. Patients with *chronic schizophrenia*, in contrast, tend to have essentially normal sleep patterns and, interestingly, can distinguish their dreams from hallucinations.

Depression, as is commonly noted, is associated with insomnia and EDS. PSG studies show characteristic REM abnormalities. In depression, a typically short REM latency (less than 60 minutes) is followed by an abnormally long, intense REM period. Subsequent REM periods occur in relatively quick succession, leaving the latter half of the night virtually devoid of REM sleep. Although the total amount of REM sleep is approximately the same as in normal individuals, the reduction in total sleep time is extracted from slow-wave sleep. Thus, the depressed person's sleep is insufficiently restorative and sleepiness persists into the following day.

Depressed individuals, in addition, have neuroendocrine abnormalities related to their sleep alterations. Their body temperature nadir occurs several hours earlier than normal. Likewise, they have an earlier excretion of cortisol and the norepinephrine metabolite MHPG. Overall, the earlier onset of so many features of sleep—the first REM period, the bulk of REM sleep, the temperature nadir, and nocturnal hormone excretion—is the result of the forward movement of the normal circadian rhythm (a phase advance). When depressed people fall asleep, they seem to skip into the middle of the normal sleep and neuroendocrine cycle. Sleep disturbances are such an integral part of depression that when it recedes spontaneously or responds to medication, sleep disturbances are one of the last symptoms to improve.

In *mania*, sleep latency can be excessive (seemingly infinite), REM sleep can be abolished, and total sleep time can be reduced markedly. Although *PTSD* causes hypervigilance and difficulty falling and staying asleep, its hallmark is nightmares and other recollections of the trauma. The recurrence of essentially the same nightmare sets PTSD apart from many other conditions characterized by nightmares.

Alcoholism is also associated with insomnia and EDS. In the first half of the night, alcoholic individuals generally have a short sleep latency, less REM sleep, and increased slow-wave sleep, as though they were collapsing into stupor. In the second half, they have increased REM and periods of wakefulness, as though they emerged into delirium. The net effect is decreased total sleep time and decreased slow-wave sleep. Alcohol withdrawal, which is similar to withdrawal from other hypnotic substances, produces insomnia and REM rebound.

Neurologic Disorders

Dementia.   Dementia from Alzheimer's disease and other disorders (see Chapter 7), at least in its moderate stages, disrupts patient's sleep-wake cycle and produces nighttime thought and behavioral disturbances. During the night, patients tend to become confused, agitated, and disoriented, especially in new surroundings. Alzheimer's disease patients characteristically wander at night. They walk about the house and may actually leave it.

PSGs show increased stage 1 NREM sleep, fragmentations, and decreased efficiency. Patients with dementia typically take many long naps during each day. Patients, taking multiple naps each day are said to have "polyphasic sleep."

Despite an expectation that decreased cholinergic activity in Alzheimer's disease would lead to decreased and delayed REM activity, the PSGs do not substantiate such a pattern. Moreover, PSGs do not correlate with any particular etiology of dementia.

Providing daytime exercise, exposure to sunlight, and restricted naps may reduce sleep disturbances in Alzheimer's disease. Nevertheless, early evening administration of tranquilizers, sedatives, or other medications may still be required.

Parkinson's Disease.   During sleep, the major physical problems of *Parkinson's disease* (see Chapter 18)—tremor, rigidity, and bradykinesia—characteristically disappear, but thought disorders and hallucinations emerge or become more pronounced. Sleep disorders are an integral part of Parkinson's disease possibly because the disease depigments the locus ceruleus, as well as the substantia nigra. Once Parkinson's disease is moderately advanced, sleep disorders affect most patients. The majority of families concede that sleep-related mental disturbances are the most disruptive aspect of the illness and the reason that they place patients in a nursing home.

The primary sleep problem is a combination of nocturnal hallucinations, nightmares, and agitated confusion. Part of the sleep problem is iatrogenic. In particular, dopamine-enhancing (dopaminergic) medications produce vivid dreams that evolve into visual hallucinations. Surprisingly, a dopamine agonist, pramipexole (Mirapex) induces somnolence.

For most patients, reducing the number and dosage of dopaminergic medications and administering them earlier in the evening will probably reduce nocturnal behavioral disturbances, agitation, and hallucinations; however, that strategy may worsen the physical problems in the morning and possibly for the entire day. Typical neuroleptics may reduce nighttime hallucinations and agitation, but they also worsen the physical symptoms and lead to sedation. Clozapine, which produces little or no parkinsonism, is indicated for serious nocturnal thought and behavioral disturbances.

The other Parkinson's sleep problems are manifestations of the disease itself. These problems include dementia with "sleep reversal" (sleeping during the day and being awake at night); fragmented sleep; insomnia or hypersomnia; REM sleep behavior disorder; and depression, which also interferes with sleep.

Other Movement Disorders.   As with Parkinson's disease, other basal ganglia–related involuntary movements, such as athetosis and chorea, typically disappear during sleep. In contrast, several involuntary movements are primarily or exclusively sleep-related, such as periodic limb movements, restless leg syndrome, and hypnic jerks (see above). Disorders commonly evident during the day that continue in sleep, especially during partial arousals, are tics, generalized dystonia, and focal dystonias, including blepharospasm and hemifacial spasm (see Chapter 18). These disorders, which have little in common, cannot be attributed to basal ganglia pathology. In fact, in many cases, their cause is unknown. Although partial arousals may elicit the movements, most of them are not confined to a particular sleep stage.

Fatal Familial Insomnia.   A recently described illness, *fatal familial insomnia,* is characterized by an inherited tendency to develop a progressively severe insomnia that is refractory to medicine. The insomnia, which appears on the average at 50 years of age, is accompanied by neuropsychologic impairments, including inattentiveness, amnesia, sequencing problems, and confusion. As the disease progresses, patients develop hyperactive ANS activity (tachycardia, hyperhidrosis, for example), endocrine abnormalities (elevated catecholamine and other hormone levels), and "motor abnormalities" (myoclonus, ataxia). It follows a relentless downhill course that is fatal in 6 to 36 months.

Fatal familial insomnia is closely related to Creutzfeldt-Jakob's disease (see Chapter 7). Both illnesses present with mental status changes in individuals 50 years old, which is younger than when Alzheimer's disease usually first appears. Moreover, both are prion diseases in that they result from accumulation of abnormal prion protein (PrP^{Sc}). Cerebral biopsies show spongiform cerebral cortical changes.

In contrast to Creutzfeldt-Jakob's and Alzheimer's diseases, in fatal familial insomnia, the thalamus undergoes atrophy. Moreover, fatal familial insomnia depends entirely on a well-delineated genetic abnormality. Individuals who are homozygous, compared to those who are heterozygous, for the disease tend to run a fulminant course characterized by severe sleep disturbances and ANS dysfunction. Heterozygous individuals run longer courses in which motor abnormalities predominate.

Epilepsy.   Many seizures, depending on the variety, occur primarily in sleep or on awakening (see Chapter 10). About 45% of patients with primary generalized epilepsy have seizures predominantly during sleep. These seizures typically develop within stages 1 and 2 of NREM sleep—during the first two hours of sleep. They also tend to occur at the other end of the sleep cycle—on awakening. REM sleep, in contrast, remains relatively seizure-free.

Compared to primary generalized seizures, partial seizures occur less frequently during sleep. In addition, when partial seizures occur during sleep, they are less restricted to NREM sleep. When a partial seizure, especially a frontal lobe seizure, develops during sleep, it may masquerade as a sleep-related disorder, such as a parasomnia, REM sleep behavioral disorder episode, or a nocturnal panic attack. A PSG with extra EEG electrodes is often necessary to distinguish between these nocturnal behavioral disturbances and seizures.

Sleep deprivation routinely precipitates seizures in individuals with epilepsy, and sometimes in those without a history of epilepsy. For example, medical house officers who have worked all night are susceptible to tonic-clonic seizures throughout the next day. Obtaining an EEG after enforced sleep deprivation elicits sharp waves and a variety of spike-and-sharp wave activity in more than one third of epileptic patients who have no such abnormalities on routine, daytime EEGs.

Another aspect of epilepsy and sleep is that, even at therapeutic blood concentrations, antiepileptic drugs (AEDs) can lead to EDS and mood changes. On the other hand, among their many actions, AEDs promote normal sleep. They raise the efficiency of sleep by reducing arousals and increasing slow-wave sleep.

Headaches.   Vascular headaches, particularly migraines and cluster headaches (see Chapter 9) are closely associated with sleep. REM sleep seems to precipitate migraine and, even more so, cluster headaches. In some people, these headaches appear only during REM periods, but in most, they begin during early morning intense REM sleep and continue after awakening. Thus, excessive sleep or other conditions that increase REM sleep are associated with these headaches. As would be predicted, medications that suppress REM sleep reduce the headaches. Paradoxically, naturally occurring or medication-induced sleep will abort migraines in many individuals.

Other Disorders.   Of the various medical conditions that are precipitated by sleep, cardiovascular disorders are the most important. Angina pectoris and myocardial infarctions take place much more often during REM sleep, when pulse and blood pressure are often elevated and erratic, than during NREM sleep. Thrombotic strokes are also more frequent during NREM sleep, when pulse and blood pressure are relatively low. Typically, strokes are discovered disproportionately on awakening.

Attacks of asthma, exacerbation of chronic obstructive lung disease, gastroesophageal reflux, and peptic ulcer disease tend to develop during sleep. Some of these problems may be related to the patient's sleeping position, but the attacks occur with equal frequency in either sleep phase. All these nighttime disturbances interrupt sleep and lead to EDS. In cases of "nocturnal asthma," physicians must overlook the alternative diagnosis of nocturnal panic attacks.

Sleep-related violence has been attributed to NREM and REM sleep and to neurologic and psychiatric conditions that emerge during sleep. Some form of violence is potentially a manifestation of REM sleep behavior disorder, nocturnal partial seizures, head-banging, sleepwalking and other parasomnias, or dementia-induced wandering. In these cases, the violent activity ordinarily consists of poorly directed or self-inflicted flailing or banging but almost never purposeful violence directed at another individual (i.e., aggression) (see Chapter 10). It begins abruptly, has a duration of several minutes or less, and does not leave a substantial residual memory.

INSOMNIA

Insomnia is a widespread and almost always nonspecific symptom. Moreover, when the patient's primary or exclusive symptom is insomnia, neurologists do not consider it a neurologic disorder. For example, insomnia may be a manifestation of sleep disorders, medical illnesses, substance abuse, other psychiatric disorders, or, in individuals older than 65 years, a normal variant. Thus, this book appends a brief discussion of its treatment that has neurologic implications.

Treatment of Insomnia.   Nonpharmacologic treatments may alone be sufficient and should be included, for the most part, in the initial treatment plan. Individuals should practice good "sleep hygiene." They should usually exercise on a regular basis during the day but avoid exercise in the evening; avoid stimulants, particularly caffeine; take, at most, only a brief early afternoon nap; and use the bed only for sleeping. In addition, behavior therapies, including relaxation techniques, sleep restriction, and stimulus reduction, might be helpful.

If possible, insomnia-causing medications should be discontinued. Several have been mentioned (see above). Those that neurologists are apt to prescribe include β-blockers, caffeine-containing migraine medications (see Table 9–1), dopamine precursors and agonists (see Chapter 18), and steroids.

Nonprescription hypnotics are commonly used but are usually less effective and undesirably longer-lasting than prescription hypnotics. These medicines can cause sleepiness and confusion the following day. Moreover, they carry several potential worrisome side effects. For example, antihistamines—especially in children—can produce delirium, confusion, nightmares, and dystonic reactions. Alcohol, when used for its hypnotic effect, may cause a stuporous sleep that is followed by REM rebound and early morning awakening.

Tryptophan was popular in the past because it is the "active ingredient" in warm milk and a precursor of melatonin. However, tryptophan was an ineffective hypnotic, and one batch of contaminated tryptophan pills caused the eosinophilia-myalgia syndrome (see Chapter 6).

On the other hand, melatonin promotes sleepiness. It decreases sleep latency and increases total sleep time and duration of REM sleep. Moreover, it seems to improve the restfulness of sleep. Unlike other hypnotics, melatonin does not lead to daytime sleepiness or confusion. Melatonin might be useful in the delayed sleep phase syndrome, jet lag, and age-related insomnia.

Benzodiazepines, despite their potential complications, are effective and remain a mainstay of treatment. They increase total sleep time and reduce fragmentation.

Their benefits are surprising in view of the facts that the increase in total sleep time is only about 10% and they decrease valuable slow-wave NREM sleep.

Benzodiazepines' potential complications prevent their widespread use. Depending on their duration of action and if the patient is elderly, benzodiazepines can cause anterograde amnesia, confusion, insomnia in the early morning, and then EDS. In some cases, they cause patients to fall, which often results in hip fractures. If benzodiazepines are abruptly stopped, patients may experience rebound insomnia and are placed at risk for withdrawal seizures.

Newer medications, such as zolpidem (Ambien) and zaleplon (Sonata), may replace benzodiazepines for treatment of transient insomnia. Zolpidem binds to the gamma-aminobutyric acid (GABA)-chloride channel with the benzodiazepine receptor, and zaleplon binds to the $GABA_A$ benzodiazepine receptor (see Chapter 21). These medicines have a short half-life and do not cause grogginess in the morning. They have minimal effect on sleep architecture. Because they do not suppress REM sleep, REM does not rebound when they are stopped.

Both tricyclic and SSRI antidepressants have a hypnotic effect. Curiously, fluoxetine causes extensive, prominent ocular movements during NREM sleep that may persist after the medicine has been discontinued. Fluoxetine-induced ocular movements might be mistaken for REM-induced ocular movements. SSRIs may also cause myoclonus that is more prominent at night.

TABLE 17–5. *Salient Historical Features of Patients with Insomnia and Other Sleep Disorders**

A. Nighttime sleep
  1. What are the usual times that you try to fall asleep, actually fall asleep, and awaken?
  2. Do you awaken during the night? How often? How long? What do you do when awake?
  3. When asleep, do you have any of the following interruptions?
     Nightmares or night terrors, sleepwalking, bed-wetting
     Loud or irregular snoring
     Cessation of breathing
     Restless or painful legs
     Leg or other limb movements
     Headaches, chest pain, or other medical symptoms
  4. Was the nighttime sleep restful?
B. Daytime sleep
  1. Do you take afternoon or evening naps?
     Are they restful?
     Are they irresistible?
     Do they occur at inappropriate times?
  2. Do you lose bodily tone or have episodic muscle weakness?
     Do you suddenly weaken, especially after laughter or excitement?
     Does a single muscle group, such as those in the jaw or knees, suddenly weaken?
C. If left to your own schedule:
  1. Would you be more alert in the morning or night?
  2. How much sleep would you get?
D. General health
  1. Do you suffer from medical, neurologic, or psychiatric illness?
  2. Do you take any prescription or over-the-counter medications or drugs?
  3. Do you use alcohol?
  4. Do you use coffee or other caffeine-containing beverage?

*A reliable history may be obtained only from a bed partner who, as in other conditions, may be suffering more than the patient.

REFERRAL FOR A POLYSOMNOGRAM

For most patients who have sleep disorders, a thorough medical-psychiatric evaluation might be sufficient (Table 17–5). Physicians must accept restrictions in referring patients for a PSG because it is expensive and useful in few disorders. A PSG is usually necessary in cases of suspected sleep apnea and abnormal behavior during sleep (REM behavior disorder, periodic limb movements, and potentially injurious parasomnias). In addition, it is useful for detecting neurologic disorders, particularly seizures, that develop exclusively during sleep. On the other hand, a PSG is not cost-effective in evaluating patients with insomnia unless it is treatment-resistant, induces mental aberrations, or endangers the patient's health.

Sleep latency tests are indicated in the preliminary evaluation of individuals suspected of having narcolepsy where REM activity emerges at the onset of the naps. The expense is justifiable because amphetamines and other powerful medications would be used to treat the disorder. Sleep latency tests may also suggest sleep apnea and periodic limb movements, but the diagnosis of those disorders rests on PSG findings.

REFERENCES

Abramowicz M (ed): Modafinil for narcolepsy. Med Lett *41*: 30–31, 1999
Aldrich MS: Diagnostic aspects of narcolepsy. Neurology *50* (Suppl 1): S2–S7, 1998
Aldrich MS: Diagnostic aspects of narcolepsy. Neurology *50* (Suppl 1): 34–43, 1998
Alvarez B, Dahitz MJ, Vignau J, et al: The delayed sleep phase syndrome. J Neurol Neurosurg Psychiatry *55:* 665–670, 1992
American Sleep Disorders Association: The International Classification of Sleep Disorders Diagnostic and Coding Manual. Rochester, MN, American Sleep Disorders Association, 1990
Brezezinski A: Melatonin in humans. N Engl J Med *336:* 186–196, 1997
Broughton RJ, Shimizu T: Sleep-related violence: A medical and forensic challenge. Sleep *18:* 727–730, 1995
Kavey NB, Whyte J, Resor SR, et al: Somnambulism in adults. Neurology *40:* 749–752, 1990
Kupfer DJ, Reynolds CF: Management of insomnia. N Engl J Med *336:* 341–346, 1997
Mignot E: Genetic and familial aspects of narcolepsy. Neurology *50* (Suppl 1): S16–S22, 1998
Moldofsky H, Gilbert R, Lue FA, et al: Sleep-related violence. Sleep *19:* 731–739, 1995
National Center on Sleep Disorders web site *http://search.info.nih.gov*
Penev PD, Zee PC: Melatonin: A clinical perspective. Ann Neurol *42:* 545–553, 1997
Rossi G, Macchi G, Porro M, et al: Fatal familial insomnia. Neurology *50:* 688–692, 1998
Strollo PJ, Rogers RM: Obstructive sleep apnea. N Engl J Med *334:* 99–104, 1996
Tandberg E, Larsen JP, Karlsen K: A community-based study of sleep disorders in patients with Parkinson's disease. Move Dis *13:* 895–899, 1998
US Modafinil in Narcolepsy Multicenter Study Group: Randomized trial of modafinil for the treatment of pathological somnolence in narcolepsy. Ann Neurol *43:* 88–97, 1998
Walters AS, Hening WA, Chokroverty S: Review and videotape recognition of idiopathic restless legs syndrome. Move Dis *6:* 105–110, 1991
Wise MS: Childhood narcolepsy. Neurology *50* (Suppl 1): S37–S42, 1998

QUESTIONS and ANSWERS: CHAPTER 17

1–15. Is the statement true or false?

1. Normal sleep begins with the first stage of NREM sleep and progresses through the four NREM stages before the first period of REM sleep occurs.

2. Since REM sleep usually begins about 90 to 120 minutes after the onset of sleep, normal REM latency is 90 to 120 minutes.

3. The bulk of REM sleep occurs in the early night, whereas the bulk of NREM sleep occurs in the early morning.

4. The normal sequence of NREM-REM sleep recurs with a periodicity of about 90 minutes.

5. REM sleep is a period of decreased physical and mental activity.

6. Stages 3 and 4 of NREM sleep, which are called slow-wave, delta, or deep sleep, provide great physical restfulness.

7. Sleep always begins with stage 1 of NREM sleep.

8. Aside from the artifact caused by eye movement, the REM sleep EEG is similar to the one found in wakefulness.

9. The EEG during NREM sleep is characterized by slow activity.

10. The proportion of REM sleep remains constant from birth to old age.

11. Most people's sleep-wake schedules are determined by social and occupational factors, rather than by internal, physiologic mechanisms.

12. The percent of time in slow wave NREM sleep increases with increasing age.

13. Some productive, vigorous, and well-rested people sleep as little as 5 hours nightly.

14. When an activity, such as falling asleep, tends to occur earlier in the daily cycle, the change in time is said to be a *phase advance*.

15. Infant boys have penile erections during REM sleep.

> **ANSWERS:** 1-True, 2-True, 3-False, 4-True, 5-False, 6-True, 7-False, 8-True, 9-True, 10-False, 11-True, 12-False, 13-True, 14-True, 15-True

16. In the night following sleep deprivation, which of the following cannot be expected to occur?

a. Sleep may begin with a period of REM activity.
b. Epileptiform discharges may emanate from the temporal lobe of a patient with partial complex seizures.
c. Total sleep time will increase.
d. There will be an increase in time spent in REM sleep.
e. Stages 1 and 2 of NREM sleep will increase more than slow-wave sleep.

> **ANSWER:** e. Once allowed to sleep, sleep-deprived individuals will first recoup slow-wave and REM sleep.

17–24. Which of the following characteristics are associated with (a) sleep terrors, (b) nightmares, (c) both, or (d) neither?

17. Onset during stages 1 and 2 of NREM sleep

18. Onset during slow-wave sleep

19. Onset during REM sleep

20. A variety of common dreams

21. Amnesia for any content

22. May be precipitated by loud noises during first NREM period

23. Cannot be interrupted by parents

24. Are associated with somnambulism

> **ANSWERS:** 17-d, 18-a, 19-b, 20-b, 21-a, 22-a, 23-a, 24-a

25–42. Which of the following phenomena typically occur during (a) REM sleep, (b) NREM sleep, (c) either phase, or (d) neither phase?

25. Sleepwalking (somnambulism)

26. Areflexic DTRs

27. EEG delta waves

28. Bed-wetting (enuresis)

29. Sleep terrors

30. Cluster headache

31. REM sleep behavior disorder

32. Asthma

33. Nightmares

34. Bruxism

35. Restless leg movements

36. Parkinson tremor

37. Muscular contraction (tension) headaches

38. Hemiballismus

39. Body repositioning

40. Tics

41. Low-voltage, fast EEG activity

42. K complexes

ANSWERS: 25-b, 26-a, 27-b, 28-b, 29-b, 30-a, 31-a, 32-c, 33-a, 34-c, 35-c, 36-d, 37-d, 38-d, 39-b, 40-c, 41-a, 42-b

43–47. Is each statement true or false?

43. Narcolepsy typically begins in middle age when normal afternoon fatigue becomes prominent.

44. Sleep apnea is a disorder only of adults.

45. Sleep apnea is associated with morning headaches and cardiovascular disorders.

46. Sleep apnea sometimes leads to cognitive impairments and poor school performance.

47. Hypnopompic refers to phenomena that occur on awakening, and hypnagogic refers to phenomena that occur on falling asleep.

> **ANSWERS:**
> 43. False. About 90% of cases develop between adolescence and age 25 years.
> 44. False. Children and teenagers, especially ones with nasopharyngeal abnormalities, have the disorder.
> 45. True
> 46. True
> 47. True

48. Which of the following statements concerning melatonin is false?

a. It is synthesized in the pineal gland.
b. Serotonin is a precursor in its synthesis.
c. Its maximum secretion coincides with the brightest time of the day.
d. Selective serotonin reuptake inhibitors increase melatonin plasma concentration.

> **ANSWER:** c. Light suppresses melatonin secretion. Darkness provokes melatonin synthesis and secretion.

49. In the synthesis of melatonin, what is the meaning of X?

tryptophan $\rightarrow$ X $\rightarrow$ *N*-acetyl-X $\rightarrow$ melatonin

a. Catecholamine   c. An amino acid
b. An indolamine   d. A steroid

> **ANSWER:** b. X is serotonin, which is an indolamine. Melatonin is synthesized in the pineal gland through the following pathway: tryptophan $\rightarrow$ serotonin $\rightarrow$ *N*-acetyl-serotonin $\rightarrow$ melatonin.

50. A 58-year-old man has excessive daytime sleepiness that results from irregular movements of his legs during the night. He explains that they move because they burn. If he arises from bed and walks 10 times around the room, he can go to sleep. However, even when he falls asleep, his wife reports that for the next hour his legs have a jerking movement about every 30 seconds. She, as well as her husband, has daytime sleepiness. He takes no medication. He has no underlying medical illnesses. Of the following, which category is the drug of choice?

a. Anticholinergic
b. Opioid
c. Typical neuroleptic

d. Benzodiazepine
e. Dopamine agonist
f. Hypnotic

> ANSWER: e. He has the combination of restless leg syndrome and periodic limb movements. About 80% of cases of restless leg syndrome are associated with periodic limb movements. Many cases are manifestations of peripheral neuropathy. Dopamine precursors, as well as dopamine agonists, are effective. He does not have akathisia because the movements occur predominantly when he is in bed and seem to respond to dysesthesias rather than a psychologic urge to move. In addition, he has had no exposure to dopamine-blocking neuroleptics.

51. Which characteristic is common to the sleep patterns of both depression and sleep following sleep deprivation?

a. Increased sleep latency
b. Shortened REM latency

c. Sleep terrors
d. Interruptions in sleep

> ANSWER: b

52. Which four conditions are characterized by short sleep latency?

a. Alcohol- and drug-induced sleep
b. Narcolepsy
c. Sleep apnea
d. Sleep deprivation

e. Depression
f. Delayed phase syndrome
g. Anxiety
h. Parkinson's disease

> ANSWER: a, b, c, d. As could be anticipated, disorders associated with excessive daytime sleepiness are generally associated with short sleep latency.

53. Which condition is not associated with sleep onset REM periods (SOREMPs)?

a. Restless leg syndrome
b. Alcohol and hypnotic withdrawal
c. Depression

d. Narcolepsy
e. Sleep apnea
f. Sleep deprivation

> ANSWER: a

54. Which three physiologic changes are associated with REM sleep?

a. Absent respirations
b. Lower pulse and blood pressure
c. Increased intracranial pressure

d. High-voltage, slow EEG activity
e. Absent limb and chin EMG activity
f. Erections

> ANSWER: c, e, f

55. In depressed patients, which two of the following are the most typical sleep-related changes?

a. Delay in the nighttime body temperature nadir
b. Advance of REM activity
c. Advance of cortisol secretion
d. Delay in MHPG secretion

> ANSWER: b, c

56. Which one of the following is not a usual consequence of alcohol withdrawal?

a. Hallucinations
b. Excessive dreaming
c. Increased REM sleep

d. Tendency to have seizures
e. Insomnia
f. Sleep terrors

> ANSWER: f

57. Which one of the following conditions usually does not begin before the age 25 years?

a. Delayed sleep phase syndrome
b. Kleine-Levin syndrome
c. Sleep apnea syndrome
d. Narcolepsy
e. REM behavior disorder

ANSWER: e. REM behavior disorder occurs most commonly in men older than 65 years and almost never in middle-age and younger adults. More important, the other conditions commonly affect teenagers and young adults.

58. Which two of the following are the most effective treatments for the delayed sleep phase syndrome?

a. Continually advancing the bedtime
b. Continually delaying the bedtime
c. Light therapy (phototherapy)
d. Stimulants

ANSWER: b, c

59. In which two conditions will the Multiple Sleep Latency Test (MSLT) show SOREMPs?

a. Nightmares
b. Sleep terrors
c. Narcolepsy
d. Sleep apnea
e. REM sleep disorder

ANSWER: c, d

60. Which is the most important factor in determining most individual's sleep schedule?

a. Early learning
b. Social and occupational demands
c. Cerebral cortical "time clocks"
d. Melatonin secretion
e. Suprachiasmatic nucleus of the hypothalamus

ANSWER: b. The biologic clock is the hypothalamus' suprachiasmatic nucleus. However, social and occupational demands and exposure to light in the environment determine most individuals' behavior. A ready example of external factors overriding the biologic clock is the schedule of people who work at night and then sleep during the day.

61. Which is the least likely consequence of hypnotic medication withdrawal?

a. Insomnia
b. Excessive daytime sleepiness
c. REM suppression
d. Heightened awareness
e. Vivid dreams
f. Seizures

ANSWER: c. REM rebound (excessive REM) is one of the most common and troublesome effects of hypnotic withdrawal.

62. Almost all narcolepsy patients have a major histocompatibility complex antigen in the HLA group. Which one of the following statements regarding this finding is *false?*

a. It indicates that narcolepsy has a genetic basis.
b. The short arm of the chromosome 6 is implicated.
c. Almost all people with this antigen have narcolepsy.
d. The association of narcolepsy and certain HLA groups is one of the closest in medicine.
e. Most monozygotic twins are discordant for narcolepsy.
f. Only 1% of narcolepsy patients has an affected first-degree relative.
g. The HLA antigen is associated with narcolepsy when it occurs with cataplexy but not necessarily when narcolepsy occurs without cataplexy.

ANSWER: c. Of the general population, about 25% has the antigen but less than 1% has narcolepsy. Of those with narcolepsy, almost all have the antigen. When a monozygotic twin is affected, only about 25% of the pairs have narcolepsy. Therefore, although the antigen is almost a prerequisite for developing narcolepsy-cataplexy, it alone does not cause the illness.

63. A 50-year-old man with excessive daytime sleepiness, restless nighttime sleep, and loud snoring undergoes polysomnography (PSG). The PSG shows numerous microarousals when the blood oxygen concentration falls. What is the best treatment for the daytime sleepiness?

a. Continuous positive airway pressure (CPAP)
b. Tracheostomy
c. Uvula surgery
d. Stimulants

ANSWER: a. The patient has sleep apnea. CPAP is probably the most effective and least invasive treatment. If possible, he should lose weight.

64. Which feature distinguishes the daytime sleepiness of sleep deprivation from narcolepsy?

a. Falling asleep when sitting and bored
b. Daytime naps are refreshing.
c. REM at onset of sleep
d. Falling asleep during the day can occur in potentially dangerous situations.
e. Sleep paralysis on awakening from daytime sleep

ANSWER: b. Daytime naps are refreshing for sleep-deprived individuals but not for those with narcolepsy. The daytime sleepiness in narcolepsy is also sudden in onset but gradual in sleep deprivation. The other features are common to both forms of daytime sleepiness. The defining feature of narcolepsy is the presence of cataplexy.

65. Which two sleep changes represent beneficial effects of benzodiazepines?

a. Increase in total sleep time of 10%
b. Increase in total sleep time of 30%
c. Increase in total sleep time of 50% or more
d. Reduced fragmentation
e. Increase in slow-wave NREM sleep

ANSWER: a, d

66. Which one of the following is not a benzodiazepine side effect?

a. Hip fractures from an increased tendency to fall
b. Anterograde amnesia
c. With long-acting preparations, daytime sleepiness
d. With short-acting preparations, insomnia in the morning and daytime anxiety
e. Lowered seizure threshold
f. Exacerbation of sleep apnea syndrome and chronic obstructive lung disease

ANSWER: e. Benzodiazepines have a mild to moderate anticonvulsant effect.

67. In which stage of sleep are K complexes seen on the PSG?

a. Stage 1 NREM
b. Stage 2 NREM
c. Stage 3 NREM
d. Stage 4 NREM
e. REM

ANSWER: b. K complexes on the EEG leads of the PSG distinguish stage 2 NREM.

68. In which direction is travel most likely to produce jet lag?

a. East-to-west
b. West-to-east
c. North-to-south
d. South-to-north
e. None of the above

ANSWER: b. The "lag" is greater following eastward travel because individuals cannot as easily advance as delay their sleep schedule. In other words, when going from Los Angeles to New York, most people cannot easily go to sleep 3 hours earlier than their bodily clock; however, when returning, most people can relatively easily delay going to sleep by the 3 hours. Travelers who suffer from jet lag should prepare for their trip by starting to change their sleep-wake schedule to their destination's schedule several days before the trip. After arriving, they should immediately follow the local time schedule and expose themselves to sunlight in the morning. Eastward travelers can take a hypnotic to facilitate their falling asleep earlier than normal.

69. Which statement concerning sleep apnea in children is incorrect?

a. Affected children have a normal weight.
b. The most common cause is enlarged tonsils and adenoids.
c. The disorder can cause paradoxical hyperactivity.
d. It often causes inattention and academic difficulties.
e. The diagnosis requires children to have excessive daytime sleepiness.

> *ANSWER:* e. Sleep deprivation in children has different manifestations than it has in adults. In children, sleep deprivation often causes inattention, paradoxical hyperactivity, school difficulties, and behavioral disturbances rather than merely excessive daytime sleepiness. Unlike affected adults, children with sleep apnea usually have enlarged tonsils and adenoids, which cause the problem, and normal weight.

70. By what age do children usually control their bladder during the night?

a. 3 years
b. 5 years
c. 7 years
d. 9 years

> *ANSWER:* b. Children usually stop wetting their bed between ages 2 and 4 years.

71. Which one of the following disorders interfere with falling asleep but do not interrupt sleep once it begins?

a. Delayed sleep phase syndrome
b. Sleep apnea
c. Alcohol abuse
d. Seizures
e. Night terrors

> *ANSWER:* a. Delayed sleep phase syndrome is relatively common in young adults.

72. Many high-functioning, productive individuals, such as chairs of departments, exist on relatively little sleep. In general, how do they adjust to 5 to 6 hours of sleep each night?

a. They increase the proportion of their REM sleep.
b. They increase the proportion of their stage 1 and 2 NREM sleep.
c. They increase the proportion of their stage 3 and 4 NREM sleep.
d. They virtually eliminate REM sleep.

> *ANSWER:* c. Adults who are accustomed to relatively little sleep have an increased proportion of deep, slow-wave NREM sleep. In other words, the duration of their slow-wave NREM sleep tends to be preserved at the expense of their REM and light stages of NREM sleep.

73. Which of the following features of involuntary leg movements indicate (a) periodic limb movements, (b) restless leg syndrome, (c) both, or (d) neither?

a. Associated with cognitive impairment
b. Irregular nocturnal movements
c. Seem to occur in response to burning paresthesias
d. Cause(s) excessive daytime sleepiness
e. Associated with periodic EEG activity
f. Involuntary leg movements during wakefulness as well as sleep
g. Associated with periodic EMG activity

> *ANSWERS:* a-d, b-b, c-b, d-c, e-d, f-b, g-a

74. The sleep of depressed patients is characterized by all except which one of the following?

a. A prolonged, intense initial REM period that occurs soon after sleep begins
b. Excessive slow-wave sleep periods that extend until morning awakenings, which are typically early
c. Fragmented sleep with early awakenings
d. Restless sleep followed by excessive daytime sleepiness
e. Early morning awakenings

> *ANSWER:* b. Depressed patients typically have an early onset of slow-wave (stages 3 and 4) sleep; however, their total slow-wave time is markedly reduced.

75. As individuals age, which of the following changes in their sleep pattern is most apt to occur?

a. Increase in REM, slow-wave, and total sleep time
b. Although a decrease in total sleep time, an increase in REM and slow-wave sleep
c. Decrease in REM, slow-wave, and total sleep time
d. None of the above

> **ANSWER:** c. As individuals age, they have decreased REM, slow-wave, and total sleep time. Moreover, their sleep is phase-advanced and interrupted by frequent awakenings. The early morning awakenings of older people are a manifestation of the normal phase advance. Therefore, early morning awakenings, by themselves, are not an indication of depression.

76. By what age do children consolidate their sleep into nighttime and give up their afternoon nap?

a. 2 years
b. 4 years
c. 6 years
d. 8 years

> **ANSWER:** c. Although variability may exist, children give up their afternoon nap by 5 to 6 years old. If they remain sleep-deprived, they may be irritable or hyperactive rather than overtly sleepy.

77. An 18-year-old college freshman who also works part-time as a waiter has symptoms that are essentially excessive daytime sleepiness. On careful questioning, she reveals that she has "irresistible" urges to sleep about twice daily, a tendency to become weak when laughing "hysterically," and is "sometimes totally paralyzed" when attempting to wake for her morning classes. The MSLT recorded two naps with sleep latencies of less than 3 minutes. One of them had a REM period after a latency of about two minutes. Which one of the following is the least advisable next step for her physicians?

a. A therapeutic trial of methylphenidate
b. Repeating the MSLT after she has three full nights of sleep
c. Checking her urine or blood for signs of alcohol and drug use
d. HLA typing
e. PSG

> **ANSWER:** a. Her history suggests, in a somewhat overstated fashion, several symptoms of narcolepsy: excessive daytime sleepiness, cataplexy, and sleep paralysis. However, she does not nap at inopportune times and her MSLT results were equivocal. Although narcolepsy begins in teenagers and young adults, the entire tetrad rarely develops in such young individuals. She is more likely to have sleep onset REM periods from the most common cause among young adults—sleep deprivation. In addition, she might have one of several other common problems in her age group, including abuse of alcohol, using recreational drugs, or depression. She should have a PSG and repeat MSLT after three full nights of sleep.

78. Which of the following is the best treatment for an elderly man who, during REM sleep, flails his arms and frequently strikes his wife. Sometimes he also kicks her during these episodes. His abusive behavior is restricted to REM sleep. He has mild cognitive impairment but no psychosis. Which is the best treatment for this disorder?

a. Clonazepam
b. Phenytoin
c. Carbamazepine
d. Tricyclic antidepressants

> **ANSWER:** a. Several disorders can interrupt sleep and cause violent behavior: REM sleep behavior disorder, partial seizures, head-banging, sleepwalking, other parasomnias, and dementia-induced wandering. Psychotic disturbances, other psychiatric disorders, and purposeful violence can also occur at night. This patient has REM sleep behavior disorder. Clonazepam is the best treatment. In contrast, tricyclic antidepressants, SSRIs, and monoamine oxidase inhibitors are ineffective. Even though these medicines might suppress REM sleep, they may exacerbate the problem during remaining REM sleep.

79. Which stage of sleep is most resistant to interruption?

a. Stages 1 and 2 NREM
b. Stages 3 and 4 NREM
c. REM

ANSWER: b. Individuals in stages 3 and 4 NREM sleep—deep or slow-wave sleep—require the greatest stimulus to be awakened.

80. A 50-year-old man is brought for psychiatric consultation by his wife because he has become "distant, inattentive, and confused" during the previous several months. He began to develop severe insomnia 4 months before the consultation. A variety of hypnotics, antidepressants, and other psychotropic medicines did not alleviate the insomnia. The patient's older sister died after an 18-month course of a similar condition. The psychiatrist found that the patient had personality impairment, cognitive deficits, and subtle myoclonus; he also had tachycardia and labile hypertension. Of the following, which is the most likely illness?

a. Creutzfeldt-Jakob's disease
b. Fatal familial insomnia
c. Iatrogenic sleep disorder
d. Lewy body disease
e. Drug or alcohol abuse

ANSWER: b. He has fatal familial insomnia because he and his sister have had refractory insomnia, dementia, myoclonus, and autonomic nervous system (ANS) dysfunction. This disorder, like Creutzfeldt-Jakob's disease, is a prion disease that is characterized by accumulation of PrP^{Sc}.

81. The patient in the preceding question undergoes further evaluation. Which of the following features is unlikely to be found?

a. Lewy bodies in the cerebral cortex and the basal ganglia
b. Hyperhidrosis
c. Atrophy of the thalamus
d. Spongiform cerebral cortical changes
e. Elevated catecholamines and other endocrine abnormalities

ANSWER: a. Widely distributed Lewy bodies indicate diffuse Lewy body disease. This patient has fatal familial insomnia, which causes ANS and endocrine system hyperactivity, myoclonus, and other motor abnormalities. The brain would show characteristic pathologic changes: atrophy of the thalamus and a spongiform appearance of the cerebral cortex.

82. When used to treat cataplexy, which is the mechanism of action of chlorimipramine, imipramine, and protriptyline?

a. They enhance dopamine activity.
b. They act as alpha-1 adrenergic agonists.
c. They inhibit adrenergic reuptake.
d. None of the above.

ANSWER: c. Tricyclics are helpful in cataplexy because they increase adrenergic activity by inhibiting its reuptake.

83. When used to treat narcolepsy, which is the mechanism of action of methylphenidate and amphetamine?

a. They enhance dopamine activity.
b. They act as α-1 adrenergic agonists.
c. They inhibit adrenergic reuptake.
d. None of the above.

ANSWER: a

18

Involuntary Movement Disorders

The involuntary movement disorders consist of a group of conditions, such as tremor, rather than specific illnesses. These disorders, which can be caused by different illnesses, are important because many occur frequently, provide instructive clinical-anatomic correlations, and can be induced by psychiatric medications. Moreover, dementia and depression are closely associated with several disorders and may precede or overshadow the movements. On the other hand, certain disorders cause extraordinary physical disabilities but little or no dementia or depression.

This chapter briefly reviews the anatomy and physiology of the basal ganglia, which are affected in most movement disorders. It then describes the classic disorders that are attributable to basal ganglia abnormalities: Parkinson's disease, athetosis, chorea, hemiballismus, Wilson's disease, and generalized dystonia. Next, it describes disorders that do not conform to classic patterns and for which origins are not established: focal dystonias, tremors, tics, Tourette's syndrome, and myoclonus. It concludes with a review of neuroleptic-induced and psychogenic conditions.

Several themes run through discussions of movement disorders. Diagnosis of several remains entirely clinical because no laboratory confirmation is available. As with neurocutaneous disorders, "diagnosis by inspection" prevails. Dementia or depression accompanies certain involuntary movements. Certain disorders are inherited.

THE BASAL GANGLIA

The basal ganglia are essentially composed of five subcortical, macroscopic nuclei (Figs. 18–1 and 18–2):

- The *caudate nucleus* and the *putamen,* which constitute the *corpus striatum (striatum)*
- The *globus pallidus*
- The *subthalamic nucleus (corpus Luysii)*
- The *substantia nigra*

Intricate tracts link the basal ganglia to each other and to thalamic nuclei, conjugate oculomotor circuits, and the frontal lobe. Projections from the basal ganglia constitute the *extrapyramidal system* or *"tract,"* which is complementary to the *pyramidal* or corticospinal *tract* (see Chapter 2). Although both the pyramidal and extrapyramidal tracts are intimately involved with motor activity, the extrapyramidal tract influences the corticospinal tract only indirectly—through the thalamus. In addition, the extrapyramidal tract is confined to the brain and does not descend into the spinal cord.

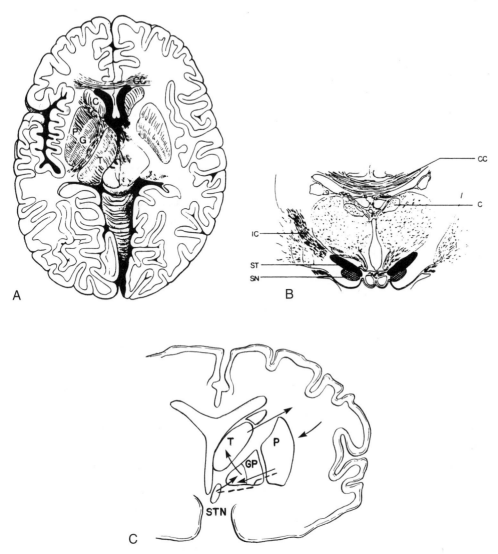

FIGURE 18–1. **A,** In this axial view, which is the plane shown in CT and MRI studies, the basal ganglia can be seen in relation to the brain. The heads of the caudate nuclei (C) indent the anterior horns of the lateral ventricles. The caudate and putamen (P) are considered the *corpus striatum* or *striatum.* The globus pallidus (G), which has internal and external segments, and the putamen form the *lenticular nucleus,* named for its resemblance to an old-fashioned lens. The lenticular nucleus is separated from the thalamus (T) by the posterior limb of the internal capsule (IC). **B,** In this coronal view of the diencephalon, the substantia nigra (SN) and the subthalamic nuclei (ST) are below the thalamus. In fresh specimens, all the nuclei are large enough to be readily identified, and the substantia nigra is black. **C,** This schematic rendition illustrates a coronal view of the major extrapyramidal circuits. The putamen sends a direct and an indirect dopamine tract to the internal segment of the globus pallidus (GP) (see Fig. 21–4). The direct tract originates in the putamen and predominantly innervates D_1 receptors on the GPi. The indirect tract goes through the subthalamic nucleus (STN) and returns to innervate the D_2 receptors on the GPi. The GPi innervates a lobe of the thalamus, which innervates a portion of the motor cortex. The cortex, completing a circuit, innervates the putamen. The putamen also has reciprocal innervations with the substantia nigra.

Of the various basal ganglia tracts, the most important one, from a clinical viewpoint, is the *nigrostriatal tract* (Fig. 18–3). As its name suggests, the nigrostriatal tract extends from the substantia nigra to the corpus striatum (striatum). It provides dopamine innervation to the striatum. Originating in the striatum, direct and indirect pathways innervate the globus pallidus internal segment (GPi) (see Fig. 21–4). The indirect pathway travels to the globus pallidus via the subthalamic nucleus.

One of the main differences between dopamine receptors is that dopamine-receptor interaction stimulates adenyl cyclase activity, but dopamine–D_2 receptor interaction inhibits adenyl cyclase activity. Parkinson's disease is characterized by a profound dopamine deficiency.

While the pyramidal tract generates voluntary movements, the extrapyramidal tract helps select, promote, inhibit, and sequence the movements. It also maintains appropriate muscle tone and adjusts posture. As with other injuries of the brain (except for those in the cerebellum), unilateral injuries of the basal ganglia induce clinical abnormalities in the contralateral limbs. In most cases, basal ganglia injuries produce involuntary movements, rigidity or dystonia, impaired postural reflexes, and slowed or absent movement (*bradykinesia* or *akinesia*).

GENERAL CONSIDERATIONS

The involuntary movement disorders have several common clinical features. Anxiety, exertion, fatigue, and stimulants, including caffeine, increase the movements. Intense concentration suppresses them. In addition, relaxation and, in some cases, biofeedback decreases them. With a few exceptions—myoclonus, tics, focal dystonias, and specific sleep-related disorders (see Chapter 17)—they are absent during sleep.

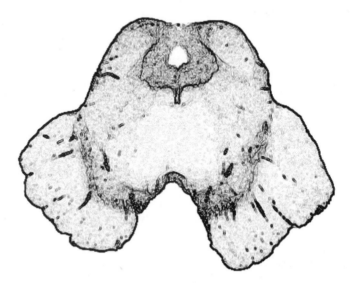

FIGURE 18–2. This figure is a computer-generated rendition of the midbrain that should be compared to a photograph (see Fig. 2–9), functional drawings (see Figs. 4–8 and 4–9), and an idealized sketch (see Fig. 21–1). The midbrain, which lies just caudal to the diencephalon (Fig. 18–1*B*), contains in its lower third the pair of horizontal, elongated, stippled pigmented nuclei—the substantia nigra. In Parkinson's disease, these and other pigmented nuclei lose their pigment. The midbrain also contains the prominent aqueduct of Sylvius, which is the dorsal structure surrounded by the periaqueductal gray matter. Cerebrospinal fluid (CSF) passes from the third ventricle, through the aqueduct, and then to the fourth ventricle. The periaqueductal gray matter is subject to microscopic hemorrhages in the Wernicke-Korsakoff syndrome.

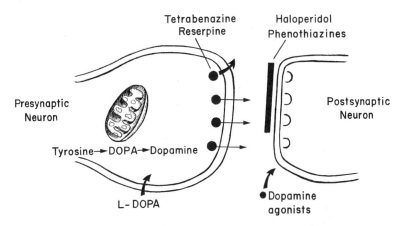

FIGURE 18–3. In the presynaptic nigrostriatal neuron, tyrosine is converted to dopa and then to dopamine, which is the neurotransmitter. In Parkinson's disease, the nigrostriatal tract degenerates, but the dopamine receptors remain intact. An absence of tyrosine hydroxylase results in insufficient dopa and then markedly reduced synthesis of dopamine. L-dopa (levodopa), which is given as an oral medication, penetrates the barrier and substitutes for endogenous dopa in dopamine synthesis. (D-dopa is useless because it does not cross the blood-brain barrier.) Dopamine can be depleted from its presynaptic sites by reserpine or tetrabenazine, which is an experimental drug in the United States. These dopamine-depleting drugs are useful in refractory cases of hyperkinetic movement disorders, including chorea, tardive dyskinesia, and Tourette's syndrome; however, presumably because they drain a vital neurotransmitter, dopamine depletors often produce drowsiness and parkinsonism.

Dopamine agonists—bromocriptine, pergolide, pramipexole, and ropinirole—also provide a dopamine-like effect on the postsynaptic dopamine receptors; however, their effect is less potent than L-dopa's. Agonists act directly on the D_2 receptor and to a lesser extent on other postsynaptic dopamine receptors. (The typical neuroleptics block D_2 receptors in proportion to their antipsychotic activity.)

In many disorders, when only extrapyramidal damage occurs, patients do not have either signs of pyramidal (corticospinal) tract damage—paresis, spasticity, hyperactive reflexes, and Babinski signs—or signs of cerebral cortex damage (dementia and seizures). Instead, patients with such disorders may be debilitated by uncontrollable movements and inarticulate speech, but they remain fully alert, intelligent, and, possibly by using unconventional techniques, able to communicate.

Another important concern is that patients with movement disorders are liable to be misdiagnosed as having psychogenic disorders (see below and Chapter 3). The error is usually made when the movements are bizarre, apparent only during anxiety, or readily suppressed by concentration, hypnosis, or amobarbital. An erroneous diagnosis is apt to occur especially when dementia is a component of the illness, in which case both movements and dementia may appear psychogenic.

PARKINSON'S DISEASE

Of the numerous involuntary movement disorders, Parkinson's disease is the most important. It has served as the prototypical basal ganglia disorder. Studies of Parkinson's disease have revealed the underlying neurophysiology of the basal ganglia and opened the door to understanding other disorders. Although the second most common disorder, it causes the greatest disability.* Treatments are effective largely because they are based on established neurophysiology principles.

---

*The most common involuntary movement is essential tremor.

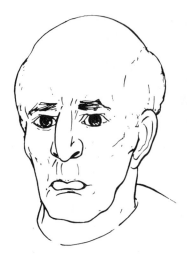

FIGURE 18–4. The facial akinesia of Parkinson's disease patients is characterized by decreased blinking and facial expression. In addition, their widened palpebral fissures and lack of head motion give them a "stare." This facial appearance has been called a "masked facies," Latin for *"face"* or *"countenance,"* but the term *masked face* has become more widely used.

There are Three Cardinal Features of Parkinson's Disease:

- Tremor
- Rigidity
- Bradykinesia

The initial and ultimately most disabling physical feature of Parkinson's disease is bradykinesia or, in the extreme, akinesia. The poverty of movement results in the classic *masked face* (Fig. 18–4), paucity of trunk and limb movement (Figs. 18–5 and 18–6), and impairment of activities of daily living, such as eating, dressing, and bathing.

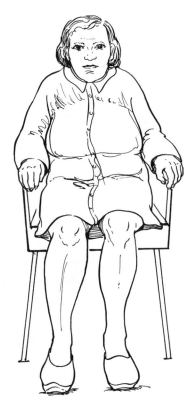

FIGURE 18–5. Parkinson's disease patients typically sit motionless with their legs uncrossed and their feet flat. Their arms, which are rarely used for normal gesturing, remain on the chair or in their lap. In contrast to normal individuals and especially those with chorea, Parkinson's disease patients do not shift their weight from one hip to another or make any unnecessary movements.

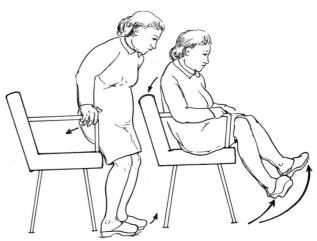

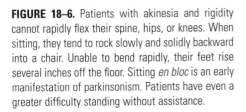

FIGURE 18–6. Patients with akinesia and rigidity cannot rapidly flex their spine, hips, or knees. When sitting, they tend to rock slowly and solidly backward into a chair. Unable to bend rapidly, their feet rise several inches off the floor. Sitting *en bloc* is an early manifestation of parkinsonism. Patients have even a greater difficulty standing without assistance.

Bradykinesia is usually accompanied by *cogwheel rigidity* (Fig. 18–7). Rigidity is also a manifestation of other extrapyramidal disorders. It should not be confused with spasticity, which is a sign of corticospinal tract disease (see Chapter 2).

The Parkinson's disease tremor is usually the most conspicuous feature of the illness. However, it is the least debilitating symptom and least associated with dementia. The tremor has a regular rate and primarily involves the hands and feet. Because the tremor is most evident when patients sit quietly with their arms supported, it is called a *resting tremor* (Fig. 18–8). This tremor differs from cerebellar and essential tremors (see below).

In Parkinson's disease, as opposed to most other movement disorders, the symptoms typically develop in an asymmetric or unilateral pattern, called *hemiparkinsonism*. As the disease progresses, its symptoms may remain largely or entirely unilateral for years before appearing bilaterally. Even when Parkinson's disease patients develop bilateral symptoms, the side initially involved always displays more pronounced symptoms.

As Parkinson's disease progresses, patients lose their *postural reflexes,* which are neurologic compensatory mechanisms that adjust muscle tone in response to change in position. Loss of postural reflexes, in combination with akinesia and rigidity, results in a gait impairment, called *marche à petit pas* or *festinating gait,* that is charac-

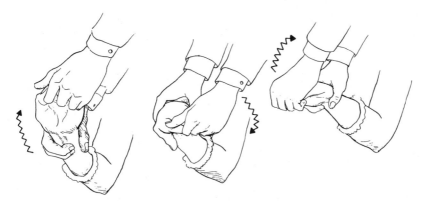

FIGURE 18–7. Cogwheel rigidity, which can be elicited by rotating the patient's wrist, is characterized by increased tone in all directions of movement and superimposed ratchetlike resistance.

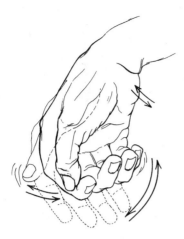

FIGURE 18–8. The *resting tremor*—a cardinal feature of Parkinson's disease—is a relatively slow (4- to 6-Hz) to-and-fro flexion movement of the wrist, hand, thumb, and fingers that is most apparent when patients sit comfortably. The cupped hand's appearance of shaking pills gave rise to the name "pill-rolling" tremor. The tremor is exaggerated or sometimes apparent only when patients are anxious. However, it may be momentarily reduced during voluntary movement or by intense concentration. It is absent during sleep. Rigidity and akinesia almost always accompany the resting tremor of Parkinson's disease.

terized by a tendency to lean forward and accelerate the pace (Fig. 18–9A). In the *pull test*, patients with impaired postural reflexes take an excessive number of steps backward. Mildly affected patients will have *retropulsion* when pushed or pulled by the examiner. More severely affected patients will rock stiffly backward with little flexion or other compensatory movement. Unless these patients are caught, they will fall *en bloc* (Fig. 18–9B). Parkinson's disease patients are eventually unable to walk because of their gait abnormality and impaired postural reflexes. They frequently fall and fracture a hip. Eventually they are confined to a wheelchair or bed.

During the progression of the illness, patients' handwriting becomes *micrographic*, that is, small and tremulous (Fig. 18–10). Similarly, their voice often becomes *hypophonic* (low in volume), tremulous, and *monotonous* (devoid of the normal fluctuations in pitch and cadence).

Parkinson's disease patients characteristically develop several sleep disturbances because of their illness, age usually greater than 60 years, medications, and other factors (see Chapter 17). Their sleep latency is prolonged. Then their sleep is interrupted by multiple awakenings; vivid, disconcerting dreams that reach the level of hallucinations; and involuntary limb movements. Their sleep is also subject to REM sleep behavior disturbances. Following their restless night, patients usually have excessive daytime sleepiness (EDS).

Some of these sleep disturbances, particularly fragmented sleep and EDS, are common in individuals in this age group. The features peculiar to Parkinson's disease are that the locus ceruleus, which governs sleep through noradrenergic activity, undergoes gross degeneration, and the medications often cause nocturnal hallucinations and EDS.

A final aspect of Parkinson's disease is that treatment with L-dopa (levodopa) reverses the symptoms and signs for several years. In practice, because there is no readily available confirmatory laboratory test, a positive response to L-dopa serves as a defining feature of the illness and the best confirmation of the diagnosis of Parkinson's disease. Similarly, absence of a response should force the clinician to reconsider the diagnosis.

Dementia and Other Mental Status Changes

Dementia.   Dementia is not an initial symptom of Parkinson's disease. Patients throughout the first 5 years of the illness typically continue to work (even as physicians), manage a household, and participate in leisure activities. Even in an incapacitating stage of the disease, some patients, who must be carefully identified, retain their full cognitive capacities.

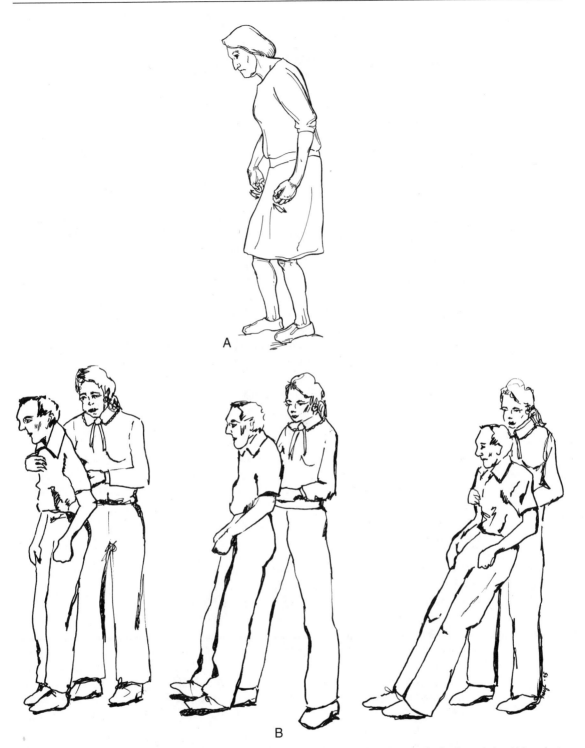

FIGURE 18–9. **A,** Parkinson' disease beyond the initial stages of the illness often produces a *festinating gait,* in which patients take short, shuffling steps and accelerate their pace. When walking, they move *en bloc,* in that they do not swing their arms, look about, or have other normal accessory movements. Likewise, when turning *en bloc,* they simultaneously move their head, trunk, and legs. **B,** The *pull test* consists of the physician gently pulling or pushing a patient. People will normally compensate by taking one or two steps backward. Parkinson's disease patients with impaired postural reflexes will take many steps backward, that is, have *retropulsion,* because they are unable to stop by righting themselves. In pronounced cases, as the one pictured here, patients unable to alter their posture will tilt backwards en bloc and fall into the physician's hands.

FIGURE 18–10. The neurologist has asked the Parkinson's disease patient to write "George Washington" and then draw a spiral. The patient's script shows a progressive decrease in height. The spiral is constrained. The small, constrained size is a characteristic of Parkinson's disease, micrographia. The handwriting also has a superimposed tremor.

As Parkinson's disease progresses and patients age, dementia is an increasingly common complication. It affects about 20% of all Parkinson's disease patients and 40% of those older than 70 years. Dementia most commonly occurs when Parkinson's disease develops in patients older than 65 years and has a rapid progression. It increases in proportion to physical impairments, especially bradykinesia.

The dementia is sometimes labeled "subcortical" (see Chapter 7) because patients have inattention, poor motivation, difficulty shifting mental sets, gait impairment, and (especially) slowed thinking, *bradyphrenia*, which is the cognitive counterpart of bradykinesia. Unlike in most other illnesses, dementia in Parkinson's disease fluctuates throughout the day, probably because medications lead to intermittent confusion.

Depression frequently coexists with dementia in Parkinson's disease. In such cases, dementia is more pronounced but not qualitatively different than when it occurs without depression.

Although Parkinson's disease medications alleviate the motor disturbances, they do not improve cognitive impairment. In fact, they frequently cause confusion, exacerbate dementia, and precipitate a toxic-metabolic encephalopathy that can be expressed as a psychosis (see below).

The cause of dementia is unclear. Unlike motor disabilities, it is not attributable to dopamine deficiency. One clue to its origin is that the majority of Parkinson's disease patients with dementia have cerebral cortex changes indicative of Alzheimer's disease. Other patients, despite seeming to have typical Parkinson's disease, have Lewy bodies in their cortex, which serves as the hallmark of diffuse Lewy body disease (see below).

Psychosis. At least 10% of Parkinson's disease patients exhibit psychotic thought and behavior. In them, psychosis is closely associated with dementia, older age, longstanding illness, physical disability, and excessive levels of antiparkinson medications. Its most common manifestations consist of visual hallucinations (see Table 12–3), delusions, and chronic confusion, but rarely auditory hallucinations. Patients can become abusive and develop paranoid ideation that extends to their physicians.

The psychosis fluctuates throughout the day and is worse during the nighttime in almost all patients. Major physical and cognitive impairments notwithstanding, hallucinations and delusions, which tend to occur during the night, impose the greatest stress on caregivers. They are the chief reason that families place Parkinson's disease patients in nursing homes.

Medications play a crucial role in Parkinson's disease psychosis. Often visual hallucinations arise independently from psychotic thoughts but in close proximity to medication administration. In addition, psychosis may be accompanied by physical manifestations of excessive medication, such as dyskinesias. Sleep disturbances often exacerbate or produce mental status changes.

Because antiparkinson medications routinely cause mental status changes, the first step in treatment is to reduce their number and dose. Physicians should taper and discontinue medications, weighing their toxicity and benefit: first anticholinergic medications, then selegiline (*deprenyl* [Eldepryl]), then dopamine agonists, and lastly L-dopa. Medications should not be given during the late evening or night. Although reducing medicines may worsen physical impairments, patients are usually more comfortable with rigidity than psychosis. However, abruptly stopping them with a "drug holiday" might lead to irreversible motor deterioration, neuroleptic-malignant syndrome, and complications of immobility.

Physicians should avoid administering typical dopamine antagonist neuroleptics because they worsen physical impairments. Instead, they should administer *atypical* neuroleptics, such as clozapine and quetiapine, which affect serotonin, as well as dopamine transmission. At relatively small doses, they control psychosis without exacerbating physical impairments or interfering with antiparkinson medications. In addition, they reduce anxiety, depression, sleep disturbances, and some involuntary motor activity.

Depression.   For the first several years after Parkinson's disease is diagnosed and before incapacity develops, patients' mood reflects their failing health, physical disabilities, isolation from coworkers and friends, reduced income, and loss of independence. As the disease progresses, unequivocal depression affects almost 50% of patients. It is closely associated with a history of depression, dementia, and physical disability, and less closely with the patient's age, duration of illness, and antiparkinson medications.

Depression in Parkinson's disease produces or worsens cognitive impairments, interferes with sleep, and accentuates physical disabilities. Nevertheless, it does not lead to a high suicide rate. Even though depression in Parkinson's disease is common, clinicians must be careful in making that diagnosis. Parkinson's disease even without depression produces lack of facial expression, a hypophonic voice, sleep disturbances, and lack of independence. These and other manifestations common to Parkinson's disease and depression invalidate certain items on the Beck Depression Inventory and the Hamilton Rating Scales.

In contrast to the frequent comorbidity of dementia and depression with Parkinson's disease, manic-depressive illness and schizophrenia are rarely comorbid. Nevertheless, the rare coexistence of Parkinson's disease and schizophrenia is important clinically and because it belies the classic "dopamine hypothesis" of schizophrenia, which predicted that these two conditions, one from decreased dopamine activity and the other from increased dopamine activity, would be mutually exclusive.

Treatment of Depression in Parkinson's Disease.   Psychological support, social services, and rehabilitation are often helpful, but psychopharmacology is almost always necessary. Keep in mind that because most patient-members of support groups are in an advanced stage of the illness, prospective members initially are often psychologically devastated.

Physicians should first optimize the standard antiparkinson medications because insufficient dosages leave the patient incapacitated and discouraged, but excessive dosages or poorly timed administration lead to agitation, sleep disturbances, and hallucinations. The physician should use mild hypnotics or stronger medicines, if necessary, to assure restful sleep for patient and caregivers. (Physicians should keep in mind that caregivers are prone to develop symptoms of depression, especially if the patient is depressed.)

Tricyclic antidepressants and trazodone are beneficial in improving patients' mood and in restoring restful sleep. However, their anticholinergic side effects may impair patients' memory.

Fluoxetine (Prozac) and other selective serotonin reuptake inhibitors (SSRIs) have received mixed reviews in Parkinson's disease patients. Moreover, SSRIs administered in conjunction with selegiline can theoretically cause serotonin syndrome because SS-RIs prevent serotonin reuptake, while the monoamine oxidase (MAO) inhibitor selegiline prevents its breakdown (see Chapter 6). However, incidence of serotonin syndrome is very low.

Electroconvulsive therapy (ECT) has been effective and safe for depression in Parkinson's disease. In addition, ECT improves the illness' physical impairments for several weeks.

Pathology of Parkinson's Disease

In Parkinson's disease, nigrostriatal tract neurons, which are presynaptic, slowly degenerate and lose their tyrosine hydroxylase (Fig. 18–3). In the absence of tyrosine hydroxylase, which is the rate-limiting enzyme in dopamine synthesis, tyrosine is not converted to DOPA:

$$\text{Phenylalanine} \xrightarrow{\text{phenylalanine hydroxylase}} \text{Tyrosine} \xrightarrow{\text{tyrosine hydroxylase}}$$
$$\text{DOPA} \xrightarrow{\text{DOPA decarboxylase}} \text{Dopamine}$$

Once 80% of the nigrostriatal tract neurons degenerate, they produce insufficient dopamine, and symptoms appear. As a temporary treatment, the medication L-dopa penetrates the blood-brain barrier and substitutes for DOPA. L-dopa inserts itself into the synthetic chain and undergoes decarboxylation to form dopamine:

$$\text{L-dopa} \xrightarrow{\text{DOPA decarboxylase}} \text{Dopamine}$$

Bypassing the tyrosine hydroxylase deficiency, L-dopa provides a substrate for dopamine synthesis. It is an effective strategy until virtually all the nigrostriatal tract neurons have undergone degeneration.

In contrast to the degenerating presynaptic neurons, the postsynaptic nigrostriatal neurons, which are coated with dopamine receptors, remain intact. The receptors respond to naturally synthesized dopamine, dopamine synthesized from L-dopa, and dopamine substitutes (agonists).

The characteristic neuropathologic finding of Parkinson's disease, which is immediately evident on gross examination of the brain, is loss of normal pigment in certain nuclei: the substantia nigra, locus ceruleus, and vagus motor nuclei. Another finding is that the depigmented nuclei's neurons contain microscopic intracytoplasmic inclusions, *Lewy bodies*. They appear as round, eosinophilic dense cores surrounded by loose fibrillary forms.

The biochemical defect is not confined to dopamine synthesis. Serotonin concentrations are reduced in the brain and CSF.

Positron emission tomography (PET) using fluorodopa reveals decreased dopamine activity in the basal ganglia. These changes are detectable in presymptomatic individuals, as well as in those with established Parkinson's disease. However, PET is not suitable for clinical practice (see Chapter 20). Other tests, such as magnetic resonance imaging (MRI), computed tomography (CT), and routine serum and CSF tests, fail to reveal consistent, readily identifiable abnormalities. The diagnosis therefore remains based on the patient's clinical features and response to treatment.

Causes of Parkinson's Disease

A worldwide epidemic of encephalitis during 1917 and 1918 produced innumerable cases of Parkinson's disease. Until about 1960, "postencephalitic Parkinson's disease" constituted most cases that physicians encountered. Epidemiologic studies of subsequent cases have suggested various industrial and environmental toxins. For example, Parkinson's disease is relatively prevalent in manganese miners, farmers, and other workers chronically exposed to herbicides and insecticides. Episodes of either cyanide and carbon monoxide intoxication, if not fatal, can destroy the basal ganglia and cause signs of Parkinson's disease. Curiously, despite producing various gases, cigarette smoking is inversely related to the development of Parkinson's disease.

The most notable toxin that causes Parkinson's disease, which was a landmark discovery in the 1970s, is *methyl-phenyl-tetrahydro-pyridine (MPTP)*. This substance was a by-product of the illicit manufacture of meperidine (Demerol) or another narcotic. It caused fulminant and often fatal Parkinson's disease in dozens of drug abusers who unknowingly administered it to themselves. MPTP is highly toxic to nigrostriatal tract neurons and is used to produce the standard laboratory animal model of Parkinson's disease.

On the other hand, Parkinson's disease does not result from cerebrovascular infarctions (strokes). The old term, "arteriosclerotic Parkinson's disease," in other words, no longer denotes a recognized entity. Also, unless head trauma causes coma or is repetitive, as with prizefighters (see below), it has no role.

One unequivocal risk factor is age. The mean onset of the illness is approximately 60 years. Although children might develop Parkinson's disease, pediatricians must first eliminate several other conditions that produce similar features (see below). Studies comparing monozygotic and dizygotic twins, where one member was affected, showed that in typical Parkinson's disease that developed when the individual was 50 years or older, genetic (chromosomal) factors played no role. However, when the illness developed earlier, genetic factors were significant.

One major line of investigation into alternative explanations centers on mitochondrial abnormalities, which have already been found to underlie numerous neurologic illnesses (see mitochondrial myopathies [Chapter 6] and Appendix 3). Mitochondrial abnormalities would explain why many familial cases do not follow a genetic pattern.

Defective mitochondria in Parkinson's disease patients, according to the *oxidative stress* theory, cannot detoxify potentially lethal endogenous or environmental oxidants. Endogenous oxidants, which are normal metabolic by-products, include hydrogen peroxide and *free radicals*, such as superoxide and nitric oxide. The active metabolic product of MPTP, methylphenylpyridinium (MPP^+), generates intracellular free radicals. Free radicals are atoms or molecules that are highly unstable because they contain a single, unpaired electron. To complete their electron pairs, free radicals snatch away electrons from neighboring atoms or molecules. Loss of electrons, which oxidizes cells, is fatal to tissue.

MPTP, when oxidized by the naturally occurring enzyme MAO, produces MPP^+. The resultant free radicals inhibit the mitochondrial electron transport chain, which causes oxidant stress. To abort this reaction, administering MAO inhibitors prevents MPP^+ formation and subsequent tissue oxidation. Pretreatment of laboratory animals with MAO inhibitors prevents MPTP-induced Parkinson's disease.

Despite the attractiveness of these theories, none has been proven. The inexplicable loss of neurons in Parkinson's disease and other illnesses has given rise to the term "neurodegenerative disease." Amyotrophic lateral sclerosis (ALS), Alzheimer's disease, and other illnesses also fall into this category.

Parkinsonism

Parkinson's disease's physical features constitute the clinical condition called *parkinsonism*. When distinguishing between parkinsonism and Parkinson's disease, physicians must be aware of similar physical features. For example, when neuroleptic treatment produces tremor, rigidity, and bradykinesia, the patient has parkinsonism rather than Parkinson's disease.

In some diseases characterized by parkinsonism, dementia appears at the onset rather than after a delay of approximately 5 years. For example, in diffuse Lewy body disease, dementia pugilistica (see Chapter 22), and several uncommon illnesses, dementia is often the first and most prominent symptom.

Diffuse Lewy Body Disease.   From a clinical perspective, *diffuse Lewy body disease* seems to be a hybrid of Parkinson's and Alzheimer's diseases (see Chapter 7). Rigidity and other signs of Parkinson's disease are prominent, but dementia is the initial and most prominent feature. Thus, this illness, which is the second most common cause of dementia, is sometimes called "dementia with Lewy body disease." The dementia fluctuates and is typically accompanied by visual hallucinations and a labile affect.

Patients with diffuse Lewy body disease are unusually sensitive to dopamine-blocking neuroleptics. On a histologic level, this disease is diagnosed by Lewy bodies scattered throughout the cortex rather than, as in Parkinson's disease, confined to the basal ganglia.

Medication-Induced Parkinsonism.   The most common cause of parkinsonism is probably the administration of *typical* dopamine-blocking neuroleptics, such as phenothiazines and haloperidol. Their tendency to induce parkinsonism is related to their affinity for (tendency to block) D_2 dopamine receptors. In addition, at least in neuroleptic-naïve patients, risperidone (Risperdal) in moderate doses (more than 6 mg) causes parkinsonism and other extrapyramidal side effects as frequently as the typical neuroleptics. In contrast, clozapine and quetiapine, which have little or no affinity for D_2 receptors, do not produce parkinsonism.

Numerous nonpsychiatric medications, such as metoclopramide (Reglan), cisapride (Propulsid), trimethobenzamide (Tigan), prochlorperazine (Compazine), and promethazine (Phenergan), also block D_2 receptors and produce parkinsonism. In addition, they can produce other sequelae of dopamine blockade, such as neuroleptic-malignant syndrome, oculogyric crisis, and akathisia.

The clinical similarity between Parkinson's disease and iatrogenic parkinsonism is so great that the examination cannot easily distinguish them. However, one helpful feature is that medication-induced parkinsonism causes symmetric, bilateral signs from the onset rather than hemiparkinsonism. Another feature is that medications often induce face and limb dyskinesia and akathisia, as well as parkinsonism.

Parkinsonism induced by typical antipsychotic medications is related to the medication's dose and antipsychotic strength, as well as its D_2 affinity. Trying to counteract parkinsonism with anticholinergics remains controversial because of their side effects. If anticholinergics are given, they should be withdrawn after 3 months to determine if they are still necessary. L-dopa should not be given because it can precipitate a toxic psychosis.

Neuroleptic-induced parkinsonism may persist for months after the medication has been discontinued. Of patients with persistent symptoms, at least 10% are harboring Parkinson's disease. In them, the neuroleptics merely unveiled the disorder. That group also includes patients who actually have diffuse Lewy body disease, which is unusually sensitive to typical neuroleptics.

Multisystem Atrophy.   A group of neurodegenerative illnesses—loosely termed *Parkinson plus* diseases or the *multisystem atrophies*—share Parkinson's disease rigidity and bradykinesia. The group also shares a predominantly subcortical dementia, but its frequency, severity, and time of onset are variable.

These illnesses are characterized by other disturbances, including ataxia *(olivopontocerebellar degeneration)*, autonomic dysfunction *(Shy-Drager syndrome)*, and limited oculomotor movements and axial rigidity *(progressive supranuclear palsy)*. In contrast to Parkinson's disease, several are caused by loss of nigrostriatal *postsynaptic* neurons.

Parkinsonism in Children and Young Adults.   Although Parkinson's disease can begin in individuals younger than 21 years, such early onset is rare. As will be discussed below, other illnesses that cause parkinsonism are more common in this age group. In many, as in the following examples, dementia, psychosis, depression, a personality disorder, or other psychiatric symptom regularly accompanies or even overshadows the parkinsonism:

- Dopamine-responsive dystonia
- Juvenile Huntington's disease
- Parkinson's disease
- Side effects of medications or illicit drugs
- Wilson's disease

Therapy of Parkinson's Disease

Medication.   The current medical treatment for Parkinson's disease attempts to maintain normal dopamine activity by enhancing dopamine synthesis, retarding dopamine metabolism, and providing dopamine agonists. Enhancing dopamine synthesis, usually the initial treatment, consists of substituting orally administered L-dopa for the reduced concentrations of DOPA (Fig. 18–3). This "precursor replacement" strategy is highly effective for the first 3 to 5 years of the illness, when sufficient nigrostriatal neurons (more than 20%) remain intact and are still able to convert L-dopa to dopamine.

To preserve dopamine concentration by retarding its metabolism, L-dopa treatment is supplemented by medications that inhibit its metabolism by two different enzymes, *dopa decarboxylase* and *catechol-O-methyltransferase (COMT)*. One enzyme-inhibiting medication, *carbidopa*, which is combined with L-dopa as *Sinemet,* inactivates dopa decarboxylase. Entacapone (Comtan) and others inhibit COMT (Fig. 18–11). Because these enzyme-inhibiting medications do not cross the blood-brain barrier in significant concentrations, they do not interfere with the normal nigrostriatal conversion of L-dopa to dopamine. In addition, they reduce dopamine's systemic side effects.

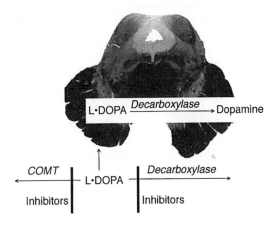

FIGURE 18–11. Inhibitors of COMT, such as entacapone, and inhibitors of decarboxylase, such as carbidopa, markedly increase systemic L-dopa concentrations. Because these enzyme inhibitors do not cross the blood-brain barrier, nigrostriatal tract decarboxylase still converts L-dopa to dopamine.

As Parkinson's disease progresses to destroy more than 80% of neurons, dopamine production—even supplemented by L-dopa—falls to inadequate levels. At that point, dopamine agonists are necessary (Fig. 18–3). These medications stimulate D_2 receptors and have a variable effect on other dopamine receptors.

L-dopa and dopamine agonists, despite their remarkable effectiveness, almost inevitably lead to treatment-limiting "dopamine toxicity." With high doses, they cause nausea, presumably because they stimulate the dopamine-sensitive emesis (vomiting) center in the medulla. The L-dopa and carbidopa combination Sinemet (Latin, *sine* without, *em* vomiting), is superior to L-dopa administration alone because it allows lower L-dopa systemic concentrations to be effective, thereby producing less nausea and vomiting.

Other side effects occur after 5 years of Parkinson's disease, when presynaptic neurons cannot properly store and release dopamine. Then L-dopa and dopamine agonists often cause dyskinesias, sleep disturbances, and mental status changes. The dyskinesias consist of buccal-lingual movements, chorea, akathisia, dystonic postures, and rocking. Some of these movements are similar to tardive dyskinesia. Despite the problems with dyskinesias, most patients prefer overstimulation, which allows them to walk and move about, to understimulation with its rigidity and immobility.

Anticholinergics may reduce tremor in Parkinson's disease and other forms of parkinsonism, presumably by compensating for the dopamine depletion or blockade (Fig. 18–12). On the other hand, they routinely produce anticholinergic side effects—dry mouth, constipation, and urinary retention. More important, the anticholinergic side effects can exacerbate the memory impairments of Alzheimer's disease, possibly hasten the development of tardive dyskinesia, and, in patients with cognitive impairment, precipitate delirium.

Amantadine *(Symmetrel)* produces a temporary, modest improvement in rigidity and bradykinesia. Through unknown actions, it enhances dopamine activity and may also antagonize glutamate. Amantadine rarely produces confusion or hallucinations unless the patient has underlying dementia, is also being treated with anticholinergics, or has renal insufficiency.

Another strategy is administering selegiline for its "neuroprotective" effect, as well as its MAO-B inhibition. Selegiline reduces free radical formation and forestalls cell death through its antioxidant effect. According to some studies, which are controver-

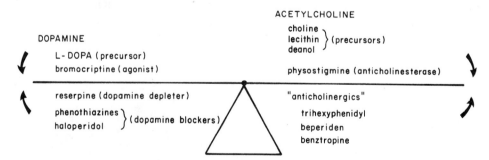

FIGURE 18–12. In a classic but somewhat limited model, the countervailing effects of dopamine and acetylcholine can be pictured as a balanced scale. The left side of the scale would be pulled upward when there is dopamine depletion, as in Parkinson's disease. It would be realigned by dopamine precursors, dopamine agonists, or anticholinergics—Parkinson's disease treatments. In conditions where excessive dopamine activity is postulated, such as chorea, the left side would be pushed further downward. Substances that either antagonize dopamine or enhance acetylcholine could restore the balance. Although helpful for understanding Parkinson's disease and chorea, this model is not useful for dystonia, tics, and several other conditions.

sial, selegiline might slow the progression of Parkinson's disease. In any case, selegiline improves patients' symptoms. It enhances dopamine activity because it preserves both naturally occurring and medically derived dopamine. As an added benefit, it diverts some dopamine metabolism to create amphetamine, which provides a mild antidepressant benefit.

MAO inhibitors used for depression are type A or mixed A and B. Selegiline is a MAO type-B inhibitor, which if administered in routine dose (10 mg daily), does not leave patients vulnerable to hypertensive crises. However, as previously noted, combinations of selegiline and SSRI can lead to the rare, but potentially fatal serotonin syndrome.

Alpha tocopherol (vitamin E) is an antioxidant and free radical scavenger that should theoretically protect dopamine from destruction by free radicals and other toxins. However, a major study showed that tocopherol either alone or combined with selegiline did not slow progression of Parkinson's disease.

Surgery. Several innovative neurosurgical techniques have provided extraordinary therapeutic benefits in Parkinson's disease and revealed aspects of the underlying physiology of the basal ganglia. In addition, similar techniques have been applied successfully in other movement disorders, particularly dystonia and essential tremor.

For Parkinson's disease surgery, the techniques fall into three groups—*ablative procedures, deep brain stimulation,* and *transplantation.* The targets consist of two regions—specific thalamic nuclei and the GPi. In ablative procedures, surgeons place minute lesions in either the thalamus *(thalamotomy)* or GPi *(pallidotomy),* under MRI-guided trajectories. In deep brain stimulation, they insert electrodes in the subthalamic nucleus or thalamus. They also implant a pacemaker-like device in the chest, which stimulates the desired area through the electrodes. The stimulation deactivates the basal ganglia regions by saturating them with high-frequency pulses. In transplantation, embryonic mesencephalic (fetal midbrain) cells or autologous cells genetically engineered to synthesize tyrosine hydroxylase are implanted in the basal ganglia.

For hemiparkinsonism, surgeons perform the procedure on the contralateral side of the brain. Bilateral symptoms require bilateral surgery.

Ablative procedures and deep brain stimulation of the thalamus control the tremor but have little effect on bradykinesia, which then emerges as the most disabling symptom. Early reports indicate that transplanting fetal cells or deep brain stimulation of the subthalamic nucleus may help bradykinesia. In other words, surgical procedures do not uniformly help each of the cardinal features of the illness.

The potential complications, especially with bilateral procedures, are worrisome. Inserting the probes can cause cerebral hemorrhage or unintended lesions, particularly in adjacent visual tracts. Bilateral procedures may cause pseudobulbar palsy and cognitive impairment. Procedures involving the subthalamic nucleus, as might be anticipated, have been complicated by hemiballismus (see below).

Transplanted cells have produced only inconsistent benefits in Parkinson's disease. In fact, fetal cell transplantation is more successful in MPTP-induced parkinsonism than in Parkinson's disease. Although the blood-brain barrier shields transplanted cells from immunologic rejection (the brain is an "immunologically privileged site"), transplanted cells usually survive less than 6 months.

ATHETOSIS

Athetosis consists of slow, regular, continual twisting movements that are typically bilateral and symmetric and predominantly affect the distal parts of limbs (Fig.

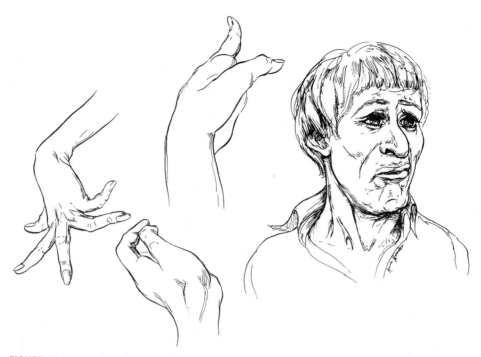

FIGURE 18–13. In athetosis, the face has incessant grimacing and fractions of smiles that alternate with frowns. Neck muscles contract and rotate the head. Laryngeal contraction and irregular chest and diaphragm muscle movements cause dysarthria that has an irregular cadence and nasal pitch. Fingers writhe constantly and tend to assume hyperextension postures while the wrists rotate, flex, and extend. These movements prevent writing, buttoning, and other fine hand movements, but they usually permit gross shoulder, trunk, and hip movements.

18–13). Athetosis, choreas, and hemiballismus comprise a spectrum where movements are progressively greater in amplitude and irregularity. The distinction between them is entirely clinical.

Although not apparent in infants, athetosis usually originates in congenital brain injuries, such as *cerebral palsy* (see Chapter 13). The movements, which are sometimes punctuated by chorea *(choreoathetosis)*, become apparent in early childhood. The underlying cause is a combination of perinatal hyperbilirubinemia (kernicterus), hypoxia, and prematurity. Genetic factors are unimportant.

Because athetosis originates in congenital brain injuries, it is closely associated with seizures and mental retardation. However, when damage is confined to the basal ganglia, some patients have normal intelligence, despite disabling movements and a garbled voice. These individuals represent one of the outstanding examples of patients retaining their cognitive capacity despite devastating neurologic problems.

Dopamine antagonists suppress the movements, but their long-term use may lead to complications. The new neurosurgical procedures may be effective for athetosis, as well as Parkinson's disease.

CHOREA

Huntington's Disease

The best known cause of chorea is Huntington's disease, which was previously called "Huntington's chorea." Huntington's disease is an autosomal dominant genetic illness characterized by chorea and dementia. The mean age when patients' symptoms first become apparent is approximately 37 years. However, approximately 10% of patients develop symptoms in childhood and 25% when they are older than 50 years. Adults with the illness succumb to aspiration and inanition 1 to 2 decades after the diagnosis, but children die twice as rapidly.

Between 2 and 6 out of 100,000 persons suffer from Huntington's disease, making it a relatively frequent cause of dementia in middle-aged adults. Although individuals from all races and ethnic backgrounds have been diagnosed with Huntington's disease, patients in the United States have been traced to several 17th-century English immigrants.

The world's largest group of people with Huntington's disease lives in a Venezuelan village, where more than 100 affected individuals have shared the same genetic pool, environment, and lack of exposure to potential toxins. Extensive studies have described affected children, heterozygous individuals (carriers) in the presymptomatic state, and patients who are homozygous for the disorder. (Homozygous and heterozygous patients are phenotypically indistinguishable.)

Clinical Features.   In contrast to athetosis, distinguished by slow, writhing movements, chorea consists of random, discrete, brisk movements that jerk the pelvis, trunk, and limbs (Fig. 18–14). Likewise, the face intermittently frowns, grimaces, and smirks (Fig. 18–15). When affected individuals attempt to walk, irregular, unpredictable movements give the gait an irregular, jerky pattern (Greek, *chorea*, "dance") (Fig. 18–16).

In its earliest stage, chorea is often so subtle that it mimics the nonspecific movements observable in anxiety, restlessness, discomfort, or clumsiness. It may then consist of only excessive face or hand gestures, frequent weight shifting, continual leg crossing, or twitching fingers (Fig. 18–17). The movements interrupt tasks and cause *motor impersistence*, which impairs the ability to grasp an object firmly or extend the hand or tongue for more than 10 seconds.

Huntington's disease also characteristically interferes with normal eye movements (see Chapter 12). In particular, it impairs *saccades*, which are the rapid, almost re-

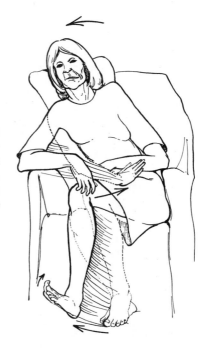

FIGURE 18–14. Patients with chorea, such as this woman who has Huntington's disease, have intermittent and random involuntary movements. Although chorea usually consists of brisk pelvic, trunk, and limb movements, it can be merely a wrist flick, then a forward jutting of the leg, and then a shrugging of the shoulder. Patients with chorea are sometimes said to have movements that are *choreiform*, which is the adjective.

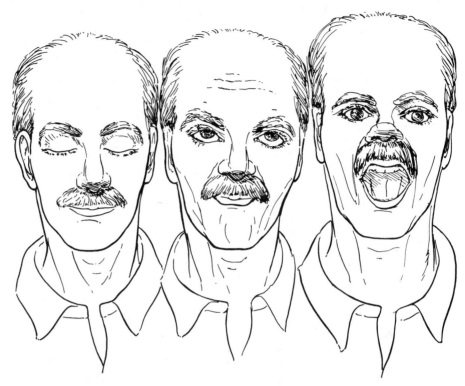

FIGURE 18–15. Huntington's disease patients have unexpected, inappropriate, and incomplete facial expressions, including frowns, eyebrow raising, and smirks.

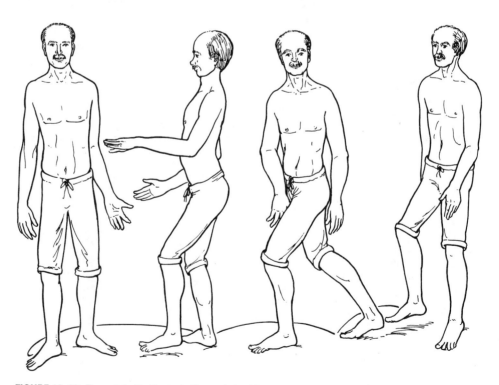

FIGURE 18–16. The gait in Huntington's disease is lurching and contorted and neither rhythmic nor graceful. The gait abnormality results from intermittent, unexpected trunk and pelvic motions, spontaneous knee flexion, lateral swaying, and a variable cadence.

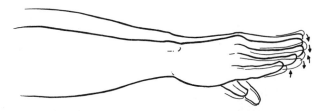

FIGURE 18–17. When Huntington's disease patients arms and hands are extended, they make fidgety "piano playing" choreiform movements that consist of momentary finger and wrist flexion and extension. Motor impersistence, another sign, can be demonstrated by a patient intermittently squeezing if asked to grasp two of the examiner's fingers ("milk maid's sign") or by the patient intermittently, involuntarily withdrawing the tongue when attempting to protrude it for 30 seconds ("Jack-in-the-box tongue"). These classic, graphic terms reflect 200 years of physicians' diagnoses based solely on clinical manifestations.

flexive, conjugate eye movements that people normally use to glance from one object to another. In Huntington's disease, patients cannot make a sudden, smooth, or accurate shift of their gaze toward an object that suddenly enters their visual field. Patients sometimes must first blink or jerk their head to initiate the saccade. However, these abnormalities are not peculiar to Huntington's disease. For example, patients with schizophrenia characteristically have abnormal saccades.

Huntington's disease also interferes with *pursuit movements*, which are the normal, relatively slow conjugate eye movements used in following (tracking) moving objects, such as a baseball thrown into the air. Patients have irregular, particularly slow, and inaccurate pursuit movements.

In adults, the dementia typically begins one year either before or after the appearance of the chorea. Even before dementia appears, patients often display inattentiveness, erratic behavior, apathy, personality changes, and impaired judgment. Especially in view of the gait abnormality, the dementia is often categorized as subcortical. However, this description of the dementia in Huntington's disease is another example of the questionable validity of the cortical/subcortical classification: bedside testing, mental status testing, neuropsychologic evaluation, and pathologic examination often all reveal cortical, as well as subcortical, abnormalities.

Almost as an integral part of the disease, approximately 50% of patients have a change in affect. Most of them have a single episode of depression or recurrent unipolar depression. Some have occasional, transient manic periods. Patients are prone to commit suicide for several reasons: depression, impaired judgment, impetuous behavior, or a lucid understanding of their fate.

A preliminary diagnosis of Huntington's disease can be based on the patient having chorea, dementia, and a relative with a similar disorder. DNA testing, which is definitive, is available for patients and potential carriers, including a fetus. However, DNA testing cannot predict the age when symptoms will develop in carriers unless the degree of abnormality is so great that it indicates juvenile Huntington's disease (see below).

Dopamine-blocking neuroleptics or dopamine depletors, such as tetrabenazine, may reduce chorea. Antipsychotics may suppress some bizarre thinking and abnormal behavior. Antidepressants, mood stabilizers, and lithium may also be helpful for particular symptoms. However, no treatment affects the dementia.

Juvenile Huntington's Disease. In 10% of Huntington's disease cases, dementia and personality changes appear before age 15. This *juvenile variety* of Huntington's disease is characterized not by chorea but by rigidity, dystonia, and akinesia. These symptoms mimic Parkinson's disease and other illnesses that cause Parkinsonism in Children and Young Adults (see above). The juvenile variety, unlike the adult variety, is transmitted predominantly from the child's father, causes seizures, and leads rapidly to death. Despite important clinical differences, its underlying genetic abnormality differs quantitatively—not qualitatively—from the adult variety's abnormality (see below).

Genetics.   The abnormality underlying juvenile and adult varieties of Huntington's disease—as with myotonic dystrophy, fragile X syndrome, and several other genetically transmitted diseases—is a gene containing *excessive trinucleotide repeats* (see Chapter 6 and Appendix 3D). The *Huntington gene,* which is responsible for Huntington's disease, is located on the short arm of chromosome 4. The gene consists of 37 to more than 121 repeats of the trinucleotide base CAG, compared to the normal 11 to 30 repeats. In general, the more numerous the repeats in the Huntington gene, the younger the clinical onset. The gene responsible for juvenile Huntington's disease consists of 60 or more trinucleotide repeats. The abnormally long CAG repeat encodes *huntingtin* that contains an abnormal polyglutamine sequence.

As with other genes containing expanded trinucleotide sequences, the Huntington gene is unstable and tends to expand further in successive generations. The progressive expansion of the Huntington gene, *amplification,* explains why carriers of the illness show signs at progressively younger ages in successive generations (*anticipation,* see Chapter 6). In addition, the gene's trinucleotide sequences are characteristically more likely to expand further in sperm than in eggs. Thus, affected fathers are more likely than affected mothers to transmit a Huntington gene that is amplified enough to cause the juvenile variety.

Pathology.   In Huntington's disease, glutamate and other excitatory amino acids excessively stimulate *N*-methyl-D-aspartate *(NMDA)* receptors. When overstimulated, NMDA receptors become "excitotoxic" (see Chapter 21): they allow calcium to flood neurons, which leads to their death.

Cell death in Huntington's disease and in several other neurologic illnesses differs from the more common form of cell death, *necrosis,* that occurs in strokes, trauma, and many other brain injuries. Cell death in Huntington's disease, *apoptosis,* unlike necrosis, is programmed, sequential, and requires energy. In addition, on a histologic level, apoptosis is characterized by absence of inflammation, which is prominent in necrosis.

Apoptosis rather than necrosis is also responsible for cell death in Alzheimer's disease, ALS, and other neurodegenerative illnesses. In addition, normal maturation proceeds by apoptosis. For example, apoptosis allows for closure of the neonatal patent ductus arteriosus and involution of the thymus gland.

Huntington's disease, on a biochemical level, is characterized by degeneration of corpus striatum neurons that produce gamma-aminobutyric acid (GABA). In the caudate nuclei, where the changes are most pronounced, the GABA concentrations are reduced to less than 50% of normal.

The characteristic gross pathologic finding is atrophy of the caudate nuclei, which roughly correlates with the severity of dementia. The loss of the caudate nuclei permits the lateral ventricles to balloon outward and become so voluminous that they are called "bat wing ventricles" (see Fig. 20–12). As the illness progresses, the cerebral cortex undergoes profound atrophy. PET studies demonstrate caudate hypometabolism early in the illness. CTs and MRIs also show the caudate atrophy.

Other Varieties of Chorea

Sydenham's Chorea.   Sydenham's chorea (St. Vitus' dance), a "major diagnostic criterion" of rheumatic fever, begins 2 to 6 months after the carditis and has an average duration of 2 months. It almost exclusively affects children between the ages of 5 and 15 years. Of children older than 10 years, girls are affected twice as frequently as boys. The chorea often seems to strike healthy children because it develops months after the carditis. With the decreasing incidence of rheumatic fever and development of various public health measures, Sydenham's chorea has been confined to small outbreaks in lower socioeconomic strata.

Sydenham's chorea nevertheless remains an important condition. It is sometimes the only sign of carditis, which is a life-threatening illness. In addition, it is one of the neurologic causes of hyperactivity in children, which include the following: attention deficit hyperactivity disorder (ADHD), dystonia, Sydenham's chorea, tics and Tourette's syndrome, and withdrawal-emergent dyskinesia.

The chorea begins insidiously as grimaces and limb movements (Fig. 18–18). It is usually preceded or accompanied by the nonspecific symptoms of an acute, febrile illness in a child, such as listlessness, irritability, and emotional lability. According to several reports, the antiepileptic drug valproate suppresses the chorea.

Obsessive-compulsive symptoms or obsessive-compulsive disorder (OCD) accompanies the chorea in many—possibly the majority—of children with Sydenham's chorea. However, they do not appear in children with rheumatic fever uncomplicated by Sydenham's chorea. During the 1- to 2-month duration of most cases, OCD parallels the onset and resolution of the chorea. (The reverse may also hold: about one-third of children with OCD have *choreiform movements* [mild chorea or related movements].)

Some children reportedly have evidenced learning disabilities following Sydenham's chorea; however, in many cases their premorbid educational status, which had

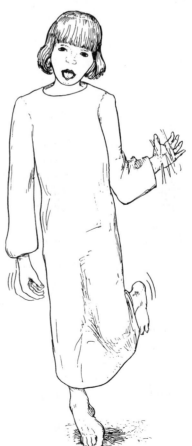

FIGURE 18–18. Children with Sydenham's chorea may appear to have coy smiles and brief grimaces. They seem to walk with a playful sashay. However, the chorea can be made obvious if the children attempt to hold a fixed position, such as standing at attention or standing on the ball of one foot. The chorea has a duration of several weeks, but sedating dopamine antagonists can suppress it and give the child some rest.

TABLE 18–1. *Causes of Chorea*

Basal ganglia lesions
    Perinatal injury (e.g., anoxia, kernicterus)
    Cerebrovascular accidents
    Tumors, abscesses, toxoplasmosis*
Genetic disorders
    Huntington's disease
    Wilson's disease
Metabolic derangements
    Hypocalcemia
    Hepatic encephalopathy
Drugs
    Oral contraceptives†
    L-dopa compounds, precursors, and agonists
    Cocaine, amphetamine, methylphenidate
    Neuroleptics
Inflammatory conditions
    Sydenham's chorea
    Systemic lupus erythematosus (SLE)

*Acquired immunodeficiency syndrome (AIDS) causes chorea when toxoplasmosis involves the basal ganglia.
†Estrogens from contraceptives or pregnancy (chorea gravidarum) cause chorea.

not been determined, may have been impaired by their lower socioeconomic status. In any case, despite the serious, extensive nature of the illness, Sydenham's chorea is not complicated by frank cognitive impairment.

Sydenham's chorea's carditis, involuntary movements, and behavioral symptoms recur under certain circumstances. Additional attacks of rheumatic fever give rise to chorea and obsessive-compulsive symptoms in about 20% of patients. Women who had Sydenham's chorea in childhood may have a recurrence of chorea if they start to take oral contraceptives or conceive (see below). In addition, close relatives of Sydenham's chorea patients are liable to develop the illness.

According to the classic explanation of Sydenham's chorea, group A β-hemolytic streptococcal (GABHS) infections trigger inflammation of the basal ganglia. In a dramatically revised, more inclusive theory, Sydenham's chorea represents the prime example of a *pediatric autoimmune neuropsychiatric disorder associated with streptococcal infections (PANDAS)*. These illnesses probably result from the body producing antibodies to antigens shared by the brain and the bacteria, which is called "molecular mimicry." The criteria for PANDAS, which are entirely clinical, consist of the following:

1. Presence of OCD or a tic disorder

2. Onset between age 3 years and puberty

3. Abrupt onset of symptoms or a course characterized by dramatic exacerbations

4. Symptoms related to GABHS infections

5. During exacerbations, presence of hyperactivity, chorea, tics, or other neurologic abnormalities

Estrogen-Related Chorea. *Oral contraceptive-induced chorea* is a rare reaction to oral estrogen-containing contraceptives. This disorder develops in teenage women several months after starting a contraceptive and resolves after the contraceptive is stopped. It is not associated with mental abnormalities.

Chorea gravidarum, another rarely occurring disorder, develops virtually only in young primigravidas in the first two trimesters of their pregnancy. Many patients or their close relatives have had Sydenham's chorea, oral contraceptive-induced chorea, or a prior episode of chorea gravidarum. Women with chorea gravidarum frequently become so exhausted that they have a spontaneous abortion or must undergo a therapeutic one. All symptoms resolve within several days after the pregnancy is terminated.

Many other common causes of chorea have been described (Table 18–1). In most of them, structural lesions, metabolic derangements, or inflammatory conditions, such as systemic lupus erythematosus (SLE), have injured the basal ganglia. In some, increased dopamine activity probably causes chorea. For example, cocaine, which increases dopamine and other neurotransmitter activity (Chapter 21), leads to incessant foot and hand movements ("crack dancing").

HEMIBALLISMUS

Hemiballismus consists of intermittent, gross movements of one side of the body. The movements are similar to chorea, except that they are unilateral and consist of a flinging (ballistic) motion (Fig. 18–19). Classic papers indelibly associated hemiballismus with lesions in the (contralateral) subthalamic nucleus, but contemporary studies have found that the responsible lesion may instead be located in the caudate nucleus or other basal ganglia. In any case, because the responsible lesions are small and located nowhere near the cerebral cortex, cognitive impairment, paresis, or other corticospinal tract signs do not accompany hemiballismus.

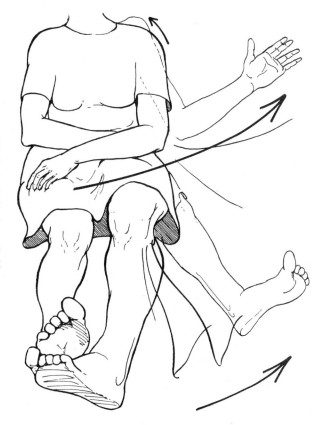

FIGURE 18–19. In this case, hemiballismus is sudden and large-scale movements of the limbs on one side of the body. In many other cases, the movements are more modest. Patients often attempt to suppress them by pressing their body or unaffected limbs against the involuntarily moving ones. They also attempt to camouflage the involuntary movements by converting them into apparently purposeful movements. For example, if this woman's arm were to fly upward, she might incorporate the movement into a gesture, such as waving to someone.

The most common etiology in individuals older than 65 years is an occlusion of a small perforating branch of the basilar artery. In individuals infected with human immunodeficiency virus (HIV), toxoplasmosis lesions have a predilection to develop in the basal ganglia and produce hemiballismus. Similarly, vasculitis can affect the basal ganglia and cause hemiballismus.

Treatment options are sparse. Dopamine-blocking neuroleptics can suppress the movements until either specific medications take effect or until the movements spontaneously resolve. Neurosurgical procedures may be used for refractory cases.

WILSON'S DISEASE

Wilson's disease *(hepatolenticular degeneration)* is an autosomal recessive genetic illness caused by a defect on chromosome 13. It is characterized by the development of dementia, minor and major psychiatric disturbances, and a variety of involuntary movements in older children and young adults. If the symptoms are diagnosed and treated early enough, they are all reversible. The cause is insufficient copper excretion that leads to destructive copper deposits in the brain, liver, cornea, and other organs. As its formal name implies, the liver and the brain's lenticular nuclei suffer the brunt of the illness (Fig. 18–1A).

Symptoms become evident at the average age of 16 years. Dementia, which may begin before the movements, can be overshadowed by personality changes, conduct disorders, mood disturbances, or thought disorders. The movements, which are likewise variable, usually consist of rigidity, akinesia, dystonia, or the characteristic *wing-beating tremor* (Fig. 18–20). Other manifestations can be a Parkinson-like tremor and ataxia. The various movements tend to occur in combination and be accompanied by corticospinal or corticobulbar tract signs.

With its various neurologic manifestations, Wilson's disease is one of the foremost causes of Parkinsonism in Children and Young Adults (see above). In addition, it is well known as a "correctable cause of dementia," especially in young adults.

Nonneurologic signs are often as prominent as neurologic ones. For example, liver involvement leads to cirrhosis, and copper deposition in the cornea produces *a Kayser-Fleischer ring* (Fig. 18–21).

Physicians should test for this illness, despite its infrequent occurrence (1 per 100,000 persons), in most older children and young adults who develop a wide variety of conditions, including tremor, parkinsonism, dystonia, atypical psychosis, dementia, dysarthria, or chronic hepatitis. Because the Kayser-Fleischer ring is deposited

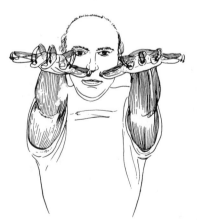

FIGURE 18–20. Although Wilson's disease may induce parkinsonism, dystonia, and dysarthria, it characteristically produces a *wing-beating tremor,* which is coarse and centered on the shoulders. Patients with this tremor, as its name implies, move their arms as though they were attempting to fly.

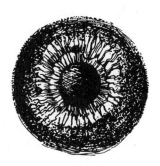

FIGURE 18–21. The Kayser-Fleischer ring is pathognomonic of Wilson's disease affecting the brain; however, its absence does not preclude the presence of Wilson's disease. The ring is a green-brown pigment in the periphery of the cornea. It is most obvious at the superior and inferior margins of the cornea where it obscures the fine structure of the iris. In the early stages of Wilson's disease, when the Kayser-Fleischer ring is forming, it can be seen only with an ophthalmologist's slit lamp.

in virtually all Wilson's disease patients with neurologic symptoms, suspected individuals should undergo a slit-lamp examination. A diagnostic finding, even when the illness does not affect the brain, is a very low concentration of serum ceruloplasmin (the serum copper-carrying protein). A chelating agent, such as penicillamine, when administered early enough, can reverse the mental deterioration, movement disorders, and nonneurologic manifestations.

DYSTONIA

Dystonia consists of involuntary twisting or turning (torsion) movements, sustained at the height of muscle contraction. It can affect one muscle group *(focal dystonia)* or virtually all muscles *(generalized dystonia)*. In generalized dystonia, patients' limb (appendicular) muscles and neck, trunk, and pelvis (axial) muscles simultaneously contract and force patients into grotesque dystonic postures. Although focal dystonia usually remain limited to the originally affected region, generalized dystonia becomes progressively more extensive over years. As a rule, primary and several secondary generalized dystonias (see below) result from genetic abnormalities, but focal dystonias do not.

Compared to other involuntary movements, dystonia usually has several unusual aspects. It can be suppressed briefly by "tricks," such as skipping, walking backward, dancing (with or without music), or pressing against the affected body part. In addition, it tends to trigger compensatory movements, which sometimes make the patients' appearance bizarre. Probably more frequently than with any other involuntary movement disorder, physicians misdiagnose dystonia as a psychogenic disturbance because the movements are so unusual but still controllable by the patient's tricks (see below, Psychogenic Movements). Patients with either focal or generalized dystonia may become physically incapacitated; however, their cognitive capacity remains intact.

Generalized Dystonias

Early Onset Primary Dystonia.   Generalized dystonia is found predominantly among Ashkenazic (Eastern European) Jews. In them, torsion of a hand or foot typically develops in 8- to 14-year-old children (Fig. 18–22), but in almost all cases by the age of 28 years. During the several years after the onset, it spreads to the other limbs, pelvis (tortipelvis), trunk, and neck (torticollis; Fig. 18–23).

Early onset primary dystonia or *idiopathic torsion dystonia*, which was previously called dystonia musculorum deformans, results from the abnormal gene *DYT1* that is located on chromosome 9. In contrast to genes characterized by excessive trinucleotide repeats, this gene results from deletion of the trinucleotide GAG. The illness is inherited in an autosomal dominant pattern but penetrance is only 30% to 40%.

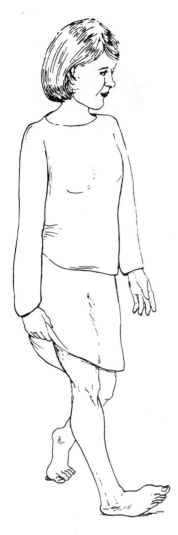

FIGURE 18–22. Patients with early onset primary dystonia typically first have involuntary inturning (torsion) of one foot. In this case, because of torsion of the right ankle and hip, the girl's foot slowly twists inward and onto its side when she walks. Although the movement is momentary and incomplete, she limps when walking. Using one of her "sensory tricks," she corrects her limp by skipping, dancing, or walking backward. Physicians can overlook or misinterpret such subtle dystonic postures and patients' tricks.

The mechanism by which the DYT1 gene produces the illness remains unknown. The only clue is that, unlike in other movement disorders, studies of CSF and autopsy material have suggested norepinephrine metabolism abnormalities.

DNA testing for the DYT1 gene can establish the diagnosis. Various tests—blood chemistry, MRI or CT, PET, and brain tissue analysis—reveal no consistent abnormality. Anticholinergics, baclofen, and carbamazepine provide only inconsistent benefit. For severe cases, thalamotomy or pallidotomy, which would have to be performed bilaterally, might be worth the risk.

Dopa-Responsive Dystonia. An illness described by Segawa and his Japanese colleagues and often named after them, *dopa-responsive dystonia* (DRD) causes dystonia in children who, on the average, are 8 years old. The dystonia fluctuates in a diurnal pattern: it is virtually absent in the morning but pronounced by the late afternoon and evening. As with the DYT1 variety of dystonia, DRD first affects children's gait and then progresses to become generalized. Another feature of DRD is that parkinsonism is often superimposed on the dystonia.

As its name indicates, L-dopa in small doses ameliorates DRD. Since the discovery of DRD, neurologists routinely give a therapeutic trial of small doses of L-dopa to children who have developed dystonia. If children improve, genetic testing is undertaken to confirm the diagnosis. Unlike in Parkinson's disease, where the L-dopa dose must be increased, in DRD the L-dopa dose remains small but constant throughout life.

Children with DRD may be misdiagnosed as having developed primary DYT1 dystonia, cerebral palsy, or mental retardation. The therapeutic trial of L-dopa and genetic testing should prevent such a misdiagnosis. Making a diagnosis of cerebral palsy developing in a child older than 5 years could be a blunder.

DRD is not restricted to the Japanese or any other population. It results from a genetic abnormality carried on chromosome 14 and inherited in an autosomal dominant pattern with incomplete penetrance. The genetic abnormality impairs the synthesis of tetrahydrobiopterin, which is a cofactor for both phenylalanine hydroxylase and tyrosine hydroxylase. The tetrahydrobiopterin deficiency eventually leads to a dopamine deficiency that is more pronounced after dopamine stores have been depleted each afternoon.

Secondary Generalized Dystonia.   Generalized dystonia can also be a prominent manifestation of several neurologic illnesses, including Wilson's disease, juvenile Huntington's disease, tardive dyskinesia, and some rare neurodegenerative illnesses. When dystonia is a symptom of one of these illnesses, it is called *secondary* or *symptomatic dystonia*.

One of the illnesses, *Lesch-Nyhan syndrome,* is notable because of its unusual symptoms and well-established biochemical deficit. Lesch-Nyhan syndrome is a sex-linked

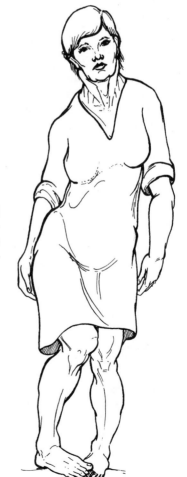

FIGURE 18–23. As dystonia encompasses the remaining limb and axial musculature, patients develop surreal, dystonic postures. Muscles hypertrophy because they continually contract. Patients lose their subcutaneous fat from all the exertion. The postures in this condition are similar to those in Wilson's disease and tardive dystonia.

recessive genetic condition in which 2- to 6-year-old children develop dystonia, self-mutilation, mental retardation, corticospinal tract signs, seizures, and hyperuricemia. The basic abnormality is a deficiency of an enzyme required for urea metabolism, hypoxanthine-guanine phosphoribosyl transferase (HGPRT).

Focal Dystonias

In contrast to generalized dystonia, *focal dystonias* typically occur sporadically, develop in middle-aged and older adults, and involve muscles in one region of the body: the face or head *(cranial dystonia)*, neck *(cervical dystonia)*, or arm *(limb dystonia)*. They are often *task-specific* in that only particular actions, such as writing, precipitate the dystonic movements.

Many focal dystonias have been attributed to either psychogenic factors or tardive dyskinesia because the movements are bizarre, follow administration of dopamine-blocking neuroleptics, or appear similar to neuroleptic-induced movements. In fact, most patients with focal dystonias have had no exposure to neuroleptics. Also, as with primary generalized dystonia, patients' mental abilities remain intact. Except for one condition, hemifacial spasm, the cause is unknown.

Another common feature of focal dystonias is that injections of *botulinum A toxin* (Botox) into affected muscles dramatically reduce the involuntary movements (Fig. 18–24). Botulinum can also be used in generalized dystonia but only to treat isolated, troublesome muscle groups. Systemic medications provide little benefit, especially compared to their side effects.

Cranial Dystonias.   *Blepharospasm*, which is easily recognizable and frequently occurring, consists of bilateral, simultaneous contractions of the orbicularis oculi (eyelid) and sometimes the frontalis (forehead) muscles (Fig. 18–25). Patients unconsciously learn "sensory tricks" that temporarily suppress the contractions (Fig. 18–26). As with other focal dystonias, botulinum injections reduce or abolish blepharospasm.

Meige's syndrome includes blepharospasm but is more extensive. It consists of contractions of the lower as well as the upper facial muscles (Fig. 18–27). Because

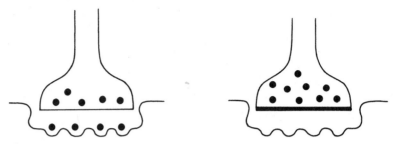

FIGURE 18–24. *Left,* At the normal neuromuscular junction, acetylcholine (ACh) vesicles (the black dots) are released from the presynaptic membrane, bind to postsynaptic membrane receptors, and trigger muscle contractions. In focal dystonias, which are characterized by intense muscle contractions, the neuromuscular system seems to be hyperactive. *Right,* Botulinum A toxin (Botox) injected into muscles binds irreversibly onto the presynaptic membrane of the neuromuscular junction. It interferes with the release of the ACh packets and thereby weakens the injected muscle. The injections reduce dystonic contractions for about 3 months. During that period, the injected muscles may be weak but they usually function normally. Afterwards, botulinum A toxin injections must be repeated. Physicians also inject small doses of botulinum to relax the facial muscles that cause undesirable furrows and wrinkles of the forehead, eyebrow ("frown lines"), lateral canthus ("crow's feet"), and other areas of the face and neck.

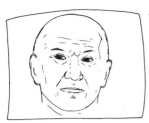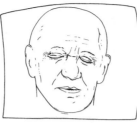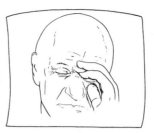

FIGURE 18–25. This elderly man has blepharospasm. His orbicularis oculi muscles have unprovoked, prolonged (average duration, 5 seconds) bilateral contractions. During the contractions (spasms), his vision is blocked and he must resort to prying open his eyelids.

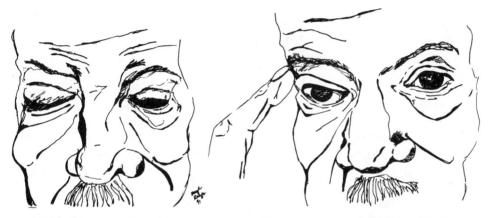

FIGURE 18–26. *Left,* A 70-year-old man, during periods of blepharospasm, cannot open his eyelids. His contracted, elevated forehead muscles show that he is making an attempt to open them. *Right,* He has instinctively learned the sensory trick of pressing one eyebrow (a *geste antagoniste*), which alleviates the spasms for several minutes.

FIGURE 18–27. This patient with Meige's syndrome has blepharospasm accompanied by comparable lower face and mouth muscle contractions. Meige's syndrome movements differ from the oral-buccal-lingual movements of tardive dyskinesia in that they are symmetric, predominantly involve the upper face, and do not cause tongue protrusions.

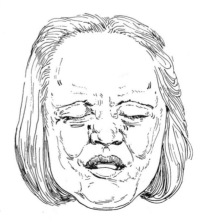

Meige's syndrome involves oral-buccal dyskinesias, it is usually considered in the differential diagnosis of tardive dyskinesia.

Hemifacial spasm, a completely different cranial dystonia, consists of spasms of the muscles on one side of the face (Fig. 18–28). These muscles are all innervated by the ipsilateral facial nerve (the seventh cranial nerve). In this disorder, the spasms occur irregularly 1 to 10 times per minute and disfigure the face. Unlike generalized and other focal dystonias, and classic movement disorders, hemifacial spasms routinely persist into stages 1 and 2 of NREM sleep and occasionally into deeper stages.

Another unique feature of hemifacial spasm is that abnormalities of a cranial nerve rather than a structural or biochemical abnormality of the basal ganglia cause it. For example, most cases are caused by an aberrant vessel or other structural lesion compressing the facial nerve at its origin from the pons (see Fig. 4–13). In addition, misdirected regrowth of the facial nerve after virtually any injury, including Bell's palsy, causes some cases.

Neurosurgeons can alleviate hemifacial spasm when it is caused by an aberrant blood vessel by performing a *microvascular decompression*, which consists of inserting a cushion between the vessel and nerve. (In a similar procedure, microvascular decompression of the trigeminal nerve [the fifth cranial nerve] provides dramatic relief of trigeminal neuralgia [see Fig. 9–5]. Trigeminal neuralgia patients, who are in severe pain, will much sooner undergo neurosurgery than hemifacial spasm patients, who are disfigured.)

Cervical Dystonias.   *Spasmodic torticollis* is a focal dystonia in which the sternocleidomastoid and adjacent neck muscles undergo involuntary, painful contractions that rotate and tilt the patient's head and neck (Figs. 18–29 and 18–30). The contractions have an initial duration of several seconds to several minutes. As the disease progresses, the head and neck continuously turn and develop a superimposed tremor.

Although it usually occurs alone, spasmodic torticollis occasionally serves as a component of primary dystonia. About 10% of cases are familial. Chronic dopamine-blocking neuroleptics can produce a variety of spasmodic torticollis, tardive dystonia (see below), in which the primary movement is posterior (retrocollis) rather than rotatory. Head and neck injuries, especially "whiplash" from motor vehicle accidents, have allegedly produced isolated cases of spasmodic torticollis and other varieties of focal dystonia.

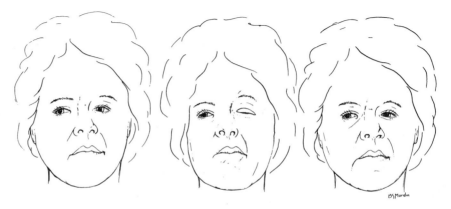

FIGURE 18–28. This 53-year-old woman with hemifacial spasm has left-sided facial muscle contractions that have a long duration (average duration 7 seconds) and variable forcefulness. They repetitively squeeze shut her left eyelids and pull her mouth to her left side.

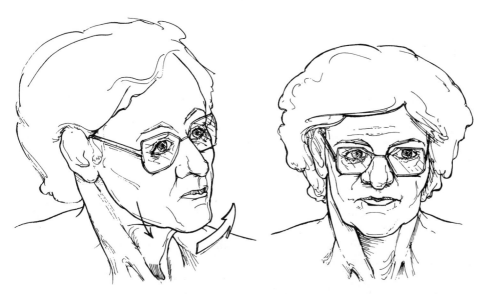

FIGURE 18–29. In spasmodic torticollis, most patients have a rotation of their head in a downward and lateral sweep because of continuous contraction of the sternocleidomastoid muscle. Lateral neck movements are accompanied by shoulder elevation, as though the head and shoulder were being pulled toward each other. Continuous contractions also result in muscle hypertrophy and pain. Most head and neck movements are predominantly lateral, but sometimes they are backward (in extension, *retrocollis*) or forward (in flexion, *anterocollis*). Nevertheless, movement in any direction is considered torticollis.

Spasmodic dysphonia, previously called "spastic dysphonia," is a distinctive speech abnormality caused by a sudden, involuntary contraction of the laryngeal muscles when patients speak. Their voice is intermittently and abruptly strained—as if they were trying to speak while being strangled. Nevertheless, they can shout, sing, and whisper because these varieties of speech bypass the larynx and rely on the lips, mouth, and tongue. Likewise, patients can normally use neighboring muscles to swallow and breathe.

Spasmodic dysphonia is often accompanied by other cranial and cervical dystonias and head tremors. Clinical evaluation can distinguish it from related conditions, such as psychogenic voice disorders, vocal cord tumors, and pseudobulbar palsy (see

FIGURE 18–30. The involuntary rotation of spasmodic torticollis can be overcome by a concerted voluntary effort. As with blepharospasm and other focal dystonias, spasmodic torticollis patients instinctively learn sensory tricks, such as applying slight counterrotational pressure against the chin, which temporarily stops the movement. This maneuver, which is common, not only camouflages the involuntary movements but also strikes a studious pose.

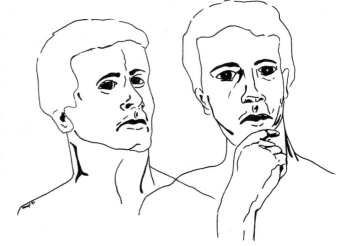

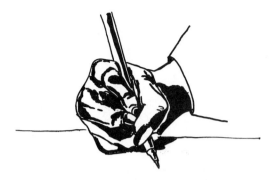

FIGURE 18–31. An author with a writer's cramp develops finger and hand muscle spasms within minutes after starting to write. However, when she uses the same hand to type, eat, or button clothing, she does not have cramps. Writer's cramp is a classic task-specific or occupational dystonia. It differs from fatigue-induced cramps, which occur after hours of performing the task and prohibit the limb from being used for other purposes. Because this author can dictate the material that she cannot write, she does not have the psychologic phenomenon of "writer's block.".

Chapter 4). Spasmodic dysphonia is treated effectively by electromyography-guided botulinum injections through the front of the throat directly into the larynx.

Some investigators have suggested that *stuttering* may be a variety of vocal dystonia. Although proponents were able to cite several similarities, conditions differ considerably. However valid the comparison, treatment with botulinum produced only a hoarse or hypophonic voice without alleviating the stuttering.

Limb Dystonias.   Limb dystonias usually affect the arms rather than the legs. *Occupational spasms* or *cramps* are hand muscle contractions that begin shortly after engaging in a repetitive activity that is often the basis of the patient's livelihood. Patients can perform routine functions with their affected hand despite the spasms related to their occupation. The cramps may or may not be painful. The best example of an occupational spasm is *writer's cramp* (Fig. 18–31). Other artistic or creative professionals are often afflicted: musicians develop *pianist's* or *violinist's cramps.* However, workers in more mundane occupations, bricklayers for example, can also be affected.

ESSENTIAL TREMOR

Patients with *essential tremor* have fine oscillations (6 to 9 Hz) of their wrist, hand, or fingers. Certain actions or postures characteristically elicit the tremor (Fig. 18–32). As in other varieties of tremor, the oscillations are usually in a single plane. In addition to patients having a tremor in their hands, many of them have head shaking (titubation), usually in a "yes" or "no" pattern, and a tremor in their voice.

Essential tremor, which is the most common involuntary movement disorder, usually develops in young and middle-aged adults. It usually follows a pattern of autosomal dominant inheritance with variable penetrance. About 30% of patients have a family history of the disorder. When multiple family members are affected, they are often said to have *benign familial tremor*. The tremor acts similarly when it develops in people older than 65 years, but it is then sometimes called *senile tremor.*

In about 50% of affected individuals, alcohol-containing beverages suppress the tremor. In almost all of them, as in many other neurologic conditions, anxiety intensifies it. These and other circumstances alter the amplitude of the tremor but not its frequency.

No completely effective treatment is available. However, β-adrenergic blockers, such as propranolol (Inderal), can suppress essential tremor in most cases.* Response to these medicines suggests that essential tremor results from excessive β-adrenergic ac-

---

*Propranolol blocks both β-1 and β-2 adrenergic sympathetic nervous system receptor sites. Metoprolol (Lopressor), which also suppresses the tremor, blocks β-1 adrenergic sites.

tivity. Primidone (Mysoline), an antiepileptic drug closely related to phenobarbital, also often suppresses the tremor. Its effect may be the result of sedation.

Recent advances offer a surgical treatment for essential tremor. Deep brain stimulation of the ventral intermediate nucleus of the thalamus, while seemingly highly invasive, is dramatically effective and carries minimal risk. Curiously, the same procedure reduces Parkinson's disease tremor.

Other Tremors. Several similar tremors also probably originate in excessive adrenergic system activity. These tremors, which also respond to β-blockers, result from anxiety, stage fright (performance anxiety), hyperthyroidism, excessive caffeine, and many medications, such as steroids; β-adrenergic stimulating agents, such as isoproterenol and epinephrine; and psychotropics, including amitriptyline, lithium, valproate, and sertraline. In addition, withdrawal from a variety of substances—alcohol, benzodiazepines, or opiates—produces tremor.

In contrast, the Parkinson's disease tremor occurs so characteristically at rest that it is the quintessential "resting tremor." It also differs from essential tremor by being "pill rolling," diminished by movements, and relatively slow (Fig. 18–8). Cerebellar

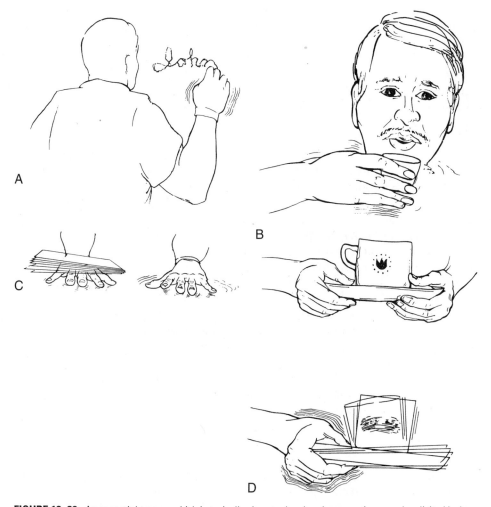

FIGURE 18–32. An essential tremor, which is typically absent when hands are resting, may be elicited by having a patient **A,** write his name, **B,** drink from a filled glass, **C,** support an envelope on his outstretched hand, or **D,** transfer a cup and saucer from one hand to the other.

dysfunction causes an intention tremor that is coarse, irregular, and elicited by movements (see Fig. 2–11). Tremors of Wilson's disease remain difficult to categorize, especially because they can appear similar to those of Parkinson's disease, cerebellar disease, or essential tremor. In young adults who develop a tremor, physicians should probably first consider Wilson's disease.

Palatal tremor, which was until recently called *palatal myoclonus,* consists of uninterrupted symmetric, rhythmic contractions of the soft palate. The frequency—120 to 140 times per minute—is consistent from patient to patient. Unlike most other movement disorders, the palate movement persists during sleep or coma. It often results from small brainstem infarctions that involve the medulla's inferior olivary nucleus (see Fig. 2–9).

TICS

Tics are repetitive, patterned, and purposeless—*stereotyped*—movements of functionally related muscle groups. Although movements that can constitute a tic are myriad, most consist of only a few stereotyped movements. Tics may be *simple* or *complex, motor* or *vocal. Simple motor tics* include a head toss, prolonged eye blink, shoulder jerk, and asymmetric smile. *Complex motor tics* are complete movements that employ several muscle groups, such as touching or hitting oneself, jumping, stomping, or skipping. *Simple vocal tics* are short, inarticulate sounds, such as throat clearing, grunting, and sniffing. *Complex vocal tics* range from words to phrases and include coprolalia (see below). Other tics can involve the patient moving in response to an uncomfortable sensation (sensory tics), repeating words (echolalia), or mimicking movements (echopraxia or echokinesis).

Often, tics occur in rapid succession or in combination, usually with lightning-like rapidity. Various tic combinations can persist for several seconds and generate complex movements. After several months, one tic may recede or be replaced by another.

Tics share many characteristics with other movement disorders. Excitement, anxiety, and fatigue increase their intensity, but their appearance does not change. Affected individuals consciously or subconsciously use various tricks to hide tics. Intense concentration may suppress tics completely for minutes to hours—in fact, more than in any other involuntary movement disorder. Afterward, however, tics rebound in a flurry. Like breathing, they are unnoticed by the individual and can be briefly suppressed at will, but afterward return forcefully.

An almost unique characteristic of tics is that patients have a "psychic urge" to have them that is so strong as to be called a compulsion. For example, patients with essential tremor do not feel that they need to shake, but patients with tics describe an irresistible need to move or make sounds. Suppressing their tics creates the anxiety of an unfulfilled need. Other characteristics setting tics apart from the classic movement disorders are stereotyped movements and persistence during all stages of sleep (see Chapter 17).

Simple motor tics develop in about 5% of school-aged children but, by the end of adolescence, most undergo spontaneous remission. Boys are affected three times more often than girls. A disproportionate number of children with tics have a close relative with one or more tics.

Tics in Adults. Adults may have tics as a chronic disorder that began in childhood or as a newly arising condition. Compared to tics in children, which usually tend to involve only the head or neck, those in adults involve the chest, diaphragm, entire trunk, and limbs, that is, the more caudal structures. In addition, they tend to have a longer duration, be more complex, and occur in combination with other tics.

Tics in adults may be a symptom of various neurologic illnesses: encephalitis, Parkinson's disease, neuroleptic treatment (tardive tics), and the use of cocaine or other psychoactive substances. Even dramatic bursts of obscenities—complex vocal tics ordinarily found in only severe cases of Tourette's syndrome—may result in adults from nondominant hemisphere injury or the disordered, frustrated speech of someone with aphasia (see Chapter 8).

Gilles de la Tourette's (Tourette's) Syndrome

The criteria in the *Diagnostic and Statistical Manual of Mental Disorders (DSM-IV)* for Tourette's Disorder require that the patient display both motor and vocal tics but not necessarily simultaneously; tics are sudden and rapid; the disturbance causes distress or significant functional impairment; and development occurred before age 18 years. (The Tourette Syndrome Association has criticized those criteria on several grounds [see Erenberg and Fahn in References].) The *DSM-IV* also sets criteria for *Chronic Motor or Vocal Tic Disorder,* which allows for either motor *or* vocal tics, but requires that the tic cause distress or significant functional impairment before age 18 years. Its criteria for *Transient Tic Disorder* are similar, except that duration is 4 weeks to 12 months.

Neurologists, as well as psychiatrists, require a *combination* of vocal and multiple motor tics that develops before the age of 18 years and lasts longer than 1 year for a diagnosis of Tourette's syndrome (Fig. 18–33). It affects boys two to three times more frequently than girls, becomes apparent on average at age 7 years, and is present in 90% of patients by age 13 years. In affected children, the tics are often greatest at the beginning of the school year and least during the summer months. By the time they are adults, about 30% of patients undergo a complete remission, and another 30%

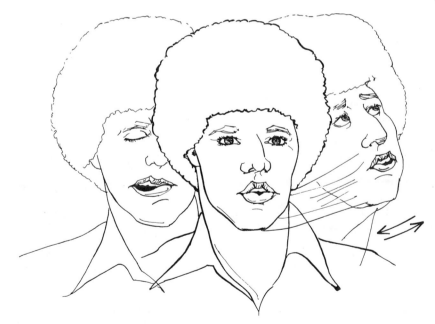

FIGURE 18–33. In a typical Tourette's syndrome, a young man has multiple motor tics, including head jerking (head toss), grimacing of the right side of his mouth (half-smile), and depression of his forehead (frowning). His motor tics are accompanied by vocal tics of throat clearing and a short blowing sound. Tics continue throughout the day and are only slightly affected by conversation, eating, and social situations. They also appear briefly during all stages of sleep.

substantial improvement. As Tourette's syndrome persists, patients display various tics that change in distribution, vary in intensity, and undergo transient remissions. The "repertoire" of their tics changes yearly.

An essential feature of Tourette's syndrome is vocal tics, which are repetitive, stereotyped sounds that the patients blurt rapidly, irresistibly, and compulsively. Throughout the course of the illness, most patients' vocal tics are simple. They usually consist of inarticulate sounds, such as sniffing, throat clearing, or clicks; however, many patients eventually make loud and disconcerting noises, such as grunting, snorting, or honking. When vocal tics become complex, they can culminate in unprovoked outbursts of obscene words, *coprolalia*. Although most explosions contain only fractions of obscene words, such as "shi" or "fu," some consist of strings of unequivocal obscenities. Coprolalia is often accompanied by intrusions of obscene thoughts, *mental coprolalia*, or involuntary obscene movements or gestures, *copropraxia* (Fig. 18–34).

Ever since the original description of the illness, physicians and the public have overemphasized coprolalia. It is not a diagnostic criterion for the illness. Less than 10% of patients have it. Moreover, in cases involving coprolalia, it appears about 6 years after motor tics begin.

Although the relationship remains unclear, Tourette's syndrome is closely associated with attention deficit hyperactivity disorder (ADHD) and obsessive-compulsive disorder (OCD) or symptoms of OCD. For example, ADHD and OCD may be conditions that are comorbid with Tourette's syndrome or they may all be manifestations of an underlying, common disorder. In any case, ADHD and OCD each add tremendously to the burden of Tourette's syndrome and may overshadow the tics.

Between 30% and 70% of Tourette's syndrome patients have OCD or at least obsessive-compulsive symptoms. One explanation for the variability is that complex tics, such as touching, mimic compulsions. Another explanation is that both tics and obsessive-compulsive symptoms stem from caudate nucleus or other basal ganglia dysfunction. Whatever the site of basal ganglion dysfunction, accepting OCD as a manifestation of a brain disorder represents a major revision in psychiatric theory.

In addition to those patients with OCD or merely obsessive-compulsive symptoms, approximately 50% of Tourette's syndrome patients have at least elements of ADHD. Whereas adults with Tourette's syndrome tend to have OCD, children with Tourette's syndrome tend to have ADHD. In them, school difficulties in Tourette's syndrome have been attributed to ADHD as much as to tics. According to some au-

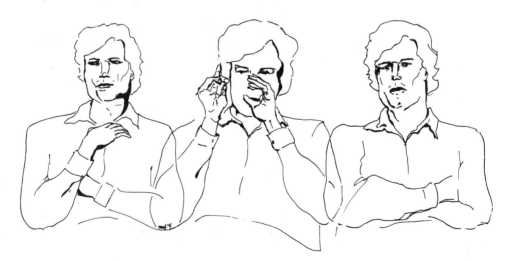

FIGURE 18–34. Copropraxia is typically furtive and compulsive but not sexual or aggressive.

thors, tics in as many as one-third of ADHD–Tourette's syndrome children have been provoked or exacerbated by methylphenidate (Ritalin), amphetamines, or pemoline (Cylert)—stimulants that block the re-uptake of norepinephrine and dopamine. However, other authors found no causal relationship and suggested that the natural progression or fluctuation in the disease activity accounted for any tic increase following stimulant use.

The original descriptions of Tourette's syndrome differ from the current experience. Children with Tourette's syndrome have normal intelligence and no propensity toward psychosis. About 50% of patients have soft neurologic signs and 13% to 50% have minor, nonspecific electroencephalogram (EEG) abnormalities. CT, MRI, and PET do not reveal a consistent, specific abnormality. However, some studies have found increased dopamine (D_2) receptor activity in the caudate nucleus.

As with many other movement disorders, diagnosis remains in the hands of clinicians. They should be able to diagnose Tourette's syndrome when tics are subtle and do not include coprolalia.

Etiology. Studies have indicated that a single autosomal dominant gene makes children vulnerable to Tourette's syndrome. Penetrance is almost complete (100%) in boys, but only about 50% to 70% in girls. With the concordance for Tourette's syndrome in monozygotic twins far less than 100%, nongenetic factors must be important.

In view of various serologic abnormalities in patients, one potential nongenetic cause of Tourette's syndrome in susceptible individuals is group A β-hemolytic streptococcal infection, which is the cause of Sydenham's chorea. Several studies have indicated that Tourette's syndrome, like Sydenham's chorea, represents an example of PANDAS.

Whatever the underlying etiology, dopamine hypersensitivity seems to be the immediate cause of the tics. Dopamine-blocking neuroleptics, particularly haloperidol, suppress them. Similarly, dopamine-enhancing substances, such as cocaine, exacerbate or provoke tics. In Tourette's syndrome patients, as if a feedback loop senses excessive dopamine stimulation, the spinal fluid contains reduced concentrations of the dopamine metabolic product homovanillic acid (HVA). Dopamine's other metabolic products are within normal limits. Autopsy studies have been inconclusive.

Treatment. Medications are usually not indicated for children with single tics, and guidelines are not established for adults with either single or multiple motor tics without vocal tics. In fact, many Tourette's syndrome patients have mild manifestations that do not require medications.

Dopamine (D_2) receptor antagonists, such as haloperidol, fluphenazine, and pimozide, suppress the vocalizations and most motor tics in about 80% of patients. Although these dopamine antagonists often cause transient dystonia and gynecomastia in young men, they rarely induce tardive dyskinesia. Tetrabenazine—the dopamine-depleting agent—has other drawbacks, but it has been effective in refractory cases. An α-adrenergic agonist, clonidine (Catapres), has been a popular treatment carrying few side effects, but its purported usefulness has been challenged. Botulinum injections might be used for single, particularly bothersome motor tics.

Treatment of other symptoms, particularly OCD and ADHD, requires different medications supplemented by nonmedical therapy. The treatment should be aimed at the most pressing symptom. Treatment of obsessive-compulsive symptoms often requires medications that act on the serotonin system rather than on the dopamine receptors. SSRIs may alleviate those symptoms, but they do not suppress tics. Although stimulants *possibly* precipitate or exaggerate tics, they may be necessary and worth this risk in treating ADHD in the presence of Tourette's syndrome.

Applying the theory that Tourette's syndrome has as immunologic etiology, at least one study has shown that plasma exchange and administration of intravenous immunoglobulin reduce tic disorder in children.

Related Conditions

Stereotyped movements *(stereotypies)* tend to be complex, rhythmic, slower than tics, and performed in place of routine activities. Some authors include several commonplace, possibly anxiety-induced activities, such as leg shaking and hair curling. Generally accepted examples are the blind or mentally retarded individuals' rocking motions, which may serve to alleviate sensory deprivation. Classic neurologic examples include the incessant hand washing motions of Rett's syndrome (see Fig. 13–18) and the various movements—hand shaking, body rocking, and face slapping—associated with pervasive developmental disorder (autism). Amphetamine use can also lead to stereotypies and other movement disorders (see Chapter 21). Some stereotypies may even mimic tardive dyskinesia. There is no common denominator or effective treatment.

MYOCLONUS

In several respects, myoclonus differs from the classic movement disorders. It consists of irregular, shocklike, and generalized or focal muscle contractions. It originates in motor neuron abnormalities of the cerebral cortex, brainstem, or spinal cord rather than the basal ganglia. Myoclonus persists when patients are asleep or comatose. Sometimes patients' voluntary movements can elicit *action myoclonus. Stimulus-sensitive myoclonus* can be elicited by the examiner's stimulating the patient with noise, touch, or light.

Not all myoclonus reflects pathology. Benign forms include hiccups, which are merely physiologic shocklike contractions of the diaphragm, and hypnic jerks, which are sudden, generalized muscle contractions that occur at the start of sleep.

When myoclonus results from extensive cerebral cortex damage, which is common, it is associated with dementia, delirium, and seizures. For example, myoclonus is occasionally a manifestation of the AIDS-dementia complex and Alzheimer's disease. In addition, it is the most prominent physical manifestation of both subacute sclerosing panencephalitis (SSPE) and Creutzfeldt-Jakob disease, which are characterized by a triad of myoclonus, dementia, and periodic EEG complexes (see Chapters 7 and 10). Myoclonus also commonly results from toxic-metabolic encephalopathy due to anoxia, uremia, or toxic levels of medications, including penicillin, meperidine (Demerol), and SSRIs. Clonazepam or sometimes valproate can suppress myoclonus.

MOVEMENT DISORDERS FROM DOPAMINE-BLOCKING NEUROLEPTICS

Both *typical* dopamine-blocking neuroleptics and nonpsychiatric dopamine-blocking medications cause parkinsonism and the neuroleptic-malignant syndrome (see Chapter 6), lower the seizure threshold, alter the EEG (see Chapter 10), and produce retinal abnormalities (see Chapter 12). In addition, they can cause a variety of striking involuntary movement disorders that are often called "extrapyramidal reactions."

Neurologists divide most dopamine-blocking disorders into two major groups—*acute* and *tardive dyskinesias* (Table 18–2). Acute dyskinesias develop within days of ini-

TABLE 18–2. *Neuroleptic-Induced Movement Disorders*

Acute dyskinesias
    Oculogyric crisis and other dystonias
    Parkinsonism
    Akathisia
Tardive dyskinesias
    Oral-buccal-lingual dyskinesia*
    Dystonia
    Akathisia
    Tics
    Tremor
    Stereotypies
Neuroleptic-malignant syndrome
Serotonin syndrome
Withdrawal emergent dyskinesias

*Commonly referred to as tardive dyskinesia.

tiating or increasing the dose of the medication and subside spontaneously or in response to decreasing the neuroleptic dose. Tardive dyskinesias develop late—as their name indicates. By definition, the interval must be at least 6 months after initiating the neuroleptic. They rarely subside spontaneously and are resistant to treatment.

Acute Dyskinesias

Acute Dystonias. Acute dystonic reactions consist of abruptly developing limb or trunk dystonic postures, repetitive jaw and face muscle contractions, tongue protrusion, torticollis, or oculogyric crisis (Fig. 18–35). These movements may occur alone or in combination. Unlike other movement disorders, acute dystonic reactions are painful.

Compared to middle-aged and older individuals, adolescents and young adults seem to be more susceptible to forceful, dramatic trunk, neck, and limb extension with prominent retrocollis. Physicians must keep in mind that several serious neurologic disorders—seizures, meningitis, and tetanus—can cause similar postures and psychosis.

Prophylactic use of oral anticholinergics may prevent acute dystonic reactions. Once these reactions have begun they can be aborted by intravenous anticholinergic

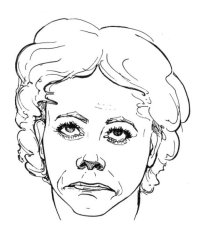

FIGURE 18–35. During an oculogyric crisis, the patient's eyes roll upward or sidewards. The ocular movements are often accompanied by jaw and neck muscle contractions. When these movements follow the administration of dopamine-blocking neuroleptics, they usually can be aborted by anticholinergics.

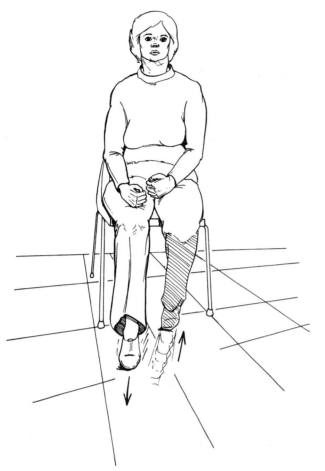

FIGURE 18–36. Akathisia usually consists of continual, fairly regular, to-and-fro sliding leg movements, repeated leg crossings, or lateral knee movements. Leg movements are especially prominent when a neuroleptic causes akinesia of the upper trunk, arms, and face, as in this case. Akathisia can also lead to repetitive arms movements, such as scratching, hair smoothing, and rubbing.

or antihistamine medications, such as diphenhydramine (Benadryl) 50 to 100 mg or trihexyphenidyl, 2 mg IV, followed by oral anticholinergics for several days.

Several explanations have been proposed. The beneficial response to anticholinergics indicates that acute dystonic reactions most likely result from excessive cholinergic activity. On the other hand, they may result from brief, excessive dopamine activity when the dopamine blockade initially stimulates dopamine receptors. Another explanation is that, as the initial neuroleptic dose falls off, dopamine receptors are left completely exposed and oversensitive.

Parkinsonism.   Neuroleptic-induced parkinsonism was differentiated from Parkinson's disease in the previous section.

Akathisia.   Akathisia is continual, almost regular leg movements while lying, sitting, or standing (Fig. 18–36). As with tics, akathisia is partly a response to a psychic urge. Patients complain of having a need or compulsion to move, restlessness, and an intense desire to walk. Because the desire to move can exceed the movements, akathisia may reasonably be mistaken for anxiety, agitated depression, or an insufficiently treated psychiatric disturbance. In this case, the psychiatrist is confronted with the problem of whether to increase the psychiatric medications or institute treatment for akathisia, which might include reducing the medications.

The leg movements resemble those induced by fluoxetine, cocaine, or excessive L-dopa. Although they also mimic restless leg syndrome, patients' lack of paresthesias distinguishes akathisia.

As neuroleptic treatment continues, akathisia recedes. It can be alleviated by reducing the neuroleptic dosage or, according to some reports, by propranolol and benzodiazepines.

Tardive Dyskinesias

Oral-Buccal-Lingual Variety. The *oral-buccal-lingual, choreic,* or *orofacial syndrome* variety is so common that it has become the generic term for all tardive dyskinesias; however, physicians should recognize several varieties of tardive, as well as acute, dyskinesias (Table 18–2). It consists of the well-known tongue, jaw, and lower face movements that are either stereotyped or irregular (Fig. 18–37). They can properly be labeled as either stereotypies or chorea. They are painless and are not provoked by urges to move.

Incidence remains constant throughout neuroleptic exposure, which results in an increasing prevalence with increasing age. In other words, most patients have the same chance of developing tardive dyskinesia during the first year as during the fifth year of neuroleptic treatment. Prevalence is greater among women than men, especially for individuals older than 65 years. Those with preexisting brain disease are also particularly at risk.

Causes. Despite its limitations, the *dopamine receptor hypersensitivity theory* remains popular and is consistent with several of tardive dyskinesia's major clinical features (Fig. 18–38). For example, tardive dyskinesias begin only a relatively long time (6 months) after typical dopamine-blocking neuroleptics are instituted, when denervation hypersensitivity would be expected to develop. The dyskinesias are similar, although not identical, to those produced by excessive L-dopa. They are worsened by maneuvers that expose the postsynaptic neuron to increased dopamine concentrations, such as reducing the dosage of these neuroleptics, stopping them (withdrawal-emergent syndrome, see below), or adding L-dopa. Likewise, tardive dyskinesias are suppressed by increasing the neuroleptic dosage, which would reduce dopamine receptor exposure. In addition, many months after the neuroleptics are discontinued,

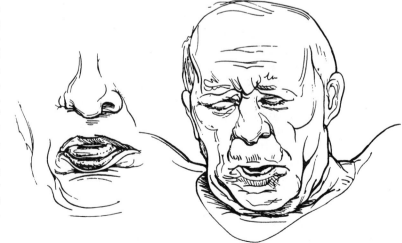

FIGURE 18–37. The oral-buccal-lingual variety of tardive dyskinesia consists of repetitive tongue movements accompanied by continual jaw and facial muscle contractions, that is, chorea of the tongue, jaw, and lower face. The movements, which may be stereotyped, typically include tongue darting, lip smacking, kissing, lip puckering, chewing, and sometimes blepharospasm. Note that in this variety of tardive dyskinesia, unlike chorea and cranial dystonias, tongue movements are prominent and tongue enlargement (macroglossia) may develop.

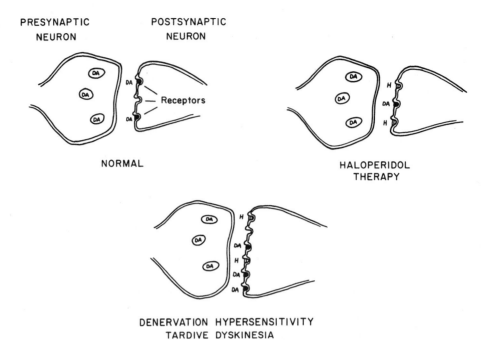

FIGURE 18–38. The denervation hypersensitivity theory proposes that when postsynaptic (D$_2$) dopamine receptors are occupied by typical neuroleptics, such as haloperidol, dopamine receptor blockade leads to physiologic denervation. In response, postsynaptic receptor sites eventually become more numerous and more sensitive (hypersensitive). Once hypersensitivity is established, minute quantities of dopamine—either released from the presynaptic neuron, able to evade the blockade, or present in the ambient fluid—can trigger receptors.

some cases spontaneously remit, which suggests that dopamine sensitivity can revert to normal. Finally, the theory is consistent with reports that clozapine and other atypical neuroleptics, which do not block D$_2$ dopamine receptors, are uncomplicated by parkinsonism or tardive dyskinesias.

An alternative theory attributes the disorder to abnormal GABA activity in the striatum. Another one is that the glutamate system triggers excitotoxicity through the NMDA receptors.

Treatment.   In recent studies, clozapine reportedly suppressed tardive dyskinesia; however, this effect may take months to appear. Switching to this atypical neuroleptic at least spares the patient continued exposure to D$_2$ receptor blockade.

The traditional approach has aimed at reducing dopamine activity. Dopamine depletors, such as reserpine, α-methylparatyrosine, and tetrabenazine, have been helpful in some cases. Tetrabenazine is consistently effective in tardive dyskinesias, as in other hyperkinetic disorders. However, dopamine-depleting medications frequently cause hypotension, depression, sleep disturbances, or parkinsonism.

Along the same line, but as a last resort, physicians have reinstituted the dopamine receptor blockade by increasing the dosage of a typical dopamine-blocking neuroleptic, substituting a more potent neuroleptic, or restarting the neuroleptic if it had been discontinued. This strategy may create a vicious cycle in which recurrence of the dyskinesia again requires additional medication.

A different strategy has been to counterbalance enhanced dopamine activity with enhanced acetylcholine (ACh) activity. However, except for brief periods, physostigmine, which prolongs ACh activity, and ACh precursors, such as deanol (Deaner), lecithin, or choline, have all failed to help. The opposite approach, giving anticholinergics, also does not help.

Medications that affect other neurotransmitters have also not been helpful. For example, GABA agonists, such as valproate (Depakote) and baclofen (Lioresal); a calcium channel blocker, diltiazem (Cardizem); lithium; opiates; and clonazepam do not consistently alleviate the movements.

Botulinum toxin injections cannot yet be administered for dyskinesias that involve the tongue. Injecting its main muscles (genioglossus and geniohyoid) would require a needle to pass through the upper part of the neck, which contains vital structures. Moreover, the medication would entail a risk of throat weakness and the tongue slipping back to occlude the airway.

Tardive Dystonia.   A related condition, *tardive dystonia* consists of sustained, powerful, twisting, and predominantly extensor postures (Fig. 18–39). The increased tone of the neck extensor muscles produces its characteristic feature, retrocollis. Tardive dystonia can develop after a relatively short neuroleptic exposure, sometimes as brief as 3 months, but its incidence is constant on a year to year basis.

As with many of the tardive dyskinesias, tardive dystonia is often accompanied by other neuroleptic-induced movements, including oral-buccal-lingual dyskinesia, blepharospasm, and akathisia. Tardive dystonia is otherwise similar to the dystonia seen in Wilson's disease, generalized dystonia, focal dystonia (spasmodic torticollis), and juvenile Huntington's disease.

Tardive dystonia, in contrast to choreic oral-buccal-lingual dyskinesia, partially responds to anticholinergics and sometimes to dopamine depletors. Botulinum toxin injections, a more readily available and less risky treatment of this condition, alleviate the dystonia in affected muscles groups. In clinically perplexing cases—such as where neck movements might represent either spasmodic torticollis or tardive dystonia—botulinum toxin injections are effective whatever the underlying cause.

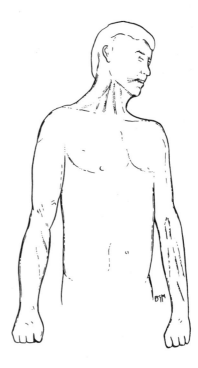

FIGURE 18–39. Tardive dystonia in a 35-year-old man who has been receiving neuroleptic treatment for several years consists of prolonged twisting and extension of his arms, extension of his head and neck (retrocollis), and arching of his back. This variety of tardive dyskinesia is accompanied in the majority of cases by choreiform oral-buccal-lingual movements, blepharospasm, or other varieties of tardive dyskinesia. Tardive dystonia differs from idiopathic or torsion dystonia by its tendency for retrocollis rather than torticollis and by the simultaneous appearance of other tardive dyskinesias.

Other Tardive Dyskinesias.   *Tardive akathisia*, which appears similar to the acutely developing disorder, persists long after initiation of neuroleptic therapy. It may appear only after the neuroleptic is withdrawn. Oral choreiform movements and other tardive dyskinesias often accompany tardive akathisia. To emphasize that tardive akathisia, like acute akathisia, stems from uncomfortable sensations, one neurologist quipped that patients with tardive dyskinesia are distressed because they move, but those with tardive akathisia move because they are distressed.

Opioids, benzodiazepines, and propranolol sometimes can alleviate tardive akathisia. Reported benefits from reserpine, tetrabenazine, amantadine, anticholinergics, and other medications remain unconfirmed.

Patients may have *tardive tics* that involve vocalization and breathing, such as grunts and loud, irregular gasping. They can have *tardive oculogyric crises, tardive tremors,* and other tardive movements. As with tardive dystonia and akathisia, all these dyskinesias are typically accompanied by oral choreiform movements.

Withdrawal-Emergent Syndrome

Withdrawal-emergent syndrome (WES) consists of involuntary movements that appear after the abrupt cessation of prolonged neuroleptic administration. The movements consist of mild to moderately severe chorea with motor impersistence and restlessness. WES characteristically lasts less than 6 weeks. It typically affects children and mimics Sydenham's chorea, except for OCD or ADHD symptoms.

WES lasting longer than 6 months probably represents tardive dyskinesia. For intolerable dyskinesias, physicians might have to reinstitute the neuroleptic and then slowly withdraw it.

MOVEMENT DISORDERS FROM OTHER PSYCHIATRIC MEDICATIONS

Atypical Neuroleptics

Probably because they have little or no affinity for the D_2 receptors, atypical neuroleptics are less likely than typical neuroleptics to cause extrapyramidal movement disorders. Risperidone and olanzapine, at very low doses, carry a low incidence of parkinsonism; however, at therapeutic doses, risperidone induces dose-dependent parkinsonism at a rate comparable to haloperidol-inducing parkinsonism. Neither of these neuroleptics is particularly suitable for treatment of psychosis in either Parkinson's or diffuse Lewy body diseases.

Clozapine and quetiapine rarely cause acute extrapyramidal reactions, such as parkinsonism or neuroleptic malignant syndrome. Moreover, not only is clozapine unlikely to cause tardive dyskinesia, it may also suppress dyskinesias when they are caused by a typical neuroleptic. Nevertheless, abruptly discontinuing clozapine can produce a WES.

SSRIs

As SSRIs elevate a patient's mood, they may also increase motor activity to abnormal levels, inducing "shakiness," tremor, leg movements that resemble akathisia, or myoclonus. In addition, some patients have developed "complex movements" that involve myoclonus.

As discussed previously, SSRIs may exacerbate motor symptoms of Parkinson's disease. A greater concern is that they will interact with MAO inhibitors or other medications and cause the serotonin syndrome. Despite these caveats, reports of serious adverse reactions to SSRIs refer to a small proportion of patients. The serious reactions usually occurred when SSRIs were administered in high doses, combined with other psychiatric medications, or patients had a preexisting movement disorder.

Other Medications. Tricyclic antidepressants, because of their anticholinergic properties, cause ocular accommodation impairment (see Fig. 12–4), narrow angle glaucoma (see Fig. 12–7), and urinary hesitancy or retention (see Fig. 15–5). In addition, about 10% of patients taking them develop a fine tremor that appears similar to essential tremor and also responds to propranolol. The antidepressant amoxapine, which has dopamine antagonist properties, can induce parkinsonism; however, almost no other antidepressant causes parkinsonism or other sign of extrapyramidal dysfunction.

Lithium, at high therapeutic serum concentrations, can induce a fine, rapid tremor that mimics essential tremor. At toxic concentrations, it produces a severe, coarse intention tremor that is often accompanied by ataxia of the trunk—signs of cerebellar dysfunction. Sometimes lithium toxicity causes extrapyramidal signs. Although adding propranolol may suppress a mild tremor, reducing the lithium dose would usually be the preferable treatment.

Antiepileptic drugs often cause tremors, ataxia, and sometimes asterixis, but generally only at serum concentrations greater than necessary for their therapeutic effect. In addition, phenytoin at those levels may cause athetosis or chorea. One exception is that valproate may cause a tremor that may not be dose-related.

Non-Iatrogenic Movements. Abnormal tongue, jaw, and facial movements are, of course, not peculiar to tardive dyskinesia. In fact, stereotyped movements of the face, mouth, or tongue have been observed in schizophrenic patients who have never received neuroleptics. *Buccolingual dyskinesia of the elderly* is observable in individuals considerably older than 65 years, especially those with dementia. Toothless older individuals may develop *edentulous orofacial dyskinesia.* In this dyskinesia, the absence of teeth presumably deprives the tongue of its expected proprioceptive feedback. Properly fitting dentures will stop the tongue movements.

The *Abnormal Involuntary Movement Scale (AIMS)* is a suitable device to record the presence or absence of abnormal movements (Fig. 18–40). However, this scale has several drawbacks. It attempts to assess dyskinesias that fluctuate in intensity during the day; the measurements are gross; it does not recognize akinesia (lack of movement), which is as important as hyperkinesia; and it does not distinguish among chorea, dystonia, tics, and stereotypies.

PSYCHOGENIC MOVEMENTS

Commonly accepted indications of a psychogenic movement are (1) the absence of movements when patients believe themselves to be unobserved; (2) relief with non-pharmacologic treatment, such as placebos, psychotherapy, or physical therapy; (3) incongruency (a variable location, intensity, or occurrence of the movements); (4) coexistence of psychogenic weakness or sensory loss, a somatization disorder, or other relevant psychiatric condition; and (5) outstanding litigation.

Virtually every variety of movement disorder has been considered psychogenic, but dystonia, tremor, and myoclonus are most commonly diagnosed as psychogenic. In psychogenic dystonia, movements tend to be bizarre, inconsistent in location, incongruent, paroxysmal, and associated with psychogenic weakness and sensory loss.

		DEPARTMENT OF HEALTH AND HUMAN SERVICES	PATIENT NUMBER	DATA GROUP	EVALUATION DATE

DEPARTMENT OF HEALTH AND HUMAN SERVICES
PUBLIC HEALTH SERVICE
Alcohol, Drug Abuse, and Mental Health Administration
NIMH Treatment Strategies in Schizophrenia Study

ABNORMAL INVOLUNTARY MOVEMENT SCALE (AIMS)

PATIENT NUMBER   DATA GROUP   EVALUATION DATE

— — — —   aims   M M   D D   Y Y

PATIENT NAME

RATER NAME

RATER NUMBER

— — —

EVALUATION TYPE *(Circle)*

1 Baseline	4 Start double-blind	7 Start open meds	10 Early termination
2 2-week minor	5 Major evaluation	8 During open meds	11 Study completion
3	6 Other	9 Stop open meds	

INSTRUCTIONS: Complete Examination Procedure (reverse side) before making ratings.
MOVEMENT RATINGS: Rate highest severity observed.

Code: 1 = None
2 = Minimal, may be extreme normal
3 = Mild
4 = Moderate
5 = Severe

			(Circle One)
FACIAL AND ORAL MOVEMENTS:	**1.** Muscles of Facial Expression e.g., movements of forehead, eyebrows, periorbital area, cheeks; include frowning, blinking, smiling, grimacing	1 2 3 4 5
	2. Lips and Perioral Area e.g., puckering, pouting, smacking	1 2 3 4 5
	3. Jaw e.g., biting, clenching, chewing, mouth opening, lateral movement	1 2 3 4 5
	4. Tongue Rate only increase in movement both in and out of mouth, NOT inability to sustain movement	1 2 3 4 5
EXTREMITY MOVEMENTS:	**5.** Upper *(arms, wrists, hands, fingers)* Include choreic movements, (i.e., rapid, objectively purposeless, irregular, spontaneous), athetoid movements (i.e., slow, irregular, complex, serpentine). Do NOT include tremor (i.e., repetitive, regular, rhythmic)	1 2 3 4 5
	6. Lower *(legs, knees, ankles, toes)* e.g., lateral knee movement, foot tapping, heel dropping, foot squirming, inversion and eversion of foot	1 2 3 4 5
TRUNK MOVEMENTS:	**7.** Neck, shoulders, hips e.g., rocking, twisting, squirming, pelvic gyrations	1 2 3 4 5
GLOBAL JUDGMENTS:	**8.** Severity of abnormal movements	None, normal 1 Minimal 2 Mild 3 Moderate 4 Severe 5
	9. Incapacitation due to abnormal movements	None, normal 1 Minimal 2 Mild 3 Moderate 4 Severe 5
	10. Patient's awareness of abnormal movements Rate only patient's report	No awareness 1 Aware, no distress 2 Aware, mild distress 3 Aware, moderate distress 4 Aware, severe distress 5
DENTAL STATUS:	**11.** Current problems with teeth and/or dentures	No 1 Yes 2
	12. Does patient usually wear dentures?	No 1 Yes 2

ADM 117
Rev. 11-85

FIGURE 18–40. The *Abnormal Involuntary Movement Scale (AIMS)* guides the examiner through inspection for dyskinesias of the face, jaw, tongue, trunk, and limbs. The physician is asked to record observations when the patient is at rest, extending the tongue or limbs or performing certain activities, such as finger tapping, standing, or walking. In addition, the examiner is asked to check for rigidity. This revision of the original (Guy, 1976) requests that patients remove their shoes and socks, and it does not rate as less severe those movements that are activated. However, tests for akinesia, tremor, and dysarthria are omitted.

EXAMINATION PROCEDURE

Either before or after completing the Examination Procedure observe the patient unobtrusively, at rest (e.g., in waiting room).

The chair to be used in this examination should be a hard, firm one without arms.

1. Ask patient to remove shoes and socks.

2. Ask patient whether there is anything in his/her mouth (i.e., gum, candy, etc.) and if there is, to remove it.

3. Ask patient about the current condition of his/her teeth. Ask patient if he/she wears dentures. Do teeth or dentures bother patient now?

4. Ask patient whether he/she notices any movements in mouth, face, hands, or feet. If yes, ask to describe and to what extent they currently bother patient or interfere with his/her activities.

5. Have patient sit in chair with hands on knees, legs slightly apart, and feet flat on floor. (Look at entire body for movements while in this position.)

6. Ask patient to sit with hands hanging unsupported. If male, between legs, if female and wearing a dress, hanging over knees. (Observe hands and other body areas.)

7. Ask patient to open mouth. (Observe tongue at rest within mouth.) Do this twice.

8. Ask patient to protrude tongue. (Observe abnormalities of tongue movement.) Do this twice.

9. Ask patient to tap thumb, with each finger, as rapidly as possible for 10-15 seconds; separately with right hand, then with left hand. (Observe facial and leg movements.)

10. Flex and extend patient's left and right arms (one at a time). (Note any rigidity.)

11. Ask patient to stand up. (Observe in profile. Observe all body areas again, hips included.)

12. Ask patient to extend both arms outstretched in front with palms down. (Observe trunk, legs, and mouth.)

13. Have patient walk a few paces, turn, and walk back to chair. (Observe hands and gait.) Do this twice.

FIGURE 18–40. *Continued*

TABLE 18–3. *Commonly Cited Movement Disorders that Begin in Childhood or Adolescence*

Early Childhood
    Athetosis or choreoathetosis
    Lesch-Nyhan syndrome*
Childhood
    Dopa-responsive dystonia*
    Dystonia associated with DYT1 gene*
    Myoclonus from subacute sclerosing panencephalitis (SSPE)
    Parkinson's disease
    Sydenham's chorea
    Tourette's syndrome*
    Withdrawal emergent dyskinesia
Adolescence
    Essential tremor*
    Huntington's disease (juvenile Huntington's disease)*
    Medication- and drug-induced movements
    Tardive dyskinesia
    Wilson's disease*

*Genetic transmission is established.

Psychogenic tremor characteristically develops abruptly, oscillates in two or more planes, and has a variable frequency. In addition, because of fatigue, it has a diminishing amplitude during long examinations. When a psychogenic tremor affects one arm, it often switches sides when the physician restrains the affected arm. It may not interfere with activities requiring the same muscles. Patients with a psychogenic tremor typically display a "selective disability."

Psychogenic myoclonus is almost random regarding the affected muscle groups, velocity of muscle contraction, and fluctuations in intensity. When generalized, psychogenic myoclonus goes away after a few minutes because patients get tired, but it returns after a rest period.

Some disorders, by definition, assume that underlying neurologic illnesses have been excluded. For example, *catatonia* is diagnosed by its three cardinal features: immobility, mutism, and refusal to eat or drink. Optional, secondary diagnostic criteria include waxy flexibility, staring, and rigidity. A therapeutic trial of benzodiazepine may confirm the diagnosis. An EEG should be normal. Assuming that physicians have excluded medication or drug use, juvenile Huntington's disease, and other neurologic illnesses, catatonia is more likely to be a manifestation of a mood disorder than schizophrenia.

Instead of being psychogenic in the usual sense, some movements seem culturally determined. For example, the "Jumping Frenchmen of Maine," a group of otherwise healthy individuals of French-Canadian descent, respond to unexpected loud noises by leaping upward, screaming, or throwing any object that they might be holding.

On the other hand, making a diagnosis of psychogenic movement disorder is perilous. As discussed previously (see above and Chapter 3), neurologic movement disorders may be misdiagnosed when they are bizarre, complicated by compensatory movements, or modified by tricks. Many may be self-limited or reduced by various interventions, including concentration, reduced anxiety, or solitude. The most commonly cited examples are tics, Parkinson's tremor, and focal dystonias.

Another problem is that in patients with primarily psychiatric disorders, medications may be responsible for bizarre yet partly controllable movements, such as acute dystonic reactions, tardive dystonia, and akathisia. The movements may exacerbate the psychiatric disturbances so much that the entire situation is deemed psychiatric.

Further reason for caution in diagnosing psychogenic movement disorders is that, outside of referral centers, they are actually rare. As with the high incidence of psychogenic seizures reported by epilepsy centers (see Chapter 10), the high incidence of psychogenic movement disorders is partly attributable to these centers attracting unique or bizarre cases, having the clinical experience and technology to diagnosis or exclude various movement disorders, and being willing to make a probably unwelcome diagnosis. In addition, few patients have seen movement disorders that might serve as a model for psychogenic behavior. Even fewer patients have the strength and determination to sustain movements. (Try it yourself.)

SUMMARY

Many involuntary movement disorders are still diagnosed exclusively by their clinical features, family history, patient's age at onset (Table 18–3), presence or absence of dementia (Table 18–4), or exposure to neuroleptics (Table 18–2). Laboratory or genetic tests are available for Huntington's and Wilson's diseases, SSPE, Lesch-Nyhan syndrome, and early onset dystonia. Patients with involuntary movement disorders have benefited from many major recent medical advances: new medications and surgical treatments for Parkinson's disease; identification of the DNA trinucleotide repeat in Huntington's disease, the DYT1 gene in early onset dystonia, and genetic abnormality in other illnesses; the concept of PANDAS; and botulinum toxin treatment for focal dystonias. Although tardive dyskinesia treatment remains largely ineffective, atypical neuroleptics may avoid producing it and can possibly alleviate many cases.

TABLE 18–4. *Movement Disorders Associated with Cognitive Impairment**

Young children
    Athetosis or choreoathetosis[†]
    Lesch-Nyhan syndrome
    Rett's syndrome
Older children and adolescents
    Huntington's disease
    Subacute sclerosing panencephalitis
    Sydenham's chorea[‡]
    Wilson's disease
Adults
    AIDS[§]
    Creutzfeldt-Jakob disease, rarely Alzheimer's disease[||]
    Huntington's disease
    Parkinson's disease

*Dementia, depression, or psychotic behavior.
[†]Despite severe movement disorders, many choreoathetosis patients will not have mental abnormalities (see Chapter 13).
[‡]Possible learning disabilities.
[§]Depending on presence of encephalitis or toxoplasmosis, can cause parkinsonism, chorea, tremor, or myoclonus.
[||]Myoclonus.

REFERENCES

Parkinson's Disease and Parkinsonism

Bandmann O, Marsden CD, Wood NM: Genetic aspects of Parkinson's disease. Move Dis 13: 203–211, 1998

Friedman A, Sienkiewicz J: Psychotic complications of long-term levodopa treatment of Parkinson's disease. Acta Neurol Scand 84: 111–113, 1991

Goetz CG: New lessons from old drugs. Neurology 50: 1211–1212, 1998

Goetz CG, Stebbins GT: Risk factors for nursing home placement in advanced Parkinson's disease. Neurology 43: 2227–2229, 1993

Hallett M, Litvan I: Evaluation of surgery for Parkinson's disease: A report of the Therapeutics and Technology Assessment Subcommittee of the American Academy of Neurology. Neurology 53: 1910–1921, 1999

Jankovic J: New and emerging therapies for Parkinson's disease. Arch Neurol 56: 785–790, 1999

Jankovic J: Video Atlas of Movement Disorders. San Diego, Arbor Publishing Co., 1999

Lang AE, Lozano AM: Parkinson's disease. N Engl J Med 33: 1044–1053 and 1130–1143, 1998

Lieberman A: Managing the neuropsychiatric symptoms of Parkinson's disease. Neurology 50 (Suppl 6): S33–S38, 1998

Moellentine C, Rummans T, Ahlskog JE, et al: Effectiveness of ECT in patients with parkinsonism. J Neuropsychiatry 10: 187–193, 1998

Papka M, Rubio A, Schiffer RB: A review of Lewy body disease, an emerging concept of cortical dementia. J Neuropsychiatry 10: 267–279, 1998

The Parkinson's Study Group: Low-dose clozapine for the treatment of drug-induced psychosis in Parkinson's disease. N Engl J Med 340: 757–763, 1999

Pate DS, Margolin DI: Cognitive slowing in Parkinson's and Alzheimer's disease patients: Distinguishing bradyphrenia from dementia. Neurology 44: 669–674, 1994

Tanner CM, Ottman R, Goldman SM, et al: Parkinson disease in twins: An etiologic study. JAMA 281: 341–346, 1999

Trosch RM, Friedman JH, Lannon MC, et al: Clozapine use in Parkinson's disease. Mov Disord 13: 377–382, 1998

Troster AI, Stalp LD, Paolo AM, et al: Neuropsychological impairment in Parkinson's disease with and without depression. Arch Neurol 52: 1164–1169, 1995

Wolters EC: Dopaminomimetic psychosis in Parkinson's disease patients. Neurology 52 (Suppl 3): S10–S13, 1999

Lewy Body Disease

Kalra S, Bergeron C, Lang AE: Lewy body disease and dementia: A review. Arch Int Med 156: 487–493, 1996

Papka M, Rubio A, Schiffer RB: A review of Lewy body disease, an emerging concept of cortical dementia. J Neuropsychiatry 10: 267–279, 1998

Chorea

Folstein SE: The psychopathology of Huntington's disease. Assoc Res Nerv Ment Dis 69: 181–191, 1991

Garvey M, Giedd J, Swedo SE: PANDAS: The search for environmental triggers of pediatric neuropsychiatric disorders. Lessons from rheumatic fever. J Child Neurol 13: 413–423, 1998

Kremer B, Goldberg P, Andrew SE, et al: A worldwide study of the Huntington's disease mutation: The sensitivity and specificity of measuring CAG repeats. N Engl J Med 330: 1401–1406, 1994

LaSpada AR, Paulson HL, Fischbeck KH: Trinucleotide repeat expansion in neurologic disease. Ann Neurol 36: 814–822, 1994

Lipe H, Schultz A, Bird TD: Risk factors for suicide in Huntington's disease: A retrospective case controlled study. Am J Med Genet 48: 231–233, 1993

Martin JB: Molecular basis of the neurodegenerative disorders. N Engl J Med 34: 1970–1980, 1999

Penny JB, Young AB, Shoulson I, et al: Huntington's disease in Venezuela: 7 years of follow-up on symptomatic and asymptomatic individuals. Mov Disord 5: 93–99, 1990

Swedo SE, Leonard HJ, Garvey M: Pediatric autoimmune neuropsychiatric disorders associated with streptococcal infections: Clinical description of the first 50 cases. Am J Psychiatry 155: 264–271, 1998

Tian JR, Zee DS, Lasker AG, et al: Saccades in Huntington's disease. Neurology 41: 875–881, 1991

Wilson's Disease

Akil M, Brewer GJ: Psychiatric and behavioral abnormalities in Wilson's disease. Adv Neurol 65: 1717–1718, 1995

Brewer GJ, Yuzbasiyan-Gurkan V: Wilson disease. Medicine 71: 139–164, 1992

Rathbun JK: Neuropsychological aspects of Wilson's disease. Int J Neurosci 85: 221–229, 1996

Dystonia (Nonneuroleptic)

Bandmann O, Valente EM, Holman P, et al: Dopa-responsive dystonia: A clinical and molecular genetic study. Ann Neurol 44: 649–656, 1998

Bressman SB, de Leon D, Raymond D, et al: Secondary dystonia and the DYT1 gene. Neurology 48: 1571–1577, 1997

Kaufman DM: Facial dyskinesias. Psychosomatics 30: 263–268, 1990

Kiziltan G, Akalin MA: Stuttering may be a type of action dystonia. Mov Disord 11: 278–282, 1996

Krauss JK, Trankle R, Kopp KH: Posttraumatic movement disorders after moderate or mild head injury. Mov Disord 12: 428–431, 1997

Lee MS, Rinne JO, Ceballos-Bauman A, et al: Dystonia after head trauma. Neurology 44: 1374–1378, 1994

Molho ES, Feustel PJ, Factor SA: Clinical comparison of tardive and idiopathic cervical dystonia. Mov Disord 3: 486–489, 1998

Nygaard TG, Wooten GF: Dopa-responsive dystonia. Neurology 50: 853–855, 1998

Therapeutics and Technology Assessment Subcommittee of the American Academy of Neurology: Assessment: The clinical usefulness of botulinum toxin-A in treating neurologic disorders. Neurology 40: 1332–1336, 1990

Essential Tremor

Deuschl G, Bain P, Brin M, et al: Consensus statement of the Movement Disorder Society on tremor. Mov Disord 13: 2–23, 1998

Koller WC, Busenbark K, Miner K, et al: The relationship of essential tremor to other movement disorders: Report on 678 patients. Ann Neurol 35: 717–723, 1994

Lou JS, Jankovic J: Essential tremor: Clinical correlates in 350 patients. Neurology 41: 234–238, 1991

Schuurman PR, Bosch DA, Bossuyt PMM, et al: A comparison of continuous thalamic stimulation and thalamotomy for suppression of severe tremor. N Engl J Med 342: 461–468, 2000

Wasielewski PG, Burns JM, Koller WC: Pharmacologic treatment of tremor. Mov Disord 13 (Suppl 3): 90–100, 1998

Tics, Tourette's Syndrome, and Related Disorders

Abwender DA, Como PG, Kurlan R: School problems in Tourette's syndrome. Arch Neurol 53: 509–511, 1996

Erenberg G, Fahn S: Tourette syndrome. Arch Neurol 53: 588, 1996

Garvey MA, Giedd J, Swedo SE: PANDAS: The search for environmental triggers of pediatric neuropsychiatric disorders. Lessons from rheumatic fever. J Child Neurol 13: 413–423, 1998

Goldenberg JN, Brown SB: Coprolalia in younger patients with Gilles de la Tourette syndrome. Mov Disord 9: 622–625, 1994

Jankovic J, Fahn S: The phenomenology of tics. Mov Disord 1: 17–26, 1986

Kurlan R: Tourette's syndrome and 'PANDAS': Will the relation bear out? Neurology 50: 1530–1534, 1998

Leckman JF, Cohen DJ: Tourette's Syndrome Tics, Obsessions, Compulsions: In Developmental Psychopathology and Clinical Care. New York, John Wiley, 1999

Perlmutter SJ, Leitman SF, Garvey MA, et al: Therapeutic plasma exchange and intravenous immunoglobulin for obsessive-compulsive disorder and tic disorders in childhood. Lancet 354: 1153–1158, 1999

Schuerholz LJ, Baumgardner TL, Singer HS, et al: Neuropsychological status of children with Tourette's syndrome with and without attention deficit hyperactivity disorder. Neurology 46: 958–965, 1996

Singer HS, Walkup JT: Tourette syndrome and other tic disorders. Medicine 70: 15–32, 1991

Tan A, Salgado M, Fahn S: The characterization and outcome of stereotypic movements in nonautistic children. Mov Disord 12: 47–52, 1997

Tourette Syndrome Classification Study Group: Definitions and classifications of tic disorders. Arch Neurol 50: 1013–1016, 1993

Wojciezek JM, Lang AE: Gestes antagonistes in the suppression of tics: "tricks for tics." Mov Disord 10: 226–228, 1995

Medication-Induced and Related Movement Disorders

Bharucha KJ, Sethi KD: Complex movement disorders induced by fluoxetine. Mov Disord 11: 324–326, 1996

Burke RE, Fahn S, Jankovic J, et al: Tardive dystonia: Late-onset and persistent dystonia caused by antipsychotic drugs. Neurology 32: 1335–1346, 1982

Burke RE, Kang UJ, Jankovic J, et al: Tardive akathisia: An analysis of clinical features and response to open therapeutic trials. Mov Disord 4: 157–175, 1989

Cardoso FEC, Jankovic J: Cocaine-related movement disorders. Mov Disord 8: 175–178, 1993

Factor S, Friedman JH: The emerging role of clozapine in the treatment of movement disorders. Mov Disord *12:* 483–496, 1997

Guy W: Abnormal Involuntary Movement Scale (AIMS). In: ECDEU Assessment Manual for Psychopharmacology. U.S. Department of Health, Education, and Welfare, pp. 534–537, 1976

Jankovic J, Beach J: Long-term effects of tetrabenazine in hyperkinetic movement disorders. Neurology *48:* 358–362, 1997

Kang UJ, Burke RE, Fahn S: Natural history and treatment of tardive dystonia. Mov Disord *1:* 193–208, 1986

Kaufman DM: Use of botulinum toxin injections for spasmodic torticollis of tardive dyskinesia. J Neuropsychiatry Clin Neurosci *6:* 50–53, 1994

Leo RJ: Movements disorders associated with the serotonin selective reuptake inhibitors. J Clin Psychiatry *57:* 449–454, 1996

Rosebush PI, Mazurek MF: Neurologic side effects in neuroleptic-naïve patients treated with haloperidol or risperidone. Neurology *52:* 782–785, 1999

Stacy M, Jankovic J: Tardive tremor. Mov Disord *7:* 53–57, 1992

Tarsy D, Kaufman D, Sethi KD, et al: An open-label study of botulinum toxin A for treatment of tardive dystonia. Clin Neuropharm *20:* 90–93, 1997

Wojcik JD, Falk WE, Fink JS, et al: A review of 32 cases of tardive dystonia. Am J Psychiatry *148:* 1055–1059, 1991

Psychogenic Movement Disorders

Deuschl G, Koster B, Lucking CH, et al: Diagnosis and pathophysiological aspects of psychogenic tremors. Mov Disorders *13:* 294–302, 1998

Fahn S, Williams DT: Psychogenic dystonia. Adv Neurol *50:* 431–455, 1988

Koller WC, Biary NM: Volitional control of involuntary movements. Mov Disord *4:* 153–156, 1989

Lang AE: Psychogenic dystonia: A review of 18 cases. Can J Neurol Sci *22:* 136–143, 1995

Owens DG: Dystonia—a potential psychiatric pitfall. Br J Psychiatry *156:* 620–634, 1990

Rosebush PI, Mazurek MF: Catatonia: Re-awakening to a forgotten disorder. Mov Disord *14:* 395–397, 1999

Saint-Hilaire MH, Saint-Hilaire JM, Granger Luc: Jumping Frenchmen of Maine. Neurology *36:* 1269–1271, 1986

QUESTIONS and ANSWERS: CHAPTER 18

1–5. Complete the sentence.

1. In general, movement disorders:

a. Are present intermittently 24 hours a day.
b. Are absent during sleep.
c. May be suppressed by intense voluntary effort.
d. Are made worse by anxiety.
e. Are associated with dementia.

   ANSWER: b, c, d

2. Gilles de la Tourette's (Tourette's) syndrome is characterized by:

a. Multiple motor tics.
b. Single motor tics.
c. Vocal tics.
d. Variation of the pattern and intensity of tics over many months or years.
e. Constant pattern of verbal and motor tics.
f. Frequent obsessive-compulsive traits.
g. Frequent attention deficit disorders.
h. Progressive cognitive impairment.
i. Family members with a similar or less pronounced condition.

   ANSWER: a, c, d, f, g, i

3. Obscenities in Tourette's syndrome are:

a. Present in all cases.
b. Clearly present in less than 25% of patients.

c. Usually develop as an initial symptom.
d. A late manifestation when they occur.
e. Occasionally expressed by gestures (copropraxia).

ANSWER: b, d, e

4. Tourette's syndrome develops:

a. Usually before 5 years of age.
b. Usually before 13 years of age.
c. Predominantly in white Anglo-Saxon Protestants.
d. In girls more than boys.

ANSWER: b

5. By which two methods is dopamine deactivated?

a. Decarboxylation
b. Oxidation
c. Re-uptake
d. Hydroxylation
e. Reduction

ANSWER: b, c. Most dopamine undergoes re-uptake, but some of it is metabolized by monoamine oxidase (MAO) and other enzymes.

6–9. Match the tremor (6–9) with the examination (a–d) that will elicit it.

6. Essential tremor

7. Cerebellar tremor

8. Parkinson's disease tremor

9. Lithium-induced tremor

a. Finger-nose test
b. Psychologic stress
c. Extending arms and hands
d. Observing the patient's hands when they are at rest

ANSWERS: 6-c, 7-a, 8-d, 9-c. (Psychologic stress exacerbates most neurologic disorders, including tremors.)

10–15. Match the tremor (10–15) with an effective therapy (a–f).

10. Essential

11. Cerebellar

12. Parkinson's disease

13. Stage fright

14. Hyperthyroidism

15. Delirium tremens

a. L-dopa
b. Propranolol (Inderal)
c. Amantadine (Symmetrel)
d. Trihexyphenidyl (Artane)
e. Primidone (Mysoline)
f. None of the above

ANSWERS: 10-b, e; 11-f; 12-a, c, d (L-dopa may be less effective than anticholinergics); 13-b; 14-b; 15-f

16–20. Pick three correct answer(s).

16. Spasmodic torticollis:

a. May consist of retrocollis and anterocollis as well as torticollis.
b. Develops in childhood.
c. May be relieved by sectioning the sternocleidomastoid and adjacent muscles.

 d. May be resisted by applying slight pressure to the chin.
 e. Whether a manifestation of tardive dystonia or an idiopathic condition, may respond to botulinum toxin injections.

   ANSWER: a, d, e

17. A psychiatrist is asked to evaluate an immobile, mute, 21-year-old woman who stares straight ahead and has waxy flexibility. She has an unsubstantiated history of a mood disorder. Before making a diagnosis of catatonia, the psychiatrist must do all except which one of the following?

 a. At the least, exclude medication and drug use, juvenile Huntington's disease, Wilson's disease, and partial complex status epilepticus.
 b. Give a therapeutic trial of a benzodiazepine.
 c. Obtain an EEG, which should be normal.
 d. Establish a diagnosis of schizophrenia.

   ANSWER: d. Catatonia is more likely to be a manifestation of a mood disorder than schizophrenia. Numerous neurologic conditions can produce the symptoms of catatonia. Catatonia responds dramatically to benzodiazepine.

18. Which statement is false regarding early onset primary dystonia, which was previously called "torsion dystonia" or "musculorum deformans."

 a. Patients eventually have involvement of the trunk and neck muscles, but the illness usually first affects the lower limb muscles.
 b. At its onset, the disorder may be confused with Wilson's disease.
 c. Patients may present with tortipelvis.
 d. The inheritance is mostly autosomal dominant with relatively low penetrance.
 e. The disease is prevalent among Eastern European (Ashkenazic) Jews.
 f. Like Huntington's disease, early onset primary dystonia results from excessive trinucleotide repeats.
 g. Affected individuals have no cognitive impairment, despite sometimes devastating physical impairment.

   ANSWER: f. The abnormal gene, DYT1, results from deletion of a trinucleotide.

19. Which feature is least closely associated with childhood Huntington's disease?

 a. Chorea
 b. Rigidity
 c. More trinucleotide repeats than the adult variety
 d. More rapid demise than the adult variety

   ANSWER: a

20. Chronic dystonia of the head and neck muscles in young adults may result from:

 a. Early onset primary (torsion) dystonia
 b. Wilson's disease
 c. Huntington's disease
 d. Neuroleptic medications (i.e., tardive dystonia)

   ANSWER: a, b, c, d

21. Which of the following statements concerning the oxidative stress hypothesis of Parkinson's disease is false?

 a. Hydrogen peroxide is an oxidant.
 b. Free radicals are oxidants.
 c. Giving MAO inhibitors immediately after MPTP injections will prevent the development of Parkinson's disease in animals.
 d. Oxidants have one or more unpaired electrons and seek to acquire electrons.
 e. Oxidation is fatal to tissue.
 f. Normal cellular metabolism produces oxidants.

   ANSWER: c. MAO inhibitors must be administered before MPTP injections to prevent the formation of free radicals.

22. Which two statements are true concerning D_2 receptors?

a. Parkinsonism from classic, typical dopamine-blocking neuroleptics is related to their blocking D_2 dopamine receptors in the caudate nucleus.
b. Anti-Parkinson dopamine agonists block both D_1 and D_2 receptors.
c. Anti-Parkinson dopamine agonists activate D_2 receptors but not necessarily D_1 receptors.
d. D_2 receptors are found primarily in the nigrostriatal tract but are identifiable throughout the CNS.

ANSWER: a, c

23. With which factor is depression in Parkinson's disease least closely associated?

a. History of depression
b. Dementia
c. Physical disability
d. Duration of illness

ANSWER: d. Depression is associated with dementia, physical disability, and a history of depression. The patient's age, antiparkinson medications, and duration of illness are less close associations.

24. Which one of the following is not a multisystem atrophy?

a. Olivopontocerebellar degeneration
b. Shy-Drager syndrome
c. Progressive supranuclear palsy
d. MPTP-induced parkinsonism

ANSWER: d. A group of several illnesses—loosely termed "Parkinson plus" or "multisystem atrophies"—are syndromes that include Parkinson's cardinal features but are characterized by other disturbances. Olivopontocerebellar degeneration is characterized by ataxia, Shy-Drager syndrome by hypotension and incontinence, and progressive supranuclear palsy by ocular motility limitations. MPTP-induced parkinsonism is a relatively pure disorder. Neither it nor Parkinson's disease is considered multisystem.

25. An 8-year-old girl, who had been entirely well, began to develop dystonic movements of her legs that interfered with her athletic activities most afternoons. Then she had gait impairments every evening. She remained undiagnosed for 2 years. At that time, the dystonia was present almost throughout the day, but it remained worse in the afternoon. In the mornings, she had almost an entirely normal examination. No family member has a similar problem. Of the following, which is the most likely illness that has affected her?

a. Duchenne's muscular dystrophy
b. Dopa responsive dystonia
c. Cerebral palsy
d. Early onset primary (torsion) dystonia

ANSWER: b. Dopa responsive dystonia (DRD), unlike primary dystonia, is characterized initially by dystonia that interferes with gait and that has diurnal fluctuations. Small doses of L-dopa correct the gait impairment and involuntary movements. DRP mimics athetosis or other varieties of cerebral palsy (CP). Duchenne's muscular dystrophy affects only boys.

26. What is the biochemical deficiency in dopamine responsive dystonia?

a. Loss of the cofactor for synthesis of tyrosine hydroxylase
b. Loss of dopa-decarboxylase
c. Absence of the substrate phenylalanine
d. Abnormal DOPA

ANSWER: a. Dopamine responsive dystonia is due to insufficient synthesis of tetrahydrobiopterin, which is an essential cofactor for phenylalanine and tyrosine hydroxylases.

27. Which statement is correct regarding the development of oral-buccal-lingual dyskinesia from typical antipsychotic agents?

a. The incidence is greater in the first year of use.
b. The incidence is greater in the fifth year of use.
c. The incidence is equal in the first and fifth years.

ANSWER: c. The annual rate of the development of this complication for each person at risk (the incidence) is constant. With time, the individual patient is more likely to have developed the complication. In addition, the proportion of people at risk who develop the condition (prevalence) increases.

28. A psychiatrist is asked to evaluate a 70-year-old man who has developed visual hallucinations. His vision was normal, but he had cognitive impairments that fluctuated from day to day. He also had mild slowness and generally increased tone. His neurologic examination was otherwise normal. The psychiatrist prescribed small doses of haloperidol. One week later, the patient was rigid, akinetic, and unable to speak or eat. Of the following, which is the most likely underlying pathology?

a. He simply had too much haloperidol because older patients require smaller doses of neuroleptics.
b. He had Parkinson's disease that was made overt by the dopamine-blocking neuroleptic haloperidol.
c. He probably has an illness that causes excessive cerebral cortex plaques and tangles.
d. He probably has an illness that causes cerebral cortex Lewy bodies.

ANSWER: d. He probably has diffuse Lewy body disease, which causes fluctuating cognitive impairment early in the illness. Because one hallmark of the disease is dementia, the illness is sometimes called dementia with Lewy body disease. The patient had another hallmark, visual hallucinations. This patient developed severe parkinsonism after treatment with neuroleptics because the illness makes patients unusually sensitive to dopamine-blocking neuroleptics.

29. Which one of the following enzymes increases the concentration of dopa?

a. COMT
b. MAO
c. Decarboxylase
d. Tyrosine hydroxylase

ANSWER: d. Tyrosine hydroxylase converts tyrosine to dopa, but the other enzymes metabolize dopa.

30. Which one of the following is a characteristic of necrosis that is not found in apoptosis?

a. Energy requiring
b. Programmed
c. Necrosis
d. Normal mechanism of development for some organs
e. Cell death

ANSWER: c. Both apoptosis and necrosis are a form of cell death. Apoptosis is programmed cell death, which occurs in the normal development of certain organs, such as the thymus gland, as well as in several degenerative illnesses, such as Huntington's disease and ALS. It is sequential, energy requiring, but devoid of inflammation, which is a characteristic of necrosis.

31. A 70-year-old man is comatose one week after sustaining a brainstem infarction. Among other abnormalities, his soft palate contracts regularly and symmetrically 120 times per minute. The palate elevates, as though the patient were saying "ah." Which feature is untrue?

a. As the coma lightens, the movements will persist during sleep as well as wakefulness.
b. The inferior olivary nuclei, the paired scalloped-shaped structures in the medulla, have sustained damage.
c. The regular movements in one plane define the disorder as a tremor.
d. The disorder is really a variety of myoclonus.

ANSWER: d. He has palatal myoclonus, which has been reclassified as a tremor because it consists of regular, rhythmic movements in a single plane. The movements result from lesions in the medulla that involve the inferior olivary nuclei. Unlike most movement disorders, palatal myoclonus persists during sleep and coma.

32–35. Match the description (32–35) with the illness (a–d).

a. Huntington's disease
b. Sydenham's chorea
c. Wilson's disease
d. None of the above

32. Recessive sex-linked inheritance

33. Autosomal recessive inheritance

34. Autosomal dominant inheritance

35. May develop in children

ANSWERS: 32-d; 33-c; 34-a; 35-a, b, c

36. One strategy in the treatment of hyperkinetic movement disorders, such as the oral-buccolingual variety of tardive dyskinesia, is the depletion of dopamine from the presynaptic neurons. In this context, which medication does tetrabenazine mimic?

a. Carbidopa
b. COMT inhibitors
c. Reserpine
d. Risperidone

ANSWER: c. Both tetrabenazine and reserpine deplete dopamine from the storage vesicles of the presynaptic neurons. Carbidopa blocks the synthesis of dopamine from DOPA. Because it does not cross the blood-brain barrier, it would be ineffective in reducing basal ganglia dopamine stores. Tetrabenazine is effective, despite serious risks, in treatment of chorea, hemiballismus, and Tourette's syndrome, as well as the oral-buccolingual variety of tardive dyskinesia.

37. What is the implication of a patient falling backward during the pull test?

a. Basal ganglia dysfunction
b. Gait apraxia
c. Gait ataxia
d. Impaired postural reflexes

ANSWER: d. A patient having retropulsion during the test has the same significance as falling. Whichever the specific abnormality, impaired postural reflexes is a manifestation of basal ganglia disease. The finding is a typical sign of moderately advanced Parkinson's disease.

38. Depletion of which of the following neurotransmitters is most closely associated with depression in Parkinson's disease?

a. Acetylcholine
b. Dopamine
c. Norepinephrine
d. Serotonin

ANSWER: d. Although the motor symptoms of Parkinson's disease are attributable to a dopamine deficiency, depression is attributable to a serotonin deficiency. The cognitive and mood changes in Parkinson's disease reflect more than the prominent degeneration dopaminergic system.

39. A 30-year-old woman, who is a recovering cocaine addict, has suddenly developed incessant feet movements that force her, she describes, to walk incessantly. She has similar but less severe movements in her hands. She is belligerent but has no cognitive impairment. Which of the following is the most likely cause of her movements and walking?

a. Sydenham's chorea
b. Obsessive-compulsive disorder
c. Huntington's chorea
d. Tourette's syndrome
e. Active cocaine use

ANSWER: e. She has "crack dancing," which are movements in the feet and hands triggered by an urge to walk. Cocaine provokes release of dopamine from presynaptic storage sites and thus increases dopamine activity. Chorea, akathisia, and the restless leg syndrome may also cause movements of the feet.

40. Which is the rate-limiting step in dopamine synthesis?

a. Phenylalanine to tyrosine
b. Tyrosine to DOPA
c. Tyrosine to dopamine
d. DOPA to dopamine
e. Dopamine to norepinephrine
f. None of the above

ANSWER: b. The rate-limiting step in dopamine synthesis is dependent on tyrosine hydroxylase, which converts tyrosine to DOPA.

41–49. Match the underlying abnormality (41–49) with the condition (a–h).

41. Cerebral cortical anoxia or uremia

42. Toxoplasmosis

43. Perinatal kernicterus

44. Low serum ceruloplasmin

45. Infarction of the subthalamic nucleus

46. Nigrostriatal depigmentation

47. Probably caused by an infectious agent

48. Atrophy of the caudate heads

49. Cavitary lesions of the globus pallidus and putamen

a. Huntington's disease
b. Wilson's disease
c. Hemiballismus
d. Creutzfeldt-Jakob disease

e. Choreoathetotic cerebral palsy
f. Parkinsonism
g. Myoclonus
h. SSPE

ANSWERS: 41-g; 42-c; 43-e; 44-b; 45-c; 46-f; 47-d, h; 48-a; 49-b

50–53. Are these statements true or false?

50. Only one neuroleptic-induced movement disorder may occur at a time.

51. Tetrabenazine and reserpine deplete dopamine from the presynaptic neurons.

52. Phenothiazines induce oculogyric crises and other acute dystonias only when used as an antipsychotic medication.

53. Tardive dyskinesia rarely develops when haloperidol is used for Tourette's syndrome.

ANSWERS: 50-F, 51-T, 52-F, 53-T

54–55. A 29-year-old man has been hospitalized intermittently for the previous 3 years for progressively severe schizophrenia. He has been readmitted because of paranoid hallucinations. His treatment has been resumed with dopamine-blocking neuroleptics. Several weeks later, a visiting physician notices that the patient has intermittent, forceful contractions of all the head and neck muscles that last several seconds. His neck tends to retrovert (extend). Likewise, his limbs involuntarily extend forward. His tongue protrudes intermittently for several seconds. The patient remains alert during these movements, which appear bizarre and "psychotic" to the neurologists.

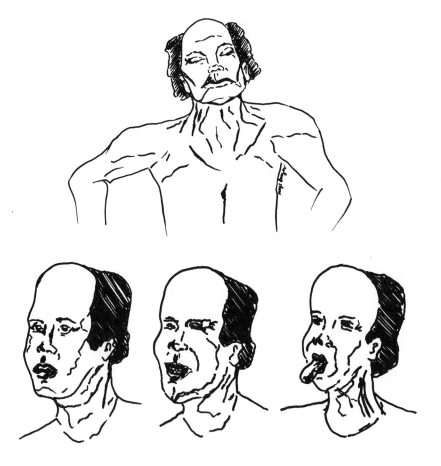

54. Which single condition is unlikely to cause dystonia in this individual?

a. Wilson's disease
b. Chronic neuroleptic use (tardive dystonia)
c. Early onset primary (torsion) dystonia
d. Multiple sclerosis

ANSWER: d. Multiple sclerosis only rarely produces a movement disorder. The other choices can each produce dystonia with bizarre features. Wilson's disease and tardive dystonia are associated with mental abnormalities.

55. Which of the conditions listed in Question 54 is associated with forceful, prolonged tongue movements?

ANSWER: b. Tardive dystonia is often accompanied by classic, choreiform buccolingual dyskinesia. Classic oral-buccal-lingual tardive dyskinesia tongue movements are brief and irregular (i.e., choreiform).

56. Which single statement is true regarding the trinucleotide (CAG) repeats in Huntington's disease?

a. The pathologic sequence is located on chromosome 4.
b. Normal individuals do not have trinucleotide (CAG) repeats.
c. The repeats in affected individuals are stable.
d. An affected mother's gene would be more unstable than an affected father's.

ANSWER: a. Normal individuals have about 20 repeats of the CAG trinucleotide. Huntington's disease patients have 37 or more repeats. The father's gametes are highly unstable and that instability leads to the father being more apt to have a child with juvenile Huntington's disease.

57. Which three illnesses are *not* associated with trinucleotide repeats?

a. Myotonic dystrophy
b. Depression
c. Fragile X syndrome
d. Alzheimer's disease
e. Huntington's disease
f. Duchenne's muscular dystrophy

ANSWER: b, d, f

58. What is the term applied when a genetic illness produces symptoms in younger victims in successive generations?

a. Anticipation
b. Suppression
c. Dys-inhibition
d. None of the above because it does not happen

ANSWER: a. *Anticipation* occurs in Huntington's disease, myotonic dystrophy, and several other illnesses. It results from unstable trinucleotide repeats.

59. Which disorders often develop in adolescence and are associated with dementia, which might present with personality change?

a. Creutzfeldt-Jakob disease
b. Wilson's disease
c. Choreoathetotic cerebral palsy
d. Huntington's disease
e. SSPE
f. Essential tremor

ANSWER: b, d, e

60. In which ways does the juvenile variety of Huntington's disease differ from the adult variety?

a. Children may have marked rigidity.
b. In children, the striatum is preserved.
c. The outcome is not fatal.
d. Children may appear to have parkinsonism.
e. Seizures are relatively frequent.

f. Chorea is absent or minimal.
g. Children may appear to have dystonia.
h. The affected chromosome is different.
i. Affected children are more likely to be boys, and their father is more likely to have been the affected parent.
j. Most individuals with 60 or more CAG trinucleotide repeats have juvenile rather than adult Huntington's disease.

ANSWER: a, d, e, f, g, i, j

61–65. Match the patients' description (61–65) with the neurologic disturbances (a–g) that are often initially diagnosed as psychogenic.

61. A 70-year-old man develops a high-pitched, squeaky voice that forces him to speak in a whisper. Nevertheless, he can sing in a normal volume and pitch.

62. An actor begins to have a high-pitched voice and hand tremor while on stage.

63. Continual forced bilateral eyelid closure prevents a 70-year-old man from seeing.

64. A middle-aged woman develops continual face, eyelid, and jaw contractions.

65. An author develops hand cramps when writing with a pen, but he can type, play tennis, and button his shirts.

a. Blepharospasm
b. Writer's cramp
c. Spasmodic dysphonia
d. Meige's syndrome
e. Oromandibular dystonia
f. Anxiety-induced tremor (e.g., stage fright)
g. Aphasia
h. Spasmodic torticollis

ANSWERS: 61-c, 62-f, 63-a, 64-d, 65-b. Meige's syndrome, oromandibular dystonia, and spasmodic dysphonia are varieties of cranial dystonia. Spasmodic dysphonia and spasmodic torticollis are varieties of cervical dystonia. Neuroleptic exposure often precedes the development of cranial and cervical dystonias; however, many patients have no history of medicine exposure, psychiatric illness, or other indication that their movements are a variety of tardive dyskinesia.

66. Which two structures constitute the corpus striatum?

a. Caudate
b. Putamen
c. Globus pallidus
d. Subthalamic
e. Substantia nigra

ANSWER: a, b

67. Which one of the following characteristics does not pertain to the nigrostriatal tract?

a. It links the substantia nigra to the corpus striatum.
b. The substantia nigra is normally black, but in Parkinson's disease, it is hypopigmented.
c. It produces about 80% of the dopamine of the brain.
d. Tyrosine is converted to DOPA in this tract.
e. Its origin cannot be seen with the naked eye.
f. Its major metabolic end product is HVA.
g. Degeneration of most of the presynaptic neurons leads to Parkinson's disease.

ANSWER: e

68. Sinemet is a combination of L-dopa and which other substance?

a. Carbidopa, a dopa decarboxylase inhibitor
b. Bromocriptine (Parlodel), a dopamine agonist
c. Anticholinergics

ANSWER: a

69. A 25-year-old man has had involuntary slow, twisting movements of his face, mouth, trunk, and limbs since infancy. The neck muscles have become hypertrophied. He performs poorly on standard intelligence tests. Which two of the following statements regarding his condition are true?

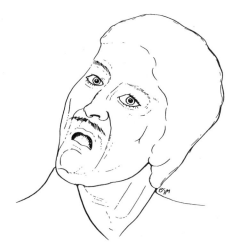

a. His children might inherit this condition.
b. He probably performs poorly, in part, because he is dysarthric and unable to use his hands.
c. He probably has lesions in the basal ganglia.
d. His condition is not associated with cognitive impairments.

ANSWER: b, c. He probably has congenital athetosis—a variety of cerebral palsy (CP) that becomes apparent between infancy and ages 2 and 4 years. It is often, but not necessarily, associated with mental retardation. Children with all forms of cerebral palsy tend to be underestimated and undereducated because of their motor impairments and dysarthria. Early onset primary dystonia (torsion dystonia or dystonia musculorum deformans), which appears in childhood, is carried on the DYT1 gene and inherited as an autosomal dominant condition. It is not associated with cognitive impairment. Dopamine responsive dystonia, which mimics cerebral palsy, becomes apparent during childhood and has a diurnal fluctuation.

70. Which of the following statements describe the Lesch-Nyhan syndrome?

a. It is characterized by the onset of dystonia and other movements in children aged 2 to 6 years.
b. It is an autosomal dominant genetic illness.
c. Brain HVA and CAT concentrations are low.
d. The basic deficit is a deficiency of HGPRT.
e. Hyperuricemia is present.

ANSWER: a, c, d, e

71. In which conditions is myoclonus found?

a. Cerebral anoxia
b. SSPE
c. Creutzfeldt-Jakob disease
d. Alzheimer's disease
e. Meperidine (Demerol) use
f. Psychogenic disturbances
g. Uremia
h. Neuroleptic use

ANSWER: a, b, c, d (rarely), e, g

72. What is the mechanism of action that permits propranolol to suppress essential tremor?

a. It slows the cardiac output.
b. It is a mild sedative.
c. It blocks both β-1 and β-2 adrenergic sympathetic nervous system receptor sites.
d. It blocks both β-1 adrenergic sympathetic nervous system receptor sites.
e. It suppresses synthesis of norepinephrine.

ANSWER: c. Propranolol is a relatively nonspecific adrenergic blocker that is useful in suppressing essential tremor and migraine headaches. However, it may precipitate asthma and congestive heart failure in susceptible individuals. Moreover, depression and cognitive impairments frequently complicate its use.

73. Which one of the following is *not* a characteristic of MPTP-induced parkinsonism?

a. MPTP provides a laboratory model of Parkinson's disease.
b. Pretreatment with monoamine oxidase inhibitors protects animals.
c. Patients respond, at least temporarily, to L-dopa replacement.
d. MPTP is toxic only if oxidized by a monoamine oxidase.
e. MPTP is a by-product of hydrocarbon manufacturing.

> **ANSWER:** e. Methyl-phenyl-tetrahydro-pyridine (MPTP), a meperidine analogue, is a by-product of illicit narcotic manufacturing. MPTP is actually not the toxin. It must be converted to MPP$^+$ by MAO. The reaction can be prevented with MAO inhibitors.

74. When botulinum A toxin is used to treat blepharospasm, Meige's syndrome, and other orofacial dyskinesias, which mechanism is involved?

a. Botulinum, like tetrabenazine, depletes dopamine.
b. Botulinum binds to the postsynaptic neuron.
c. Botulinum prevents release of ACh from the presynaptic neuromuscular junction neuron.
d. Botulinum penetrates the blood-brain barrier.

> **ANSWER:** c

75. Which is the most accurate test for Huntington's disease?

a. Genetic linkage analysis
b. Restriction length fragments
c. Measuring CAG nucleotides
d. PET

> **ANSWER:** c. DNA testing for repeats of the trinucleotide CAG is highly accurate. In general, the number of repeats cannot determine the age when symptoms will develop; however, more than 60 repeats indicate that the illness will develop in childhood.

76. Which statement is false regarding saccades?

a. The term refers to rapid, purposeful, conjugate eye movements.
b. Saccades are abnormal in Huntington's disease and schizophrenia.
c. Abnormal saccades are an early, reliable sign of Huntington's disease.
d. When abnormal, saccades might be initiated by patients jerking their heads.
e. Wernicke-Korsakoff syndrome is characterized by abnormal saccades.
f. In Huntington's disease, in addition to ocular saccades being initiated by head movement or blinks, ocular pursuit is jerky and interrupted by blinking and head movement.

> **ANSWER:** e

77. Which statement is false regarding the NMDA receptor?

a. It is a type of glutamate receptor.
b. Its inactivity is causally related to Huntington's disease.
c. It is probably causally related to neurologic damage in epilepsy and stroke.
d. It is a receptor for excitatory neurotransmitters.

> **ANSWER:** b

78. Which structure undergoes the greatest atrophy in Huntington's disease?

a. GABA-producing neurons of the striatum
b. GABA-producing neurons of the cerebral cortex
c. ACh-producing neurons of the striatum
d. ACh-producing neurons of the cerebral cortex
e. NMDA receptors

> **ANSWER:** a. The striatum consists of the caudate and the putamen. In Huntington's disease, the heads of the caudate nuclei atrophy. Also, GABA concentration in the striatum decreases by 50%.

79. An intravenous drug addict, who has been given neuroleptics, develops dystonic movements that affect his entire body. He is febrile and is found to have a deep infection in his left thigh muscles. His breathing becomes strained because of laryngeal and pharyngeal contractions. His face assumes prolonged contractions. His jaw is pulled backward. Anticholinergics and antihistamines do not correct the problem. Which conditions may have developed?

a. Acute dystonic reaction to neuroleptics
b. Seizures
c. Meige's syndrome
d. An infectious complication of drug abuse

ANSWER: d. Although neuroleptic-induced dystonia is possible, the history of his drug abuse, trismus (lockjaw), and the infection indicate that he may have classic, generalized tetanus. Drug addicts who share dirty needles are prone to tetanus. Immunization lasts for about 10 years. When it wears off, patients can develop tetanus that is either generalized or restricted to the limb with the infection, "regional tetanus." Affected limbs have spontaneous or stimulus-sensitive muscle spasms that mimic dystonia.

80. Which of the following conditions or medications elevate the serum prolactin concentration?

a. Use of clozapine
b. Use of pergolide
c. Use of haloperidol
d. Primary generalized seizures
e. Partial complex seizures
f. Petit mal seizures
g. Pituitary adenoma
h. L-dopa
i. Risperidone

ANSWER: c, d, e, g, and i. Prolactin is a pituitary hormone but not a neurotransmitter. Its secretion into the systemic circulation is normally inhibited by dopamine. Dopamine agonists as well as dopamine inhibit its secretion. In contrast, dopamine blockade, as occurs with many neuroleptics, enhances prolactin secretion, which produces elevated serum prolactin levels. Seizures that involve the limbic system also trigger a transient prolactin release. Many pituitary adenomas, prolactinomas, secrete prolactin. These adenomas can be shrunk and their prolactin secretion suppressed with bromocriptine administration.

81. A 50-year-old woman, who has been taking antidepressants for 10 years, complains that her face pulls to her left. The movements are uncomfortable but not painful, are more intense during anxiety, and last for several seconds. The eyelid closure prevents her from driving her car. Which one of the following conditions is probably causing her movements?

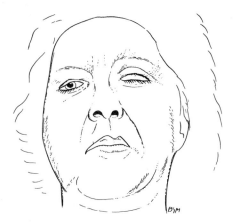

a. An aberrant blood vessel at the cerebellopontine angle
b. Partial complex seizures
c. Dopamine-blocking neuroleptics
d. Psychogenic mechanisms
e. Antidepressants

ANSWER: a. She has hemifacial spasm that is caused in most cases by an aberrant blood vessel compressing the facial nerve as it exits from the brainstem.

82. Which two structures constitute the lenticular nuclei?

a. Caudate
b. Putamen
c. Globus pallidus
d. Subthalamic
e. Substantia nigra

ANSWER: b, c

83. Which one of the following nuclei is not part of the set of the others?

a. Substantia nigra
b. Locus ceruleus

c. Dorsal motor nuclei
d. Anterior thalamic nuclei

ANSWER: d. Thalamic nuclei are not pigmented. Substantia nigra, locus ceruleus, and dorsal motor nuclei are normally pigmented but lose their color in Parkinson's disease.

84. A 72-year-old man is brought by his family for evaluation of dementia that developed along with mild rigidity and bradykinesia during the previous several months. Which one of the following statements is applicable to this case?

a. Parkinson's disease often causes dementia early in its course.
b. His cerebral cortex, as well as substantia nigra, probably contains Lewy bodies.
c. He probably has depression.
d. He probably has Alzheimer's disease.

ANSWER: b. He probably has diffuse Lewy body disease. Parkinson's disease, at its onset, usually does not cause depression or dementia. Alzheimer's disease usually does not present with either pyramidal or extrapyramidal signs.

85. In the treatment of depression in Parkinson's disease patients, which of the following statements are false?

a. Fluoxetine may cause a potentially fatal interaction with selegiline.
b. ECT is counterindicated.
c. Selegiline has an antidepressant effect.
d. Tocopherol is often helpful.

ANSWER: b, d. ECT is often indicated for depression in Parkinson's disease patients, in whom it will temporarily relieve the motor symptoms as well as the depression. Tocopherol is vitamin E, which has no benefit on either the mental or physical manifestations of Parkinson's disease. Selegiline is metabolized, in part, to amphetamine.

86. Which of the following complications is the most common reason why families place Parkinson's disease relatives in nursing homes?

a. Hallucinations and delusions
b. Depression

c. Rigidity
d. Akinesia

ANSWER: a. Psychosis, not physical incapacity or incontinence, is the most frequent reason that families place Parkinson's disease patients in nursing homes. Sleep disturbances, which usually accompany or result from hallucinations or delusion, is the other major reason.

87. Of the following dopamine receptors, with which do all dopamine agonists interact positively?

a. D_1
b. D_2

c. Both
d. Neither

ANSWER: b. Effective antiparkinson dopamine agonists stimulate D_2, but they may either stimulate or inhibit D_1.

88. With which feature of Parkinson's disease is dementia least associated?

a. Older age
b. Rapid progression of the illness
c. Poor response to dopamine medications
d. Tremor
e. Akinesia

ANSWER: d. Of the cardinal features, dementia is *least* closely associated with tremor. If dementia occurs at the onset of an illness with parkinsonism, consider diffuse Lewy body disease in individuals older than 50 years. In young adults, consider Wilson's disease, juvenile Huntington's disease, and drug abuse.

89. A 70-year-old man, under treatment for depression for 10 years, has begun to develop intermittent contractions of the orbicularis oculi. His medications were tricyclics until 2 years ago when serotonin re-uptake inhibitors were substituted. He had a good response to the change. He underwent two courses of ECT. The involuntary movements impair his ability to read and intensify the depression. What would be the best treatment?

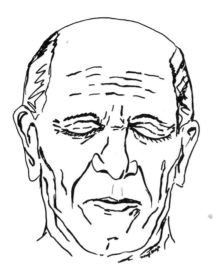

a. Return to the tricyclic antidepressants.
b. Prohibit any further ECT.
c. Reduce the dose of the serotonin re-uptake inhibitors.
d. Add anticholinergic medications.
e. None of the above.

ANSWER: e. The patient has developed blepharospasm, but it is probably not a side effect of either the antidepressants or ECT. (Although blepharospasm may follow treatment with dopamine-blocking neuroleptics, in most cases it is an idiopathic condition.) Regardless of its origin, botulinum toxin injections into the affected muscles will alleviate the blepharospasm and permit the antidepressant treatment to continue.

90–92. Match the neurotransmitter (90–92) with its metabolic product(s) (a–c).

90. Norepinephrine

91. Dopamine

92. Serotonin

a. HVA
b. 5-HIAA
c. VMA

ANSWERS: 90-c, 91-a, 92-b

93. Which one of the following movement disorders is not accompanied or preceded by an urge to move?

a. Tics
b. Akathisia
c. Tremor
d. Restless leg syndrome movements

ANSWER: c. Tremor, athetosis, hemiballismus, and most other movements are unaccompanied by sensations. However, tics, akathisia, and restless leg movements seem to stem from irrepressible, sometimes indescribable sensations, urges, or psychic tension, which is sometimes termed a compulsion. Patients can suppress these movements for several minutes, but when the movements break through, they return in a flurry.

94. Which three movements are typically preceded by sensations that compel patients to move?

a. Chorea
b. Tics
c. Restless leg syndrome
d. Akathisia
e. Dystonia
f. Resting tremor

ANSWER: b, c, d

95. Unlike typical neuroleptics, clozapine does not induce parkinsonism. The sparing of which receptor explains this freedom?

a. D_1 dopamine
b. D_2 dopamine
c. D_3 dopamine
d. NMDA
e. GABA

ANSWER: b

96. Which of the following is not a characteristic of free radicals?

a. They contain single, unpaired electrons.
b. They are stable.
c. They snatch away electrons from neighboring atoms or molecules.
d. Removal of electrons oxidizes atoms or molecules.
e. Methylphenylpyridinium (MMP^+) is a free radical.

ANSWER: b

97. Which three characteristics distinguish visual hallucinations in Parkinson's disease from those in schizophrenia?

a. In Parkinson's disease, visual hallucinations often arise independent of psychotic thought.
b. In Parkinson's disease, visual hallucinations are almost never accompanied by auditory hallucinations.
c. In Parkinson's disease, visual hallucinations are often accompanied by dyskinesias.
d. In Parkinson's disease, visual hallucinations are symptoms at the onset of the illness.

ANSWER: a, b, c. Visual symptoms in Parkinson's disease are precipitated or caused by L-dopa medications. They are typically found in older patients with long-standing disease that is complicated by dementia. Although visual hallucinations are usually not symptoms of early Parkinson's disease, they are an early manifestation of Lewy body disease.

98. Dementia frequently complicates Parkinson's disease. Which two of the following characteristics accurately describe dementia in Parkinson's disease?

a. It responds to L-dopa.
b. It responds to dopa agonists.
c. Thought processes are typically slow.
d. Patients have difficulty shifting mental sets.
e. Aphasia and apraxia are common manifestations of the dementia.

ANSWER: c, d. Bradyphrenia and lack of initiative are frequently occurring manifestations of the dementia of Parkinson's disease; however, these cognitive impairments and commonplace, generalized dementia do not respond to L-dopa or dopa agonists. The incidence of dementia in Parkinson's disease increases with age. Although the dementia conforms more to a subcortical than cortical pattern, a valid distinction is often impossible because of the frequent coexistence of Alzheimer's and Parkinson's diseases, the possibility that the illness is actually Lewy body disease, and the general unreliability of the dichotomy.

99. Which two of the following symptoms do not respond to either L-dopa or dopa agonists?

a. Dementia
b. Tremor
c. Rigidity
d. Bradykinesia
e. Depression
f. Hallucinations

ANSWER: a, e, f. Mental aberrations are unaffected by restoring dopamine activity. In fact, excessive dopamine activity precipitates hallucinations, especially in the later states of the illness.

100. A neurologic examination of a 17-year-old boy, who has had declining schoolwork, reveals dysarthria, tremor, and a brown-green ring at the periphery of each cornea. Which of the following laboratory abnormalities is most likely to be found?

a. Little or no copper-transporting serum protein
b. Metachromatic granules in the urine
c. Periodic EEG complexes
d. MPTP metabolic products in the urine

ANSWER: a. He probably has Wilson's disease, which is an autosomal recessive disorder that is also called hepatolenticular degeneration. It is associated with a marked reduction in ceruloplasmin, the copper-transporting serum protein, and visible copper deposits in the periphery of the cornea, the Kayser-Fleisher ring.

101. What is the effect of dopamine stimulating D_1 receptors?

a. The interaction stimulates adenyl cyclase activity.
b. The interaction inhibits adenyl cyclase activity.
c. The interaction has no effect on adenyl cyclase activity.

ANSWER: a. Dopamine–D_1 receptor interaction stimulates adenyl cyclase activity, but dopamine–D_2 receptor interaction inhibits adenyl cyclase activity.

102. Why do typical dopamine-blocking neuroleptics produce parkinsonism?

a. They block D_1 receptors.
b. They block D_2 receptors.
c. They stimulate D_1 receptors.
d. They stimulate D_2 receptors.

ANSWER: b. Their tendency to induce parkinsonism results from their affinity for (tendency to block) D_2 dopamine receptors.

103. In Huntington's disease and several other neurologic disorders that result from excessive trinucleotide repeats, the abnormal genetic segment can undergo amplification. Which of the following statements concerning amplification is true?

a. Amplification of trinucleotide repeats leads to the genetic abnormality appearing in additional chromosomes.
b. Amplification of trinucleotide repeats is more apt to occur in eggs than sperm.
c. Amplification leads to anticipation.
d. Amplification leads to the disease producing its symptoms at an older age.

ANSWER: c. In successive generations, the expanded trinucleotide segment expands further, that is, undergoes amplification. Because these defects are more unstable in sperm than eggs, amplification is greater when the abnormality is transmitted from the father than mother. The greater the amplification, the younger the age of onset of symptoms in the children who inherit the abnormal chromosome. When the symptoms appear at a younger age, the victims show anticipation.

104. What is the net effect of reducing dopamine activity in the corpus striatum?

a. Increased GPi activity
b. Decreased GPi activity
c. Inability to replete the deficiency with medications
d. All of the above

ANSWER: a

19

Brain Tumors and Metastatic Cancer

Because of their unpredictable onset and potentially tragic consequences, brain tumors command unique attention. They frequently develop insidiously in young and middle-aged adults in whom they may produce depression, thought disorders, or cognitive impairment without overt physical symptoms. Brain tumors epitomize an organic cause of psychiatric symptoms.

VARIETIES

Primary Brain Tumors

Primary brain tumors develop within the brain tissue *(parenchyma)* or its coverings *(meninges)* and are named after their original cell line (Table 19–1). Most of these tumors arise from the brain's numerous, mostly small, *glial cells,* which include *astrocytes* and *oligodendrocytes*. Glial cells normally form the central nervous system (CNS) connective tissue and provide its mechanical, biochemical, and immunologic support. Oligodendrocytes, in addition, produce the myelin insulation for CNS neurons. (Schwann cells produce the myelin insulation for the peripheral nervous system [PNS].) Unlike neurons, glial cells do not generate or transmit electrophysiologic signals.

If glial cells undergo malignant transformation, they form *gliomas.* This group of tumors consists mostly of the *astrocytoma,* which arises from the astrocyte, and its more malignant variety, *glioblastoma multiforme.* Astrocytomas affect children as well as adults, are relatively noninvasive, and develop in the cerebral cortex, optic nerves, and structures of the posterior fossa (cerebellum, pons, and medulla).

Astrocytomas are common brain tumors in children, in whom they tend to be cystic and located in the cerebellum and brainstem. Because cerebellar astrocytomas may

TABLE 19–1. *Primary Brain Tumors*

Gliomas
  Astrocyte tumors
    Astrocytoma
    Glioblastoma
  Oligodendroglioma
Meningioma*
Lymphoma
Medulloblastoma
Pituitary adenoma*
Acoustic neuroma*

*Relatively benign histology.

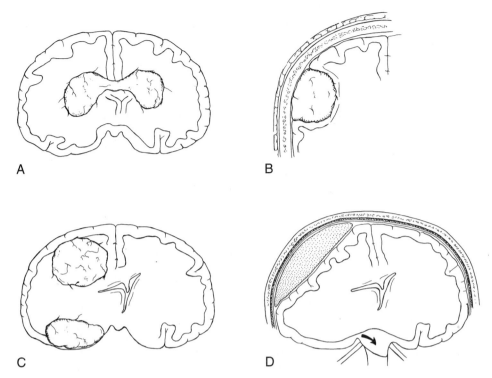

FIGURE 19–1. A, A *glioblastoma* is a highly malignant tumor that typically infiltrates along white matter tracts. Sometimes it spreads in a "butterfly pattern" from one cerebral hemisphere through the heavily myelinated corpus callosum to the other (see Fig. 20–6*A*). **B,** *Meningiomas* grow slowly from the meninges overlying the brain or spinal cord (see Fig. 20–5). They compress and irritate but do not infiltrate the CNS. **C,** *Metastatic tumors,* usually multiple and surrounded by edema, destroy large areas of brain and raise intracranial pressure (see Fig. 20–6*B*). **D,** *Subdural hematomas,* typically located over the cerebral hemisphere (see Figs. 20–10 and 20–11), compress the underlying brain. Acute, rapidly expanding subdural hematomas push the brainstem and ipsilateral oculomotor (third cranial) nerve through the tentorial notch. That process, which also occurs with epidural hematomas (see Chapter 22), *transtentorial herniation,* constitutes an immediately life-threatening condition. In contrast, small or slowly growing meningiomas and subdural hematomas cause relatively few physical symptoms because they are "extra-axial," that is, situated outside of the brain.

be totally removed in children, the cure rate is about 90%. In contrast, astrocytomas in adults usually occur predominantly in the cerebrum, infiltrate extensively, and evolve into more malignant forms, such as the glioblastoma. Total surgical removal is practical only if the surrounding brain can be sacrificed. Although cure rates are low, combined surgery and radiotherapy routinely prolong life for approximately 10 years.

Glioblastomas are highly malignant and infiltrating glial tumors, which develop almost exclusively in the cerebrum. They grow rapidly and invade across the corpus callosum (Figs. 19–1*A* and 20–6). Contrary to many physicians' expectations that brain tumors, like most other cancers, arise in the elderly, the average age of patients at the time of diagnosis of a glioblastoma is only 54 years.

Surgical excision, though often attempted, is rarely curative. Radiotherapy, steroids, and chemotherapy may reduce the growth rate of inoperable tumors and provide a brief (6 month to 1 year), physically comfortable survival. However, elderly patients, especially those with pronounced neurologic deficits, gain little or nothing from radiotherapy or chemotherapy. Moreover, in virtually all patients, persistence or recurrence of the tumor, radionecrosis (see below), and other treatments produce progressive mental deterioration.

Oligodendrocytes, the other major group of glial cells, also give rise to primary brain tumors, but their incidence is low. These cells lead to *oligodendrogliomas*, which grow slowly.

Meningiomas are tumors that arise from cells of the meninges, which forms the coverings of the CNS, rather than from those constituting actual brain or spinal cord tissue. Meningiomas are often associated with neurofibromatosis type 1 (see Chapter 13). These usually cause symptoms by compressing the underlying brain or spinal cord (Figs. 19–1*B* and 20–5), but sometimes they invade the underlying brain tissue. They grow slowly and develop almost exclusively in adults.

Small meningiomas are usually innocuous and need not necessarily be removed. Slowly growing lesions in certain areas can be asymptomatic. For example, meningiomas over the frontal lobes can grow to an extraordinary size before they cause symptoms. When necessary, most meningiomas can usually be totally removed by surgery.

Another variety of primary brain tumor is the *primary cerebral lymphoma*. In contrast to systemic lymphoma, which commonly spreads to the CNS, primary cerebral lymphoma develops exclusively within the brain. Because lymphomas are often a consequence of an impaired immunologic system, primary cerebral lymphoma typically arises in patients with the acquired immune deficiency syndrome (AIDS) and those receiving immunosuppressive therapy for renal and cardiac transplants. In AIDS patients, primary cerebral lymphomas are particularly aggressive. They are difficult to distinguish from cerebral toxoplasmosis (see Figs. 20–7 and 20–18) and cytomegalic inclusion disease because of similar clinical, computed tomography (CT), and magnetic resonance imaging (MRI) findings. Treatment of a lymphoma relies on steroids, radiotherapy, and chemotherapy. Although biopsies are performed to confirm the diagnosis, surgical excision is usually not feasible.

Metastatic Tumors

More common than primary brain tumors, metastatic tumors spread hematogenously to the brain and spinal cord. (The brain does not have a lymphatic system.) Metastatic tumors tend to be multiple, surrounded by edema, and rapidly growing, constituting a burdensome mass (Figs. 19–1*C* and 20–6*B*). The most common metastatic brain tumors originate from cancer of the lung, breast, kidney, and skin (malignant melanomas). In contrast, gastrointestinal, pelvic, and prostatic cancers spread to the brain rarely or only late in their course because the portal vein diverts metastases to the liver. Whatever the origin of the metastatic cancer, treatment modalities, such as steroids, which dramatically reduce the edema, and radiotherapy are palliative. Surgical removal of a single metastasis is often appropriate.

Approximately 15% of cancer patients develop symptoms or signs of cerebral metastases. Occasionally the discovery of a metastatic brain tumor is the first indication that a person has cancer. In addition to their problems from cerebral metastases, patients may develop neurologic problems from PNS metastases, nonneurologic metastases, remote effects of cancer, and adverse reactions to many forms of treatment.

INITIAL PHYSICAL SYMPTOMS

Compared to mental status changes, physical symptoms—seizures, headaches, and lateralized signs—occur more frequently. Seizures represent the initial symptom of cerebral tumors in approximately one-half of patients. For individuals older than 50 years, seizures are caused almost equally by brain tumors and strokes. When seizures are a manifestation of a brain tumor, they may be either partial elementary or partial complex seizures, which often undergo secondary generalization, rather than either absences (petit mal) or other primary generalized seizures (see Chapter 10).

The tendency for tumors to cause seizures relates to electroconvulsive therapy (ECT). If a patient harboring a brain tumor were to undergo ECT, the tumor might give rise to multiple, uninterrupted, life-threatening seizures *(status epilepticus)*. Another ECT complication would occur with a large brain tumor, which might even be the origin of the depression. In certain locations, a large tumor can swell and produce transtentorial herniation (Fig. 19–1*D*). Thus, before undergoing ECT, patients should have either an MRI or CT.

Brain tumors often cause headaches. On the other hand, both patients and physicians are usually overconcerned that headaches may indicate a brain tumor, even though less than 1 out of 1,000 people with headaches has a tumor. Brain tumor–induced headaches are not distinctive. They usually mimic tension-type headaches because they are diffuse, dull, relatively mild, and responsive to mild analgesics, including aspirin. Sometimes brain tumor–induced headaches mimic migraines because they may be predominantly unilateral and worse in the early morning hours, awakening patients from sleep.

With increases in intracranial pressure, tumor headaches intensify, and nausea and vomiting develop. The increased intracranial pressure also causes generalized, nonspecific cognitive impairment and personality changes. Pressure transmitted along the optic nerve to the optic disks causes *papilledema* (Fig. 19–2). The physician should bear in mind that the notorious triad of headache, vomiting, and papilledema occurs late, if at all, in the course of brain tumors. Only a minority of brain tumor victims has papilledema during an initial examination: its absence should not be taken as evidence against the presence of a brain tumor.

Tumors of the CNS also cause common physical neurologic deficits, such as hemiparesis and other lateralized signs, which follow the usual clinical correlations (see Chapters 2 and 4). In most cases, however, tumors do not initially cause readily apparent physical deficits because they may be small, slow growing, or located in "silent areas" of the brain, such as the right frontal or either of the anterior temporal lobes.

Tumors that arise from cranial nerves, although rare, result in readily recognizable deficits. For example, optic nerve gliomas cause optic atrophy and visual loss. Acoustic neuromas cause unilateral progressive hearing loss and tinnitus (see below).

Meningiomas are a special case. As discussed previously, small meningiomas are common and usually innocuous, and large meningiomas can be asymptomatic. Nevertheless, meningiomas tend to develop in certain locations and produce characteristic signs. A meningioma arising from the falx, a *parasagittal meningioma,* can compress

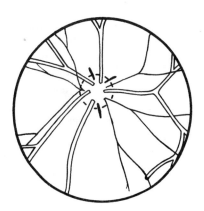

FIGURE 19–2. Papilledema is characterized by reddening of the optic disk, which loses its distinct margin, and by distention of the retinal veins. The disk is elevated and hemorrhages appear at its edge. (Compare this disk to the normal optic disk in Figure 4–3.)

the medial motor cortex and cause spastic paresis of one or both legs. Meningiomas arising from the sphenoid wing (see Fig. 20–5, top) can cause damage to the adjacent temporal lobe and, because of their proximity to the orbit, proptosis and paresis of eye movement. Likewise, *olfactory groove meningiomas* can compress the immediately adjacent olfactory and optic nerves and the overlying frontal lobe (see Foster-Kennedy Syndrome, Chapter 4). These tumors characteristically cause anosmia, unilateral blindness, and, when large, frontal lobe dysfunction (see Chapter 7).

INITIAL MENTAL SYMPTOMS

Direct Effects of Tumors

In most cases, tumor-induced mental changes consist of nonspecific personality changes and mild cognitive impairment. These symptoms, which vary tremendously, depend on the tumor's location, rate of growth, effect on intracranial pressure, and many other factors.

Frontal lobe tumors may produce a characteristic clinical picture of psychomotor retardation, emotional dulling, loss of initiative, poor insight, and reduced capacity to execute complex mental tasks. Nevertheless, despite causing these changes, these tumors occasionally spare cognitive capacity.

Sometimes, in a somewhat opposite effect, frontal lobe tumors impair normal inhibitory systems. Patients may overreact to any irritation, tend to use profanities, cry with little provocation, and jump excitedly from topic to topic.

Similarly, temporal lobe tumors also cause personality changes and memory impairment. However, parietal or occipital lobe tumors, unless they cause increased intracranial pressure, have relatively little effect on personality or memory.

Tumor-induced increased intracranial pressure (pressures exceeding 200 mm H_2O) impairs cerebral function, which often leads to personality changes and cognitive impairment. Continued increased intracranial pressure leads to headache and lethargy that overshadow cognitive symptoms, and eventually stupor and coma.

Tumors can elevate intracranial pressure through several possible mechanisms. Regardless of the site of the tumor, tumor mass and surrounding edema raise intracranial pressure because the brain is encased within the rigid skull and has almost no room to expand. Another mechanism is that metastases can obstruct flow of cerebrospinal fluid (CSF). For example, metastases in the cerebellum can obstruct CSF flow through the fourth ventricle, which results in *obstructive hydrocephalus*. In *carcinomatous meningitis*, cancer cells coat the meninges at the base of the brain and impede reabsorption of CSF, which leads to *communicating hydrocephalus*. Moreover, malignant cells can also strangle cranial and spinal nerves.

Medications and Other Treatments.   Medications, notoriously opioids, can cause delirium and other signs of toxic-metabolic encephalopathy. In an extreme example, accumulation of normeperidine, which is the metabolic product of meperidine (Demerol), results in a toxic psychosis and myoclonus. On the other hand, insufficient opioids can lead to relentless suffering, restless sleep, and drug-seeking behavior. Similarly, hypnotics—often essential for control of pain, insomnia, and anxiety in cancer patients—can cause mental dullness, confusion, and disruption of the sleep-wake cycle.

Other medications likely to induce mental status changes in cancer patients are anticonvulsants, steroids, psychotropics, and antiemetics that contain antihistamines or phenothiazines. Although physical side effects of common medications are usually predictable, mental side effects, especially in cancer patients, are sometimes unexpected. For example, patients might have undiagnosed liver metastases that slow metabolism of medications, leading to accumulation of antidepressants. Another situation is that cancer patients have often lost body mass. For example, a cachetic patient might be given a dose of a medication appropriate for a healthy, average-weight individual, but it would cause an overdose in view of the reduce body mass. When several organs are involved, various specialists are each likely to order different medications that not only cause mental status abnormalities but also interfere with each other's intended benefits.

Chemotherapy agents generally do not cause mental status changes because they cannot penetrate the blood-brain barrier. However, one exception is methotrexate, which is administered intrathecally (into the subarachnoid space, usually through a lumbar puncture [LP]) in conjunction with craniospinal radiotherapy. Although this strategy protects children from leukemic cells invading the CNS, the methotrexate often induces confusional states, learning disabilities, and permanent intellectual impairment.

Another debilitating aspect of chemotherapy is its tendency to induce nausea and vomiting (*chemotherapy-induced emesis*). Chemotherapy agents trigger the brain's *chemoreceptor zone* and the adjacent *vomiting center*. These zones are located in the *area postrema* of the medulla, which is one of the few regions of the brain unprotected by the blood-brain barrier. The absence of an overlying blood-brain barrier leaves the chemoreceptor zone freely accessible to any blood-borne substance. Morphine, heroin, and high doses of L-dopa, as well as the chemotherapeutic agents, readily activate it and trigger vomiting. On the other hand, both dopamine blocking agents and 5-HT$_3$ antagonists prevent chemotherapy-induced nausea and vomiting (see Chapter 21).

Cranial ("whole brain") radiotherapy is another cause of iatrogenic mental status changes, particularly dementia. When administered in high doses over a short period of time, radiotherapy can cause necrosis of small cerebral arteries, which leads to a series of small, strokelike cerebral infarctions, termed *radiation necrosis* or *radiation arteritis*. In an analogous complication, radiotherapy of the spine or mediastinum can cause spinal cord radiation necrosis, *radiation myelitis*.

Cerebral radiation necrosis usually begins about 6 to 18 months after a course of radiotherapy. During several months, it causes stepwise onset of cognitive impairment, hemiparesis, and dysarthria that mimics multi-infarct (vascular) dementia. Cranial radiation given to children for acute leukemia and childhood onset brain tumors can lead to mental retardation, cognitive impairment, growth retardation, and other signs of hypothalamic-pituitary deficiency. Younger children are comparatively more vulnerable to radiation-induced cognitive impairment.

Failure of Vital Organs.   Medications or metastases can also cause renal, pulmonary, or hepatic failure. The organ failure, usually in the late stages of cancer, can lead to metabolic aberrations. In addition, certain cancers produce ("ectopic") hormones that can cause metabolic aberrations. For example, excess tumor-induced parathyroid hormone production causes hypercalcemia, and inappropriate antidiuretic hormone (ADH) secretion causes hyponatremia. When severe enough, metabolic aberrations cause lethargy, confusion, disorientation, and other manifestations of a metabolic encephalopathy. However, the aberrations occasionally cause agitation, combativeness, hallucinations, and other problems that may require antipsychotics. Apart from the mental aberrations, the metabolic alterations lead to seizures, which would require additional medications, at least until a normal metabolic state is restored.

Paraneoplastic Syndromes.   Systemic cancer can induce antibody-mediated inflammatory disorders of the CNS or PNS, termed *paraneoplastic syndromes* or *remote* *effects of carcinoma.* These syndromes precede the discovery of the cancer in the majority of cases. Once they are recognized, their mental and physical symptoms parallel the exacerbations and remissions of the cancer.

The most common syndrome consists of subacute cerebellar degeneration associated with gynecologic cancers, small cell cancer of the lung, or lymphoma. A relatively common syndrome that affects the PNS and resembles myasthenia gravis is the Lambert-Eaton syndrome (see below).

An important, although rare, paraneoplastic syndrome consists of limbic system inflammation, *limbic encephalitis.* This disorder presumably results from antibodies directed toward an underlying small cell carcinoma of the lung or testicular cancer that cross-reacts with CNS neurons in the limbic system. Over several days to several weeks, affected individuals develop pronounced memory impairment combined with irritability, behavioral disturbances, and cognitive ability. Sometimes the disorder's manifestation is exclusively an amnestic syndrome. (However, because the amnesia develops slowly and persists, it cannot be included as a cause of "transient amnesia" [see Table 7–1].) MRIs in cases of limbic encephalopathy commonly show abnormalities of the mesial temporal lobes.

In general, paraneoplastic syndromes do not respond to removal of the cancer. Also, they fail to respond to administration of immunosuppressive treatments, such as steroids, plasmapheresis, or intravenous immunoglobulin.

Inflammatory and Infectious Conditions.   Cancer patients are susceptible to various bacterial infections, particularly when they have indwelling intravenous lines and urinary catheters. They are also susceptible to fungal infections, particularly from *Cryptococcus,* and other opportunistic organisms. These infections, which are espe-

TABLE 19–2. *Evaluation of Cancer Patients with Mental Aberrations*

What is the primary tumor?
  Lung, breast, kidney, malignant melanoma*
Where are metastases known to be present?
  Brain, liver, lung, spine
Does the patient have symptoms or signs of a cerebral lesion?
  Headache, seizures, hemiparesis, papilledema
What treatments have been given?
  Radiation: total dose
  Chemotherapy: medications and antiemetics
  Analgesics: daily dose, route, indication, recent changes
  Psychotropics: antidepressants, hypnotics, tranquilizers
  Others: steroids, cimetidine
What is the patient's general status?
  Pain control
  Sleep schedule and restfulness
  Nutrition, weight change, and appetite
  Temperature
What are the results of important laboratory tests?
  Complete blood count
  Liver and renal function tests
  Serum calcium concentration
  CT or MRI

*Cancers that tend to metastasize.

cially likely to develop in patients with radiotherapy- and chemotherapy-induced immunosuppression, are unaccompanied by fever and leukocytosis. Thus, lethargy, confusion, and withdrawal in cancer patients are often a manifestation of a toxic encephalopathy induced by an occult infection.

Similarly, viruses can affect patients who have received intensive chemotherapy. Several can cause a patchy loss of myelin in the brain. For example, *progressive multifocal leukoencephalopathy (PML)*, which is probably a manifestation of a papovavirus, results in dementia and variable physical impairments late in the course of an illness (see Chapter 7). Although PML complicates the course of some cancer patients, it affects AIDS patients more frequently.

For a patient known to have a brain tumor, a psychiatrist might attempt to determine how psychologic stresses, neurologic deficits, and iatrogenic factors influence the patient's mental state (Table 19–2). In addition to providing traditional supportive psychotherapy, psychiatrists might help patients, their families, and other physicians by weighing the consequences of various treatments, including withdrawal of all treatment except analgesics. They can arrange for health care proxies if patients lose their cognitive capacity. They can also advise on pain management, antidepressant treatments, and control of behavioral problems.

DIAGNOSTIC TESTS FOR BRAIN TUMORS

Even a thorough history and physical may fail to reveal brain tumors that are slowly growing, located in silent areas, or cause only nonspecific mental changes, including depression. Despite their expense, CT and MRI are reliable, ultimately cost-effective routine diagnostic procedures (see Chapter 20). They can detect virtually all of the tumors that might present with depression, psychosis, or similar mental disorders. In addition, they are usually sufficient to identify other intracranial lesions, including strokes, subdural hematomas, and arteriovenous malformations (AVMs).

Although CT is a satisfactory screening procedure, MRI is better able to detect small lesions. It is necessary to detect lesions in areas encased by bone, such as optic gliomas, acoustic neuromas, pituitary adenomas, and some posterior fossa tumors. It is also better able to detect lesions in the white matter, such as PML. If CT detects a tumor, an MRI is often necessary to determine its exact location, internal structure, and involvement of the surrounding brain. Positron emission tomography (PET) can help distinguish between cerebral radiation necrosis and tumor recurrence, but it is not a standard diagnostic test.

An electroencephalogram (EEG), especially in comparison to CT and MRI, is simply not useful for detecting tumors or other structural lesions. Even with some large meningiomas, an EEG may show few or only nonspecific abnormalities. Nevertheless, it remains a good test for toxic-metabolic encephalopathy, particularly hepatic encephalopathy.

An LP to analyze CSF is usually not performed when a brain tumor or other intracranial mass lesion is suspected. In these cases, the CSF profile is usually not diagnostic because it is usually either normal or only nonspecifically abnormal (see Chapter 20). Moreover, with large, expanding supratentorial mass lesions, an LP can precipitate transtentorial herniation (Fig. 19–3). An LP is indicated, however, when patients are suspected of having either carcinomatous or chronic infectious meningitis. For those conditions, large volumes of CSF must be examined for neoplastic cells, fungi, and *Cryptococcus* antigens.

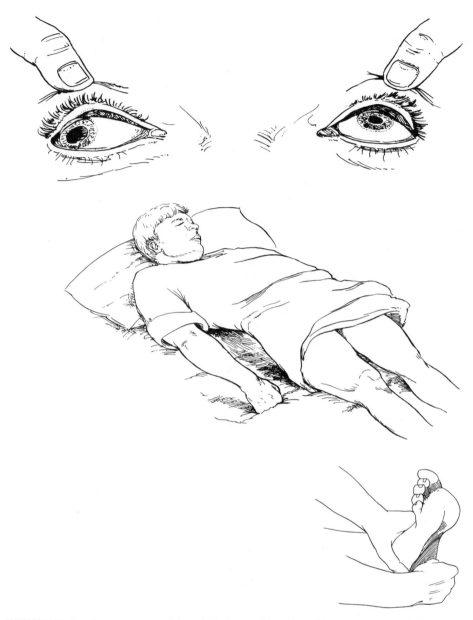

FIGURE 19–3. A patient in *transtentorial herniation* from a right-sided subdural hematoma, as in Fig. 19–1*D*, has coma, decerebrate (extensor) posture, Babinski signs, and a dilated right pupil. This catastrophe has resulted from the right temporal lobe compressing the right-sided oculomotor nerve and brainstem through the tentorial notch.

RELATED CONDITIONS

Pituitary Adenomas

Although pituitary adenomas are also considered brain tumors, their clinical manifestations, histology, and treatment are entirely different from those of the common supratentorial tumors, such as glioblastomas, astrocytomas, and meningiomas. In classic studies, the usual manifestations of pituitary adenomas included major mental, physical, and visual abnormalities; however, those symptoms resulted from massive pituitary tumors that produced extraordinary levels of hormones, expanded out of the sella to encroach on the adjacent temporal lobes and optic chiasm, and obstructed the flow of CSF through the third ventricle. Physicians now routinely diagnose pituitary adenomas early in their course, while they are "microscopic," by using MRI and hormone radioimmunoassay, which represent practical applications of two Nobel Prize–winning concepts.

Most pituitary adenomas are either *prolactinomas,* which secrete prolactin, or *chromophobe adenomas,* which are nonsecretory. Pituitary adenomas occur almost only in adults and rarely infiltrate the adjacent brain. While prolactinomas are usually microscopic, chromophobe adenomas typically grow large enough to exert pressure on surrounding structures (Fig. 19–4). Adenomas' upward pressure on the diaphragm sellae causes bitemporal or generalized headache. Their pressure on the optic chiasm, which is above the diaphragm, also causes characteristic visual field cuts: bitemporal superior quadrantanopia and, with further enlargement, bitemporal hemianopsia (see Fig. 12–9).

The early symptoms of pituitary adenomas, in addition to headache, reflect hormone irregularities: they include infertility, amenorrhea, decreased libido, and galactorrhea. Eventually pituitary hormone insufficiency results in a lack of energy, apathy, and listlessness. Patients may appear to be depressed, but their cognitive capacity is normal.

MRI reveals virtually all pituitary adenomas. The serum prolactin level is elevated in patients with prolactinomas and in most with chromophobe adenomas. Visual field testing is helpful in detecting pituitary adenomas that have expanded out of the sella. Treatment varies with tumor type, symptoms, and institutional expertise, but the usual options are radiation, transsphenoidal microsurgery, and, with prolactin-secreting tumors, a dopamine agonist, such as bromocriptine. Treatment with radiation or craniotomy, which risks damaging the temporal lobes, can lead to memory impairment and partial complex seizures.

Less common pituitary growths secrete *growth hormone,* which can cause *acromegaly,* or *adrenocorticotropin hormone (ACTH),* which can lead to *Cushing's syndrome.* These growths are not really adenomas but collections of hyperplastic cells. Their

FIGURE 19–4. Pituitary adenomas grow laterally and inferiorly against the walls of the sella turcica and upward against the *diaphragm sellae.* Large adenomas compress the optic chiasm, which causes a distinctive bitemporal hemianopsia or bitemporal superior quadrantanopia (see Fig. 12–9). Chronic pressure on the chiasm results in optic atrophy. Large pituitary tumors may first lead to pituitary insufficiency that may have an insidious onset.

Extraordinarily large pituitary tumors compress and damage the adjacent medial inferior surface of the temporal lobe. Radiotherapy directed at a pituitary tumor might also damage this area.

The suprasellar region of the brain, which is above the diaphragm sellae, contains the hypothalamus. Lesions in this area, such as craniopharyngiomas, cause diabetes insipidus as well as optic chiasm compression and pituitary insufficiency.

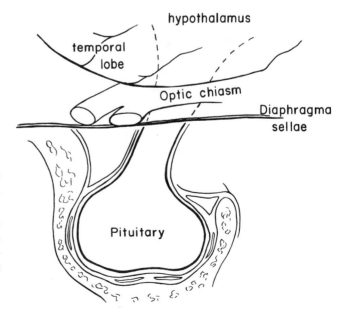

mass is insufficient to cause visual impairment or severe headache. The hormones they secrete change patients' general appearance and produce various psychologic symptoms, including depression and psychosis.

In contrast to these relatively benign pituitary lesions, *craniopharyngioma*, a tumor that occurs in children as well as in adults, is frequently fatal or severely debilitating. This tumor is a calcified, cystic, congenital lesion derived from Rathke's pouch. Unlike pituitary adenomas, the craniopharyngioma grows within the hypothalamus, located above the diaphragm sellae (Fig. 19–4). Because it disrupts endocrine function, affected children have retarded physical, sexual, and mental development; adults have symptoms of impaired libido, amenorrhea, and apathy; and both children and adults develop diabetes insipidus. Large craniopharyngiomas press downward on the optic chiasm, causing optic atrophy and visual field defects similar to those found with large pituitary adenomas. If the third ventricle is compressed, patients develop obstructive hydrocephalus, which causes papilledema with headache, nausea, and vomiting—classic signs of increased intracranial pressure.

Another condition causing pituitary insufficiency is *postpartum pituitary necrosis*, more widely known as *Sheehan's syndrome*. It is usually the result of obstetric deliveries complicated by severe hypotension, usually from massive blood loss. In overt cases, which are unmistakable, women fail to lactate, remain hypotensive, lose weight, and undergo recession of secondary sexual characteristics. In subtle cases, after several months to several years postpartum, women develop scant menses, constant fatigue, and diminished libido. Another postpartum condition, *autoimmune hypothyroidism*, can produce similar symptoms.

Women with these disorders are liable to be misdiagnosed as having psychogenic "postpartum depression." Indeed, the *Diagnostic and Statistical Manual of Mental Disorders-IV (DSM-IV)* specifies that the symptoms of an episode of Major Depressive Disorder and related conditions may have a *Postpartum Onset*. However, these disorders must have their onset within 4 weeks postpartum, which clearly distinguishes them, at any rate, from more subtle cases of Sheehan's syndrome.

Acoustic Neuromas

The covering of the acoustic (eighth cranial) nerve sometimes proliferates to form a relatively benign tumor—the *acoustic neuroma*. (The term "acoustic neuroma" is actually a misnomer because Schwann cells, not neurons, proliferate. Moreover, the growth arises in the vestibular, not acoustic, portion of the nerve.)

This tumor develops in the internal auditory canal and cerebellopontine angle where it may compress adjacent structures, particularly the fifth (trigeminal) and seventh (facial) cranial nerves. Acoustic neuromas cause hearing impairment with early involvement of speech discrimination. Subsequent symptoms—tinnitus, imbalance, and vertigo—result from eighth nerve involvement. If the acoustic neuroma compresses the fifth cranial nerve, patients can develop facial sensory loss. If it compresses the seventh cranial nerve, they can develop facial muscle weakness.

Most acoustic neuromas develop unilaterally and spontaneously. Bilateral acoustic neuromas characteristically arise in young adults with neurofibromatosis-type 2 (NF2), an autosomal dominant disorder of chromosome 22 (see Chapter 13). Gadolinium-enhanced MRI, auditory tests, and brainstem auditory evoked responses (see BAERs, Chapter 15) detect acoustic neuromas. Neurosurgeons, performing "stereotactic radiosurgery" with a gamma knife or linear accelerator, can remove acoustic neuromas while preserving a moderate degree of hearing and the adjacent facial nerve.

Spine Metastases

Lung, breast, and other cancers often metastasize to the vertebrae, where they can grow into the spinal epidural space (Fig. 19–5). *Epidural metastases* cause severe pain not only in the affected region (local pain) but also along the path of the affected nerve roots (radicular pain). For example, patients with thoracic spine metastases typically have interscapular spine pain that radiates around the chest in a bandlike pattern. Similarly, patients with lumbar spine metastases have lower back pain that radiates down the legs.

If cervical or thoracic epidural metastases continue to enlarge, they compress the spinal cord. Spinal cord compression, which is a dreadful complication of cancer, causes pain, quadriplegia or paraplegia, loss of sensation, and incontinence of urine and feces (see Chapters 2 and 16). Cognitive capacity is preserved, but depression often ensues.

Early diagnosis can prevent epidural spinal cord compression; however, once it occurs, the deficits are often permanent. MRI of the spine can detect most metastases, but CT-myelography is sometimes necessary. Therapy usually consists of steroids, radiation, and, sometimes, decompressive laminectomy.

Other Causes of Limb Weakness

Certain cancers trigger paraneoplastic inflammatory conditions that affect the PNS, as well as the CNS. For example, lung, breast, ovarian, gastric, and other solid tumors provoke *dermatomyositis*, which consists of diffuse, proximal muscle weakness, muscle tenderness, and a heliotrope rash on the face and extensor skin surfaces.

The *Lambert-Eaton syndrome* is another paraneoplastic syndrome associated with small cell lung cancer that affects the neuromuscular junction (see Chapter 6). Unlike

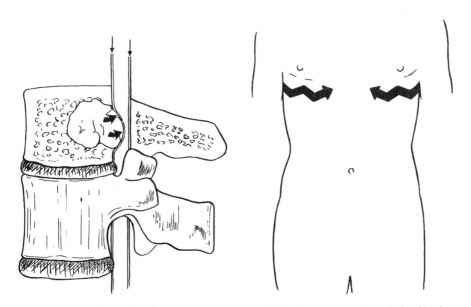

FIGURE 19–5. *Left,* Vertebral metastases typically grow posteriorly to encroach on the spinal *epidural space (arrows),* which contains the spinal cord and its nerve roots. These *epidural metastases* cause spinal cord compression, which results in paraplegia or quadriplegia, loss of sensation (hypalgesia) below the level of the lesion, and incontinence of feces and urine. *Right,* Patients have "local pain" from destruction of the vertebrae and a characteristic bandlike "radiating pain," which follows the course of the nerves *(jagged arrows).* The location of the pain and level of the hypalgesia indicate the site of an epidural metastatic tumor (see Fig. 2–15).

myasthenia gravis—the most widely known neuromuscular junction disorder—the Lambert-Eaton syndrome causes proximal limb muscle weakness, which is partially alleviated by repetitive actions. Also unlike myasthenia gravis, the Lambert-Eaton syndrome does not cause extraocular muscle palsy or dysarthria.

The Lambert-Eaton syndrome (as well as botulism and botulinum toxin) causes weakness by impairing the release of acetylcholine (ACh) from the *presynaptic* neuromuscular junction neuron. (In contrast, the weakness in myasthenia is due to abnormally rapid ACh inactivation at the *postsynaptic* site.)

Iatrogenic myopathies and neuropathies are common. Prolonged steroid use results in *steroid myopathy*. Administration of diuretics without potassium supplements results in *hypokalemic myopathies*. Various chemotherapy agents, such as vincristine, cause a generalized impairment of nerves, *polyneuropathy*, which often has a sensory component (see Chapter 5). Chemotherapy-induced neuropathy can be so sudden, profound, and extensive that it mimics metastatic spinal cord compression. In most cases, the symptoms improve several months after chemotherapy is completed.

In contrast to the generalized weakness induced by these conditions, injuries of individual peripheral nerves, *mononeuropathies*, cause paresis and sensory loss along the distribution of a single nerve (see Table 5–1). The sequence in cancer patients begins with loss of muscle bulk and subcutaneous fat. Then peripheral nerves, deprived of their protective cushion, are vulnerable to pressure as light as from the patient's own weight. The sciatic, peroneal, and radial nerves are most often injured when patients are bedridden, moved onto stretchers, or secured in wheelchairs. Sometimes misplaced injections or other accidents injure these nerves.

The most painful cancer complication is probably direct tumor infiltration of a nerve plexus. When lung and breast cancer invades the brachial plexus or pelvic cancer invades the lumbosacral plexus, patients develop excruciating pain, as well as paresis of the limb. Because the nerves are invaded, the pain is poorly responsive to routine treatments, such as radiotherapy and analgesics (see Chapter 14).

DISORDERS THAT MIMIC BRAIN TUMORS

Strokes, as well as tumors, occur predominantly in older people and cause cognitive impairment, physical deficits, and seizures. However, the course of strokes and tumors is markedly different. Strokes usually occur acutely or occasionally develop over several days, but brain tumors usually evolve over at least several weeks. In addition, even when strokes cause extensive physical and intellectual deficits, patients usually remain alert and free of headaches. For example, a patient with a stroke may be fully alert despite having a homonymous hemianopsia, hemiparesis, and hemisensory loss. To produce a comparable extensive deficit, a tumor would have to be massive and extend through an entire cerebral hemisphere. It would then increase the intracranial pressure and produce stupor. As a rule, CT and MRI can readily differentiate these conditions.

Subdural hematomas, which also occur frequently, can mimic brain tumors as well. Intracranial venous bleeding, usually initiated by head trauma, causes a hematoma in the potential space between the dura (the thick layer of the meninges) and the underlying brain (Figs. 19–1D and 20–11). Over a period of several weeks, the subdural hematoma, which may be either unilateral or bilateral, accumulates fluid and progressively enlarges. As the subdural hematoma grows, it compresses one or both cerebral hemispheres and produces generalized cerebral dysfunction (see Chapter 22).

Older individuals are especially prone to subdural hematomas because they have intracranial bleeding after minor trauma, even with no obvious head injury. The bleeding continues unchecked because an atrophied brain cannot compress the bleeding veins. Subdural hematomas typically cause headaches, personality changes, and cognitive impairment but usually not lateralized signs. They may be easily evacuated through small "twist-drill" holes. When promptly treated, cerebral function can be restored. In other words, subdural hematomas are a relatively common and correctable form of dementia.

AVMs and brain abscesses, which are other common, nonmalignant cerebral mass lesions, also begin with headaches, mental changes, lateralized signs, or seizures. AVMs are congenital abnormalities that consist of large veins and arteries directly joined without normal intervening small vessels. If they rupture, AVMs cause intraparenchymal hemorrhage, lateralized signs, and seizures.

Abscesses usually follow intravenous drug abuse, dental procedures, sinusitis, bacterial endocarditis, and immunodeficiency. In most cases, the infective organisms are bacteria, but in AIDS, *toxoplasmosis* is usually responsible. Patients with *neurocysticercosis*, which is the neurologic component of *cysticercosis*, develop multiple focal neurologic deficits, seizures, and increased intracranial pressure. Because cysticercosis is endemic in Central and South America, immigrants from these areas often harbor neurocysticercosis (see Fig. 20–7C). *Tuberculosis* causes intracerebral masses, *tuberculomas*, particularly in patients with AIDS and residents of the Indian subcontinent. CT and MRI can detect these lesions even when they are not suggested by the clinical evaluation.

In contrast to malignant and nonmalignant mass lesions, *pseudotumor cerebri* is a metabolic disturbance characterized by excessive fluid accumulation in the brain parenchyma. Pseudotumor mimics actual tumor because in it cerebral edema from interstitial fluid retention raises intracranial pressure that produces headache, papilledema, constricted visual fields, and sometimes sixth cranial nerve palsies (see Chapter 9). Although its etiology is unknown, pseudotumor cerebri predominantly affects obese young women who have menstrual irregularities. Unlike actual tumors, it does not cause stupor or coma.

In pseudotumor cerebri, the LP will disclose markedly elevated CSF pressure (300 to 600 mm H_2O) and no increase in white cells. Because the differential diagnosis of pseudotumor is tumor, neurologists suspecting this disorder still order a CT or MRI. In pseudotumor cerebri, those studies usually reveal cerebral swelling and compressed, small ventricles, but no mass lesions.

INDICATIONS FOR EVALUATION FOR BRAIN TUMORS

Physicians should consider brain tumors and related conditions without waiting for the patient to have florid physical or mental deficits. They should not rely exclusively on the mental status examination to distinguish between psychogenic disorders and brain tumors. Commonplace complaints of fatigue, weight loss, menstrual irregularity, or infertility might prompt evaluation for pituitary insufficiency or hypothyroidism.

Neurologists generally order CT or MRI of the brain, admittedly liberally, for any patient who has intellectual decline; those over 50 years who develop substantial emotional changes; and most adults with headaches that are not attributable to migraines, cluster headaches, trigeminal neuralgia, or temporal arteritis (see Chapter 9). They often also suggest CT or MRI for patients who develop any new mental illness severe enough to warrant psychiatric hospitalization. In addition, they suggest CT or MRI before depressed patients undergo ECT, not only because a tumor or other mass lesion might precipitate status epilepticus or transtentorial herniation, but also because a tumor might underlie the mental disorder. Finally, whenever the patient is worried about a brain tumor, a scan might be performed to resolve the issue and permit appropriate therapy to begin.

REFERENCES

Barry M, Kaldjian LC: Neurocysticercosis. Sem Neurol *13:* 131–143, 1993
Braunstein JB, Vick NA: Meningiomas: The decision not to operate. Neurology *48:* 1459–1462, 1997
Byrne TN: Spinal cord compression from epidural metastases. N Engl J Med *327:* 614–619, 1992
Clouston PD, DeAngelis LM, Posner JB: The spectrum of neurological disease in patients with systemic cancer. Ann Neurol *31:* 268–273, 1992
Dalmau JO, Posner JB: Paraneoplastic syndromes affecting the nervous system. Sem Oncol *24:* 318–328, 1997
Duffner PK, Horowitz ME, Krischer JP, et al: Postoperative chemotherapy and delayed radiation in children less than three years of age with malignant brain tumors. N Engl J Med *328:* 1725–1731, 1993
Martin RC, Haut MW, Kreisler KG: Neuropsychological functioning in a patient with paraneoplastic limbic encephalitis. J Int Neuropsychologic Soc *2:* 460–466, 1996
Newman NJ, Bell IR, McKee AC: Paraneoplastic limbic encephalitis: Neuropsychiatric presentation. Biol Psychiatry *27:* 529–542, 1990
Scharf D: Neurocysticercosis: Two hundred thirty-eight cases from a California hospital. Arch Neurol *45:* 777–780, 1988

QUESTIONS and ANSWERS: CHAPTER 19

1. An 8-year-old boy, with a 6-week history of progressively greater difficulty with athletic activities, develops a severe headache, papilledema, and ataxia. Of the following, which is the most likely cause?

a. Meningioma of the cerebellum
b. Glioblastoma of the cerebrum
c. Metastatic carcinoma
d. Astrocytoma of the cerebellum

ANSWER: d. Because he has ataxia as well as signs of increased intracranial pressure, the lesion is probably located in the cerebellum. It has caused obstructive hydrocephalus. In children, cerebellar astrocytomas are a common variety of brain tumor.

2. A 60-year-old man, who has smoked two packs of cigarettes daily since age 20, develops partial complex seizures. He has headaches, a left superior quadrantanopia, and mild left hemiparesis. In addition, he has right-sided dysmetria and intention tremor. Of the following conditions, which is the most likely illness?

a. Subdural hematomas
b. Metastatic carcinoma in the right temporal lobe and right cerebellar hemisphere
c. Glioblastoma of the left temporal lobe
d. CVAs in the right temporal lobe and right cerebellar hemisphere
e. Multiple sclerosis

ANSWER: b. The patient has partial complex seizures, visual field loss, and hemiparesis from a right frontal and temporal lobe lesions. He also has right-sided coordination impairments from a right cerebellar lesion. These lesions are probably manifestations of metastatic cancer, but multiple embolic CVAs or abscesses are possible. Strokes cause mild and transient headaches. Subdural hematomas rarely cause seizures or cerebellar dysfunction. In addition, although subdural hematomas often occur over both cerebral hemispheres, they rarely occur in the posterior fossa. He is too old to have developed multiple sclerosis (MS). Moreover, headaches and seizures are not initial symptoms of MS.

3. Which of the following patients is most likely to develop cerebral gliomas?

a. A 30-year-old woman with multiple café au lait spots
b. A 21-year-old woman with bilateral acoustic neuromas
c. A 21-year-old man with mental retardation, epilepsy, and adenoma sebaceum
d. A 30-year-old man with a vascular malformation in the distribution of the trigeminal nerve

ANSWER: c. The patient with the mental retardation, epilepsy, and adenoma sebaceum has tuberous sclerosis. The cerebral tubers often undergo malignant transformation into gliomas. The woman with the café au lait spots has neurofibromatosis type 1 (NF1), which is often complicated by meningiomas, as well as neuromas of peripheral nerves. The woman with the acoustic neuromas probably has neurofibromatosis type 2 (NF2). The man with the vascular malformation has Sturge-Weber syndrome, which is not complicated by neoplasms.

4. A 50-year-old woman has an impaired ability to hear while listening with the telephone receiver next to her right ear. She also has right-sided tinnitus and loss of auditory acuity, but otherwise her neurologic examination is normal. Of the following, which one is the most likely illness?

a. Left temporal lobe meningioma
b. Psychogenic factors
c. MS
d. A cerebellopontine angle tumor

ANSWER: d. Acoustic neuromas, the most common cerebellopontine angle tumor, typically cause speech discrimination impairment, tinnitus, and the gradual loss of auditory acuity. They do not cause vertigo because they develop slowly. Lesions of the cerebral hemispheres or the brainstem, such as MS, do not cause auditory disturbances. Bilateral acoustic neuromas are usually a manifestation of NF2.

5. During the previous year, a 55-year-old woman with multiple café au lait spots developed mild paresis of the left leg, which had hyperactive DTRs and a Babinski sign. Before undergoing further evaluation, she had a seizure that began with clonic movements of the left foot, then leg, and finally the arm. On examination, she has left hemiparesis, hyperactive DTRs, and a Babinski sign. Of the following, which is the most likely illness?

a. Right cerebral glioblastoma
b. Right cerebral meningioma
c. Left cerebral glioblastoma
d. Left cerebral meningioma

ANSWER: b. The evolution of a hemiparesis over a relatively long time, especially when it is accompanied by a partial (motor) seizure, suggests a cerebral tumor. In view of the chronicity of the hemiparesis and her probably having NF1, a meningioma is more likely than a glioblastoma. Moreover, meningiomas are more common in women than men.

6. Which two of the following are unlikely to cause headaches in the elderly?

a. Subdural hematomas
b. Open-angle glaucoma
c. Brain tumors
d. Pseudotumor cerebri
e. Temporal arteritis
f. Nitroglycerin and other vasodilator medications

ANSWER: b, d. Open-angle glaucoma is not associated with headaches. Pseudotumor, although it causes headaches, occurs almost exclusively in young women.

7. Brain tumors often produce headaches that are worse in the early morning, waking patients from sleep. Which four of the following headaches also typically begin in the early morning?

a. Muscle contraction tension
b. Pseudotumor cerebri
c. Migraine
d. Trigeminal neuralgia
e. Postconcussive syndrome
f. Cluster headache
g. Sleep apnea induced headache
h. Caffeine withdrawal

ANSWER: c, f, g, h. Migraine and cluster headaches characteristically develop during REM sleep, which occurs predominantly in the early morning. Hypoxia and carbon dioxide retention also cause headache.

8. An obese 22-year-old woman has moderately severe, generalized headaches. She has papilledema and paresis of abduction of her right eye but no other neurologic abnormalities. Routine blood and chemistry tests are normal. A CT shows small ventricles but no mass lesion. What would be the most appropriate next step?

a. An MRI to look for a brainstem glioma or cerebrovascular accident
b. EEG
c. Lumbar puncture (LP) to measure the pressure and withdraw CSF
d. None of the above

> **ANSWER:** c. The patient almost certainly has pseudotumor cerebri. The increased intracranial pressure stretches the sixth nerve. However, because the sixth nerve injury does not result from a mass, it is called a "false localizing sign." Given the clinical situation, an MRI is unnecessary. Instead, an LP should be performed for diagnosis and therapy of pseudotumor cerebri. It will also exclude chronic meningitis. In pseudotumor, the CSF pressure is usually above 300 mm, which is a marked elevation. Prolonged papilledema, for any reason, will lead to optic atrophy and then blindness. Pseudotumor is one of the rare situations where an LP is performed despite papilledema.

9. A 45-year-old police officer with various emotional difficulties has become obsessed with the thought that he has a brain tumor. Careful medical and neurologic examinations are normal. What would most neurologists do next?

a. Offer reassurance
b. Suggest psychotherapy
c. Give an antidepressant
d. Treat him for obsession
e. Take other steps

> **ANSWER:** e. Even though brain tumors are uncommon in middle-aged people, most neurologists would order a CT or MRI for several reasons. At the onset, about 50% of the patients with tumors have no overt physical neurologic deficits. Other structural lesions, such as an AVM or subdural hematoma, could be responsible for the patient's symptoms. Furthermore, with a normal study, a neurologist can give more secure reassurance, feel protected in the event of a medical-legal problem, and refer the patient to a psychiatrist who will probably feel more confident in accepting the patient.

10. A 60-year-old man with lung cancer develops confusion and agitation. He refuses a full neurologic examination, but physicians find that he has no obvious hemiparesis or nuchal rigidity. A noncontrast head CT is normal. Which one of the following is the least likely cause of an alteration in the mental status of such a patient?

a. Hyperkalemia
b. Pneumonia
c. Liver metastases with hepatic encephalopathy
d. Increased intracranial pressure
e. Inappropriate ADH secretion
f. Hypercalcemia
g. Liver metastases with slowed metabolism of medications

> **ANSWER:** a. All these disorders, except for hyperkalemia, are frequent complications of lung cancer that has not necessarily spread to the brain. (The superior vena cava syndrome causes increased intracranial pressure.)

11. Two months later, the man in the previous case undergoes a CT that reveals two ring-shaped lesions with surrounding lucency. When he became combative during the evaluation, a psychiatry consultation was solicited. Which two medications should be recommended?

a. A neuroleptic
b. An antidepressant
c. Steroids
d. Hypnotics
e. An anticonvulsant (antiepileptic drug)

> **ANSWER:** a, c. A neuroleptic should be given at least until the patient's behavioral disturbances subside. Because steroids, such as dexamethasone, will reduce the edema and thus the volume of the lesions, they will bring about a rapid and dramatic, although short-lived, improvement. Some neurologists would also prophylactically suggest an antiepileptic drug because cerebral metastases often cause seizures and the neuroleptic may lower the seizure threshold. The dose and duration of dexamethasone in this situation is usually insufficient to cause steroid psychosis.

12. A 65-year-old woman with the onset of dementia over 9 months has no physical or neurologic abnormalities except for frontal release signs and hyperactive DTRs. A complete laboratory and EEG evaluation reveals no specific abnormality. A CT shows atrophy and a small meningioma in the right parietal convexity. Which would be the most appropriate next step?

a. Have the tumor removed.
b. Tentatively diagnose Alzheimer's disease and repeat the clinical evaluation and CT in 6 to 12 months.
c. Obtain an MRI.

ANSWER: b. The meningioma is irrelevant to the dementia. These tumors grow so slowly that they can be followed with periodic scans. They should be removed if they are large enough to compress brain tissue or become symptomatic. An MRI will not be more helpful than a CT in confirming that the lesion is a meningioma or whether the patient has Alzheimer's disease.

13. A 75-year-old man, who has had dementia for 6 years, suddenly develops increased irritability and behavioral disturbances. He has no lateralized signs or indication of increased intracranial pressure. He is treated with a major tranquilizer. One week later, he becomes somnolent and has a seizure. He remains comatose with a left hemiparesis. No abnormalities are found on a general medical examination or routine laboratory tests, but a CT shows an extra-axial lucency with some dense regions and a shift of midline cerebral structures. Before any treatment can be instituted, the patient dies. An autopsy discloses cerebral atrophy and a large chronic subdural hematoma with recent hemorrhage. Which of the following statements concerning subdural hematomas is untrue?

a. Subdural hematomas are apt to occur in the elderly, especially in those individuals who have a history of dementia and cerebral atrophy.
b. The location of subdural hematomas is outside or overlying the brain (i.e., extra-axial).
c. Unless they are large or rapidly expanding, subdural hematomas may not cause lateralized signs or give indications of increased intracranial pressure.
d. In chronic subdurals, CT portrays blood as less radiodense than brain. With superimposed bleeding, densities appear within these lucent regions. In other words, chronic hematomas are black (radiolucent), and fresh ones are white (radiodense).
e. The trauma required to cause a subdural hematoma is usually so great that it causes loss of consciousness for 1 hour or longer.

ANSWER: e. In the elderly, little or no trauma is required. On the other hand, subdural hematomas in the elderly may be a sign of "elder abuse."

14. Which structure is *not* located in the posterior fossa?

a. Sphenoid wing
b. Chemoreceptors for vomiting
c. Vertebrobasilar artery system
d. Cerebellum
e. Fourth ventricle

ANSWER: a

15. Match the brain lesion (1–6) with the group(s) particularly at risk (a–j).

1. Chronic subdural hematoma
2. Cerebellar astrocytoma
3. Cerebral lymphomas
4. Cysticercosis
5. Tuberculosis
6. Acoustic neuromas

a. Drug addicts
b. Elderly individuals
c. Homosexuals
d. Children
e. Residents of Central America

f. Residents of India
g. Neurofibromatosis type 1
h. Neurofibromatosis type 2
i. Trisomy 21
j. AIDS patients

ANSWERS: 1-b; 2-d; 3-a, c, j; 4-e; 5-a, c, f, j; 6-h

16. Which one of the following is *not* usually indicative of a pituitary adenoma?

a. Increased serum prolactin level
b. Cognitive impairment
c. Galactorrhea
d. Bitemporal hemianopsia
e. Decreased libido

f. Menstrual irregularity
g. Headaches
h. Bitemporal superior quadrantanopia
i. Infertility

ANSWER: b

17. Which of the following pituitary conditions is most likely to emerge in a 14-year-old child and delay growth, puberty, and social maturity?

a. Chromophobe adenoma
b. Prolactinoma

c. Cushing's syndrome
d. Craniopharyngioma

ANSWER: d. Unlike other tumors that cause pituitary insufficiency, craniopharyngiomas are congenital lesions that emerge in children and adults. They are typically located in the hypothalamic region, are cystic, and contain calcium. They can be visualized on skull x-rays, CT, MRI, and histologic studies. In children, craniopharyngiomas cause delayed puberty and poor school performance. When craniopharyngiomas are large, they cause the visual impairments characteristic of pituitary tumors (e.g., bitemporal hemianopsia or superior quadrantanopia and optic atrophy). They also cause diabetes insipidus because they grow into the hypothalamus and obstructive hydrocephalus if they occlude outflow from the third ventricle.

18. Of the following statements regarding paraneoplastic syndromes, which is untrue?

a. They often appear before the underlying cancer has been detected.
b. Their symptoms parallel the exacerbations and remissions of the cancer.
c. Immunosuppression relieves the symptoms.
d. Paraneoplastic syndromes include dermatomyositis, Lambert-Eaton syndrome, pancerebellar degeneration, and limbic encephalitis.

ANSWER: c. Paraneoplastic syndromes resist treatment; however, they occasionally remit if the underlying cancer is cured.

19. A 65-year-old man with metastatic prostate carcinoma has been in agony from bone metastases. He is agitated, loud, and threatening in his demands for narcotics. He has become a major management problem, and his family is also becoming disruptive. Tests have shown that the patient has no cerebral metastases, hypercalcemia, or other metabolic aberrations. Which two steps should a psychiatry consultant take as an initial response to this situation?

a. Help the primary physician control the patient's pain with as much narcotics as he requires. Once the pain is controlled, the situation can be reassessed.
b. Stop all medications because they can be the cause of the behavioral disorder.
c. Immediately administer minor or major tranquilizers.
d. Before treating further, check with an MRI and LP for signs of cerebral metastases or opportunistic infections.

ANSWER: a and possibly c. Metastases to the brain from prostatic cancer rarely occur, but those to bone are common—and they are agonizingly painful. Bone pain from metastatic prostate cancer can be partly or fully controlled with hormone manipulation, radiotherapy, and narcotic analgesics that are titrated to the patient's level of comfort. If the pain is poorly controlled, drug-seeking behavior is expectable. Long-acting narcotics, such as methadone, and narcotics given by patch or continuous intravenous infusion are effective. "Breakthrough pain" may be alleviated by "rescue doses" of parenteral narcotics, such as morphine. Narcotics may be enhanced by steroids and nonsteroidal anti-inflammatory agents, which reduce inflammation of bone metastases. Judicious use of antidepressants and tranquilizers may provide additional analgesia, mood improvement, and restful sleep.

20. What mechanism has been proposed to explain limbic encephalitis and other paraneoplastic syndrome?

a. Antibody formation
b. Viral infection

c. Endocrine disturbance
d. Toxins secreted by the tumor

ANSWER: a. The majority of patients with pancerebellar degeneration, limbic encephalitis, and other paraneoplastic syndromes have characteristic antibodies that react with neurons.

21. Of the following lesions, which three tend to be located extra-axially?

a. Butterfly gliomas
b. Astrocytomas
c. Meningiomas

d. Epidural hematomas
e. Subdural hematomas
f. Medulloblastomas

ANSWER: c, d, e

22. Which two of the following are not functions of glial cells?

a. To provide structure for the spinal cord
b. To provide structure for the brain
c. To clear debris from infections and CVAs
d. To generate a myelin coat for CNS neurons
e. To generate a myelin coat for PNS neurons
f. To generate electrochemical potentials

ANSWER: e, f

23. Which are three functions of oligodendrocytes?

a. Occasionally become oligodendrogliomas
b. Generate myelin for the CNS
c. Generate myelin for the PNS
d. Generate action potentials
e. Act as a glial cell

ANSWER: a, b, e

24. In which three aspects do brain tumors in children differ from those in adults?

a. Childhood tumors are usually located in the cerebellum.
b. Childhood astrocytomas are usually relatively benign.
c. In children, tumors tend to present with signs of hydrocephalus.
d. Metastatic tumors in children are as common as primary brain tumors.
e. Meningiomas are relatively common in children.
f. Pituitary adenomas are relatively common in children.

ANSWER: a, b, c

25. Match the condition that causes weakness (1–6) with the impairment of ACh transmission (a–d).

1. Myasthenia gravis
2. Lambert-Eaton syndrome
3. Botulism
4. Guillain-Barré syndrome
5. Botulinum toxin
6. Dermatomyositis

a. Impaired ACh release from the presynaptic surface of the neuromuscular junction
b. Greater inactivation at the postsynaptic surface of the neuromuscular junction
c. Enhanced re-uptake
d. None of the above

ANSWERS: 1-b, 2-a, 3-a, 4-d, 5-a, 6-d

26. Which statement is untrue regarding the chemoreceptor area of the brain?

a. It is located in the superior surface of the medulla.
b. It is located in the area postrema.
c. It is unprotected by the blood-brain barrier.
d. The area is inaccessible to most chemicals.

ANSWER: d. The chemoreceptor area of the brain is almost completely susceptible to blood-borne substances.

27. Serum prolactin levels that are transiently elevated above the baseline are a useful diagnostic test for seizures. Which five of the following conditions or medicines elevate the baseline serum prolactin level?

a. Chromophobe adenoma
b. Prolactinoma
c. Phenothiazines
d. Butyrophenones
e. Estrogens

f. Bromocriptine
g. Dopamine
h. Quetiapine
i. L-dopa

ANSWER: a–e. In contrast, bromocriptine, dopamine, and L-dopa reduce prolactin secretion.

28. Which two are complications of performing ECT on a patient with an undetected meningioma?

a. Skin necrosis
b. Status epilepticus

c. Transtentorial herniation
d. Exacerbating Parkinson's disease

ANSWER: b, c. ECT will alleviate, at least temporarily, the motor impairments of Parkinson's disease.

29–31. Match the varieties of hemorrhage with the most likely cause.

29. Subarachnoid hemorrhage

30. Subdural hematoma

31. Epidural hematoma

a. Middle meningeal artery laceration
b. Rupture of a berry aneurysm
c. Trauma of bridging meningeal veins

ANSWERS:
29. b. Although trauma and mycotic aneurysms may cause a subarachnoid hemorrhage, the most frequent and important cause is a rupture of a berry aneurysm.
30. c. Subdural hematomas are usually caused by bleeding from small meningeal veins.
31. a. Epidural hematomas are usually caused by lacerations of the middle meningeal artery, which are often a consequence of skull fracture.

32. A 46-year-old woman, who has metastatic breast cancer, develops a disconcerting numbness in the skin over the right lower jaw. She has no weakness of face or jaw muscles. The remainder of her neurologic examination is normal. An x-ray of the jaw reveals a lytic lesion in the right lower mandible. What is the diagnosis?

a. Mental neuropathy
b. Mononeuritis multiplex

c. A remote effect of carcinoma
d. A facial nerve injury

ANSWER: a. She has a mental neuropathy, which is numbness of the skin over the lower lateral chin, the mental area due to injury of the mental nerve, which is a branch of the trigeminal nerve. The term "mental neuropathy" could be easily misconstrued. In this case, the mental neuropathy is due to metastases to the jaw where the mental nerve passes through the mental foramen. Trauma to the same region could also produce mental neuropathy.

33. A family brings a 59-year-old man for a consultation because he has become apathetic and markedly forgetful but intermittently and inexplicably irritable. One month before this consultation he received a diagnosis of small cell carcinoma of the lung. An examination confirms that he has amnesia and personality changes. An MRI of the head and three LPs show no sign of metastases. The results of all his clinical chemistry tests are within normal limits. However, an EEG shows focal slowing and spikes over the temporal lobes. Which is the most likely explanation for his memory deficit and other abnormalities?

a. A depressive disorder
b. An inflammatory condition affecting the temporal lobes
c. Temporal lobe metastases that have remained undetected by the MRI
d. Partial complex seizures

ANSWER: b. He has limbic encephalitis, which is a paraneoplastic syndrome associated with small cell carcinoma of the lung and testicular carcinoma. It is characterized by profound memory impairment and personality changes. It may also lead to generalized cognitive impairment and seizures.

34. Which of the following organs is most resistant to ionizing radiation?

a. Bone marrow

b. Brain

c. Gastrointestinal tract

d. Lung

ANSWER: Brain. The CNS is relatively resistant to ionizing radiation, including radiotherapy. The cerebral blood vessels are more sensitive that the parenchyma. Relatively large doses of radiation can be administered in an attempt to reduce the growth of brain tumors.

20

Lumbar Puncture and Imaging Studies

LUMBAR PUNCTURE

When patients have signs or symptoms of meningitis (headache, fever, and nuchal rigidity) or a subarachnoid hemorrhage (a suddenly developing severe headache, especially if it is the worst in the patient's life), neurologists usually examine the cerebrospinal fluid (CSF) by performing a lumbar puncture (LP).

In evaluating patients with dementia, an LP is helpful in diagnosing relatively few conditions—mostly infectious illnesses, such as acquired immunodeficiency syndrome (AIDS), neurosyphilis, Lyme disease, cryptococcal or tuberculous meningitis, and, in children, subacute sclerosing panencephalitis (SSPE). However, an LP is not indicated in patients suspected of having dementia attributable to Creutzfeldt-Jakob's disease, even though it is an infectious illness; Alzheimer's disease; vascular dementia; or Huntington's disease.

In several neurologic illnesses, the CSF sometimes reveals a characteristic abnormality. For example, in Guillain-Barré syndrome (see Chapter 5), the CSF has a high protein concentration and only a slight increase in the cell content. In multiple sclerosis (MS), it often contains oligoclonal bands and myelin basic protein (see Chapter 15). In SSPE, it contains antimeasles antibodies. Specific antigens may be detected in bacterial and fungal meningitis.

Diagnosing neurologic illnesses depends on abnormalities of the *CSF profile*, which is composed of the CSF color, white blood cell count, and concentrations of protein and glucose (Table 20–1). In most infectious or inflammatory illnesses, with the notable exception of Guillain-Barré syndrome, the CSF has *pleocytosis*, which is an increase in the white blood cell count. A rise in protein concentration parallels the CSF pleocytosis, but the profile's hallmark is a decreased glucose concentration. In bacterial meningitis that profile is accentuated: CSF pleocytosis is polymorphonuclear instead of lymphocytic. Unless antigen testing is immediately available, reliable identification of virus, fungus, and *Mycobacterium* may require 1 to 3 weeks of culture. The clinical situation and the CSF profile typically determine the patient's initial diagnosis and treatment.

Despite the potential contribution of CSF examination, an LP is sometimes counterindicated. For example, neurologists do not perform one when patients have an extensive sacral decubitus ulcer because the LP needle might drive bacteria into the spinal canal. In addition, they insert the needle only below the first lumbar vertebra, which is the lower boundary of the spinal cord, to prevent the needle from striking the spinal cord.

The most common counterindication to an LP is presence of an intracranial mass lesion. This prohibition is based on the fear that an LP could suddenly reduce pressure in the spinal canal, allowing the unopposed force of a cerebral mass to lead to

TABLE 20–1. *Cerebrospinal Fluid (CSF) Profiles**

	Color	WBC/mm	Protein (mg/100 ml)	Glucose (mg/100 ml)	Miscellaneous
Normal	Clear	0–4[†]	30–45	60–100	
Bacterial meningitis	*Turbid*	100–500[‡]	75–200	*0–40*	Gram-stain may reveal organisms
Viral meningitis	*Turbid*	*50–100*[†]	50–100	40–60	
TB and fungal meningitis[§]	*Turbid*	*100–500*[†]	100–500	40–60	Cryptococcus antigen should be ordered
Neurosyphilis	Clear	5–200[†]	45–100	40–80	VDRL positive[‖]
Guillain-Barré syndrome	Clear	*5–20*[†]	*80–200*	60–100	
Subarachnoid hemorrhage	*Bloody*[¶]	45–80	60–100		Supernatant usually xanthochromic

*Characteristic abnormalities in italics.
[†]Mostly lymphocytes.
[‡]Mostly polymorphonuclear cells.
[§]In carcinomatous meningitis, the CSF profile is similar to fungal meningitis but malignant cells may be detected.
[‖]About 40% of neurosyphilis cases have a false-negative VDRL CSF test (see Chapter 7).
[¶]White and red cells are in same proportion as in blood (1:1,000).

transtentorial herniation (see Fig. 19–3). Moreover, a CSF examination would not be helpful in diagnosing most mass lesions, such as brain tumors, strokes, subdural hematomas, and toxoplasmosis abscesses, because their CSF profiles are not distinctive. Unless neurologists suspect acute bacterial meningitis or subarachnoid hemorrhage, in which case rapid diagnosis is crucial, they usually do not perform an LP or they postpone it until after computed tomography (CT) or magnetic resonance imaging (MRI) excludes an intracranial lesion.

COMPUTED TOMOGRAPHY

CT generates images using beams of ionizing radiation. It displays the brain, skull, other tissues, and various abnormalities along a black-to-white scale. The normal brain's image is adjusted to gray. Structures that are increasingly *more* radiodense than brain—tumors, blood, bone, and calcifications—are increasingly closer to white. Structures that are increasingly *less* radiodense than the brain, particularly the ventricles, which are filled with CSF, are increasingly closer to black. Common lesions that are virtually black are cerebral infarctions, chronic subdural hematomas, cystic lesions, and edema surrounding tumors.

When iodine-containing contrast solutions are administered intravenously, blood-filled structures become more radiodense and thus more white. This phenomenon, *contrast enhancement*, highlights vascular structures, such as arteriovenous malformations (AVMs), glioblastomas, and the membranes around chronic subdural hematomas.

Ionizing radiation from a CT is slightly greater than from a conventional x-ray skull series. Even though that dose is still relatively small and confined to the head, CTs should be avoided in pregnant women. In addition, because the contrast solution can provoke a reaction in individuals who are allergic to iodine-containing substances, including shellfish, contrast solutions should be selectively administered. Nevertheless, risks of CTs are minimal compared to their benefits.

CTs are usually indispensable, cost-effective, and reliable. Neurologists even concede that in many situations CTs, and certainly MRIs, are more reliable than their neurologic examination.

CTs are routinely performed for common neurologic conditions, including dementia, delirium, aphasia, other neuropsychologic deficits, headaches in elderly individuals, and partial seizures (Figs. 20–1 to 20–12). On the other hand, they are not indicated in sleep disturbances, absence (petit mal) seizures, cluster and migraine headaches, Parkinson's disease, tics, essential tremor, or diseases of the peripheral nervous system.

Text continues on page 542

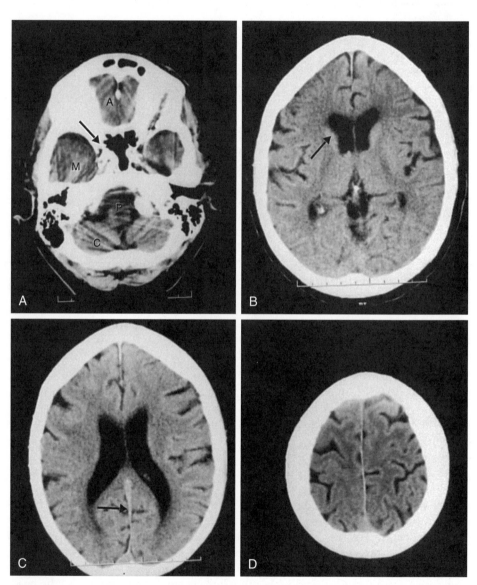

FIGURE 20–1. Four representative, progressively higher *transaxial (axial)* view CTs of a normal brain. **A,** The anterior fossae *(A)* contain the anterior frontal lobes and the olfactory nerves. The middle fossae *(M)* contain the anterior temporal lobes, which are situated behind the sphenoid wing *(arrow)*. The posterior fossa contains the cerebellum *(C)* and the medulla and pons *(P)*, which are called the bulb. The black streaks that seem to cut across the posterior fossa are artifacts from the skull. **B,** The heads of the caudate nuclei *(arrow)* indent the anterior horns of the lateral ventricles. **C,** The lateral ventricles, spread lengthwise in the hemispheres, are separated by the white, straight sagittal sinus *(arrow)*. **D,** The cerebral cortex is adjacent to the inner table of the skull. The normal gyri are separated by thin sulci.

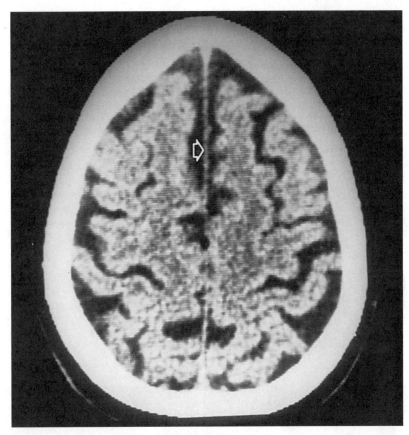

FIGURE 20–2. This CT shows cerebral atrophy (see Fig. 20–16 for MRI appearance of cerebral atrophy). The gyri are thin, and the sulci are wide. Because of the atrophy, the cerebral cortex is retracted from the inner table of the skull and from the sagittal sinus *(open arrowhead)*. Cerebral atrophy, as pictured in this CT, is a normal concomitant of old age and not necessarily associated with intellectual deterioration. However, it is closely associated with Alzheimer's disease, trisomy 21, AIDS-dementia, alcoholism, cocaine abuse, neurodegenerative illnesses, and treatment-resistant schizophrenia.

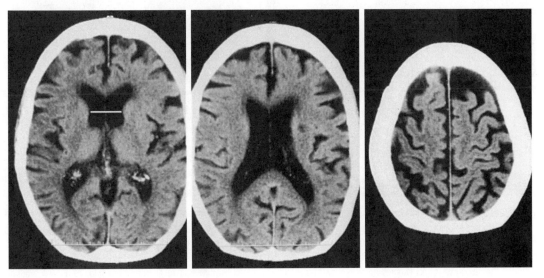

FIGURE 20–3. These three progressively higher CTs (left to right) show cerebral atrophy. The cerebral atrophy has led to expansion of the lateral ventricles and widening of the third ventricle *(line)*—hydrocephalus ex vacuo or an increased ventricular-brain ratio.

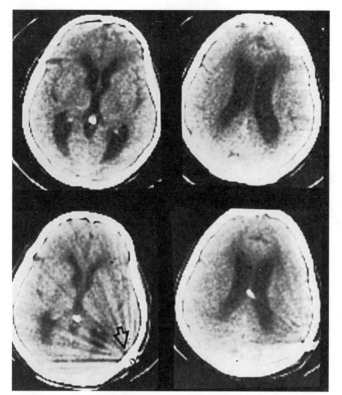

FIGURE 20–4. *Top two scans,* In normal pressure hydrocephalus (NPH), these CTs show widening of the third and lateral ventricles (see Fig. 20–15 for MRI of NPH) but little or no cerebral atrophy. *Bottom two scans,* After a shunt *(open arrow)* has been inserted into the lateral ventricles, their size has decreased. Linear artifacts emanate from the shunt. Distinctions between NPH and hydrocephalus ex vacuo, based exclusively on CT and MRI, are unreliable.

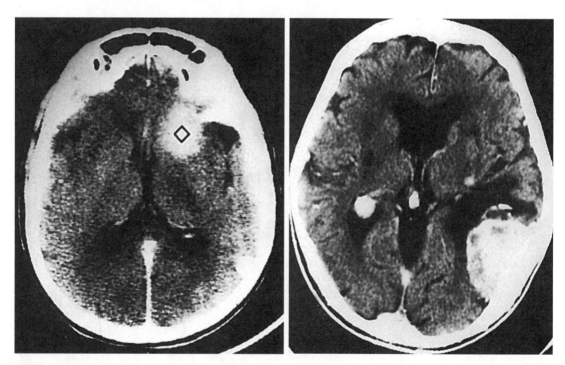

FIGURE 20–5. *Left,* This CT shows a rounded radiodense lesion *(diamond),* typical of a meningioma, arising from the right sphenoid wing. These lesions can irritate the adjacent temporal lobe and trigger partial complex seizures. They can also grow anteriorly and compress the frontal lobe and the olfactory (first cranial) nerve, that is, cause the Foster-Kennedy syndrome (see Chapter 4). *Right,* This CT shows a large radiodense meningioma that exerts relatively little mass effect on the underlying parietal lobe and its portion of the lateral ventricle. Meningiomas, in contrast to glioblastomas (Fig. 20–6A), large infarctions (Fig. 20–8A), and subdural hematomas (Fig. 20–11), develop slowly and thus may not produce symptoms until they are large. In addition, small meningiomas, which are common, do not produce any symptoms. Because meningiomas are composed of radiodense calcium and contain virtually no water, they are one of the few lesions that are more readily visualized on CT than MRI.

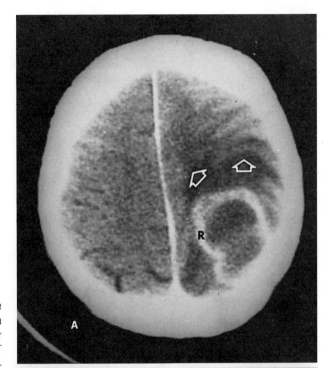

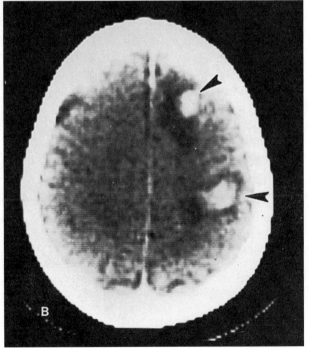

FIGURE 20–6. **A,** This CT of a glioblastoma shows the characteristic white, contrast-enhanced ring *(R)* with a black border of edema *(open arrows)*. (See Fig. 20–19 for an MRI of a glioblastoma.) **B,** This contrast-enhanced CT shows two metastatic tumors *(arrows)* in the right cerebral hemisphere. Each tumor is radiodense, relatively solid, and surrounded by edema. Distinguishing between a glioblastoma and a single metastatic lesion is often difficult.

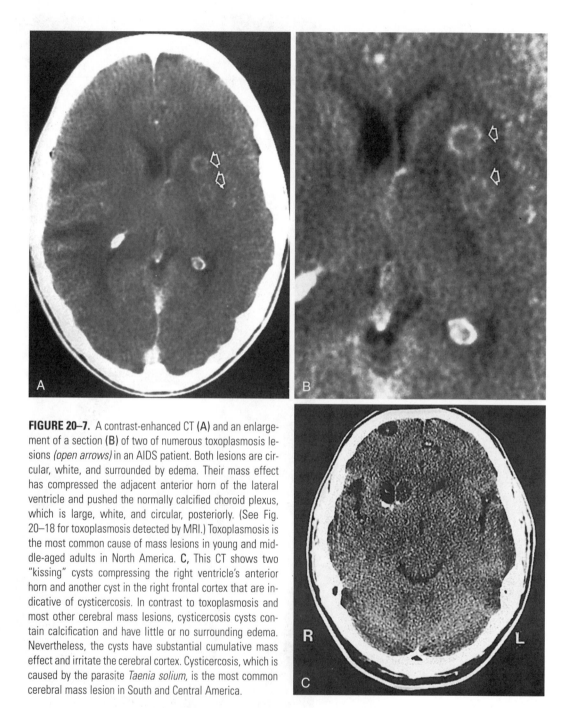

FIGURE 20–7. A contrast-enhanced CT (**A**) and an enlargement of a section (**B**) of two of numerous toxoplasmosis lesions *(open arrows)* in an AIDS patient. Both lesions are circular, white, and surrounded by edema. Their mass effect has compressed the adjacent anterior horn of the lateral ventricle and pushed the normally calcified choroid plexus, which is large, white, and circular, posteriorly. (See Fig. 20–18 for toxoplasmosis detected by MRI.) Toxoplasmosis is the most common cause of mass lesions in young and middle-aged adults in North America. **C,** This CT shows two "kissing" cysts compressing the right ventricle's anterior horn and another cyst in the right frontal cortex that are indicative of cysticercosis. In contrast to toxoplasmosis and most other cerebral mass lesions, cysticercosis cysts contain calcification and have little or no surrounding edema. Nevertheless, the cysts have substantial cumulative mass effect and irritate the cerebral cortex. Cysticercosis, which is caused by the parasite *Taenia solium,* is the most common cerebral mass lesion in South and Central America.

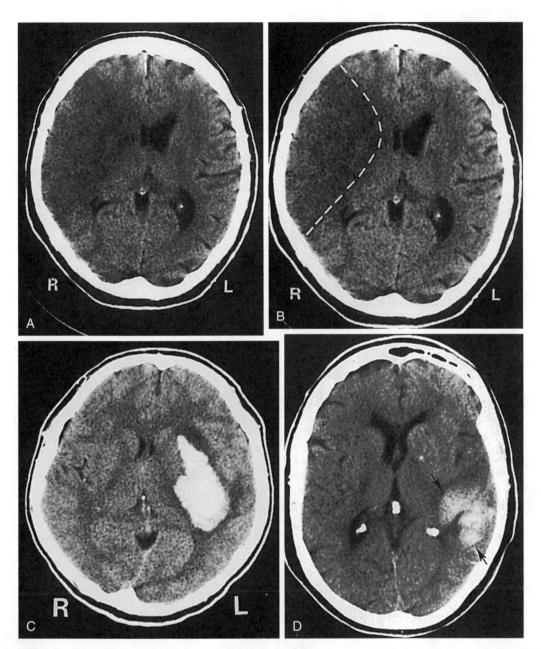

FIGURE 20–8. **A,** CTs and MRIs, by convention, display the brain with the sides reversed: look for the "R" and "L" markings. This CT shows an acute stroke from occlusion of the *right* middle cerebral artery. The stroke is darker (more hypodense) than the adjacent normal brain because it is deprived of blood, which is normally radiodense. In addition, the stroke's mass effect compresses the adjacent lateral ventricle and shifts midline structures. **B,** The stroke is outlined. Its pie-shaped area includes the lateral portion of the right cerebral hemisphere, which contains the origin of the corticospinal tract for the left face and arm. **C,** This CT shows a cerebral hemorrhage that originated in the left thalamus and extended into the lateral ventricle. The blood, denser than the brain, is seen as a white plume. **D,** This CT shows a left-sided parietal cerebral hemorrhage *(arrows)* that obliterates the occipital horn of the left lateral ventricle. The three small white areas are the normally calcified choroid plexus of the third and lateral ventricles.

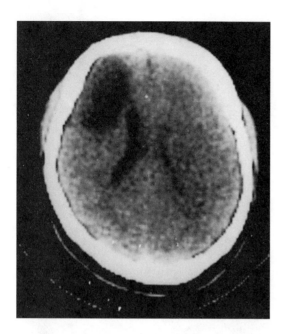

FIGURE 20–9. This CT shows a frontal lobe porencephaly, which usually represents the congenital absence of brain tissue. This porencephaly is the oval region filled with CSF. The lesion has the opposite effect of a mass lesion. The adjacent lateral ventricle and midline structures shift toward it.

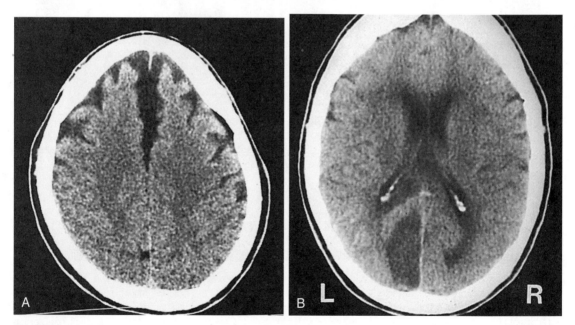

FIGURE 20–10. **A,** Frontal lobe atrophy has retracted the frontal lobes from each other and from the inner table of the skull. Other views, which are not shown, reveal temporal lobe atrophy but normal size parietal lobes. Frontal and temporal lobe atrophy is indicative of frontotemporal dementia (see Chapter 7). **B,** This CT of a patient with alexia without agraphia (see Fig. 8–4) shows a left occipital lobe stroke produced by a left posterior cerebral artery thrombosis. The stroke also included the adjacent posterior corpus callosum (not pictured).

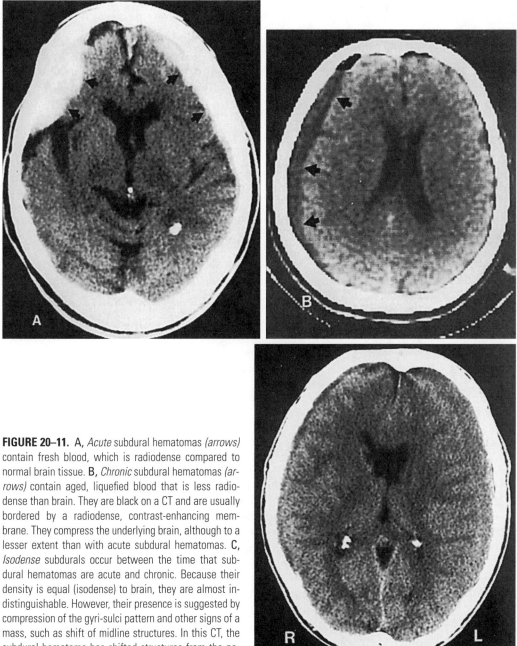

FIGURE 20–11. A, *Acute* subdural hematomas *(arrows)* contain fresh blood, which is radiodense compared to normal brain tissue. B, *Chronic* subdural hematomas *(arrows)* contain aged, liquefied blood that is less radiodense than brain. They are black on a CT and are usually bordered by a radiodense, contrast-enhancing membrane. They compress the underlying brain, although to a lesser extent than with acute subdural hematomas. C, *Isodense* subdurals occur between the time that subdural hematomas are acute and chronic. Because their density is equal (isodense) to brain, they are almost indistinguishable. However, their presence is suggested by compression of the gyri-sulci pattern and other signs of a mass, such as shift of midline structures. In this CT, the subdural hematoma has shifted structures from the patient's left to right.

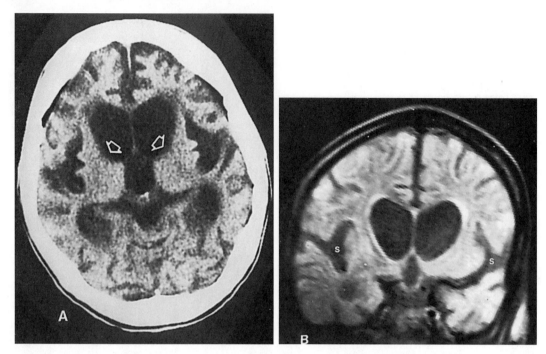

FIGURE 20–12. **A,** This CT shows the characteristic abnormality of Huntington's disease: the anterior horns of the lateral ventricles are convex because of atrophy of the caudate nuclei *(arrows).* Contrast that convex shape of the ventricles in Huntington's disease to the concave shape seen in normal individuals (Fig. 20–1*B*) and in those with hydrocephalus ex vacuo (Fig. 20–3). Huntington's disease, like many other illnesses, is associated with atrophy. The cortex is atrophied, sulci are copious, and ventricles are massively enlarged. **B,** This *coronal* view of the MRI of the same patient also shows the convex expansion of the ventricles, gigantic sulci, and sylvian fissures *(S),* as well as cerebral atrophy. Compare this scan to the coronal view of the normal brain (Fig. 20–13*B*). These MRI changes may be dramatic, but they occur long after the disease can be diagnosed on clinical grounds. Positron emission tomography in Huntington's disease may show changes earlier than the CT or MRI.

Specific criteria are still not yet established for ordering a CT or MRI for individuals who seem to have psychiatric illness. Nevertheless, their use has become commonplace for patients who have a first episode of psychosis, atypical psychosis, depression after age 50, profound depression at any age, episodic behavioral disturbances, and, in some cases, anorexia. These studies can exclude structural lesions that could account for those psychiatric symptoms. Nevertheless, relationships remain poorly defined between psychiatric symptoms and cerebral atrophy, small cerebral lesions, and congenital abnormalities.

The most consistent correlation between CT and MRI abnormalities and psychiatric illness has been shown by several studies: about 20% of chronic schizophrenic patients, compared to those with affective disorders and to control groups, have large CSF-filled lateral ventricles and small brain volume. The hydrocephalus, also called the "increased ventricular-brain ratio," is most pronounced in the temporal horns of the lateral ventricles. A large third ventricle and wide cerebral cortical sulci usually accompany the large lateral ventricles. The abnormal ventricular enlargement occurs predominantly in schizophrenic patients with severe illness, a history of perinatal complications, preponderance of negative symptoms (in most studies), greater resistance to neuroleptics, more cognitive impairments, and worse outcomes. The enlargement is not attributable to age, neuroleptic use, or electroshock therapy.

Some studies found a decreased volume of the amygdala and hippocampus (the temporal lobe components of the limbic system) in schizophrenic patients. Some children with autism have the loss of cerebral asymmetry, other dominant hemisphere abnormalities, and also relatively small cerebellar hemispheres; however, these cerebral abnormalities have been found inconsistently and were present mostly in children who also had mental retardation or congenital physical neurologic impairments.

MAGNETIC RESONANCE IMAGING

To perform an MRI, patients are placed in a strong magnet that forces protons' spin axis to be parallel with the magnetic field. Radiofrequency (RF) pulses are then applied to orient the protons' axes in the same direction. After each RF pulse, the protons resume their previous alignment ("relax") within the magnetic field and thereby emit energy. The energy forms a readily detected signal that is characteristic for the tissue. Changing relaxation times and other parameters highlight different tissues.

In the brain, the signal is emitted mostly from hydrogen nuclei (protons) in water-containing tissue. The differences in water content of the various tissues result in signals of different intensity. Sophisticated software converts these signals into images (the scans).

MRIs offer several advantages over CTs (Table 20–2). Although no physician should be a slave to photographs, the MRIs permit extraordinarily accurate diagnoses. At the least, they can offer assurance that structural lesions are not present. They display neuroanatomy in extraordinary resolution and allow physicians to see minute objects, such as the acoustic and optic nerves and the red nucleus. By manipulations of the software, rather than by having to contort the patient, MRI can view the brain from different perspectives, as well as from the three major planes: transaxial (the conventional top-down view), coronal (front-to-back view), and sagittal (side view).

Another advantage of MRI is that because most of the skull is comprised of cortical bone, which contains no water, images of the brain are free of interference from the skull (beam hardening artifact). Thus, MRI can generate detailed images of the cerebellum and other posterior fossa contents, pituitary gland, spinal cord, eyes, and other structures that are shielded from ionizing radiation by bony casings (Fig. 20–13). On the other hand, MRI may not detect lesions with little or no water content, such as some meningiomas and skull fractures.

TABLE 20–2. *Advantages of MRI over CT*

Greater imaging ability
    MRI has greater resolution: can detect smaller objects
    Distinguishes white from gray matter
    Routinely displays images in three planes: coronal, axial, sagittal
No distortion from bone
    Can display posterior fossa structures, pituitary gland, and optic nerves
    Can image the spinal cord
Does not utilize ionizing radiation
Can be applied to intra- and extracranial arteries
Can indicate certain conditions
    White matter plaques of MS and PML*
    Mesial temporal sclerosis, AVMs, and small gliomas[†]

*Progressive multifocal leukoencephalopathy.
[†]Common findings in partial complex seizures.

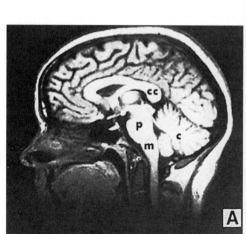
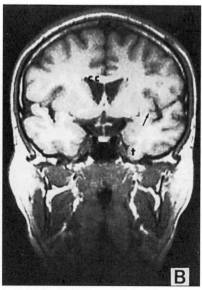

FIGURE 20–13. A, An MRI *sagittal* view of a normal brain reveals exquisitely detailed cerebral gyri and sulci, the corpus callosum *(cc)*, and the three main structures of the posterior fossa, the pons *(p)*, medulla *(m)*, and cerebellum *(c)*. In addition, it shows the cervical-medullary junction and various nonneurologic soft tissue structures. **B,** The *coronal* view reveals the corpus callosum *(cc)*, which is the "great commissure" that bridges the cerebral hemispheres. The white matter of the corpus callosum and subcortical cerebral hemispheres is distinct from the ribbon of gray matter, which constitutes the cerebral cortex. The anterior horns of the lateral ventricles, with their concave lateral borders, are beneath the corpus callosum and medial to the caudate nuclei (see Figs. 7–6 and 18–1*A*). The cerebral cortex around the left sylvian fissure *(arrow)*, including the planum temporale, is usually more convoluted than that around the right. The convolutions confer greater cortical area for language function on the dominant hemisphere. The frontal lobe is above the sylvian fissure, and the temporal lobe is below. The medial-inferior surface of the temporal lobe *(t)*, which is the origin of most partial complex seizures, is sequestered by the bulk of the temporal lobe above and the sphenoid wing anteriorly. It is far from the sites of conventional scalp electroencephalogram (EEG) electrodes.

Administration of "paramagnetic" contrast solutions, such as gadopentetate (gadolinium), can enhance intracranial abnormalities by altering the time for protons to resume their natural alignment. Although they do not cross the intact blood-brain barrier, they highlight lesions that disrupt the barrier, such as neoplasms, abscesses, active MS plaques, and acute infarctions.

In addition to detecting small intracranial and intraspinal structures, MRI can assist the diagnosis of illnesses that alter the composition of the brain tissue (Figs. 20–14 to 20–22). For example, MRI can reveal the white matter changes of MS and progressive multifocal leukoencephalopathy (PML).

With advanced equipment and software, MRI can generate images of the intracranial and extracranial cerebral vessels. This technique, magnetic resonance angiography (MRA), is most useful when it displays highly accurate images of the carotid and vertebral arteries (see Fig. 11–2). In many cases, MRA eliminates the need for conventional carotid arteriography before carotid endarterectomy, which carries considerable risk and usually requires hospitalization.

The remarkable sensitivity of MRI has led to a new technique, *functional MRI (fMRI)*, which displays metabolic activity as well as anatomy, at least grossly. fMRI exploits the small increase in blood flow and oxygenation during cerebral activity. It can highlight areas of the brain receiving sensory stimuli, initiating physical activity, imagining sensory or physical experiences, and performing cognitive processes. For example, it can detect the location of the language circuits in patients who are

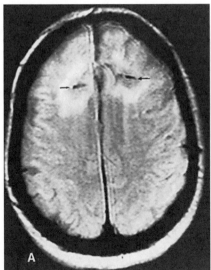
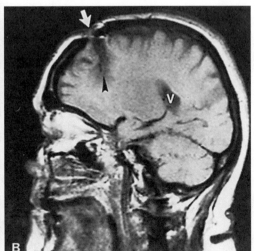

FIGURE 20–14. This MRI was performed on a patient who had undergone a frontal lobotomy. As in this case, the procedure did not involve removing the frontal lobes but drilling a hole through the skull above each frontal lobe and passing a sharp instrument through the brain immediately anterior to the motor cortex. The surgeon would attempt to sever the white matter tracts that are connections to the anterior frontal lobe; however, the incision would usually only interrupt the superior connections. **A,** The axial view shows black horizontal slits, the incisions *(arrows)*, which are surrounded by scar tissue. **B,** The sagittal view, which is through the right cerebral hemisphere, shows the skull defect *(white arrow)* and the lowermost extent of the incision *(black arrow)*, which is only about halfway down through the frontal lobe. The frontal lobe anterior to the incision is atrophied. The radiolucent area in the posterior cerebrum *(V)* is the posterior portion of the lateral ventricle.

FIGURE 20–15. This MRI shows a coronal view of the brain of a patient with normal pressure hydrocephalus. It demonstrates the classic findings: dilation of the lateral ventricles, their temporal horns *(black arrows)*, and the third ventricle *(open arrow)* but no cerebral atrophy.

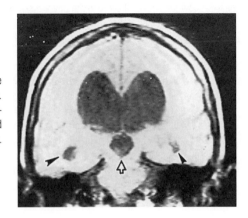

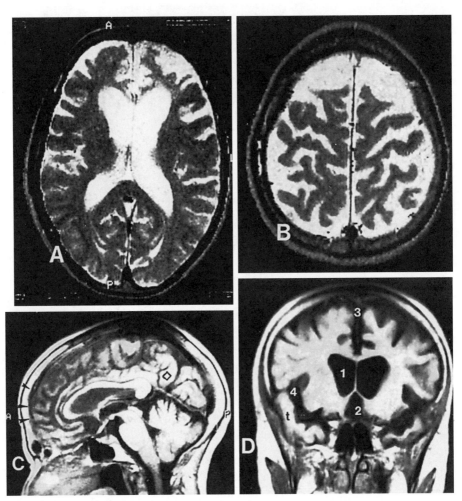

FIGURE 20–16. These MRI show four views of cerebral atrophy, which can be contrasted to the normal brain (Fig. 20–13). MRI emphasizes cerebral atrophy because it does not detect the cortical bone of the skull, which contains virtually no water. The scalp is visualized because it contains blood, fat, and other soft tissues that contain water. **A,** In an axial view through the cerebral hemispheres, the CSF is white and fills the dilated lateral ventricles and sulci. Because the frontal lobe gyri are more atrophied than those of the other lobes, the CSF fills the frontal sulci and the anterior interhemispheric fissure. **B,** In a higher axial view, the surface of the brain has thin gyri. To fill the void left by the atrophied brain, copious amounts of CSF fill the sulci and cover the cortex. **C,** In a sagittal view, where the MRI is programmed not to detect a signal from CSF, it shows thin, ribbonlike frontal lobe gyri *(arrowheads)* and the less atrophied parietal lobe gyri *(diamond)*. The corpus callosum, pons, and cerebellum are easily visualized. The tentorium, which is seen as a straight line, is above the cerebellum. **D,** As seen in this coronal view through the frontal lobes, the typical manifestations of cerebral atrophy include (1) dilated lateral ventricles, (2) an enlarged third ventricle, (3) enlargement of the anterior interhemispheric fissure because of separation of the medial surfaces of the frontal lobes, and (4) dilated sylvian fissures with the atrophic temporal lobe *(t)* below and the atrophic frontal lobe above.

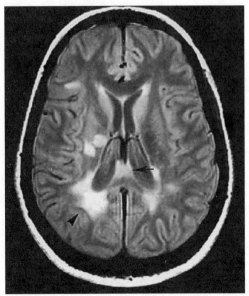

FIGURE 20–17. This MRI shows multiple cerebral plaques in a patient with MS. The lesions are typically high signal *(white)* and clustered in the white matter deep in the cerebral hemispheres, particularly in the periventricular regions. A large plaque is situated in the occipital lobe, posterior to the lateral ventricle *(arrowhead).* Another is in the posterior corpus callosum *(arrow).* Others are adjacent to the ventricle in the middle and frontal lobe on the same side.

epilepsy surgery candidates. It may replace the Wada test, which is invasive (see Chapter 8). However, persistent differences in methods and difficulty interpreting data have prevented fMRI from becoming a clinically standard test in psychiatric diagnosis. Nevertheless, some fMRI studies have revealed neurologic disturbances that were not apparent on conventional MRI studies.

Despite its greater resolution, MRI is no more effective than CT in diagnosing several major illnesses, such as Alzheimer's disease and AIDS-dementia complex. Moreover, it has some disadvantages (Table 20–3). One problem is that for 30 to 40 minutes, patients are placed entirely within the bore of the magnet, an intimidating long, narrow tunnel, with an diameter only slightly wider than their body. Even excluding individuals known to be claustrophobic, at least 10% of patients, sometimes in utter panic, will abort the procedure. Taking a benzodiazepine or wearing a sleep mask helps many anxious patients remain in the MRI tunnel.

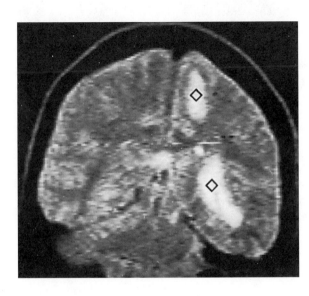

FIGURE 20–18. This MRI of a 21-year-old AIDS patient shows a coronal view of two toxoplasmosis lesions with surrounding edema *(diamonds).* Although MRI is more capable than CT in detecting small and multiple toxoplasmosis lesions, CT is better able to portray their characteristic ringlike structure (see Fig. 20–7). Neurologists often use two additional diagnostic tests before subjecting the patient to a cerebral biopsy: they give the patient a therapeutic trial of antitoxoplasmosis medicines and they obtain single photon emission computed tomography (SPECT).

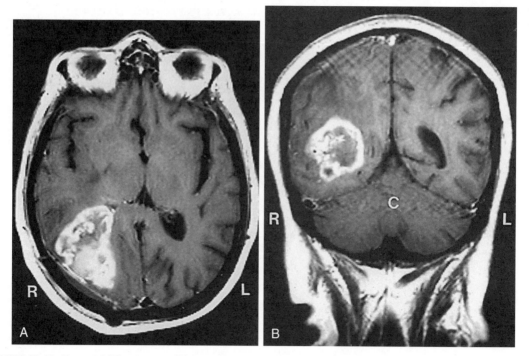

FIGURE 20–19. Transaxial (A) and coronal (B) projections of an MRI show a large, lobulated hyperintense, right-sided, posterior parietal lesion. Its mass effect has compressed the occipital horn of the lateral ventricle and shifted structures to the patient's left side. The coronal view shows the cerebellum (C). The lesion's appearance suggests a glioblastoma.

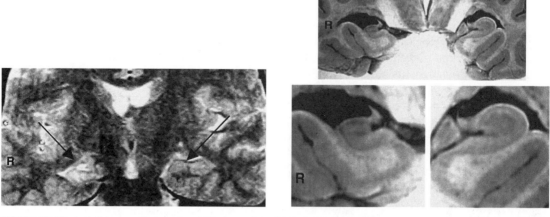

FIGURE 20–20. *Left,* This coronal view of an MRI shows right-sided mesial temporal sclerosis, which consists of shrinkage and scarring of the hippocampus and the underlying amygdala. Comparing the medial temporal lobes *(arrows)*, the patient's left-sided medial temporal lobe is round and broad but the right-sided one is contracted and poorly demarcated. Moreover, because of sclerosis, it emits a brighter *(white)* signal.

Right, The histologic specimen of the brain, at approximately the comparable section as the MRI, shows that the patient's left medial temporal lobe is normally round and has a demarcated cortex. In the enlarged sections *(below),* the patient's left medial temporal lobe appears as a duck's head facing medially. The normally rounded temporal horn of the left lateral ventricle overlies the temporal lobe. In contrast, the patient's right-sided medial temporal lobe is shrunken and contracted inferiorly and laterally. The overlying ventricle is much larger than its counterpart because the temporal lobe atrophy allowed it to expand. Most patients with partial complex seizures have mesial temporal sclerosis. It may be responsible for personality changes and memory impairments, as well as epilepsy.

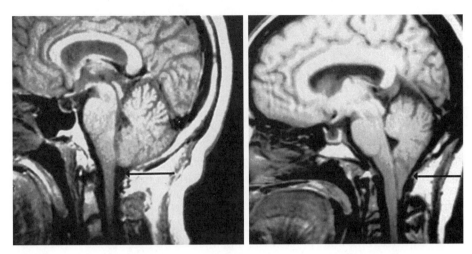

FIGURE 20–21. *Left,* In this sagittal view of the normal neuroanatomy, the cerebellum and medulla sit above the foramen magnum *(arrow).* MRI, but not CT, can display such exquisite detail in the necessary projection. *Right,* In the Arnold-Chiari malformation, the cerebellar tonsils and the medulla are located below the foramen magnum *(arrow),* as though they were pulled downward. The malformation has also caused aqueductal stenosis that will lead to hydrocephalus (not seen).

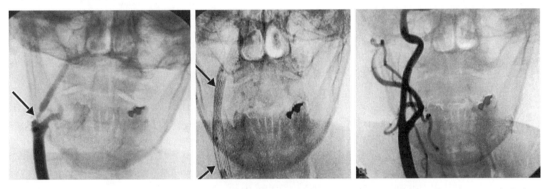

FIGURE 20–22. These studies show correction of right-sided carotid stenosis by insertion and expansion of a stent. *Left,* An angiogram shows the common carotid artery ascending and dividing into the external and internal carotid artery, which has a severe stenosis *(arrow).* *Middle,* The stent *(arrows)* has been inserted and expanded. *Right,* A follow-up angiogram shows a fully patent and smooth internal carotid artery.

TABLE 20–3. *Disadvantages of MRI over CT*

Cost is approximately two to three times greater than CT
Requires about 40 minutes, more than twice as long as CT

Being in the magnet often precipitates a claustrophobic reaction

Ferrous metal devices cannot be placed near the MRI magnet
    Patients cannot have a pacemaker, old intracranial aneurysm clips, cochlear implants, or many other implanted ferrous metal devices
    Respirators and most other life-support machinery, unless specially designed, cannot be near the magnet

CT can rapidly and easily detect acute hemorrhage from acute intracranial hematomas, subdural hematomas, and subarachnoid hemorrhage. CT is better than MRI as a screening procedure for head trauma and subarachnoid hemorrhage. Because it can be performed rapidly, CT is more suitable for patients unable to cooperate with the MRI process.

A potentially life-threatening problem with MRI is that ferrous metals are attracted or ruined by the MRI magnet. Pacemakers, implanted hearing devices, intracranial aneurysm clips, and other medical devices might be dislodged or destroyed if the patient were exposed to the intense magnetic field of an MRI study.

POSITRON EMISSION TOMOGRAPHY

In contrast to CT and MRI, which can provide exquisitely detailed images of the CNS, *positron emission tomography (PET)* provides a rough picture of the brain's metabolic activity, chemistry, and physiology. PET is based on positron-emitting, biologically active radioisotopes *(radioligands)* that must be produced in cyclotrons and incorporated into organic molecules. The radioligands, which are inhaled or injected intravenously, are metabolized in the brain and release positrons. When the positrons collide with electrons, both particles are annihilated and their masses are converted into energy. The reaction of one positron and one electron produces two photons, which are detected and transformed into images.

Most studies measure the metabolism of fluorine-18 labeled fluorodeoxyglucose (FDG), which is absorbed into the brain and metabolized as though it were glucose. Positron emission from FDG reflects the rate of cerebral glucose metabolism. Metabolism of oxygen-15 labeled water reflects cerebral blood flow. Metabolism of fluorine-18 labeled fluorodopa parallels dopamine metabolism.

Radioligands for serotonin, gamma-aminobutyric acid (GABA), and acetylcholine (ACh) permit visualization of the distribution and activity of their receptors. All these radioligands have a brief half-life. For example, oxygen-15 has a half-life of 2 minutes, and fluorine-18 less than 2 hours.

PET has been used to analyze cerebral metabolism during normal activities, administration of medications, and several illnesses. PET images have shown that in partial complex epilepsy, the affected temporal lobe is generally hypoactive in the interictal period but hyperactive during seizures. Deciding which temporal lobe is epileptogenic by this method, which is complementary to electroencephalography, is one method of determining whether temporal lobectomy would benefit a patient with intractable epilepsy (see Chapter 10).

PET is helpful in studying Parkinson's and Huntington's diseases, where PET abnormalities can appear before clinical signs or MRI abnormalities. PET studies have followed basal ganglia changes in individuals exposed to methyl-phenyl-tetrahydropyridine (MPTP) before and after they developed in parkinsonism. They can also display the progress of transplanted cells (see Chapter 18).

In Alzheimer's disease, PET shows decreased cerebral metabolism, especially in the parietal and frontal lobes' association areas. In vascular dementia, in contrast, PET studies show multiple, random areas of decreased metabolism. They are also helpful in distinguishing recurrent brain tumors from radiation necrosis.

PET has come to play a crucial role in investigations of epilepsy, neurodegenerative diseases, and cerebral ischemia. However, it remains prohibitively expensive and impractical for routine clinical neurologic diagnosis.

Of the various imaging techniques, PET has been the most informative in studying schizophrenia, depression, and obsessive-compulsive disorder. It has been even more helpful when its physiologic information has been combined with the spatial imaging data of fMRI. However, in these disorders, regional changes in cerebral metabolism or blood flow may be the result, not the cause, of the disorder. In addition, psychotropic medications undoubtedly induce changes.

SINGLE PHOTON EMISSION COMPUTED TOMOGRAPHY

Compared to PET, *single photon emission computed tomography (SPECT)*, while similar, is less precise, and its spatial resolution is relatively crude. On the other hand, it is simpler to operate, less expensive, and suitable for clinical studies.

SPECT uses readily available, stable radioligands, such as radioactive xenon, that do not require a cyclotron for preparation and have a relatively long half-life. The radioligands emit only a single photon, which is relatively easy to detect.

SPECT, like PET, portrays changes in cerebral function. It can map cerebral blood flow and, to a certain extent, neurotransmitter receptor activity. It can show changes in cerebral blood flow, which reflects metabolic activity, in strokes, seizures, migraine, recurrent brain tumors, and neurodegenerative diseases. It shows somewhat different patterns in dementia from Alzheimer's disease, Lewy body disease, and head injury. However, SPECT, like PET, should not be considered part of the routine evaluation of patients with dementia.

INTERVENTIONAL RADIOLOGY

In the past decade, neuroradiologists have introduced dramatic therapies for several neurologic diseases. For example, they offer MRI guided needle biopsies of cerebral and spinal lesions, which are often deep-seated or otherwise unapproachable. These biopsies are also suitable for lesions at the base of the skull and within vertebrae, which would also be accessible only to a highly invasive conventional surgical approach.

By borrowing catheter techniques, neuroradiologists have been able to approach small intracerebral vessels. They can float epoxy resins or particles into inoperable AVMs or aneurysms. Similarly, they can direct catheters to deliver chemotherapy to brain tumors.

One of the most helpful advances has been their inserting *stents,* which are essentially expandable tubes, into stenotic vessels. When properly seated, stents reestablish a near normal blood flow and recreate a blood vessel's smooth internal surface. They can expand stenotic carotid arteries and avoid the lengthy hospitalization and risks of a carotid endarterectomy. Stents can also be used in vertebral artery stenosis, which has been unapproachable by conventional vascular surgery.

REFERENCES

Atlas SW: MRI of the Brain and Spine on CD-ROM. Hagerstown, MD, Lippincott-Raven, 1998
Cummings JL: The neuroanatomy of depression. J Clin Psychiatry *54* (Suppl): 14–20, 1993
Gilman S: Imaging the brain. N Engl J Med *338:* 812–820, 1998
Krishnan KRR, Doraiswamy PM: Brain Imaging in Clinical Psychiatry. New York, Marcel Dekker, 1997
Levin JM, Ross MH, Renshaw PF: Clinical applications of functional MRI in neuropsychiatry. J Neuropsychiatry Clin Neurosci *7:* 511–522, 1995
Therapeutics and Technology Assessment Subcommittee of the American Academy of Neurology: Assessment of brain SPECT. Neurology *46:* 278–285, 1996
Turner R: Magnetic resonance imaging of brain function. Ann Neurol *35:* 637–638, 1994

Websites for Neuroimaging

American Academy of Neurology   http://www.aan.com
The Whole Brain Atlas   http://www.med.harvard.edu/AANLIB/home.html

Author's note: A Question and Answer section does not follow Chapter 20 because the information is included in other sections and in the Additional Review Questions section.

21

Neurotransmitters and Drug Abuse

This chapter recapitulates and expands information, introduced in previous chapters, about neurotransmitters' metabolism, anatomic pathways, receptors, and altered activity in various neurologic disorders. With a few necessary exceptions, it restricts the discussion to their role in the central nervous system (CNS) diseases and does not address psychopharmacology. This chapter reviews the following neurotransmitters:

- Monoamines: dopamine, norepinephrine, epinephrine, and serotonin
- Acetylcholine
- Gamma-aminobutyric acid (GABA)—an inhibitory amino acid
- Glutamate—an excitatory amino acid
- Neuropeptides
- Nitric oxide

MONOAMINES

Dopamine

Synthesis and Metabolism

Phenylalanine $\xrightarrow{\text{phenylalanine hydroxylase}}$ Tyrosine $\xrightarrow{\text{tyrosine hydroxylase}}$
DOPA $\xrightarrow{\text{DOPA decarboxylase}}$ Dopamine

The neurotransmitter dopamine is synthesized from phenylalanine. *Tyrosine hydroxylase* is the rate-limiting enzyme in this pathway. Both endogenously produced DOPA and L-dopa, the medication for Parkinson's disease (see Fig. 18–3), undergo decarboxylation to form dopamine.

In the CNS, several processes normally terminate dopamine activity. The primary process is dopamine re-uptake into the presynaptic neuron. In addition, dopamine is metabolized by either COMT, which is mostly an extracellular enzyme, or *monoamine oxidase (MAO)*, which is mostly an intracellular enzyme.

When dopamine is metabolized, its main product is *homovanillic acid (HVA)*. The concentration of HVA in the cerebrospinal fluid (CSF) roughly corresponds to dopamine activity in the brain.

Two Parkinson's disease medications—*carbidopa* and *entacapone* (Comtan)—inactivate enzymes that metabolize L-dopa. Both act outside the CNS because they have little ability to penetrate the blood-brain barrier. They preserve systemic L-dopa and thus restrict its conversion to dopamine to the CNS (see Fig. 18–11). Giving these enzyme-inhibiting medications along with L-dopa allows smaller doses of L-dopa to be effective. In addition, they markedly reduce systemic dopamine side effects, which include nausea, vomiting, cardiac arrhythmias, and hypotension. Carbidopa (which is combined with L-dopa in Sinemet) inhibits dopa-decarboxylase outside the CNS. Entacapone (Comtan) inhibits *catechol-O-methyltransferase (COMT)*, which usually would inactivate L-dopa by converting it to 3-O-methyldopa. Most of the effect of entacapone is outside the CNS; however, small amounts penetrate the blood-brain barrier and, to a limited extent, also inhibit CNS COMT.

Selegiline (*deprenyl* [Eldepryl]) inhibits MAO-B, one of the two major forms of MAO. (MAO inhibitors used as antidepressants inhibit both MAO-A and MAO-B or only MAO-A. In contrast, selegiline, when it is used in therapeutic doses [≤10 mg], inhibits only MAO-B.) It readily penetrates the blood-brain barrier.

Anatomy.   Three dopamine "long tracts" have the greatest clinical importance in neurology:

1. The *nigrostriatal tract*, the major component of the extrapyramidal motor system, synthesizes most of the CNS dopamine. This tract projects from the substantia nigra, the crescentic pigmented nuclei in the midbrain (Fig. 21–1), to the predominantly D_2 receptors of the striatum (the caudate nucleus and putamen [see Chapter 18]).

2. The *mesolimbic tract* projects from the ventral tegmental area, which is in the inferior medial portion of the midbrain, to the amygdala and other portions of the limbic system. The receptors are predominantly D_4. This tract probably propagates the positive symptoms of psychosis. Antipsychotics reduce these symptoms by blocking dopamine's effect on limbic structure.

3. The *mesocortical tract* also projects from the ventral tegmental area but terminates in the frontal cortex. It also terminates in the cingulate and prefrontal gyrus, creating an overlap with the mesolimbic system. The mesocortical tract probably propagates some of the expression of negative symptoms of psychosis.

In addition, several short dopamine tracts have been identified. The *tubero-infundibular tract* connects the hypothalamic region with the pituitary gland. One of dopamine's functions in this tract is to suppress prolactin secretion, thus inhibiting galactorrhea. Another short tract is confined to the retina.

Outside the brain, the adrenal medulla and several other organs synthesize dopamine. In an experiment, neurosurgeons transplanted adrenal cells to the basal ganglia of Parkinson's disease patients with the reasonable hope that they would continue to produce dopamine; however, the experiment was unsuccessful because the transplanted cells did not survive.

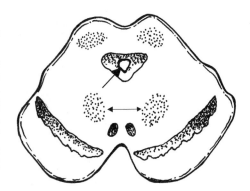

FIGURE 21–1. This sketch shows a coronal view of the midbrain (from the Greek, *meso*, middle). The midbrain gives rise to several dopamine producing tracts, including the nigrostriatal, mesolimbic, and mesocortical tracts. The nigrostriatal tract originates in the substantia nigra, the large concave semilunar black structures in the base of the midbrain (also see Fig. 18–2). Above these sit the red nuclei *(stippled oval regions, horizontal double-headed arrow)*, which receive cerebellar outflow tracts. Paired segments of the third cranial nerves are medial and inferior to the red nuclei. The upper portion of the midbrain, the tectum (from the Latin "roof," *tego*, to cover), contains the aqueduct of Sylvius *(diagonal arrow)*, which is surrounded by the periaqueductal gray matter and the superior colliculi *(stippled oval areas)*.

Receptors.   At least five dopamine receptors—D_1 through D_5—have been described. D_1 and D_2 receptors are the most important in extrapyramidal system disorders (Table 21–1). Both are found in the striatum, but D_1 receptors are more plentiful and more widely distributed. Typical antipsychotics block D_2 receptors. This blockade induces parkinsonism, raises prolactin production, and leads to tardive dyskinesia. In contrast, clozapine, which primarily blocks the D_4 receptor, exerts little or no D_2 receptor blocking effect. It does not induce parkinsonism or tardive dyskinesia. Depending on the strength of the block, these medicines are said to be "weak" or "strong" antagonists.

Conditions Due to Defects in the Dopamine Synthesis Pathway.   Several disorders result from enzyme deficiencies in dopamine's synthetic pathway. *Phenylketonuria (PKU)* results from an autosomal recessive inherited absence of the initial enzyme in the synthetic pathway, *phenylalanine hydroxylase.* Its absence results in an accumulation of phenylalanine, which is converted to phenylketones and excreted. Unless affected newborn infants are maintained on a phenylalanine-free diet, they develop mental retardation and epilepsy. Because tyrosine, a melanin precursor, cannot be synthesized, affected children lack pigment in their hair and irises, which gives them a fair complexion and eczema (see Chapter 13).

Dopamine responsive dystonia (DRD), which is a genetic deficiency in both phenylalanine hydroxylase and tyrosine hydroxylase, leads to a dopamine deficiency in children. Typically, in the afternoon, after dopamine stores have been depleted, affected children have dystonia and other abnormal involuntary movements that mimic cerebral palsy. After a night's rest, when dopamine stores are replenished, the children have no involuntary movements for several hours. The symptoms are readily corrected with relatively small amounts of L-dopa (see Chapter 18).

The classic example of dopamine deficiency remains Parkinson's disease. In its early stages, the *dopamine precursor* L-dopa corrects the dopamine deficiency (see Fig. 18–3). As long as enough nigrostriatal (presynaptic) neurons remain intact, L-dopa is converted to form sufficient quantities of dopamine. In addition, the MAO-B inhibitor, selegiline, preserves naturally occurring and medically induced dopamine by inhibiting its metabolism. When presynaptic neurons have completely degenerated and can no longer convert dopa to dopamine, dopamine's postsynaptic effects can be simulated by *dopamine agonists,* such as pramipexole (Mirapex) and ropinirole (Requip).

TABLE 21–1. *Pharmacology of D_1 and D_2 Receptors*

	D_1	D_2
Effect of stimulation on cyclic AMP production	Increased	Decreased
Greatest concentrations	Striatum, limbic system, and cerebral cortex	Striatum, substantia nigra
Effect of dopamine	Weak agonist	Strong agonist
Effects of dopamine agonists	Agonists with variable strength	Strong agonists
Effect of phenothiazines	Strong antagonists	Strong antagonists
Effect of butyrophenones	Weak antagonists	Strong antagonists
Effect of clozapine	Weak antagonist	Weak antagonist

Medication-induced parkinsonism probably results from typical antipsychotic agents' blockading the D_2 receptors. Giving L-dopa when those receptors are blocked can stimulate frontal cortex and limbic system dopamine receptors and provoke psychosis.

Conditions Due to Excessive Dopamine Activity.   Of the several mechanisms that lead to excessive dopamine activity, the most common is the dopamine precursor medication, L-dopa, pushing the synthetic pathway. Another is use of cocaine and amphetamine. These drugs provoke release of dopamine from its presynaptic storage sites and then block its re-uptake (see below). Some psychotropic medications, such as bupropion (Wellbutrin), also block dopamine's re-uptake. A different mechanism, which has been postulated to underlie some cases of tardive dyskinesia, is increased sensitivity of the postsynaptic receptors.

Whatever the cause, excessive dopamine activity often produces visual hallucinations and thought disorder that can reach psychotic proportions. Mental aberrations are commonplace in patients with Parkinson's disease who take excessive L-dopa. Another manifestation of excessive dopamine activity is hyperkinetic movement disorders, such as dystonia, chorea, and the oral-buccal-lingual variety of tardive dyskinesia. For example, individuals who have taken cocaine (see below), as well as Parkinson's disease patients taking too much L-dopa, develop chorea. With a small increase in dopamine activity, as occurs with bupropion, individuals have a sense of well-being. With greater dopamine activity, as with small doses of cocaine and amphetamine, individuals have euphoria.

Dopamine and its agonists, acting through the tubero-infundibular tract, inhibit prolactin release from the pituitary gland. Dopamine receptor blockade of the tubero-infundibular tract by typical neuroleptics and risperidone—but not clozapine or quetiapine—increases prolactin release and raises its serum concentration. In cases of pituitary adenomas, which can either secrete prolactin or stimulate other cells to secrete it, the dopamine agonist, bromocriptine, suppresses prolactin production and reduces the size of adenomas.

Norepinephrine and Epinephrine

Synthesis and Metabolism

$$\text{Dopamine} \xrightarrow{\text{dopamine } \beta\text{-hydroxylase}} \text{Norepinephrine} \xrightarrow{\text{phenylethanolamine } N\text{-methyl-transferase}} \text{Epinephrine}$$

Norepinephrine and epinephrine are synthesized through a continuation of the dopamine synthesis pathway. Along with dopamine, norepinephrine and epinephrine are classified as *catecholamines*. Tyrosine hydroxylase remains the rate-limiting enzyme in their synthesis. Their actions are terminated primarily by re-uptake and metabolism by COMT and MAO. However, most norepinephrine is metabolized outside the CNS. Its primary metabolic product, which is readily detectable in the urine, is *vanillylmandelic acid (VMA)*.

Anatomy.   The anatomy of norepinephrine and dopamine tracts differs considerably. Dopamine tracts are confined to the brain, but norepinephrine tracts project down the spinal cord, as well as within the brain. In addition, norepinephrine serves as the neurotransmitter for the sympathetic nervous system's postganglionic neurons. Norepinephrine is converted into epinephrine almost exclusively in the adrenal gland.

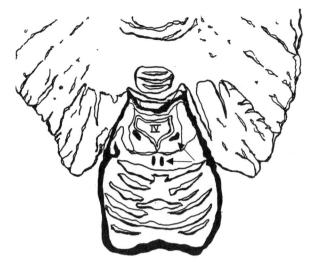

FIGURE 21–2. This sketch shows a coronal view of the pons (from the Latin *pons*, "bridge"). The pons contains the paired loci cerulei *(diagonal arrow)* and dorsal raphe nucleus *(horizontal arrow)*. The loci cerulei, which sit lateral and inferior to the fourth ventricle (IV), give rise to norepinephrine tracts. The dorsal raphe nucleus gives rise to serotonin tracts that spread to the diencephalon and cerebrum. A caudal raphe nucleus, in the pons and medulla (not pictured here), gives rise to serotonin tracts that spread to the spinal cord. The cerebellum sits above the pons.

Norepinephrine is synthesized primarily in the brain in the *locus ceruleus,* which is located in the dorsal portion of the pons (Fig. 21–2). Neurons from the locus ceruleus project to the cerebral cortex, limbic system, and reticular activating system.

Receptors.   Norepinephrine receptors are located in the cerebral cortex, brainstem, and spinal cord. The $\alpha2$ and $\beta2$ receptors, termed "autoreceptors," are situated on presynaptic neurons where they modulate norepinephrine synthesis and release (Fig. 21–3). The postsynaptic receptors are also of two types, $\alpha1$ and $\beta1$. Sympathetic nervous system receptors for norepinephrine and epinephrine produce varied and sometimes virtually opposite effects (Table 21–2).

Conditions Reflecting Changes in Norepinephrine Activity.   In Parkinson's disease, the locus ceruleus, as well as the substantia nigra, degenerates and loses its pigment. The depletion of norepinephrine neurons may lead to depression and sleep disturbances. It may also lead to orthostatic hypotension in Parkinson's disease and the related multisystem atrophies, such as the Shy-Drager syndrome (see Chapter 18).

Excessive stimulation of $\beta2$ adrenergic sites leads to tremor, bronchodilatation, and dilation of coronary, peripheral, and possibly meningeal arteries. Essential tremor's response to β-blockers suggests that it results from excessive β-adrenergic activity (see Chapter 18).

The best known example of excessive norepinephrine and epinephrine activity results from pheochromocytomas. Continually or in erratic bursts, these tumors secrete norepinephrine or epinephrine. Depending on the pattern, patients have hypertension, tachycardia, and, in a small percent of cases, convulsions.

FIGURE 21–3. In norepinephrine and epinephrine synapses, the postsynaptic neuron has the $\alpha1$ and $\beta1$ receptors. They are associated with the traditional sympathetic "flight or fight" response. The presynaptic neuron has the autoreceptors, $\alpha2$ and $\beta2$ receptors, which modulate the sympathetic response (see Table 21–2).

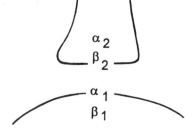

TABLE 21–2. *Pharmacology of Epinephrine and Norepinephrine Receptors*

Receptor	Effect of Stimulation	Agonists	Antagonists
α1[a]	Vasoconstriction	Phenylephrine	Phenoxybenzamine, phentolamine
α2[b]	Vasodilation, hypotension	Clonidine	Yohimbine
β1[a]	Cardiac stimulation	Dobutamine	Metoprolol
β2[b]	Bronchodilation	Isoproterenol	Propranolol

[a]Postsynaptic, see Fig. 21–3.
[b]Presynaptic, see Fig. 21–3.

Serotonin

Synthesis and Metabolism

Tryptophan

Tryptophan hydroxylase → ↓

5-Hydroxytryptophan

Amino acid decarboxylase → ↓

5-Hydroxytryptamine (5-HT, Serotonin)

MAO → ↓

5-Hydroxyindoleacetic acid (5-HIAA)

Serotonin (5-hydroxytryptamine, 5-HT), another monoamine, is an *indolamine* but not a catecholamine. Its synthesis parallels dopamine's: Hydroxylation is followed by decarboxylation. The rate-limiting enzyme in serotonin synthesis is also hydroxylation but with the enzyme tryptophan hydroxylase. In addition, availability of the substrate, tryptophan, may represent the rate-limiting factor. The actions of serotonin are also terminated by re-uptake and, to a lesser extent, by MAO metabolism.

Its primary metabolic product is 5-hydroxyindoleacetic acid (5-HIAA). Although platelets and various nonneurologic cells synthesize more than 98% of the body's *total* serotonin, CSF concentrations of HIAA reflect CNS serotonin activity. Serotonin is also metabolized to melatonin.

Anatomy.   In the brain, serotonin-producing neurons are located predominantly in the *dorsal raphe nuclei*, which are located in the midline of the dorsal midbrain and pons (Figs. 21–2 and 18–2). Their tracts project rostrally (upward) to innervate the cortex, limbic system, striatum, and cerebellum. They also innervate intracranial blood vessels, particularly those around the trigeminal nerve. Other serotonin-producing nuclei, the *caudal raphe nuclei*, are located in the midline of the lower pons and medulla. They project caudally (downward) to the dorsal horn of the spinal cord to provide analgesia (see Chapter 14).

In addition, these nuclei modulate other brainstem centers. Serotonin-producing cells are active during arousal and relatively inactive during sleep. They also modulate the "vomiting center," which is adjacent to the "chemoreceptor trigger zone," in the medulla's *area postrema*. This region is one of the few areas unprotected by the blood-brain barrier. Thus, numerous blood-borne substances, including heroin, cancer chemotherapeutic agents, and contaminated food's toxins, immediately provoke vomiting.

Receptors.   At least eight CNS serotonin receptors (5HT₁–5HT₇) and a number of subtypes have been identified. The receptors differ in their function, response to medications, effect on second-messenger systems, and capacity to be excitatory or inhibitory. Several, such as 5-HT_{1D}, are presynaptic autoreceptors that suppress serotonin synthesis or block its release. 5HT_1 promotes production of adenyl cyclase and is inhibitory. In contrast, 5HT_2 promotes production of phosphatidyl inositol and is excitatory. Other receptors are usually guanine nucleotide-binding protein (G-protein) linked and excitatory.

Several receptors are involved in headache therapy (see Chapter 9). For example, sumatriptan (Imitrex), the other "triptans," and ergotamine act primarily as agonists of 5-HT_{1D} receptors, which are located in the trigeminal nerve endings. Methysergide (Sansert) and other preventative migraine medications are 5-HT_2 antagonists.

LSD (D-lysergic acid diethylamide) probably produces hallucinations by acting as a 5-HT_2 receptor agonist. The hallucinogen "ecstasy" (methylenedioxymethamphetamine [MDMA]) is also a serotonin agonist, but it has dopaminergic activity.

A series of powerful antiemetics, including dolasetron and ondansetron, are 5HT_3 antagonists. Presumably, by affecting the area postrema, they reduce chemotherapy-induced nausea and vomiting.

Conditions Reflecting Changes in Serotonin Activity.   Depression is the most common condition associated with low serotonin activity. Antidepressants primarily affect the 5HT_{2A} receptor, although they may also affect dopamine or norepinephrine re-uptake.

In contrast, psychosis is associated with increased activity of 5HT_2 receptors. Several atypical neuroleptics have a greater affinity for 5HT_2 than D_2 receptors.

Cases of suicide by violent means are characterized by low postmortem CSF concentrations of the serotonin metabolite HIAA. This finding, which is one of the most consistent in biologic psychiatry, indicates low CNS serotonin activity. Similarly, individuals with poorly controlled violent tendencies, even those who were not depressed, have low concentrations of CSF HIAA.

Brain serotonin levels are also decreased in individuals with Parkinson's or Alzheimer's disease. In Parkinson's disease, the decrease is more pronounced in depressed patients.

Some conditions are felt to result from low serotonin activity either because a deficiency has been found in the blood, CSF, or histologic testing or because medications that enhance serotonin activity have been helpful. For example, a serotonin deficiency has been postulated to cause or perpetuate chronic pain because, in part, small doses of serotonin-enhancing antidepressants alleviate pain (see Chapter 14).

In contrast, some medications are probably effective because they are serotonin antagonists. For example, as previously noted, several antiemetics and preventative migraine medicines are serotonin antagonists.

On the other hand, serotonin antagonism can be dangerous. For example, LSD and ecstasy, which are potent serotonin antagonists, cause psychosis and hallucinations. Excessive serotonin activity is also dangerous. For example, combinations of medicines that simultaneously block serotonin re-uptake and inhibit its metabolism produce markedly elevated serotonin levels, which causes the *serotonin syndrome* (see Chapters 6 and 18).

ACETYLCHOLINE (ACh)

Synthesis and Metabolism

$$\text{Acetyl CoA} + \text{Choline} \xrightarrow{\text{choline acetyltransferase}} \text{ACh}$$

Acetylcholine (ACh) is formed by the combination of acetyl coenzyme A and choline. The rate-limiting factor is the substrate choline. The reaction also depends on the enzyme *choline acetyltransferase (ChAT)*.

Unlike the monoamines, ACh does not undergo re-uptake. Its action is terminated in the synaptic cleft by the enzyme *cholinesterase,* which hydrolyzes ACh back to acetyl coenzyme A and choline. *Anticholinesterases,* such as edrophonium (Tensilon) and physostigmine, prolong the action of ACh by inhibiting cholinesterase (see Chapter 6 and Fig. 7–5).

Anatomy.   ACh is not only one of the primary neurotransmitters in the CNS but is also one of the major neurotransmitters in the autonomic nervous system and at the neuromuscular junctions (see Fig. 6–1). In the CNS, most ACh tracts originate in the *nucleus basalis of Meynert* (also known as the *substantia innominata*) and adjacent nuclei in the *basal forebrain* (a rostral portion of the brainstem) (Fig. 21–4). These nuclei project cholinergic neurons extensively throughout the cerebral cortex but particularly to the hippocampus, amygdala, and cortical association areas.

Receptors.   Two major types of ACh receptors have been described: *nicotinic* and *muscarinic.* Neuromuscular junctions rely on nicotinic receptors. They are excitatory and can be blocked by two poisons: curare and α-bungarotoxin.

Cerebral cortex receptors are predominantly, but not exclusively, muscarinic. They can be either excitatory or inhibitory. Atropine and scopolamine block them.

Conditions Reflecting Changes in ACh Activity.   ACh activity may be altered at the neuromuscular junction by either presynaptic or postsynaptic influences. Both can lead to fatal muscle paralysis. Botulinum toxin, whether ingested as a food poison (botulism) or received as medication for focal dystonia (see Chapter 18), impairs ACh release from the presynaptic neuron. Similarly, antibodies impair the release of ACh from presynaptic neurons and cause weakness in Lambert-Eaton syndrome, which is a paraneoplastic disorder (see Chapters 6 and 19).

On the postsynaptic side of the neuromuscular junction, curare and other poisons, and antibodies, such as found in myasthenia gravis, block ACh receptors. Administering anticholinesterases, such as edrophonium and pyridostigmine (Mestinon), as in treatment of myasthenia gravis, briefly increases ACh activity enough to overcome muscle weakness.

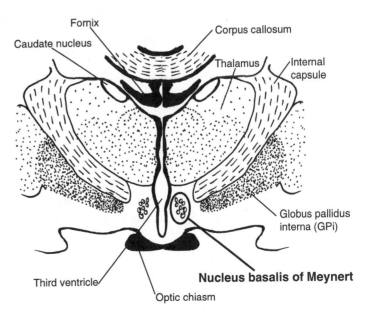

FIGURE 21–4. This coronal view of the diencephalon shows the nucleus basalis of Meynert, which is situated adjacent to the third ventricle and the hypothalamus.

In Alzheimer's disease, the cerebral cortex has markedly reduced cerebral ACh concentrations, ChAT activity, and muscarinic receptors (see Chapter 7). In addition, some nicotinic receptors are depleted. Reduced ACh concentrations are also found in trisomy 21 and Parkinson's disease. To counteract the ACh deficiency in Alzheimer's disease, neurologists have administered ACh precursors, such as choline and lecithin (phosphatidylcholine). However, the dementia did not respond. A complementary strategy has been to administer long-acting anticholinesterases that cross the blood-brain barrier. Although physostigmine does not help, tacrine tetrahydroaminoacridine [THA, Cognex] and donepezil [Aricept]) might provide benefit (see Chapter 7).

Scopolamine and other drugs that block muscarinic ACh receptors interfere with memory and learning—even in normal individuals. In particular, medicines that are specifically anticholinergic, such as those for Parkinson's disease, as well as those with merely anticholinergic side effects, can produce cognitive impairment.

Typical neuroleptics, to a greater or lesser degree, block muscarinic ACh receptors and cause anticholinergic side effects, such as accommodation paresis (see Chapter 12), confusion, drowsiness, dry mouth, urinary hesitancy, and constipation. Neuroleptics with the greatest tendency to produce anticholinergic side effects have the least tendency to produce extrapyramidal side effects, such as parkinsonism. Conversely, neuroleptics with the least anticholinergic side effects have the greatest extrapyramidal side effects.

Another experimental therapy has centered on *nerve growth factor (NGF)*. NGF is a trophic substance that promotes survival and helps maintain neurons. Because NGF may preserve or restore damaged cholinergic neurons, it is an experimental medication for several neurodegenerative conditions, including Alzheimer's disease.

GAMMA-AMINOBUTYRIC ACID (GABA)—AN INHIBITORY AMINO ACID NEUROTRANSMITTER

Synthesis and Metabolism

$$\text{Glutamate} \xrightarrow{\text{glutamate decarboxylase}} \text{GABA}$$

GABA is formed by the decarboxylation of glutamate by the enzyme *glutamate decarboxylase (GAD)*. (GAD requires vitamin B_6 [pyridoxine] as a cofactor.) The actions of GABA are terminated by re-uptake or metabolism by several enzymes. GABA and, to a lesser extent, glycine are the brain's major inhibitory neurotransmitters.

Anatomy.   Reflecting the widespread and important role of inhibition, GABA is distributed throughout the entire CNS. Its highest concentrations are in the striatum, hypothalamus, spinal cord, and temporal lobe.

Receptors.   The two GABA receptors, $GABA_A$ and $GABA_B$, are complex molecules. $GABA_A$ is more numerous and important. It has binding sites for benzodiazepines, barbiturates, alcohol, and convulsants. Flumazenil, a benzodiazepine antagonist, blocks the actions of GABA at its receptor and reverses benzodiazepine-induced sedation or stupor. It can briefly reverse hepatic encephalopathy, presumably by displacing false, benzodiazepine-like neurotransmitters from GABA receptors (see Chapter 7).

$GABA_A$ receptor activity opens chloride channels, which permits flow of negatively charged chloride ions (Cl^-) into the cell. The influx of this negative charge lowers (makes more negative) the neurons' resting potential, which is normally -70 mV. Lowering the neurons' resting potential has an inhibitory effect because it hyperpolarizes their membrane. The rapidity of this hyperpolarization has allowed GABA to be considered a "fast" neurotransmitter. In contrast, monoamines are "slow" neurotransmitters.

The GABA$_B$ receptor is a G-protein linked to calcium and potassium channels. It is also inhibitory. Baclofen (Lioresal) binds to the GABA$_B$ receptor. However, the large numbers of ligands that bind to the GABA$_A$ receptor do not bind to the GABA$_B$ receptor.

Conditions Reflecting Changes in GABA Activity. GABA deficiency, which is roughly equivalent to lack of inhibition, leads to excessive neurologic activity. Sometimes chorea and seizures may be manifestations of GABA deficiency. In Huntington's disease, GABA concentrations are decreased in the basal ganglia and CSF. Diets deficient in pyridoxine, the cofactor for GAD, impair GABA synthesis and cause seizures. Similarly, overdose of isoniazid (INH), which interferes with pyridoxine, leads to seizures. In both cases, intravenous pyridoxine aborts the seizures.

Preliminary work indicates that several antiepileptic medicines are effective, in part, because in some way they increase GABA activity. Divalproex (Depakote) increases brain GABA concentration. Tiagabine (Gabitril) inhibits GABA re-uptake. Topiramate (Topamax) enhances GABA$_A$ receptor activity. Vigabatrin (Sabril)* increases GABA concentrations by reducing GABA-transaminase. Although gabapentin (Neurontin) does not interact with GABA receptors, it is structurally related to GABA.

GLUTAMATE—AN EXCITATORY AMINO ACID NEUROTRANSMITTER

Synthesis, Metabolism, and Anatomy

$$\text{Glutamine} \xrightarrow{\text{glutaminase}} \text{Glutamate}$$

Glutamate or glutamic acid, a simple amino acid synthesized from glutamine, is one of the brain's most important excitatory neurotransmitters. Its actions are terminated mostly by re-uptake into presynaptic neurons and adjacent support cells. To a lesser extent, it undergoes nonspecific metabolism. Its tracts project throughout the brain and spinal cord.

Aspartate is another excitatory amino acid. However, its anatomy and clinical importance are not established.

Receptors. A multimolecular complex, N-methyl-D-aspartate *(NMDA)*, constitutes the major glutamate receptor. This receptor, which is modulated by the inhibitory neurotransmitter glycine, regulates the patency of a calcium channel. In its interactions with the NMDA receptor, glutamate is a fast neurotransmitter. The NMDA also has binding sites for glycine, phencyclidine (PCP), and a PCP congener, ketamine (see below).

Conditions Reflecting Changes in NMDA Activity. In contrast to its vital functions at normal levels of activity, excessive NMDA activity floods the neuron with lethal concentrations of calcium and sodium. Through this process, termed *excitotoxicity*, glutamate-NMDA interactions lead to neuron death. Excitotoxicity may be intimately involved in the pathogenesis of epilepsy, stroke, Parkinson's disease, Huntington's disease, head trauma, and, conceivably, schizophrenia.

---

*Vigabatrin is remains an investigational drug in the U.S.

Several experimental medications that block glutamate-NMDA interaction provide a "neuroprotective" effect that lessens neuron damage from strokes and other injuries. Several medications that interfere with glutamate activity help certain neurologic illnesses. For example, lamotrigine (Lamictal), which is an antiepileptic drug, and riluzole (Rilutek), which slows the progress of amyotrophic lateral sclerosis (ALS), decrease glutamate activity but may not necessarily affect the NMDA receptor. Deficient NMDA can also be deleterious. For example, PCP (see below) blocks the NMDA calcium channel.

NEUROPEPTIDES

Endorphins, enkephalins, and substance P, which are situated in the spinal cord and brain, primarily provide endogenous analgesia in response to painful stimuli (see Chapter 14). Other neuropeptides are somatostatin, cholecystokinin, and vasoactive intestinal peptide (VIP). Substance P and, to a lesser degree, other neuropeptides are depleted in Alzheimer's disease.

NITRIC OXIDE

Synthesis and Metabolism

$$\text{Arginine} + \text{Oxygen} \xrightarrow{\text{nitric oxide synthase}} \text{Nitric oxide} + \text{Citrulline}$$

Nitric oxide (NO), which is synthesized in a complex reaction, is an important neurotransmitter. It also has important roles in endothelial cells and the immunologic system.

NO should not be confused with nitrous oxide (N_2O), which is an anesthetic gas ("laughing gas"). N_2O, when inhaled daily as a form of drug abuse, results in peripheral neuropathy and spinal cord damage.

Anatomy.   NO inhibits platelet aggregation, dilates blood vessels, boosts host defenses against infections and tumors, and functions in diverse CNS roles. For a neurologic viewpoint, its main functions are in regulating cerebral blood flow and facilitating penile erections.

Receptors.   NO diffuses into cells and interacts directly with enzymes and iron-sulfur complexes; however, it has no specific membrane receptors. In the CNS, NO may have a neuroprotective effect.

Conditions Reflecting Changes in NO Activity.   The best-known role of NO is in generating erections (see Chapter 16). With sexual stimulation of the penis, parasympathetic neurons produce and release NO. NO then promotes the production of cyclic guanylate cyclase monophosphate (cGMP), which dilates the vascular system and creates an erection. Sildenafil (Viagra) slows the metabolism of cGMP and increases blood flow. The pressure generated by the increased blood flow strengthens and prolongs erections.

NEUROLOGIC ASPECTS OF DRUG ABUSE

Many neurologic aspects of drug abuse can be attributed to specific neurotransmitter abnormalities. Neurologists classify an individual's episode of drug use as "recreational" when the drug is taken in its usual route and quantity, and produces the intended results. They classify an episode as an "overdose" when it leads to exaggerated or untoward results. Overdoses are much more likely than recreational doses to lead to neurologic complications and death.

The *Diagnostic and Statistical Manual of Mental Disorders-IV (DSM-IV)* classifies the neurologic complications of the several drugs discussed below as Substance-Induced Disorders. Intoxications, according to the *DSM-IV*, can be complicated by Perceptual Disturbances, which consist of either hallucinations with preserved reality testing or special sensory illusions without underlying delirium. Depending on the drug, Substance-Induced Disorders can include such subcategories as Delirium, Psychotic Disorder, Mood Disorders, Anxiety Disorder, Sexual Dysfunction, Sleep Disorder, and Withdrawal.

Cocaine

Pharmacology.   Both cocaine and amphetamine (see below) are primarily CNS stimulants through sympathomimetic mechanisms. They block the re-uptake of dopamine, norepinephrine, and serotonin. Cocaine also provokes a discharge of dopamine from presynaptic storage vesicles and then blocks its re-uptake. The combination of the forced dopamine discharge and its blocked re-uptake greatly increase synaptic dopamine concentration. The increased synaptic dopamine concentration results mostly from blocked re-uptake. Dopamine receptors, especially D_4 mesolimbic system receptors, are overstimulated. An alternative but a less well-supported theory is that cocaine primarily enhances serotonin activity.

In addition to affecting the CNS, cocaine also blocks peripheral nerve impulses. Thus, when cocaine is applied or injected at a specific site, it produces local anesthesia.

Abusers sometimes inject cocaine, but usually they smoke the solid alkaloid form *(crack)*. When cocaine is inhaled through the nostrils (snorted), the effects are similar to crack, but the neurologic consequences are less likely to occur. Except during attempts to elude capture, cocaine users or traffickers do not swallow it; however, when they do swallow it or packets break open in their intestines, they absorb massive amounts of the drug. Routine cocaine effects may be enhanced and confounded by mixing it with alcohol or other illicit drugs.

Before being metabolized by plasma and liver cholinesterases, cocaine has a half-life of about 30 minutes to 1 hour. This relatively short half-life provides only a brief, although intense, period of intoxication. Urine toxicology screens may detect cocaine's metabolic products for about 2 days.

Clinical Effects.   The immediate effect of recreational doses of cocaine is typically euphoria accompanied by a sense of increased sexual, physical, and mental power. When using cocaine, individuals are fully alert—even hypervigilant. Their heightened awareness is a prominent exception to the general rule that patients in delirium or a toxic-metabolic encephalopathy are lethargic or stuporous and have a fluctuating level of consciousness (see Chapter 7). Routine cocaine use also produces sympathomimetic effects, such as pupillary dilation, hypertension, and tachycardia.

Stimulants reduce sleep. They particularly suppress rapid eye movement (REM) sleep, often to the extent of eliminating it. When stimulants are stopped, abusers usually have a rebound in their REM sleep (see Chapter 17).

Overdose.   With greater than their usual dose, cocaine users typically become agitated, irrational, and paranoid. They often experience delusions and hallucinations. Moreover, cocaine's sympathomimetic and dopaminergic effects may produce permanent neurologic damage.

Cocaine-induced strokes usually occur within 2 hours of cocaine use. Many such strokes are nonhemorrhagic ("bland") cerebral infarctions. However, most are cerebral hemorrhages related to cocaine-induced hypertension and underlying aneurysms. Other causes of strokelike brain damage in cocaine users are vasoconstriction, vasculitis, bacterial endocarditis, AIDS-related infections, emboli of foreign particles, and head trauma.

Cocaine-induced seizures, another complication, also occur within 2 hours after drug use. They disproportionately follow first-time cocaine use and are often fatal. Most seizures are generalized and are not associated with either an abnormal CT (computed tomogram) or interictal EEG (electroencephalogram). Seizures that are focal or followed by hemiparesis may be a manifestation of an underlying stroke.

(In contrast, seizures associated with alcohol, barbiturates, or benzodiazepines usually occur after withdrawal from chronic high-dose use. They rarely occur in the midst of an overdose. Seizures related to those substances constitute a marker of dependency. In practical terms, the development of a seizure in a young adult should prompt an investigation for drug abuse.)

Other neurologic complications from excessive cocaine use include involuntary movement disorders, such as ticlike facial movements, chorea, tremor, dystonia, and repetitive, purposeless behavior (stereotypies, see Chapter 18). When cocaine induces chorea, patients cannot stand at attention and are said to have "crack dancing." These movements are attributable to the greatly increased dopamine activity.

In addition, cocaine seems to increase sensitivity to neuroleptic-induced dystonic reactions. For example, hospitalized cocaine users, compared to other inpatients, have at least three times the incidence of dystonic reactions from neuroleptics.

The frequency, nature, and severity of cocaine-induced cognitive impairment are not established. According to some reports, individuals repeatedly using cocaine have cognitive defects that consist of impairments in attention, verbal learning, and memory. They probably result from strokelike brain damage.

Dementia has not come to be a recognized complication of cocaine use. However, CTs of habitual cocaine users show cerebral atrophy. Magnetic resonance imaging (MRI) shows demyelination, hyperintensities, and vasoconstriction. Single photon emission computed tomography (SPECT) scans show multiple patchy areas of hypoperfusion (a "Swiss cheese" pattern).

In addition to its effect on the brain, cocaine produces dangerous sympathomimetic effects. During an overdose, cocaine causes tachycardia, cardiac arrhythmias, and marked hypertension. The pupils dilate.* Cocaine users often suffer the cardiac counterpart of strokes—myocardial infarctions.

Treatment of Intoxication and Overdose.   Many behavioral and cognitive aspects of cocaine overdose are brief and respond to seclusion and the passage of time. If necessary, benzodiazepines will suppress agitation and its related symptoms. Psychosis and violent behavior will respond to dopamine-blocking neuroleptics; however, because neuroleptics, as well as cocaine itself, lower the seizure threshold, they must be used judiciously. Potentially life-threatening hypertension may require aggressive treatment with an α-blocker antihypertensive medication, such as phentolamine (Table 21–2).

Withdrawal.   When deprived of cocaine, habitual users often suddenly lose their energy and ability to appreciate their normally pleasurable activities ("crash"). They typically crave the stimulant and languish in a dysphoric mood. They develop sleep disturbances with vivid, disturbing dreams, which probably represent REM rebound.

---

*With 2% to 10% cocaine eye drops, normal pupils widely dilate because it leads to α1 stimulation.

Reflecting the lack of dopamine receptor stimulation during withdrawal, dopamine agonists and other dopamine-enhancing medications alleviate some withdrawal symptoms. Antidepressants may also help, although the mechanism is unknown.

Amphetamine

The term "amphetamine" commonly refers to dextroamphetamine (Dexedrine), methamphetamine, methylphenidate (Ritalin), and several other related substances. Like cocaine, amphetamine is sympathomimetic. Amphetamine first provokes a powerful presynaptic dopamine discharge and then blocks its re-uptake.

Amphetamine is usually taken orally but sometimes intravenously. Because the half-life of amphetamine is about 8 hours, its effects last much longer than those of cocaine.

Several amphetamines are legitimately used to treat children and adults with attention deficit hyperactivity disorder (ADHD). For example, methylphenidate (Ritalin) helps individuals with ADHD to focus their attention and ward off distractions. Paradoxically, these amphetamines, which are usually considered a stimulant, suppress physical and mental hyperactivity. One possible explanation is that they stimulate inhibitory neurons but do not affect the less sensitive excitatory neurons.

Recreational doses of amphetamines produce cocainelike effects, such as hyperalert states. Amphetamines also decrease total sleep time and suppress the proportion of rapid eye movement (REM) sleep. Although the effects of amphetamine and cocaine are similar, those of amphetamine last longer and are more apt to produce a severe sympathomimetic discharge.

Overdose. As with cocaine, the most common permanent neurologic complications are hemorrhagic and bland strokes. Although most amphetamine-induced strokes result from hypertension, some result from amphetamine-induced vasculitis. Amphetamines also cause dyskinesias and stereotypies. However, in contrast to cocaine overdose, seizures are relatively infrequent in amphetamine overdose.

During an overdose, hallucinations and thought disorders can reach psychotic proportions, which can be labeled an Amphetamine-Induced Psychotic Disorder With or Without Delusions or Hallucinations. As with chronic cocaine use, chronic amphetamine use might lead to cognitive impairment; however, evidence does not establish that it can cause dementia.

Because of their similar pharmacology, treatment of amphetamine overdose, as with cocaine overdose, relies on dopamine-blocking neuroleptics. Also, symptoms and treatment of amphetamine and cocaine withdrawal are similar.

Opioids

Pharmacology. *Opioid* is a broad term encompassing medicinal narcotics, "street" narcotics, and analgesic neurotransmitters synthesized in the CNS. It includes morphine, methadone, heroin, and endogenous opiate-like substances (see endorphins, Chapter 14). Although these opioids may affect dopamine and other neurotransmitters, their primary action is directly on several specific opioid receptors, labeled *delta, kappa,* and *mu,* in the brain and spinal cord. These receptors are G-protein linked and affect adenyl cyclase.

Several antagonists, which can successfully compete with the opioids for their receptors, prevent or reverse the effects of opioids. If these antagonists are given to someone dependent on narcotics, they may produce withdrawal symptoms. For example, the antagonist naloxone (Narcan), which is usually administered intravenously in cases of narcotic overdose, displaces opioids from their receptors and reverses many of the effects of the overdose. In addition, it can precipitate a narcotic withdrawal. Another antagonist, naltrexone (ReVia), is an oral medication used for narcotic maintenance or detoxification. It also prevents opioids from reaching their receptors and thus blocks their usual effects.

Clinical Effects.   Therapeutic opioid doses relieve pain and reduce anxiety. Higher doses, usually associated with the early stages of abuse, lead to a burst of euphoria, a sense of well-being, and then sleepiness. Sometimes they produce paradoxical agitation, psychosis, and mood changes. Intravenously administered opioids routinely lead to nausea and vomiting, which presumably result from opioids directly stimulating the medulla's chemoreceptor trigger zone. Uncomplicated intoxications usually have a duration of several hours.

Overdose.   Opioid overdose causes a characteristic triad of coma, "pin-point pupils" (miosis), and respiratory depression. The respiratory depression results from a slowed respiratory rate rather than a reduced amplitude or depth of respirations. It may reflect opioids acting on the CNS respiratory drive center, which is located adjacent to the chemoreceptor trigger zone. Opioid overdose frequently results in neurogenic pulmonary edema. An overdose can also result in cerebral hypoxia with cerebral cortex and basal ganglia damage. Compared to the complications of amphetamines or cocaine, opioid-induced vascular occlusions and cerebral hemorrhages are infrequent. Except as a manifestation of overdose-induced hypoxia, seizures rarely complicate opioid use, addiction, or withdrawal. Unlike with stimulant overdose, opioid overdose routinely leads to nerve compression from prolonged, static positioning of the body (see Table 5–1).

If an overdose leads to cerebral hypoxia, it can result in cognitive impairment. However, formal studies have failed to demonstrate cognitive impairment with chronic, well-controlled opioid use. For example, individuals on methadone maintenance programs, patients given narcotics for chronic pain, and well-known intellectuals who abused narcotics, including Sigmund Freud, have not developed cognitive decline. As a general rule, in the absence of overdose or other complication, chronic opioid use does not cause dementia.

Treatment of Overdose.   The life-threatening aspect of the overdose is the respiratory depression. While physicians establish a patent airway and support vital functions, they usually administer a narcotic antagonist, such as naloxone. During an overdose, patients are usually comatose and do not require any psychotropic medications. However, an opioid antagonist, as previously noted, may precipitate withdrawal symptoms that require psychotropic medications.

Withdrawal from Chronic Use.   Symptoms of opioid withdrawal usually consist of intense drug- or medication-seeking behavior, dysphoric mood, lacrimation, abdominal cramps, piloerection, and autonomic hyperactivity. In general, heroin withdrawal symptoms begin in several hours after the last dose and peak at 1 to 3 days. Methadone withdrawal symptoms begin after 1 to 2 days and peak at about 6 days after the last dose. Clonidine, the $\alpha2$ norepinephrine agonist, may alleviate some narcotic withdrawal symptoms.

Other Clinical Aspects.   Several apparently unrelated facts are important. Physicians, dentists, nurses, and other health care workers are particularly at risk for surreptitious opioid abuse. They are prone to abuse meperidine (Demerol) and fentanyl (Sublimaze), which are highly addictive.

Administration of a synthetic analogue of meperidine, MPTP, routinely induces parkinsonism (see Chapter 18). Phenytoin (Dilantin), which enhances methadone metabolism, can precipitate opioid withdrawal symptoms.

Compared to morphine, heroin more readily penetrates the blood-brain barrier. It does not have a specific receptor but attaches to the mu receptor and produces the same effects as other opioids. Contrary to some popular pronouncements, aside from acting rapidly, heroin holds no distinguishable advantage as a treatment for cancer patients or other individuals in pain.

Phencyclidine (PCP)

Phencyclidine (PCP) is simultaneously a central analgesic, depressant, and hallucinogen. It is usually either swallowed or smoked with marijuana or tobacco. As with cocaine, PCP blocks the re-uptake of dopamine, serotonin, and norepinephrine. In its primary mechanism of action, PCP binds to the NMDA receptor and prevents glutamate from activating it. The PCP-NMDA interaction prevents the influx of calcium that glutamate would ordinarily provoke.

In small doses, PCP causes symptoms and signs similar to alcohol intoxication, such as euphoria, dysarthria, nystagmus, and ataxia. At higher doses, it causes disorganized thinking, negativism, bizarre thinking, and visual hallucinations. These symptoms sometimes lead to violence.

Not only does PCP cause delusions, paranoia, and hallucinations (the positive symptoms of schizophrenia) but it also causes psychomotor retardation and emotional withdrawal (negative symptoms of schizophrenia). The ability of PCP to produce the full range of schizophrenia symptoms sets it apart from LSD and other psychomimetic drugs, which usually produce only the positive symptoms. PCP intoxication has thus become a laboratory model of schizophrenia.

Overdose.   PCP overdose causes combinations of muscular rigidity, vertical nystagmus (which is a characteristic), stereotypies, and a blank stare. The muscle rigidity may evolve into rhabdomyolysis and high fevers, which mimic the neuroleptic malignant syndrome (see Chapter 6). Individuals who have taken an overdose have been described as being in "coma" with their eyes open and oblivious to pain. Overdoses often cause seizures that progress to status epilepticus; however, PCP rarely causes strokes. Another important aspect of PCP overdose is that the psychotic behavior often leads to violent incidents, such as motor vehicle accidents, confrontations with police, and drowning.

Multiple exposures to PCP, according to individual reports, may produce chronic cognitive impairment characterized by memory impairment and confusion. One study found that about one-fourth of individuals who experienced a PCP-induced psychosis returned in about one year with schizophrenia. However, in general, chronic PCP use is not associated with dementia.

Treatment.   Unlike the specific antagonists for opioids, no particular medicine acts as an antagonist for PCP. Treatment usually includes seclusion, sedation with benzodiazepines for mild intoxications, and other symptomatic treatments. Patients may need muscle relaxants, such as dantrolene, to prevent rhabdomyolysis and benzodiazepines for seizures.

Ketamine

Ketamine is a legitimate general anesthetic that is frequently used in veterinary surgery. It has a chemical structure similar to PCP and also binds to the NMDA receptor but does not block dopamine re-uptake. Ketamine produces many of the same effects as PCP. However, probably because ketamine does block dopamine re-uptake, it is less likely than PCP to cause hallucinations, thought disturbances, agitation, or violence.

Marijuana

Marijuana (cannabis) is a cannabinoid that contains several psychoactive ingredients. The most potent is Δ9-THC. The cerebral cortex, basal ganglia, hippocampus, and cerebellum all contain specific Δ9-THC receptors.

Marijuana is usually smoked, but sometimes it is swallowed. It produces euphoria, and pleasantly altered perceptions, but it slows thinking and impairs judgment. Its effects usually last 1 to 3 hours, but heavy use can cause changes from 1 to 2 days. As with other drugs, marijuana reduces REM sleep.

Overdose.   Marijuana overdoses can cause severe anxiety or psychosis. Benzodiazepines or, if necessary, antipsychotic agents can control these symptoms. Unlike overdoses of other drugs of abuse, marijuana overdoses are not fatal. Moreover, they rarely if ever cause acute neurologic problems, such as seizures or strokes.

Initial reports of cerebral atrophy have been unconfirmed. As with other drugs of abuse, individual reports have linked marijuana use to permanent inattention, word fluency problems, and impaired executive functions. However, it has not been linked to dementia. For most marijuana users, cognitive impairments are either transient or mild.

Social Considerations.   Marijuana possesses several properties that have served as the springboard for attempts to legalization. It possesses mild anticonvulsant activity, reduces intraocular pressure, and suppresses chemotherapy-induced vomiting, in addition to its mood-elevating properties.

On balance, the value of its medicinal benefits is often overstated. Conventional medicines are more effective for all these purposes. For example, D_2 dopamine and $5HT_3$ serotonin antagonists are much more effective than marijuana in reducing chemotherapy-induced nausea and vomiting.

It also has some unequivocal deleterious effects. Marijuana is involved in an inordinate number of motor vehicle accidents. High doses can induce hallucinations and delusions. A related problem is that drug enforcement agencies spray toxic chemicals (herbicides) on marijuana plants to kill them. Residual herbicides, which are inhaled along with the marijuana smoke, may be harmful.

Nicotine

Nicotine affects CNS nicotinic receptors, which represent a minority of cerebral cortex cholinergic receptors. They are located in the mesolimbic dopamine pathway, where they have the capacity to provide pleasure and modulate affect.

Virtually all individuals who use nicotine obtain it from cigarettes, which, as the tobacco industry has acknowledged, are primarily a nicotine delivery system. The nicotine probably stimulates the release of mesolimbic dopamine. As with other drugs of abuse, increased dopamine activity is pleasurable; however, with cigarettes, the pleasure is often subliminal. The nicotine in cigarettes has no appreciable cognitive effect.

The main drive to chronic tobacco use is more to suppress withdrawal symptoms—anxiety, restlessness, weight gain, tremulousness, and craving—than to provide pleasure. Individuals going through withdrawal may have temporary cognitive impairment because of anxiety, poor concentration, and preoccupation with their lack of cigarettes.

During attempts to stop cigarette smoking, some withdrawal symptoms may be suppressed by substituting other nicotine delivery systems. For example nicotine chewing gum, nasal spray, and transdermal patches can provide blood nicotine concentrations equal to or greater than those from cigarettes. As an alternative or supplement, bupropion (Wellbutrin) or sustained-release bupropion (Zyban) may help because, like nicotine, these medications increase dopamine concentration in the mesolimbic system.

REFERENCES

Neurotransmitters

Ackerman MJ, Clapham DE: Ion channels—Basic science and clinical disease. N Engl J Med *336:* 1575–1586, 1997

Cooper JR, Bloom FE, Roth RH: The Biochemical Basis of Neuropharmacology. (7th ed). New York, Oxford University Press, 1996

Dawson TM, Dawson VL, Synder SH: A novel neuronal messenger molecule in brain: The free radical, nitric oxide. Ann Neurol *32:* 297–311, 1992

Doble A: The pharmacology and mechanism of action of riluzole. Neurology *47* (Suppl 4): S233–S241, 1996

Greenamyre JT, Porter RHP: Anatomy and physiology of glutamate in the CNS. Neurology *44* (Suppl): S7–S13, 1994

Lipton SA, Rosenberg PA: Excitatory amino acids as a final common pathway for neurologic disorders. N Engl J Med *330:* 613–622, 1994

Stahl SM: Essential Psychopharmacology: Neuroscientific Basis and Clinical Applications. Cambridge, Cambridge University Press, 1996

Drug Abuse

Abramowicz M (ed): Acute reactions to drugs of abuse. Med Lett *38:* 43–46, 1996

Bolla KI, McCann UD, Ricaurte GA: Memory impairment in abstinent MDMA ("ecstasy") users. Neurology *51:* 1532–1537, 1998

Burst JCM: Neurologic Aspects of Substance Abuse. Boston. Butterworth-Heinemann, 1993

Brust JCM: Substance abuse, neurology, and ideology. Arch Neurol *56:* 1528–1531, 1999

Cardoso FE, Jankovic J: Cocaine-related movement disorders. Movement Disord *8:* 175–178, 1993

Daras M, Koppel BS, Atos-Radzion E: Cocaine-induced choreoathetoid movements ("crack dancing"). Neurology *44:* 751–752, 1994

Derlet RW, Rice P, Horowitz BZ, et al: Amphetamine toxicity: Experience with 127 cases. J Emerg Med *7:* 157–161, 1989

Foley KM: Opioids: Neurologic complications of drug and alcohol abuse. Neurol Clin *11:* 503–522, 1993

Galanter M, Kleber HD: Textbook of Substance Abuse Treatment. (2nd ed). Washington, DC, American Psychiatric Press, 1999

Holland RW, Marx JA, Earnest MP, et al: Grand mal seizures temporally related to cocaine use: Clinical and diagnostic features. Ann Emerg Med *21:* 772–776, 1992

Hollister LE: Health aspects of cannabis. Pharmacol Rev *38:* 1–20, 1986

Levine SR, Burst JCM, Futrell N, et al: A comparative study of the cerebrovascular complications of cocaine: Alkaloidal versus hydrochloride—a review. Neurology *41:* 1173–1177, 1991

McCarron MM, Schulze BW, Thompson GA, et al: Acute phencyclidine intoxication: Incidence of clinical findings in 1,000 cases. Ann Emerg Med *10:* 237–242, 1981

Pascual-Leone A, Dhuna A, Anderson DC: Cerebral atrophy in habitual cocaine abusers: A planimetric study. Neurology *41:* 34–38, 1991

Pope HG, Yurgelum-Todd D: The residual cognitive effects of heavy marijuana use in college students. JAMA *275:* 521–527, 1996

Qureshi AI, Akbar MS, Czander E, et al: Crack cocaine use and stroke in young patients. Neurology *48:* 341–345, 1997

Sanchez-Ramos JR: Psychostimulants: Neurologic complications of drug and alcohol abuse. Neurol Clin *11:* 535–553, 1993

Spivey WH, Euerle B: Neurologic complications of cocaine abuse. Ann Emerg Med *19:* 1422–1428, 1990

QUESTIONS and ANSWERS: CHAPTER 21

1. Which features are characteristic of opioid administration?

a. Blocks re-uptake of dopamine into presynaptic neurons
b. Agitation
c. Hypertension
d. Slowed respiratory rate

e. Stimulation of the area postrema
f. Miosis
g. Blockade of dopamine re-uptake
h. Chorea in some cases

ANSWER: d, e, f

2. Which features are common complications of opioid administration?

a. Cerebral hemorrhage
b. Cerebral ischemia
c. Seizures
d. Radial nerve palsy
e. Tics
f. Stereotypies
g. Psychotic thinking
h. Pulmonary edema

ANSWER: b, d, h

3. Which three causes of seizures are disproportionately more common in 15- to 50-year-old individuals than in older adults?

a. Marijuana use
b. Head trauma
c. Drug and alcohol abuse
d. Sleep deprivation
e. Brain tumors
f. Strokes

ANSWER: b, c, d

4. Which substance's primary active ingredient is Δ9-THC?

a. Cocaine
b. Phencyclidine (PCP)
c. Amphetamine
d. Cannabis
e. Heroin

ANSWER: d. Cannabis is marijuana.

5. Which neurotransmitter is deficient when the patient has unilateral miosis, ptosis, and anhidrosis?

a. Acetylcholine
b. Dopamine
c. Norepinephrine
d. Serotonin

ANSWER: c. The patient has Horner's syndrome, which is a manifestation of sympathetic denervation.

6. A former heroin addict, who is being maintained on methadone, develops a seizure for which he is hospitalized and treated with phenytoin (Dilantin). A psychiatry consultation is solicited when the patient becomes combative. The psychiatrist finds that the patient has piloerection, muscle cramps, nausea, and abdominal pain. A CT and EEG have not been performed, but the clinical chemistry and hematology laboratory results are normal. Which should be the course of action?

a. Add a minor tranquilizer.
b. Add a major tranquilizer.
c. Increase the anticonvulsant.
d. Increase the methadone.
e. Demand a CT.
f. None of the above.

ANSWER: d. Opioid addicts often undergo withdrawal when hospitalized and given inadequate methadone. In addition, when phenytoin is administered to an individual enrolled in a methadone program, the metabolism of methadone will increase. The usual dose of methadone will have to be increased to compensate for its increased metabolism.

7. Which is probably the primary mechanism of action of acute cocaine administration?

a. It enhances dopamine activity.
b. It enhances serotonin metabolism.
c. It diverts serotonin innervation.
d. It leads to reduced gamma-aminobutyric acid (GABA) levels.

ANSWER: a. Cocaine enhances dopamine activity by triggering its release from presynaptic nerve endings and then blocking its re-uptake.

8. Which is not a sign of excessive sympathetic activity?

a. Tachycardia
b. Angina
c. Hypertension
d. Miosis
e. Anxiety

ANSWER: d. With excessive sympathetic activity, pupils dilate.

9. Which one of the following is not a manifestation of amphetamine use?

a. Weight loss
b. Insomnia
c. Psychosis similar to cocaine-induced psychosis
d. Parkinsonism
e. Stereotypies

ANSWER: d. Use of synthetic narcotics, particularly MPTP, but not amphetamines, has been routinely complicated by parkinsonism. MPTP destroys nigrostriatal neurons.

10. A college student is brought to the emergency room in a coma. He has a weak and thready pulse, infrequent and shallow respirations, and miosis. A chest x-ray shows pulmonary edema. The physicians secure an airway. Of the following, which should be the next treatment?

a. Inject naloxone.
b. Give thiamine.
c. Obtain a CT scan of the head.
d. Inject glucose.

ANSWER: a. He probably has a narcotic overdose, which typically causes coma, depressed respirations, and miosis. In severe cases, it causes pulmonary edema. Naloxone is a narcotic antagonist. Because its half-life is often shorter than the half-life of narcotics, repeated naloxone injections are often required. In addicts, it may precipitate narcotic withdrawal.

11. Which statement is false regarding vomiting?

a. Opioids typically induce it.
b. Marijuana reduces nausea and vomiting induced by chemotherapy.
c. The blood-brain barrier protects the brain's vomiting center.
d. Lesions located in posterior fossa structures are more apt to induce vomiting than those in the other parts of the brain.

ANSWER: c. Vomiting is induced by stimulation of the chemoreceptor trigger zone (CTZ), which is located in the area postrema of the medulla. This region is unprotected by the blood-brain barrier. D_2 dopamine blockers and $5HT_3$ antagonists are antiemetic medications. Marijuana weakly suppresses nausea and vomiting.

12. After a 29-year-old man is revived from an opioid overdose, physicians find that he has paresis of his right wrist extensor muscles and impairment of his ability to make a fist but no abnormalities in his legs. He is alert and has normal mental and language ability. Babinski signs are absent. Where is the most likely site of his injury?

a. Left cerebral hemisphere
b. Left internal capsule
c. Near the right humerus spiral groove
d. Near the right wrist

ANSWER: c. He has a "wrist drop" because he has compressed the right radial nerve as it winds around the spiral groove of the humerus. He cannot make a fist because the wrist must be extended to make a fist. Radial nerve and other nerve compressions, known as "pressure palsies," are a frequent complication of alcohol and drug overdose. The absence of aphasia and hemiparesis indicate that the problem is unlikely to be a cerebral lesion.

13. Which is the metabolic product of dopamine that is measurable in the CSF?

a. Monoamine oxidase (MAO)
b. Homovanillic acid (HVA)
c. Catechol-O-methyltransferase (COMT)
d. Vanillylmandelic acid (VMA)

ANSWER: b

14. Which is the rate-limiting enzyme in the synthesis of dopamine?

a. DOPA decarboxylase
b. Tyrosine hydroxylase
c. MAO
d. COMT
e. Dopamine β-hydroxylase

ANSWER: b

15. Of the enzymes listed in Question 14, which converts dopamine to norepinephrine?

ANSWER: e

16. Of the choices listed in Question 14, which is the rate-limiting enzyme in the synthesis of norepinephrine?

ANSWER: b

17. Which two statements about stimulating D_1 and D_2 dopamine receptors are correct?

a. Stimulation of the D_1 receptor increases ATP to cyclic AMP production.
b. Stimulation of the D_2 receptor decreases ATP to cyclic AMP production.
c. Stimulation of the D_1 receptor decreases ATP to cyclic AMP production.
d. Stimulation of the D_2 receptor increases ATP to cyclic AMP production.

ANSWER: a, b. A characteristic difference between these two receptors is that D_1 receptor activity increases ATP to cyclic AMP production through adenyl cyclase.

18. Which dopamine tract is responsible for the elevated prolactin levels induced by many antipsychotic agents?

a. Nigrostriatal
b. Mesolimbic
c. Tubero-infundibular
d. None of the above

ANSWER: c. The tubero-infundibular tract is the connection between the hypothalamus and the pituitary gland. Dopamine and dopamine agonists inhibit this tract and suppress prolactin release. Dopamine blockade provokes prolactin release, which is the basis of elevated serum prolactin levels.

19. Which is the primary site for conversion of norepinephrine to epinephrine?

a. Locus ceruleus
b. Striatum
c. Adrenal medulla
d. Nigrostriatal tract

ANSWER: c

20. Which is the major pathway for serotonin metabolism?

a. Metabolism by COMT to 5-hydroxyindoleacetic acid (5-HIAA)
b. Metabolism by MAO to 5-HIAA
c. Metabolism by decarboxylase to HVA
d. Metabolism by HVA to 5-HIAA

ANSWER: b. Although most serotonin undergoes re-uptake, the remainder is subject to metabolism by MAO, which converts serotonin to 5-HIAA.

21. Where is the main site of serotonin production?

a. Dorsal raphe nuclei
b. Regions adjacent to the aqueduct in the midbrain
c. Striatum
d. None of the above

ANSWER: d. Almost all serotonin is produced in platelets and various nonneurologic cells. Within the brain, which generates less than 2% of the total, serotonin-producing neurons are located predominantly in the *dorsal raphe nuclei*, which are adjacent to the aqueduct in the dorsal midbrain.

22. A 48-year-old man, with a history of major depression, commits suicide by igniting several sticks of dynamite. Which is the most likely neurotransmitter abnormality that would be found on postmortem examination?

a. Low concentrations of CSF HVA
b. Low concentrations of CSF HIAA
c. Low GABA concentrations in the basal ganglia
d. High dopamine concentrations

ANSWER: b. Low concentrations of CSF HIAA, which reflect decreased CNS serotonin activity, characterize violent suicides. Low GABA concentrations in the basal ganglia are characteristic of Huntington's disease.

23. Which two statements are false regarding ACh receptors in the cerebral cortex?

a. They are predominantly muscarinic.
b. They are predominantly nicotinic.
c. Atropine blocks muscarinic receptors.
d. Scopolamine, which antagonizes muscarinic receptors, induces memory impairments that mimic Alzheimer's disease dementia.
e. Botulinum toxin penetrates the blood-brain barrier to block cholinergic receptors and cause memory impairments.

ANSWER: b, e. Cerebral cortex ACh receptors are predominantly muscarinic. Blocking CNS muscarinic receptors causes memory impairments, even in normal individuals. Botulinum toxin, which impairs release of ACh from the presynaptic neuron at the neuromuscular junction, neither penetrates the blood-brain barrier nor causes memory impairments.

24. In the reaction, acetyl-CoA + choline to acetylcholine, which is the rate-limiting factor?

a. Choline acetyltransferase (ChAT)
b. Acetyl CoA
c. Choline
d. None of the above

ANSWER: c

25. Which two comparisons of Lambert-Eaton syndrome and myasthenia gravis are true?

a. Lambert-Eaton syndrome is a paraneoplastic syndrome, whereas myasthenia gravis is an autoimmune disorder.
b. Lambert-Eaton syndrome is associated with decreased ACh production, whereas myasthenia gravis is associated with excess ACh production.
c. Lambert-Eaton syndrome is characterized by impaired presynaptic ACh release, whereas myasthenia gravis is characterized by defective ACh-receptor interaction.
d. Lambert-Eaton syndrome is alleviated by botulism, whereas myasthenia gravis is alleviated by anticholinesterases.

ANSWER: a, c.

26. When gamma-aminobutyric acid (GABA) interacts with postsynaptic $GABA_A$ receptors, which four events can be anticipated?

a. Sodium channels are opened.
b. Chloride channels are opened.
c. The electrolyte shift depolarizes the neuron.
d. The electrolyte shift hyperpolarizes the neuron.
e. Hyperpolarization leads to inhibition.
f. The electrolyte shift in polarization leads to excitation.
g. Glutamate provokes a similar response.
h. Glycine provokes a similar response.

ANSWER: b, d, e, h. The $GABA_A$ receptor is a ubiquitous, multifaceted complex that is sensitive to benzodiazepines and barbiturates, as well as GABA. When stimulated, the $GABA_A$ receptor permits the influx of chloride. The electrolyte shift hyperpolarizes the neuron's membrane and inhibits depolarization. Glycine, like GABA, is an inhibitory amino acid neurotransmitter.

27. Which is the approximate normal resting potential of neurons?

a. +100 mV
b. +70 mV
c. 0 mV
d. –70 mV
e. –100 mV

ANSWER: d. The normal resting potential is –70 mV. When the resting potential is –100 mV, the neuron is hyperpolarized and thereby inhibited.

28. Which two roles does glycine play?

a. Glycine is an inhibitory amino acid neurotransmitter.
b. Glycine modulates the *N*-methyl-D-aspartate (NMDA) receptor.
c. Glycine is the rate-limiting substrate in glutamate synthesis.
d. Glycine raises the resting potential (i.e., makes it less negative).

ANSWER: a, b. Glycine is an inhibitory amino acid neurotransmitter that modulates the NMDA receptor. Inhibitory neurotransmitters generally make the resting potential more negative.

29. Which two roles do nitric oxide (NO) play?

a. It leads to cerebral vasodilation and, when the penis is stimulated, generates erections.
b. Like aspirin (ASA), it promotes platelet aggregation.
c. Excessive NMDA activity leads to increased NO activity, which leads to neuron death.
d. When used excessively, NO causes a peripheral neuropathy.

ANSWER: a, b. NO bypasses secondary messengers and binds with enzymes and sulfur or iron-containing molecules. Both NO and ASA inhibit platelet aggregation. Nitrous oxide (N_2O) is a gas anesthetic that, when used daily, causes a peripheral neuropathy.

30. Which neurotransmitter is confined almost entirely to the brain?

a. Dopamine
b. ACh
c. Glycine
d. Norepinephrine
e. Serotonin
f. Glutamate

ANSWER: a. Dopamine is found in the adrenal medulla, but its primary tracts are confined to the brain. The other neurotransmitters are found in high concentrations in the spinal cord, as well as in the brain.

31. Which are two effects of glutamate-NMDA activity?

a. Intracellular neuron calcium concentration increases.
b. Inhibition occurs through hyperpolarization.
c. Excitation occurs under normal circumstances.
d. Excitotoxicity occurs under normal circumstances.
e. Inhibition occurs under normal circumstances.

ANSWER: a, c. Glutamate, the principal CNS excitatory neurotransmitter, interacts with the NMDA and other receptors to open calcium channels. With excessive activity, the calcium influx raises intracellular concentrations to lethal levels. This process is termed "excitotoxicity."

32. Of the following, which is the best treatment for atropine poisoning?

a. Scopolamine
b. Edrophonium
c. Neostigmine
d. Physostigmine

ANSWER: d. Atropine is an inhibitor of muscarinic cholinergic receptors. Physostigmine crosses the blood-brain barrier and increases the acetylcholine concentration.

33. In Alzheimer's disease, which of the following receptors is most severely depleted?

a. Muscarinic acetylcholine
b. Nicotinic acetylcholine
c. Nigrostriatal dopamine
d. Frontal dopamine

ANSWER: a. In Alzheimer's disease, muscarinic acetylcholine receptors are depleted, especially in the limbic system and association areas. Although they are also found in the brain, nicotinic acetylcholine receptors are found predominantly in the spinal cord and the neuromuscular junction.

34. Which one of the following diverts dopamine metabolism to amphetamine?

a. Haloperidol
b. Selegiline (deprenyl)
c. Amitriptyline
d. Bromocriptine

ANSWER: b. Although the neuroprotective role of selegiline (deprenyl) remains controversial, it provides an antidepressant effect partly through diverting dopamine metabolism to amphetamine.

35. What effect does tetrabenazine have on dopamine transmission?

a. It stimulates dopamine transmission by acting as a precursor.
b. It substitutes for dopamine by acting as an agonist.
c. It interferes with dopamine transmission by blocking D_2 receptors.
d. It reduces dopamine transmission by depleting dopamine from its presynaptic storage sites.

ANSWER: d. Tetrabenazine, like reserpine, depletes dopamine from its presynaptic storage sites and reduces involuntary movements. Both tetrabenazine and reserpine are useful to a limited extent, in the treatment of hyperkinetic movement disorders, such as chorea, Tourette's syndrome, and oral-bucco-lingual tardive dyskinesia.

36. A 50-year-old man is hospitalized for alcohol-withdrawal. Clonidine and a β-blocker are administered prophylactically. Which of the following complications will be unaffected?

a. Tachycardia
b. Tremor
c. Agitation
d. Seizures
e. Hypertension

ANSWER: d. These medicines will suppress cardiovascular and some psychological manifestations of alcohol withdrawal; however, they do not prevent the development of seizures during alcohol withdrawal.

37. The man in the previous question develops a series of seizures on the third day of withdrawal. Which treatment should be administered while further evaluation and treatment is undertaken?

a. Lorazepam
b. Valproate
c. Carbamazepine
d. Phenobarbital

ANSWER: a. Lorazepam is probably the most rapidly acting, effective antiepileptic medicine in this situation. Because valproate and carbamazepine cannot be given as a "load," they require too much time to be effective in acute situations. Phenobarbital is often used, but it sedates patients and has a long half-life.

38. Which one of the following characterizes fast neurotransmitters?

a. They work through ion channels.
b. They work through G-proteins.
c. They work through second messengers.
d. They include dopamine and norepinephrine.

ANSWER: a. Fast neurotransmitters, such as GABA and glutamate, work through ion channels. Slow neurotransmitters, such as the catecholamines, work through G-proteins and second messengers, such as adenyl cyclase.

39. Excessive glutamate–NMDA interactions lead to which process?

a. Hyperpolarization
b. Excitotoxicity
c. Apoptosis
d. Involution

ANSWER: b. In excitotoxicity, excessive glutamate–NMDA interactions lead to flooding of the neurons with lethal concentrations of calcium.

40. Which of the following is false regarding serotonin?

a. Serotonin is a monoamine but not a catecholamine.
b. Depending on the receptor class, serotonin interactions may lead to increased adenyl cyclase activity.
c. Serotonin is a slow neurotransmitter that works through G-proteins and second messengers.
d. Depending on the receptor class, serotonin interactions may be inhibitory or excitatory.
e. The antimigraine medications, "triptans," are $5\text{-}HT_{1D}$ receptors antagonists.

ANSWER: e. In one of neurology's most effective therapies, sumatriptan and other trip-tans, which are 5-HT_{1D} receptor agonists, consistently abort migraines. Serotonin is not a catecholamine, but it is a monoamine that is either a slow inhibitory or excitatory neurotransmitter. It works through G-proteins and second messengers.

41. Which one of the following statements concerning neurotransmission is false?

a. Glutamate-NMDA interactions are fast and excitatory.
b. Glutamate-NMDA interactions affect the calcium channel.
c. Benzodiazepine-$GABA_A$ receptor interactions are fast and inhibitory.
d. Benzodiazepine-$GABA_A$ receptor interactions affect the chloride channel.
e. Benzodiazepine-$GABA_A$ receptor interactions, which promote the influx of chloride, reduce the polarization of the resting potential.

ANSWER: e. Benzodiazepine-$GABA_A$ receptor interactions promote the influx of chloride, but the resting potential is made more negative. Hyperpolarized neurons are refractory to stimulation (inhibited).

42. Which of the following is a second messenger?

a. Phosphatidyl inositol
b. Serotonin
c. DNA
d. Thyroid hormone
e. Prolactin

ANSWER: a. Phosphatidyl inositol and cyclic AMP are two common second messengers.

43. Which dopamine tract is most likely responsible for positive symptoms in psychosis?

a. Nigrostriatal
b. Mesolimbic
c. Tubero-infundibular
d. Mesocortical

ANSWER: b

44. Which dopamine tract is most likely responsible for negative symptoms in psychosis?

a. Nigrostriatal
b. Mesolimbic
c. Tubero-infundibular
d. Mesocortical

ANSWER: d

45. Which of the following pairs are inhibitory amino acid neurotransmitters?

a. GABA and glycine
b. Glutamate and aspartate
c. Epinephrine and norepinephrine
d. L-dopa and carbidopa

ANSWER: a. GABA and glycine are inhibitory amino acid neurotransmitters. Glutamate and aspartate are excitatory amino acid neurotransmitters.

46–51. Match the medication (46–51) with the enzyme (a–e) that it inhibits.

46. Deprenyl

47. Carbidopa

48. Entacapone

49. Edrophonium

50. Selegiline

51. Pyridostigmine

a. Dopa decarboxylase
b. COMT
c. MAO-B
d. Acetylcholinesterase
e. MAO-A

ANSWERS: 46-c, 47-a, 48-b, 49-d, 50-c, 51-d

52–56. Match the illness (52–56) with the enzyme(s) (a–d) that is (are) deficient.

52. Phenylketonuria

53. Parkinson's disease

54. Dopamine responsive dystonia

55. Alzheimer's disease

56. Huntington's disease

a. Phenylalanine hydroxylase
b. Tyrosine hydroxylase

c. Glutamate decarboxylase
d. Choline acetyltransferase

ANSWERS: 52-a, 53-b, 54-a and b, 55-d, 56-c

57. Which of the following is not a characteristic of nicotinic ACh receptors?

a. They are neuromuscular junction receptors.
b. Curare and α-bungarotoxin block them.
c. They are inhibitory.
d. They are one of two main ACh receptors in the nervous system.

ANSWER: c. They are excitatory.

58. Which of the following is not a characteristic of muscarinic ACh receptors?

a. Cerebral cortex ACh receptors are predominantly muscarinic.
b. They are entirely inhibitory.
c. Atropine and scopolamine block them.
d. They are depleted in Alzheimer's disease.

ANSWER: b. They can be excitatory as well as inhibitory.

59. Which of the following is not an effect of increased GABA-GABA$_A$ receptor activity?

a. Chloride ions flow into the channel.
b. The resting potential, which is normally -70 mV, is further lowered (made more negative).
c. Calcium ions flow into the channel.
d. Lowering their resting potential hyperpolarizes neurons.
e. The speed of the reaction has allowed GABA to be termed a "fast neurotransmitter."

ANSWER: c. Calcium influx characterizes NMDA activity.

60. Which of the following is false regarding the GABA$_B$ receptor?

a. GABA$_B$ receptors are more numerous and more widely distributed than GABA$_A$ receptors.
b. GABA$_B$ receptors are G-protein linked channel inhibitors.
c. Baclofen binds to GABA$_B$ receptors.
d. Compared to the number and diversity of ligands that bind to GABA$_A$ receptors, relatively few bind to GABA$_B$ receptors.
e. Like GABA$_A$ receptors, GABA$_B$ receptors are complex molecules.

ANSWER: a

61. A 40-year-old man has been under treatment for major depression for several years. After he contracted tuberculosis (TB), isoniazid (INH) was prescribed. The TB began to respond. However, he took an overdose of the INH and developed status epilepticus. Which would be the most specific, effective treatment?

a. Phenytoin
b. Thiamine
c. Lorazepam
d. Pyridoxine (B$_6$)
e. Topiramate

ANSWER: d. Pyridoxine-deficient states lead to seizures. For example, infants fed pyridoxine-deficient diets develop seizures. In this case, INH interferes with pyridoxine, which is the cofactor for glutamate decarboxylase. Glutamate decarboxylase is a crucial enzyme in GABA synthesis. Toxic concentrations of INH cause profound GABA deficiency, which causes seizures. Intravenous pyridoxine will abort seizures caused by pyridoxine-deficiency. Patients given INH should also be given pyridoxine. Topiramate enhances GABA$_A$ receptor activity, but it is ineffective without GABA.

62. Which is a false statement regarding the NMDA receptor?

a. The NMDA receptor has binding sites for ketamine as well as phencyclidine.
b. Excessive NMDA receptor activity leads to excitotoxicity, which purportedly causes cell death in Huntington's disease, stroke, and possibly schizophrenia.
c. Lamotrigine and riluzole decrease glutamate activity but not necessarily at the NMDA receptor.
d. Excessive NMDA activity floods the neuron with excessive concentrations of chloride.
e. The NMDA receptor's activity is modulated by glycine, which is an inhibitory neurotransmitter.

ANSWER: d. Excessive NMDA activity floods the neuron with excessive concentrations of calcium.

63–67. Match the neurotransmitter (63–67) with the region of the nervous system (a–e) where it is synthesized.

63. Dopamine

64. Norepinephrine

65. Epinephrine

66. Serotonin

67. Acetylcholine

a. Locus ceruleus
b. Adrenal medulla
c. Dorsal raphe nuclei

d. Substantia nigra
e. Nucleus basalis of Meynert

ANSWERS: 63-d, 64-a, 65-b, 66-c, 67-e

68–73. Match the site of neurotransmitter synthesis (68–73) with the region(s) of the nervous system (a–e) where it is located.

68. Locus ceruleus

69. Dorsal raphe nuclei

70. Adrenal medulla

71. Substantia nigra

72. Nucleus basalis of Meynert

73. Caudal raphe nuclei

a. Basal forebrain bundle
b. Midbrain
c. Pons

d. Medulla
e. Adrenal gland

ANSWERS: 68-c, 69-b and c, 70-e, 71-b, 72-a, 73-c and d

74. A woman, who is 5 months pregnant, asks for methadone maintenance because her heroin supply has been cut off. Which would be the best course of action?

a. Do not accept her into the methadone maintenance program until after she delivers.
b. Have her only undergo heroin detoxification to avoid exposing the fetus to methadone.
c. Enroll her in the methadone maintenance program as soon as possible.
d. None of the above.

ANSWER: c. The fetus, as well as the mother, is probably addicted to heroin. Attempting to stop the mother's opioid use would probably be futile, but she probably could be switched from heroin to methadone. After she delivers, both the mother and infant can be detoxified.

75. To which site do ketamine and PCP bind?

a. Dopamine
b. Norepinephrine
c. Serotonin

d. $GABA_A$
e. NMDA

ANSWER: e. Ketamine and PCP affect ion channels at the NMDA receptor.

76. What is the effect of ketamine and PCP binding on the NMDA receptor?

a. Inhibition of the influx of calcium

b. Promotion of the influx of calcium

c. Inhibition of the influx of chloride

d. Promotion of the influx of chloride

e. None of the above

ANSWER: a. Ketamine and PCP inhibit the influx of calcium, which is usually provoked by interactions of glutamate or aspartate with the NMDA receptor.

77. Which is the common mechanism of action of LSD and MDMA (ecstasy)?

a. Promote dopamine release and then block its re-uptake

b. Block re-uptake of serotonin

c. Inhibit NMDA

d. Promote GABA-NMDA reactions, just short of excitotoxicity

e. Promote norepinephrine release and then block its re-uptake

ANSWER: b. LSD and MDMA block re-uptake of serotonin, which probably accounts for these drugs often elevating the mood during intoxication and for depression during withdrawal.

78. Of the following dopamine receptors, which is most stimulated by cocaine?

a. D_1

b. D_2 mesocortical

c. D_2 mesolimbic

d. D_3

ANSWER: c. Cocaine affects the D_2 mesolimbic receptors.

79. Which is the best treatment for cocaine-induced psychosis and violent behavior?

a. Dopamine-blocking neuroleptics

b. Benzodiazepines

c. Seclusion and, if necessary, restraints

d. None of the above

ANSWER: a. Because the main effect of cocaine is to increase dopamine activity by blocking its re-uptake, the best treatment for excessive dopamine activity is dopamine-blocking neuroleptics. However, these neuroleptics must be used with caution in this situation because most of them, as well as cocaine, lower the seizure threshold.

80. Which is rarely a neurologic complication of cocaine use?

a. Nonhemorrhagic strokes

b. Hemorrhagic strokes

c. Seizures during withdrawal

d. Seizures during overdose

e. Increased incidence of neuroleptic-induced dystonic reactions

ANSWER: c. Seizures are apt to complicate withdrawal from alcohol, barbiturates, and benzodiazepines. With cocaine, seizures complicate withdrawal only from chronic, frequent, high-dose use. However, seizures are a common complication of cocaine intoxication and may signify an underlying stroke. Hemorrhagic strokes, which stem from hypertension, are much more common than nonhemorrhagic strokes.

81. Which is the best treatment for cocaine-induced severe hypertension?

a. A diuretic

b. A calcium channel blocker

c. An ACE inhibitor

d. Phentolamine

ANSWER: d. An α-blocker, such as phentolamine, will be the most rapid and effective antihypertensive therapy. It may forestall a cerebral hemorrhage.

82. Which is the effect of amphetamines on sleep?

a. Decreases proportion of NREM stages 1 and 2

b. Decreases proportion of NREM stages 3 and 4

c. Decreases proportion of REM

d. Displaces REM from nighttime to daytime

ANSWER: c. Total sleep time is reduced. The proportion of REM sleep particularly is reduced.

83. What is the effect of opioids on respiration?

a. They reduce the respiratory rate.

b. They reduce the depth of respirations.

c. They increase the rate but reduce the depth.
d. They reduce the depth but increase the rate.

ANSWER: a. Opioids reduce the respiratory rate. In severe overdoses, they lead to pulmonary edema.

84. What is the effect of the PCP-NMDA interaction?

a. A PCP-NMDA interaction stabilizes the ion channel.
b. It leads to an influx of negatively charged chloride ions, which hyperpolarizes the neuron.
c. It triggers an influx of calcium, which leads to excitotoxicity.
d. It prevents the influx of calcium that glutamate would ordinarily trigger.

ANSWER: d

85. Which of the following is a common effect of marijuana?

a. A fatal reaction to overdose
b. Seizures
c. Strokes
d. Reduced REM sleep

ANSWER: d

86. Which of the following statements concerning nicotine is false?

a. It affects CNS cholinergic receptors.
b. Its receptors are located in the mesolimbic pathway.
c. Bupropion (Wellbutrin) may help smokers through withdrawal because, like nicotine, it increases dopamine concentrations.
d. Nicotinic receptors are the predominant CNS receptors.

ANSWER: d. Although both muscarinic and nicotinic receptors are present in the CNS, muscarinic receptors are predominant. Nicotinic receptors predominate at the neuromuscular junction.

87. Which features are characteristic of cocaine use?

a. Blocks re-uptake of dopamine into presynaptic neurons
b. Agitation
c. Hypertension
d. Slowed respiratory rate
e. Stimulation of the area postrema
f. Miosis
g. Blockade of dopamine re-uptake
h. Chorea in some cases

ANSWER: a, b, c, g, h

88. Which features are common complications of cocaine administration?

a. Cerebral hemorrhage
b. Cerebral anoxia
c. Seizures
d. Radial nerve palsy
e. Tics
f. Stereotypies
g. Psychotic thinking
h. Pulmonary edema

ANSWER: a, c, e, f, g

89. In comparing heroin to morphine in terms of their use in cancer-induced pain, which of the following are heroin's advantages?

a. Like benzodiazepine, heroin has its own receptor.
b. Because it more rapidly penetrates the blood-brain barrier, it has a more rapid onset of action.
c. It does not induce vomiting.
d. It improves affect to a greater degree.

ANSWER: b. Compared to morphine, heroin penetrates the blood-brain barrier more rapidly. However, it attaches to the mu receptor, which is a common opioid receptor. Its effects are virtually indistinguishable from morphine's.

22

Traumatic Brain Injury

MAJOR HEAD TRAUMA

The severity and nature of head trauma determine the manifestations of *traumatic brain injury (TBI)*. In a somewhat arbitrary separation, neurologists distinguish major from minor head trauma (see below). Major head trauma results in at least 1 hour of posttraumatic unconsciousness and then permanent residual neurologic deficits. Motor vehicle accidents (MVAs) are the most common cause of major head trauma in civilians, particularly 15- to 24-year-old males. Within this group, alcohol use plays a major role because it impairs drivers' judgment, coordination, and ability to remain awake. The other common causes of major head trauma are falls, work-related accidents, sports-related injuries, and gunshot wounds (GSWs).

Neurologists divide major head trauma into *penetrating* injuries, such as a GSW, and *blunt* or *nonpenetrating* injuries, such as falls. However, this division is not always clear-cut. Blunt head trauma can lead to penetrating injury, as from a depressed skull fracture.

How Does Trauma Cause Brain Injury?

In the simplest case, a blow to the head disrupts the underlying delicate brain tissue (the *parenchyma*) by its direct mechanical force (a *coup* injury). As the force throws the brain against the opposite inner surface *(inner table)* of the skull, that cerebral lobe is injured (a *contrecoup* injury). Reciprocal injuries *(coup-contrecoup injuries)* are most likely to injure the temporal lobe and anterior-inferior surface of the frontal lobes because they abut the sharp surfaces of the skull's anterior and middle fossae (Fig. 22–1). Whether the blows are direct or indirect, frontal and temporal lobe injuries characteristically lead to memory impairment and personality changes.

One exception to the damage pattern of countercoup injuries is that frontal trauma rarely leads to countercoup occipital lobe injuries because the occipital skull is relatively flat and smooth. Thus, TBI rarely causes long-lasting visual impairments.

In another process that leads to brain injury, *diffuse axonal shearing,* the force of blunt trauma stretches the brain's long, delicate axons. The sudden stretching disrupts their function. If the force is great enough, it can sever ("shear") them. The long subcortical white matter neurons are particularly susceptible to shear injuries. Diagnosis of diffuse axonal shearing requires a postmortem inspection. It can only be postulated in survivors of TBI.

Moderately severe blunt trauma, such as being struck with a baseball bat, causes intraparenchymal hematomas and petechiae, especially in the brainstem. These hemorrhages are not only injurious to affected brain areas, they also cause diffuse *cerebral edema*, which increases intracranial pressure. The increased pressure is as life-threatening as other injuries. The hematomas within the brain and over its surface cause

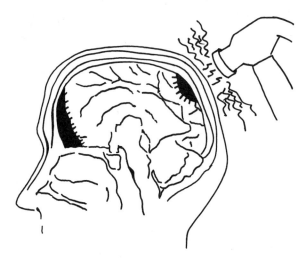

FIGURE 22–1. A *coup* refers to the brain injury immediately underlying a blow. In a *contrecoup* injury, the rebound damages the opposite side of the brain. In this drawing, a hammer blow to the back of the head inflicts a coup injury to the occipital region and through the contrecoup, a more extensive injury to the tips of the frontal and temporal lobes.

extensive damage. If they expand beyond a certain size, they lead to transtentorial herniation (see below).

In addition to direct effects of trauma, GSWs and other penetrating injuries leave bone, shrapnel, and other foreign bodies in the brain. These foreign bodies are a potential nidus for seizures and a potential site for brain abscesses.

Head injury, ruptured aneurysms, and other conditions can cause bleeding in the spaces named after the meninges (coverings of the brain and spinal cord). The meninges consist of three layers—PAD (innermost to outermost):

- *Pia mater*, the innermost layer, is a thin, almost transparent, vascular membrane adherent to the cerebral gyri. It follows the gyri into the sulci.

- *Arachnoid mater*, also thin, is the middle layer of the meninges. It goes over the tops of gyri, covering the sulci. The space between the pia mater and arachnoid mater, the *subarachnoid space*, contains the cerebrospinal fluid (CSF). The subarachnoid space over the brain continues downward to cover the spinal cord and cauda equina. It descends to the sacrum. Lumbar puncture (LP) needles are inserted into the subarachnoid space to sample CSF for the diagnosis of meningitis or subarachnoid hemorrhage (see Table 20–1).

- *Dura mater*, the outermost of the meninges, is a thick fibrous tissue that is adherent to the interior surface of the skull. The dura mater forms two thick structures that support the brain and hold some of its venous drainage: the *falx* and *tentorium*. The space between the skull and the dura, "exterior to or above the dura," is the *epidural space*. The space immediately "inferior to or below" the dura is the *subdural space*. Major head trauma often causes both subdural and epidural hematomas.

Epidural hematomas, which typically follow temporal bone fractures with concomitant middle meningeal artery lacerations, are rapidly expanding, high-pressure masses of fresh blood (Fig. 22–2). They compress the underlying brain and force it through the tentorial notch, that is, they produce *transtentorial herniation* (see Fig. 19–3). Unless surgery can immediately arrest the bleeding and evacuate epidural hematomas, they are usually fatal.

In contrast, *subdural hematomas* are common, usually not fatal, and result from either small or large veins bleeding into the subdural space. Because intracranial venous pressure is low, rate of bleeding is slow and veins are easily compressed. The dark, venous blood generally oozes into the extensive subdural space until the expanding hematoma encounters the underlying brain. The brain usually resists further expansion and arrests the bleeding (see Fig. 20–11). However, if the hematoma continues to expand, it may permanently damage the underlying brain and lead to transtentorial herniation.

Chronic subdural hematomas are hematomas that have spread diffusely in the subdural space and have persisted for weeks. They typically give rise to an insidious onset of headaches, change in personality, and dementia. Curiously, however, they cause minimal physical deficits (see Chapters 19 and 20). Surgical evacuation readily reverses their symptoms. Thus, subdural hematomas are often cited as a correctable cause of dementia.

People older than 65 years are especially susceptible to chronic subdural hematomas for several reasons. Mild head trauma, which has occurred so long ago that it is forgotten, can fracture their frail vessels. They have a tendency to fall. They are also often taking anticoagulants and other medications that greatly increase their tendency to bleed. Their age-related cerebral atrophy enlarges the subdural space: the capacious space allows hematomas to reach considerable size before they encounter the resistance of the underlying brain. Other individuals susceptible to subdural hematomas are those with neoplasms, chronic renal failure, and bleeding disorders.

Immediate Posttraumatic Delirium

Following head trauma, patients' level of consciousness can be classified as *alert, lethargic, stuporous,* or *comatose.* Neurologists and neurosurgeons measure their level of consciousness using the *Glasgow Coma Scale (GCS),* which is an assessment of three readily apparent neurologic functions: eye opening, speaking, and moving (Table 22–1). In major head trauma, the GCS has a good correlation with survival and neurologic sequelae; however, in minor head trauma, the GCS has a poor correlation with neurologic sequelae.

Of patients whose GCS scores are 3, which is the lowest possible score, on the first day, 90% have a fatal outcome and most of the rest never regain consciousness. Major head trauma victims can remain in coma for only several days to three weeks: by then, comatose patients have either improved, died, or evolved into the vegetative state (see below).

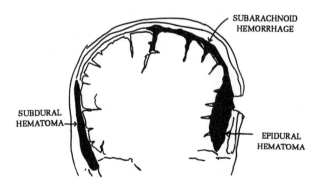

FIGURE 22–2. Arterial bleeding, which generally results from blows forceful enough to cause skull fractures, causes *epidural hematomas.* Venous bleeding, which is usually slower and less forceful, causes *subdural hematomas.* Both hematomas cause potentially fatal mass effects, including compression of the gyri and shift of midline structures. Ruptured aneurysms and major head trauma cause subarachnoid hemorrhage (SAH). With a SAH, blood may spread through the subarachnoid spaces at the base of the brain, over the convexities, between the gyri, into the interhemispheric fissure, and typically down, into the spinal canal, where it can be found by doing an LP.

TABLE 22–1. *The Glasgow Coma Scale (GCS)*

Category		Score
Eyes opening	Never	1
	To pain	2
	To verbal stimuli	3
	Spontaneously	4
Best verbal response	None	1
	Incomprehensible sounds	2
	Inappropriate words	3
	Disoriented and converses	4
	Oriented and converses	5
Best motor response	None	1
	Extension*	2
	Flexion†	3
	Flexion withdrawal	4
	Patient localizes pain	5
	Patient obeys	6
Total		3–15

*Decerebrate rigidity (Fig. 19–3).

†Decorticate rigidity (Fig. 11–5).

This standard scale indicates the level of consciousness, with the lowest scores indicating less neurologic function. Scores lower than 9 indicate coma.

Adapted, with kind permission, from: Teasdale G, Jennett B: Assessment of coma and impaired consciousness: A practical scale. Lancet 2: 81–84, 1974.

During this period, as major TBI patients emerge from coma or stupor, their course fluctuates and is frequently stormy. Patients are intermittently confused, disoriented, agitated, and combative. Neurologists and neurosurgeons call these complications of head trauma and its aftermath *posttraumatic psychosis*. The *Diagnostic and Statistical Manual of Mental Disorders-IV (DSM-IV)* would classify them as *Delirium Due to Head Trauma*. These disturbances are often so severe that they require neuroleptics.

Physicians must keep in mind that alcohol and, less frequently, drug use cause or represent a contributing factor in innumerable MVAs and other injuries. Furthermore, chronic, prehospital use of alcohol or drugs complicates the patient's immediate posttraumatic period. Their subsequent use remains a source of continued disability.

Trauma patients who have delirium, for example, may be suffering from alcohol or drug intoxication, as well as head trauma. Similarly, alcohol or drug withdrawal may cause abnormal behavior (and seizures) during the first several days of hospitalization.

Another cause of posttraumatic delirium is that preexisting dementia has rendered patients particularly susceptible to traumatic cognitive impairment and behavioral disturbances. In addition, a variety of general medical conditions can cause delirium and other mental status abnormalities: painful extracranial injuries; adverse reactions to narcotics, antiepileptic drugs, and other medications; and complications of bodily trauma, such as hypoxia, sepsis, and fat emboli to the brain.

Physical Sequelae

TBI frequently causes focal neurologic deficits, such as hemiparesis, spasticity, ataxia, and tremors. Recovery usually reaches a maximum within 6 months after the injury. Patients can further increase their strength and mobility with physical and occupational therapy, braces, other mechanical devices, and modifications of their environment. Functional recovery is usually measured on the *Glasgow Outcome Scale (GOS)* (Table 22–2).

Damage to the special sensory organs, such as the eye, ear, or nose and their cranial nerves, although not strictly speaking "brain injury," is another debilitating aspect of TBI. Sensory organ damage leads to sensory deprivation, disfigurement, functional impairments, and other consequences. Frontal head trauma, which is probably the most common injury, lacerates the filaments of the olfactory nerves as they pass through the cribriform plate on their way to terminate in the frontal lobes. Patients sustaining frontal head trauma develop combinations of anosmia and symptoms of frontal lobe injury.

Posttraumatic Epilepsy

Cerebral scars and residual foreign bodies routinely evolve into epileptic foci. Thus, posttraumatic epilepsy, which has an overall incidence of 50%, is one of the most commonly occurring complications of major TBI. Incidence is even greater when patients use alcohol. Minor TBI, in contrast, rarely causes posttraumatic epilepsy.

Posttraumatic epilepsy takes the form of focal seizures, including partial complex seizures, which tend to undergo secondary generalization (see Chapter 10). The seizures may be debilitating and lead to further head injury. Incidence increases—rather than decreases—as time passes after the injury. It greatly increases with major compared to minor head trauma, penetrating rather than blunt trauma, and a preceding subdural hematoma. Side effects of antiepileptic drugs may exacerbate other sequelae of TBI.

Cognitive Impairment

Following severe major TBI, many patients remain with their eyes open but capable of only rudimentary bodily functions. They tend toward a flexed, decorticate (fetal) posture and lack communication, cognitive capacity, and purposeful activity. Most evolve into the *persistent vegetative state*, which carries no hope for a functional recovery (see Chapter 11).

Many who survive major TBI have devastating cognitive impairment. Whether the TBI has been one massive blow, a succession of several serious injuries, or repetitive incidents in which the individual is rendered unconscious, cognitive impairment deteriorates to the point of dementia. The *DSM-IV* classifies posttraumatic cognitive impairment as Dementia Due to Head Trauma.

Less severely injured patients usually have less pronounced cognitive impairment. Those impairments correlate with depth of coma, as measured by the GCS, and the lesion's size. They include memory impairment (see below), aphasia, apraxia, impulsivity, impaired judgment, and other neuropsychologic deficits. Surprisingly, the lesion's location, with one important exception, correlates relatively poorly with the

TABLE 22–2. *The Glasgow Outcome Scale (GOS)*

Good recovery: resumption of normal life despite minor deficits
Moderate disability: disabled but independent
Severe disability: conscious but disabled
Persistent vegetative state: unresponsive and speechless
Death

Adapted, with kind permission, from: Jennett B, Bond M: Assessment of outcome after severe brain damage. Lancet 5: 480–484, 1975.

impairments. The exception is that left temporal lobe injuries produce vocabulary deficits, which represent a variety of anomic aphasia (see Chapter 8).

In addition to structural brain damage causing cognitive impairment, medications used to treat its sequelae, such as antiepileptics, antispasmodics, and analgesics, may further impair cognitive function. Moreover, these medications, alone or in combination, may alter patients' personality, mood, sleep-wake schedule, and metabolism of other medications.

Recovery of motor and language skills usually reaches a maximum within 6 months after the injury. Intellectual recovery—to the extent that it occurs—may be delayed until 18 months. In general, older patients recover more slowly and less completely than younger ones.

TBI has been alleged to be either a direct cause or at least a risk factor for Alzheimer's disease. The main evidence stems from a statistical association between head trauma and the subsequent development of Alzheimer's disease that was found in some but not all studies. Other evidence is that severe head trauma causes a deposition in the brain of beta-A4 amyloid protein, which may serve as a nidus for amyloid plaques. In addition, head trauma in individuals with two alleles of ApoE4 has been associated in some studies with a poor outcome and increased risk of subsequently developing Alzheimer's disease by tenfold (see Chapter 7). (A confounding issue is that individuals with Alzheimer's disease are apt to cause a motor vehicle accident in which they sustain a traumatic brain injury.)

Memory impairment or *posttraumatic amnesia* is the most salient, specific neuropsychologic deficit. TBI typically causes amnesia for the trauma and events immediately preceding it (retrograde amnesia) and, less often, for memorizing newly presented information (anterograde amnesia). Posttraumatic amnesia's severity and duration are directly proportional to low GCS scores. The *DSM-IV* includes posttraumatic amnesia as an Amnesic Disorder Due to Head Trauma and calls it "transient" if the duration is shorter than 1 month and "chronic" if longer.

Posttraumatic amnesia is often accompanied by another major handicap, *slowed information processing*. Additional neuropsychologic sequelae—perseveration, inattention, cognitive inflexibility, and impaired problem solving—are frequent, partly overlapping impairments.

None of the several approaches to the psychopharmacology of posttraumatic dementia has been successful. On the theory that loss of brain tissue meant loss of neurotransmitters, physicians have attempted to restore dopamine and acetylcholine activity by administering dopamine agonists, such as bromocriptine, and cholinesterase inhibitors. They have also prescribed stimulants, such as dextroamphetamine, methylphenidate, and pemoline. Although the stimulants have helped to a limited extent in improving patients' attentiveness, daytime wakefulness, and mood, their benefit may have been more in improving patients' mood and energy than restoring their cognitive function.

Families and physicians have also tried "cognitive rehabilitation," a team attempt to overcome intellectual deficits that includes retraining and focusing attention on the task at hand. Benefit probably stem entirely from a classic rehabilitation approach: social interactions with peers; identification and treatment of depression, anxiety, and insomnia; and physical, occupational, and speech therapy.

Other Psychiatric Disturbances

Most individuals with traumatic or congenital brain damage are not violent; many are as docile as if they had undergone a frontal lobotomy. However, TBI predisposes people to *Intermittent Explosive Disorder* (previously known as "episodic dyscontrol syndrome"), consisting of dissociative states and violence. It also makes people exquisitely sensitive to alcohol, so that even small amounts precipitate violent outbursts. TBI-induced violence reportedly may be reduced by carbamazepine, propranolol, and lithium, as well as neuroleptics.

Personality changes, such as being abrupt, suspicious, and argumentative, are also common. These changes presumably result from either generalized cerebral or predominantly frontal and temporal lobe damage. In particular, damage to the frontal lobes impairs the brain's inhibitory centers. Loss of inhibition, in turn, explains a good portion of TBI patients' aggressiveness and emotional lability.

Posttraumatic depression, an ill-defined combination of depressive symptoms, occurs in about 25% of TBI patients. Its development correlates weakly with the severity of the head trauma. As with poststroke depression (see Chapter 11), posttraumatic depression has been linked to damage to the left anterior cerebral hemisphere. It is classified in *DSM-IV* as a Mood Disorder Due to a General Medical Condition. Posttraumatic depression is associated with drug and alcohol abuse, previous depression, and poor social functioning. In addition, depressed TBI patients are apt to have cognitive impairments, a low seizure threshold, and limited physical, occupational, and social skills.

Depression interferes with TBI patients' rehabilitation, compliance, and socialization. It reduces their chance of making a complete recovery. In addition to needing the full array of physical, financial, and psychologic support services, they invariably require psychopharmacology.

Trauma in Childhood

Compared to adults, TBI in children has somewhat different causes, clinical features, and sequelae. Most important, children are apt to be victims of child abuse (see below). Also, children with attention deficit hyperactivity disorder (ADHD) and related disturbances are prone to TBI. Those with ADHD are more likely to have been deliberately injured (abused), as well as to have engaged in dangerous activities, than other children. The high proportion of trauma survivors who are hyperactive partly reflects their preinjury status.

The prognosis for children, in general, is better than for adults with comparable TBI. For prognostic purposes in children, severity and extent of brain damage are important, but the GCS cannot be reliably applied to them. Another major prognostic factor is the family's socioeconomic status and psychiatric history.

As with adults, children's memory is particularly vulnerable to TBI. On intelligence measurements, TBI impairs children's performance subtests more than their verbal subtests. Also, as with adults, duration of posttraumatic amnesia correlates with ultimate cognitive impairment and behavioral disturbances. Although their cognitive impairment is important, children are often more handicapped by TBI-induced social problems, developmental delays, and behavioral disturbances.

Sometimes children's residual injuries do not appear until they confront the increasing academic and social demands of successive school years. As children "grow into their deficits," TBI may be the limiting factor in cognitive and psychosocial development.

When TBI occurs before growth spurts, affected limbs will be foreshortened. This pattern is similar to the spastic hemiparesis with foreshortened limbs seen in congenital cerebral injuries (see Fig. 13–4). When dominant hemisphere injury occurs before age 5 years, it may allow the opposite hemisphere to assume control of language. For example, a left-sided cerebral injury in a 4-year-old child will probably not result in aphasia because the plasticity of the brain allows the right cerebral hemisphere to develop language centers. Another consequence of major TBI in children is abnormal hypothalamic or pituitary hormone secretion, which may result in obesity, precocious puberty, or delayed puberty.

Child Abuse. Although children may fall backward and injure their occiput, if they fall forward, they reflexively extend their arms and shield their face and eyes. Therefore, facial, ocular, and anterior skull injuries are more suspicious than occipital injuries. Head injuries accompanied by limb injuries are particularly suspicious.

Childhood TBI from abuse often takes the form of a closed head injury unaccompanied by face or scalp abrasions, spiral fractures of any long bones, or damage to internal organs. Sometimes the head injury results from blows of a blunt object, but usually it results from a baby or child being violently shaken. In the *shaken baby syndrome*, violent throws ("shaking"), without any direct impact, injure the brain parenchyma by rotational (angular) deceleration, shearing, and contusion. Severe shaking produces hemorrhages in the brain parenchyma, subdural space, and retinae. Because the abuse is most often repetitive, physicians may discover injuries in different stages of development and resolution during any particular evaluation.

Computed tomography (CT) and magnetic resonance imaging (MRI) may reveal blood—typically of different ages—in the subdural, subarachnoid, or interhemispheric space. Plain skull x-rays may reveal skull fractures more clearly than a CT or MRI. Funduscopic examination, which is necessary, may reveal retinal hemorrhages.

Overt cases of child abuse include new and old fractures of the long bones, bruises, and scars. Children who survive abuse often have cognitive impairment, behavioral difficulties, learning disabilities, developmental delay, and seizures. Sometimes these sequelae may not be apparent for several years. As discussed above, a relatively high proportion of survivors has ADHD.

Elder Abuse

Elder abuse, child abuse's geriatric counterpart, usually comes from family members or other caregivers. Those with chronic neurologic and psychiatric disorders, particularly dementia, are most at risk. Older individuals are already at risk for falls and, even with minimal trauma, subdural hematomas. TBI from elder abuse easily leads to cognitive impairment and reduced life expectancy.

Initial theories had suggested that psychologic stress precipitates violence. However, recent studies found a stronger correlation between the caregiver's emotional and financial dependence on the patient-victim. Many cases fall into the *DSM-IV* diagnosis of Physical Abuse of Adult.

Head Trauma in Sports

In most sports, including track and field events, head injuries are rare, usually minor, and accidental. However, head injuries, despite the helmets worn by athletes, are an integral part of other sports. In boxing, hockey, and several other contact sports, athletes can sustain severe, permanent, and occasionally fatal TBI.

The most common, notable sports-related TBI is a *concussion*. Concussion, a term with both physiologic and clinical aspects, is a blow, shaking, or jarring that results in a transient alteration of mental status but not necessarily a loss of consciousness. Most commonly, a concussion results in an *impairment* of consciousness. (The *DSM-IV* suggests stricter criteria for the diagnosis of concussion [see below].) Studies have postulated shearing of neurons, damage at the gray-white matter boundary, and production of intracellular vacuoles; however, pathologic studies have revealed no consistent abnormality.

Immediately after a concussion, with or without loss of consciousness, athletes are dazed, inattentive, disoriented, uncoordinated, and amnestic. They may also have headache, nausea, and vomiting. Those same symptoms might also indicate more serious injury, such as a subdural hematoma.

A *contusion,* which is a physiologic rather than a clinical term, consists of minute bleeding into the brain and overlying meninges. The bleeding often causes scar formation, but the cerebral architecture is otherwise preserved.

Even allowing for a full recovery after a concussion, multiple concussions have a cumulative effect. Sometimes a succession of two concussions produces a catastrophe. Athletes, especially children and adolescents, are apt to sustain *second impact syndrome,* in which a second blow within days of one that caused a concussion causes severe, permanent brain damage. Thus, athletes should be prohibited from playing—for at least a week, if not for the entire season—after sustaining a concussion with or without loss of consciousness.

The intercollegiate sports with the highest incidence of concussion are ice hockey, football, and both men's and women's soccer. High school TBI rates are the highest for football but are also substantial for wrestling, boys' and girls' soccer, girls' basketball, and field hockey. The high rate of TBI in soccer, which is the world's most popular sport and one that has achieved great popularity in US suburbs, is not surprising because it is one of the few popular contact sports in which athletes do not wear helmets. Studies have shown that professional and amateur soccer players have subtle but undeniable impairments in memory, visual perception, and other higher intellectual functions, which are attributable to concussions from head-to-head collisions and falls, as well as "heading" the ball. Similarly, college football players develop neuropsychologic impairments related to multiple concussions and preexisting learning disabilities, which may have a synergistically detrimental effect.

"Soccer Moms" should consider the risks of soccer, especially compared to other sports. They should be especially protective of children with learning disabilities. They might ask soccer leagues to require protective headgear.

Dementia Pugilistica.   The consensus among neurologists is that single head injuries do not cause Parkinson's disease (see Chapter 18). Repeated injuries, however, can cause Parkinson-like symptoms. Thus, boxing is associated with TBI. Several boxers have succumbed to subdural hematomas. Also, in retrospect, many probably had second impact syndrome.

In addition, boxers sometimes develop *dementia pugilistica* ("punch drunk syndrome"), which consists of insidiously developing intellectual deterioration; dysarthria, stiffness and clumsiness, and spasticity; and characteristic Parkinson-like bradykinesia. It occurs most often in boxers who are lightweight, alcoholic, or have lost many fights. These deficits, which often herald the end of the boxer's career, may progress after retirement.

CT and MRI show white matter changes, focal contusions, and cerebral atrophy in proportion to the number of bouts. Autopsy studies reveal hydrocephalus and atrophy of the corpus callosum and cerebrum. As in Parkinson's disease, the substantia nigra is depigmented. Histologic examination shows Alzheimer-like neurofibrillary tangles and, with special stains, amyloid plaques. However, despite its similarity to diffuse Lewy body and Parkinson's diseases (see Chapter 7), dementia pugilistica does not lead to Lewy bodies. Despite dementia pugilistica, histologic changes, and occasionally fatal intracranial hemorrhages, boxing organizations have resisted demands for protective headgear in prizefights, as well as during practice.

MINOR HEAD TRAUMA

Minor head trauma, by definition, causes a loss or impairment of consciousness for less than 30 minutes and a GCS no lower than 13. Alternatively, it is sometimes given the operational definition of head trauma that does not require hospitalization. Most cases result from MVAs, occupational injuries, and sports accidents. Minor head trauma causes headache, confusion, mood changes, and a variety of other impairments. Symptoms last from several hours to as long as about 8 weeks. Individuals without prior injuries, neurologic or psychiatric conditions, substance abuse, or work-related issues generally have no permanent sequelae.

Postconcussion Syndrome

The *postconcussion syndrome* is the most important long-term consequence of minor head trauma. Although lacking a strict definition in the neurologic literature, it usually consists of several core symptoms—headache, memory impairment, and insomnia—lasting more than 2 to 3 months after a concussion. Otherwise, symptoms tend to be nonspecific, highly variable, occasionally unending, and entirely subjective. Some, such as "dizziness," are trivial and prevalent in the general population. Many times symptoms, particularly those stemming from heightened arousal, are clearly more indicative of Posttraumatic Stress Disorder (PTSD) than postconcussion syndrome.

In *DSM-IV*, Postconcussional Disorder is listed as requiring further study, and manifestations of concussion are suggested to include loss of consciousness, posttraumatic amnesia, and, "less commonly," posttraumatic seizures. These symptoms would reflect a much more severe injury than neurologists require for a diagnosis of concussion. The *DSM-IV* then offers "research criteria for Postconcussional Disorder," which are also stringent. Testing must show impairment of attention or memory. In addition, symptoms, which must last for more than three months following trauma, must consist of three or more of eight difficulties, including insomnia, easy fatigability, headache, and dizziness.

Physical neurologic examination of postconcussion syndrome patients shows no abnormality. CTs and MRIs are also normal. Neuropsychologic and physiologic test results, potentially influenced by medications, normal variations, preexisting injuries, and, in some cases, inattention, depression, exaggeration, and malingering, reveal no consistent, significant abnormality.

Proposed causes of the postconcussion syndrome include neuron shearing with diffuse axonal injury, subtle cerebral contusions, and neurochemical imbalance, especially of excitatory neurotransmitters. In addition, coexistent whiplash injury (see below) may cause headache, as well as neck pain and immobility.

Although the syndrome's existence is accepted, individual patients regularly provoke skepticism. Prolonged symptoms are associated with psychiatric and socioeconomic factors, as much as with neurologic injury. The syndrome rarely affects children, soldiers, or self-employed or professional people. Its severity and duration cannot be correlated with either estimated force of impact or the usual neurologic parameters—GCS scores and duration of retrograde or anterograde amnesia.

Duration of postconcussion syndrome is sometimes extraordinarily prolonged, especially in patients with abnormal premorbid intellectual and personality traits. For some, symptoms seem inextricably linked to potential monetary rewards and other aspects of unsettled litigation. Also noteworthy is that certain symptoms, such as headache and insomnia, appear refractory to treatment only in this syndrome and nowhere else.

To be fair, however, much data indicates that postconcussion syndrome results primarily from neurologic injury. In addition, symptoms are similar from patient to patient. The syndrome develops in many self-employed and highly motivated people, including physicians, and does not prevent most patients from returning to work. Neurologic symptoms are worse in patients with bodily injuries. In fact, contrary to long-held opinion, symptoms correlate poorly with outstanding litigation and often persist after legal claims are settled.

Many children and some stoic adults may not report these symptoms because they are unable to describe them, cannot admit to pain, or endure other symptoms. For example, rather than complaining of posttraumatic headaches, children may have somnolence, inattention, or hyperactivity. Professionals, also unable to describe their feelings, may seem unusually irritable. Finally, normal neurologic examination and laboratory test results should not exclude a neurologic diagnosis: neurologists routinely diagnose many illnesses—migraines, trigeminal neuralgia, chronic pain, and dementia—in the absence of physical and laboratory abnormalities.

Headache. The essential feature of postconcussion syndrome is dull, generalized, continuous headache. Movement, bending, work, and alcohol exacerbate it. In 50% of patients, headaches last longer than 1 year, and in 25% longer than 3 years. The headaches occur more frequently in mildly injured than in severely injured individuals. Although headaches cannot be correlated with the severity of the head trauma, the presence or duration of unconsciousness, or duration of amnesia, they are the symptom most closely associated with memory and concentration impairments.

Beware that not all headaches after trauma are merely postconcussion headaches. When they are hemicranial or throbbing, develop in a patient with a history of migraines, and are accompanied by autonomic nervous system dysfunction, headache may be predominantly *posttraumatic migraines* (see Chapter 9). In contrast, head trauma does not seem to provoke cluster headaches or trigeminal neuralgia. Other causes of posttraumatic headache are trauma to the cervical muscles, ligaments, and spine (see below, whiplash); temporomandibular joint; and supra-orbital nerve (neuralgia). Patients could also have the slow development of subdural hematomas. Another cause, partly iatrogenic, is daily use of analgesic or vasoactive medications causing "rebound or withdrawal headaches" (see Chapter 9).

Memory Impairment. A characteristic postconcussion symptom is mild or intermittent amnesia. It is typically accompanied by slowed information processing, inattention or inability to concentrate, and difficulty completing complex mental tasks. As with other postconcussion symptoms, amnesia shows little correlation with the severity of trauma.

One potential explanation for amnesia in postconcussion syndrome is that the frontal and temporal lobes were thrown against the inner surfaces of the frontal and middle fossa. Another is that PTSD has obscured events surrounding the trauma, as well as the trauma itself.

Insomnia. Postconcussion syndrome patients regularly report inability to fall or remain asleep. They also describe excessive daytime sleepiness (EDS), which forces them to nap (see Chapter 17). Neither nighttime sleep nor daytime naps are restful.

Major head trauma may damage the hypothalamus, but in postconcussion syndrome and other minor head trauma, there is no established explanation for the insomnia and EDS. One potential explanation is that patients are apt to consume excessive caffeine, alcohol, and other medications, especially opioids. In addition, as with the syndrome's other symptoms, insomnia is partially attributable to anxiety, depression, and PTSD.

Other Symptoms.   Postconcussion syndrome patients often report dizziness. In most cases, it is not authentic vertigo but a nonspecific sensation with variable, idiosyncratic meanings that include lightheadedness, anxiety, weakness, and unsteadiness. Except for patients who have vertigo because of sustained labyrinth damage from a temporal bone fracture, their dizziness is difficult to define and virtually impossible to treat.

Another common symptom is hypersensitivity to light (photophobia) and sound (phonophobia). Patients seemingly cannot tolerate routine levels of conversation, reading, or socializing. This hypersensitivity is distracting and intensifies the headaches.

In addition, patients often describe depression, anxiety, irritability, and moodiness, but rarely in so few words. They also typically report decreased desire for sex and other previously enjoyable activities.

In contrast, some may consciously or subconsciously minimize symptoms. Whether stoical or in denial, they fail to acknowledge amnesia, other cognitive deficits, and personality changes. Using poor judgment, they may attempt to fulfill all their commitments and work at demanding jobs.

Treatment and Recovery.   Neurologists attempt to educate the patient and family about the nature, extent, and course of postconcussion syndrome. Many urge patients with minor or vague symptoms to return to work, even with a reduced load or part time. With a patient refractory to treatment, neurologists often decide not to challenge the patient's and family's beliefs and, instead, to agree that symptoms exist, without necessarily accepting that they originate in permanent brain injury.

For the headaches, neurologists prescribe mild, nonaddicting analgesics similar to those used for muscle contraction headaches. Sometimes, even with only a minimal migraine component, antimigraine drugs are helpful (see Chapter 9). Neurologists also prescribe nonsteroidal anti-inflammatory drugs (NSAIDs) and tricyclic antidepressants, which are useful for insomnia and neck pain, as well as headaches. Sertraline (Zoloft) may improve certain aspects of PTSD.

In contrast, biofeedback has no demonstrable benefit, and cognitive retraining remains controversial. Psychotherapy and antidepressants in therapeutic doses may be indicated for anxiety or depression. Psychiatrists should assume the care of patients whose primary problem is PTSD rather than TBI.

Insomnia must be treated cautiously. Hypnotics can easily lead to EDS, mimic symptoms of TBI, and produce cognitive impairment. Alcohol must be forbidden because it may induce behavioral changes, insomnia, EDS, headaches, poor judgment, and fatigue.

Virtually all patients improve somewhat. About 85% fully recover. None get worse. In uncomplicated cases, recovery should take place by 3 months. However, some patients have persistent symptoms, recurrent symptoms under certain circumstances, or, in a small proportion of cases, incapacitating symptoms. Recovery from postconcussion symptoms is nonlinear, uncertain, and influenced by preexisting or apparently unrelated conditions. Risk factors for prolonged or incomplete recovery include the following:

- A history of attention deficit disorder, learning disability, or neurosis.

- Before the accident, the patient was of low socioeconomic status; an unskilled or semiskilled worker; dissatisfied with the job; or in danger of being fired.

- The concussion resulted from an MVA.

- Bodily pains accompany the postconcussion syndrome.

- The postconcussion syndrome includes numerous symptoms.

WHIPLASH

Mechanism of Action

In rear-end motor vehicle accidents, the head and neck of the driver and passengers are typically thrown backward (extended) by a sudden, unexpected large force. The neck extends beyond the normal range (hyperextends) because its anterior muscles are too weak to resist and too slow to react. The hyperextension can compress, strain, or merely momentarily pull the neck's soft tissues: ligaments, tendons, the large trapezius and paraspinal muscles, and the numerous, small, delicate muscles. Immediately afterward, as the head naturally rebounds, the neck rapidly flexes forward, and similar injuries might again ensue. This violent back-and-forth movement leads to *flexion-extension injury* or *whiplash* (Fig. 22–3).

Almost any forceful or rapid movement can aggravate degenerative spine disease (see Fig. 5–5). Large enough forces can herniate intervertebral disks. Disk fragments may compress nerve roots or even the spinal cord. Severe injuries, beyond the magnitude of whiplash, may fracture or dislocate cervical vertebrae and transect the spinal cord.

Unless the victim was not wearing a seatbelt or another unusual circumstance was present, whiplash victims usually do not sustain concomitant head trauma. Nevertheless, during the flexion and extension, the brain is thrown rapidly back and forth within the skull.

Symptoms

Symptoms are greatest when the patient is an unprepared driver or passenger of the car that was struck from behind ("rear-ended") and when the head and neck are turned or flexed at the time of impact. As in the postconcussion syndrome, whiplash symptoms' development, severity, and duration do not correlate with the speed of the MVA.

Whiplash patients describe incapacitating neck pain that is increased by either moving or holding still, as when reading or typing on a keyboard, for periods of longer than 5 to 10 minutes. Their pain radiates far beyond their neck to their head, shoulders, arms, and thoracic region. With simultaneous head trauma and whiplash, symptoms multiply.

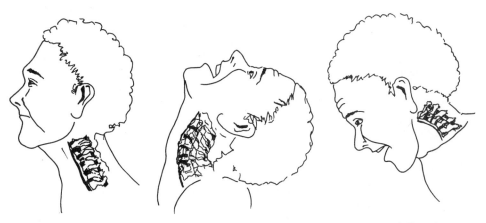

FIGURE 22–3. With rear-end collisions, the head and neck are thrown backward (extension). Then they snap forward (flexion). Flexion-extension or whiplash injuries can tear the longitudinal ligaments and other soft tissues, herniate intervertebral disks, and exacerbate cervical spondylosis (see Fig. 5–5).

When cervical intervertebral disks are herniated, patients typically have pain that radiates along the nerve roots (radicular pain), weakness, and loss of deep tendon reflexes in the arms. Herniated disks, as well as fractures and dislocations, are usually detectable with an MRI. Electromyograms (EMGs) are also helpful in establishing the injury's nature, severity, and extent. However, numerous other techniques, such as thermography, surface EMGs, and ultrasound, which have crept into the field, have no proven diagnostic reliability.

Even without head trauma, whiplash patients often have postconcussion symptoms, including cognitive impairments, mood changes, inattention, dizziness, and fatigue. In them, postconcussion symptoms are typically more extensive, prominent, and incapacitating than the neck pain and other whiplash symptoms. Despite prevalence of cognitive impairment and mood change following whiplash, the *DSM-IV*, in an apparent oversight, does not offer a description of the disorder.

Approximately 50% of patients recover by 3 months and 75% by 6 months. Still, 20% have symptoms for 2 years or longer. Risk factors for such prolonged disability include middle age, preexisting degenerative spine disease, and persistent headache and other postconcussion symptoms.

Treatment

The treatment of whiplash injury has not been subjected to rigorous examination and remains empiric and variable. Most patients improve with little or no treatment. Some respond to immobilization of their neck by rest, leisure, and wearing a soft foam rubber cervical collar. Patients with persistent symptoms usually respond to range of motion exercises, massage, and heat. However, they should avoid vigorous cervical manipulation, as occurs in chiropractic treatment, because it has led to spinal cord injury and vertebral artery damage in some cases. Medications for pain include muscles relaxants, NSAIDs, nonnarcotic analgesics, and—primarily for their analgesic and sedative effects—antidepressants. Migraine medications, according to some reports, may be helpful.

Whiplash patients (and most other adults) would probably benefit from good "neck hygiene." They should not cradle the telephone in their neck, especially when typing. If they frequently use a telephone, they should wear an expanded receiver or a headset. They should elevate the computer keyboard and monitor to a comfortable level. They should use only one pillow and should curtail tennis, golf, and other sports that strain the neck.

Although occupational, psychological, and legal issues must at least be acknowledged, effects of litigation are controversial. On one side is a landmark study by Obelieniene and others who found that rear-end MVA victims in Lithuania, a country disallowing personal injury lawsuits, described only minor, self-limited symptoms. By 1 year, victims were essentially indistinguishable from a control group. On the other side, litigating and nonlitigating patients have similar recovery rates. Moreover, most patients involved in litigation are not cured by its resolution.

REFERENCES

Annegers JF, Hauser A, Coan SP, et al: A population-based study of seizures after traumatic brain injuries. N Engl J Med *338*: 20–24, 1998

Barnes BC, Cooper L, Kirkendall DT, et al: Concussion history in elite male and female soccer players. Am J Sports Med *26*: 433–438, 1998

DeGiorgio CM, Lew MF: Consciousness, coma, and the vegetative state: Physical basis and definitional character. Issues Law Med *6*: 361–371, 1991

Cattelani R, Lombardi F, Brianti R, et al: Traumatic brain injury in childhood: Intellectual, behavioral and social outcome into adulthood. Brain Inj *12*: 283–296, 1998

Collins MW, Grindel SH, Lovell MR, et al: Relationship between concussion and neuropsychological performance in college football players. JAMA *282*: 964–970, 1999

Diaz-Olavarrieta C, Campbell J, Garcia de la Cadena C, et al: Domestic violence against patients with chronic neurologic disorders. Arch Neurology *56*: 681–685, 1999

DiScala C, Lescohier I, Barthel M, et al: Injuries to children with attention deficit hyperactivity disorder. Pediatrics *102*: 1215–1421, 1998

Friedman G, Froom P, Sazbon L, et al: Apolipoprotein E-ε 4 genotype predicts a poor outcome in survivors of traumatic brain injury. Neurology *52*: 244–248, 1999

Grafman J, Jonas BS, Martin A, et al: Intellectual function following penetrating head injury in Vietnam veterans. Brain *111*: 169–184, 1988

Jankovic J: Post-traumatic movement disorders: Central and peripheral mechanisms. Neurology *44*: 2006–2014, 1994

Jennett B, Bond M: Assessment of outcome after severe brain damage. The Lancet *5*: 480–484, 1975

Jennett B, Teasdale G, Braakman R, et al: Prognosis of patients with severe head injury. Neurosurgery *4*: 283–289, 1979

Jordan BD, Tsairis P, Warren RF (eds.): Sports Neurology. Philadelphia, Lippincott Williams & Wilkins, 1998

Kelly JP, Rosenberg JH: Diagnosis and management of concussion in sports. Neurology *48*: 575–580, 1997

Kleinschmidt KC: Elder abuse: A review. Ann Emerg Med *30*: 463–472, 1997

Levin HS, Gary HE, Eisenberg HM, et al: Neurobehavioral outcome 1 year after severe head injury. J Neurosurg *73*: 699–709, 1990

Matser EJT, Kessels AG, Lezak MD, et al: Neuropsychological impairment in amateur soccer players. JAMA *282*: 971–973, 1999

Matser JT, Kessels AGH, Jordan BD, et al: Chronic traumatic brain injury in professional soccer players. Neurology *51*: 791–796, 1998

Max JE, Robin DA, Lindgren SD, et al: Traumatic brain injury in children and adolescents: Psychiatric disorders at one year. J Neuropsychiatry and Clin Neurosci *10*: 290–297, 1998

Mayou R, Brant B, Duthie R: Psychiatric consequences of road traffic accidents. Br Med J *307*: 647–651, 1993

McCrory PR, Berkovic SF: Second impact syndrome. Neurology *50*: 677–683, 1998

Mehta KM, Ott A, Kalmijn S, et al: Head trauma and risk of dementia and Alzheimer's disease. The Rotterdam Study. Neurology *53*: 1959–1962, 1999

NIH Consensus Development Panel: Rehabilitation of persons with traumatic brain injury. JAMA *282*: 974–983, 1999

Obelieniene D, Schrader H, Bovim G, et al: Pain after whiplash: A prospective controlled inception cohort study. J Neurol Neurosurg Psychiatry *66*: 279–283, 1999

Pincus JH: Neurologist's role in understanding violence. Arch Neurol *50*: 867–868, 1993

Powell JW, Barber-Foss KD: Traumatic brain injury in high school athletes. JAMA *282*: 958–963, 1999

Quality Standards Subcommittee, American Academy of Neurology: Practice parameter: The management of concussion in sports. Neurology *48*: 581–585, 1997

Radanov BP, DiStefano G, Schnidrig A, et al: Cognitive functioning after common whiplash. Arch Neurol *50*: 87–91, 1993

Radanov BP, Sturzenegger M, DiStefano G, et al: Factors influencing recovery from headache after common whiplash. Br Med J *307*: 652–655, 1993

Roberts GW, Allsop D, Bruton C: The occult aftermath of boxing. J Neurol Neurosurg Psychiatr *53*: 373–378, 1990

Rosenthal M, Christensen BK, Ross TP: Depression following traumatic brain injury. Arch Phys Med Rehabil *79*: 90–103, 1998

Satz P, Forney DL, Zaucha K, et al: Depression, cognition, and functional correlates of recovery outcome after traumatic brain injury. Brain Inj *12*: 537–553, 1998

Schwab K, Grafman J, Salazar AM, et al: Residual impairments and work status 15 years after penetrating head injury: Report from the Vietnam Head Injury Study. Neurology *43*: 95–103, 1993

Silver JM, McAllister TW: Forensic issues in the neuropsychiatric evaluation of the patient with mild traumatic brain injury. J Neuropsychiatry *9*: 102–113, 1997

Spitzer WO, Skovron ML, Salmi LR, et al: Scientific monograph of the Quebec Task Force on whiplash-associated disorders: Redefining "whiplash" and its management. Spine *20* (Suppl 8S): 1S–73S, 1995

Teasdale G, Jennett B: Assessment of coma and impaired consciousness: A practical scale. Lancet *2*: 81–84, 1974

Volpe BT, McDowell FH: The efficacy of cognitive rehabilitation in patients with traumatic brain injury. Arch Neurol *47*: 220–222, 1990

Williams DB, Annegers JF, Kokman E, et al: Brain injury and neurologic sequelae: A cohort study of dementia, parkinsonism, and amyotrophic lateral sclerosis. Neurology *41*: 1554–1557, 1991

QUESTIONS and ANSWERS: CHAPTER 22

1. A 24-year-old man is brought to the emergency room after a motor vehicle accident (MVA). He is stuporous and has a Glasgow Coma Score (GCS) of 6. Skull x-rays show a fracture through his left temporal bone. During his transfer to a tertiary care hospital, he develops coma with decerebrate posturing and a left third cranial nerve palsy. On arrival, his GCS is 3. What is the most likely cause of his deterioration?

a. A subdural hematoma
b. Alcohol intoxication
c. Middle meningeal artery laceration
d. None of the above

    ANSWER: c. The young man has probably sustained a laceration of the middle meningeal artery from the temporal bone skull fracture. Bleeding from this artery has led to an epidural hematoma, which is a rapidly expanding, usually fatal, intracranial mass lesion. A GCS of 3 or less is associated with a fatal outcome.

2. Which two characteristics differentiate epidural from subdural hematomas?

a. Epidural hematomas originate from arterial bleeding, but subdural hematomas usually originate from venous bleeding.
b. Epidural hematomas are more likely to be fatal.
c. Epidural hematomas are more likely to be chronic.
d. Epidural hematomas are more likely to occur in the elderly.

    ANSWER: a, b. Subdural hematomas originate in venous bleeding, which is under lower pressure. Their bleeding is apt to stop spontaneously. Although subdural hematomas are usually reabsorbed slowly, they may persist and expand over weeks.

3. Which statement is untrue regarding chronic subdural hematomas?

a. On CT, they appear as a curved extra-axial lucency (black region).
b. They are a correctable cause of dementia.
c. They cause few physical deficits, such as hemiparesis, compared to nonspecific symptoms, such as headaches and personality changes.
d. The elderly are prone to subdural hematomas because they have cerebral atrophy and a tendency to fall.
e. Many chronic subdural hematomas are reabsorbed without the need for surgery.
f. On CT, they are typically radiodense.

    ANSWER: f. Acute subdural hematomas, which contain fresh blood, are radiodense.

4. Which single condition is most likely to follow in a head trauma patient with a GCS of 7?

a. Anterograde amnesia   c. Chronic neck pain
b. Postconcussion syndrome   d. Seizures

    ANSWER: a. In cases of moderately severe TBI, anterograde and retrograde amnesia is the most common residual effect. Seizures are also associated with TBI, but the association is not as close. Postconcussion syndrome and neck pains have only inconsistent associations.

5. To which injury can the term *contrecoup* apply?

a. Temporal lobe, especially the temporal tip, injury after an occipital blow
b. Blindness after an occipital lobe blow
c. Diffuse axonal injury after localized head trauma
d. Neck pain after head injury

    ANSWER: a. Head trauma that damages the opposite side of the brain is a *contrecoup* injury. These injuries can be envisioned as resulting from the brain "bouncing against the other side of the skull." They are most apparent in areas where the brain strikes rough or sharpened inner surfaces of the skull, such as in the middle fossa, which hold the temporal lobes. Temporal lobe injuries result in the characteristic posttraumatic memory impairments (amnesia).

6. Shrapnel and other foreign bodies that are retained in the brain are frequently uncorrectable sequelae of penetrating head injuries. Which two are their consequences?

a. They may act as a scar focus for posttraumatic epilepsy.
b. Depending on their position, they are associated with general cognitive impairments.
c. They may act as a nidus for a brain abscess.
d. They can cause a permanent state of coma.

> **ANSWER:** a, c. In general, posttraumatic cognitive impairments are related to the severity and extent of the brain injury, not its location. One exception is that dominant temporal lobe lesions are related to a posttraumatic aphasia and other language disorders. TBI patients may remain in coma for up to 3 weeks. After that time, if they do not succumb, their level of consciousness returns toward normal or evolves into a persistent vegetative state.

7. Which two injuries specifically suggest the "shaken baby syndrome" rather than blunt trauma?

a. Retinal hemorrhages
b. Occipital skull fracture
c. Blood in the interhemispheric fissure
d. Nasal fracture
e. Wrist fracture

> **ANSWER:** a, c. Shaken babies suffer from raised intracranial pressure and intracranial bleeding. Most shaken babies do not have skull or long bone fractures or obvious soft tissue injuries. The other injuries, of course, are signs of overt child abuse.

8. Which cognitive function is most susceptible to head trauma?

a. Judgment
b. Language function
c. Memory
d. Constructional ability

> **ANSWER:** c. Amnesia for the event is common. It is often accompanied by retrograde amnesia. With temporal and frontal lobe damage, patients have antegrade amnesia.

9. Of the following, which variety of seizure is the most common manifestation of posttraumatic epilepsy?

a. Psychogenic
b. Focal with secondary generalization
c. Petit mal
d. Primary generalized

> **ANSWER:** b. Focal (partial) seizures, including partial complex seizures, result from cerebral cortex injury. Primary generalized seizures—petit mal (absences) and tonic-clonic—do not result from head trauma.

10. Which one of the following statements regarding dementia pugilistica is untrue?

a. It mimics Parkinson's disease: tremors, rigidity, and depigmentation of the substantia nigra.
b. Histologic examination shows Alzheimer's-like cerebral plaques and tangles.
c. It occurs most frequently in lightweight boxers and alcoholics.
d. Gross examination shows atrophy of the corpus callosum and the cerebrum.
e. Histologic examination shows Lewy bodies in the basal ganglia.

> **ANSWER:** e. Although dementia pugilistica shares many clinical and histologic features with Parkinson's disease, Lewy bodies is not one of them.

11. Which are the two most reliable guidelines of the seriousness of a head injury?

a. GCS score
b. Duration of amnesia
c. Seizure on impact
d. Blood alcohol level

> **ANSWER:** a, b. The depth of coma is measured by the GCS. Both retrograde and anterograde amnesia correlate with the seriousness of head injury.

12. Which two regions of the brain are most likely to be injured in a coup-contrecoup injury?

a. Frontal lobe
b. Parietal lobe
c. Occipital lobe
d. Temporal lobe tips
e. Cerebellum
f. Brainstem

ANSWER: a, d. Coup-contrecoup injuries have their greatest impact on the temporal lobe and frontal lobes' anterior-inferior surface because those areas are rough and abut against sharp surfaces of the anterior and middle fossae.

13. Which three of the following are typically found in the subarachnoid space?

a. Cerebrospinal fluid (CSF)
b. Urine
c. Purulent CSF in cases of meningitis
d. Epidural hematomas in cases of major head trauma
e. Blood from ruptured berry aneurysms
f. Aqueous humor

ANSWER: a, c, e. The subarachnoid space, which is situated between the arachnoid and the pia layers of the meninges, normally contains CSF. The CSF becomes purulent in meningitis and bloody with subarachnoid hemorrhages from ruptured berry aneurysms and trauma. The subarachnoid space surrounds the brain and spinal cord. It extends down into the lumbar sac. Lumbar punctures (LP) needles are inserted into the subarachnoid space to sample the CSF.

14. Which of these statements is false regarding cognitive impairment following major TBI?

a. Recovery is slower and less complete in patients older than 65 years compared to younger patients.
b. Recovery of motor and language skills usually reaches a maximum within 6 months after the injury.
c. Intellectual recovery, to the extent that it occurs, takes place sooner than motor recovery.
d. Cognitive impairment correlates with low GCS scores

ANSWER: c. Intellectual recovery may be delayed until 18 months. It may be further delayed in individuals older than 65 years and by other factors (see below).

15. Which of these statements is false regarding cognitive impairment following major TBI?

a. Cognitive impairment correlates with the lesion's size.
b. Cognitive impairment correlates with the lesion's location.
c. Use of alcohol may add to posttraumatic cognitive impairment.
d. Use of antiepileptic drugs may add to posttraumatic cognitive impairment.

ANSWER: b. With one exception, the traumatic lesion's location does not correlate with the presence or severity of cognitive impairment. Left temporal lesions are associated with aphasia-like difficulties.

16. For children who survive TBI, which of these intelligence subtests will usually show the greater impairment?

a. Verbal
b. Performance

ANSWER: b. Performance subtests require intact visuomotor perception, dexterity, and attentiveness. Verbal subtests may be difficult, but they are based on a more limited set of cognitive functions.

17. Which of the following statements describes postconcussion headaches?

a. Their severity is proportional to the duration of unconsciousness.
b. Their severity is proportional to the severity of the head trauma.
c. Of the common symptoms, they are most closely associated with symptoms of memory and concentration impairment.
d. They are a risk factor for posttraumatic epilepsy.

ANSWER: c. As with the other postconcussion symptoms, headaches show little correlation with the duration of unconsciousness or severity of trauma. Concussions, including those followed by prolonged postconcussion symptoms, carry only a negligible risk for posttraumatic epilepsy.

APPENDIX 1

Patient and Family Support Groups

The following organizations provide patients and their families with educational, legal, medical, and personal assistance. However, because these groups often consist disproportionately of incapacitated patients, a personal visit may be discouraging. Some organizations provide educational materials for physicians.

A site that serves as a clearinghouse for all illnesses is www.healthfinder.gov

Acquired immune deficiency syndrome (AIDS)

Gay Men's Health Crisis
119 West 24th Street, New York, NY 10011
800-AIDS-NYC (Hotline)
212-367-1000
212-367-1220 (Fax)
Web site: www.gmhc.org

Alzheimer's disease

Alzheimer's Association
919 North Michigan Avenue, Suite 1000, Chicago, IL 60611-1676
800-272-3900
312-335-8700
312-335-1110 (Fax)
Web site: www.alz.org

Amyotrophic lateral sclerosis (ALS)

The Amyotrophic Lateral Sclerosis Association
27001 Agoura Road, Calabasas Hills, CA 91301-5104
800-782-4747
818-880-9007
818-880-9006 (Fax)
Web site: www.alsa.org

Aphasia and related disorders

American Speech-Language-Hearing Association
10801 Rockville Pike, Rockville, MD 20852
800-638-8255
301-897-5700
301-571-0457 (Fax)
Web site: www.asha.org

National Aphasia Association
156 Fifth Avenue, Suite 707, New York, NY 10010
800-922-4622
212-255-4329
Web site: www.aphasia.org

Blepharospasm

Benign Essential Blepharospasm Research Foundation
PO Box 12468, Beaumont, TX 77726-2468
409-832-0788
409-832-0890 (Fax)
Web site: www.blepharospasm.org/~bebrf

Blindness

American Foundation for the Blind
11 Penn Plaza, Suite 300, New York, NY 10001
800-232-5463
212-502-7600
212-502-7777 (Fax)
Web site: www.afb.org

Brain tumors

American Brain Tumor Association
2720 River Road, Suite 146, Des Plaines, IL 60018
800-886-2282
847-827-9910
847-827-9918 (Fax)
Web site: www.abta.org

Children's Brain Tumor Foundation
274 Madison Avenue, Suite 1301, New York, NY 10016
212-448-9494
212-448-1022 (Fax)
Web site: www.cbtf.org

National Brain Tumor Foundation
414 13th Street, Suite 700, Oakland, CA 94612-2603
800-934-CURE
510-839-9777
510-839-9779 (Fax)
Web site: www.braintumor.org

Cerebral palsy

United Cerebral Palsy Association
1660 L Street NW, Suite 700, Washington, DC 20036-5602
800-USA-5UCP
202-776-0406
202-776-0414 (Fax)
Web site: www.ucpa.org

Dystonia

Dystonia Medical Research Foundation and National Spasmodic Dysphonia Association
One East Wacker Drive, Suite 2430, Chicago, IL 60601-1905
800-377-DYST
312-755-0198
312-803-0138 (Fax)
Web site: www.dystonia-foundation.org

Epilepsy

Epilepsy Foundation of America
4351 Garden City Drive, Landover, MD 20785-2267
800-332-1000
301-459-3700
301-577-2684 (Fax)
Web site: www.epilepsyfoundation.org

Guillain-Barré syndrome

Guillain-Barré Syndrome Foundation International
PO Box 262, Wynnewood, PA 19096
610-667-0131
610-667-7036
Web site: www.webmast.com/gbs

Head injury

Brain Injury Association, Inc.
105 North Alfred Street, Alexandria, VA 22314
800-444-6443
703-236-6000
703-236-6001 (Fax)
Web site: www.biausa.org

Huntington's disease

Huntington's Disease Society of America
158 West 29th Street, 7th Floor, New York, NY 10001-5300
800-345-4372
212-242-1968
212-239-3430 (Fax)
Web site: www.hdsa.org

Migraine and headache

American Council for Headache Education
19 Mantua Road, Mt. Royal, NJ 08061
856-423-0258
856-423-0082 (Fax)
Web site: www.achenet.org

The National Headache Foundation
428 West St. James Place, Chicago, IL 60614-2750
800-843-2256 / 800-NHF-5552
773-388-6399
773-525-7357 (Fax)
Web site: www.headaches.org

Multiple sclerosis

National Multiple Sclerosis Association of America (MSAA)
706 Haddonfield Road, Cherry Hill, NJ 08002-2652
800-LEARN-MS
609-488-4500
609-661-9797 (Fax)
Web site: www.msaa.com

National Multiple Sclerosis Society
733 Third Avenue, New York, NY 10017-3288
800-FIGHT-MS
212-986-3240
212-986-7981 (Fax)
Web site: www.nmss.org

Muscular dystrophy and related disorders

Muscular Dystrophy Association, Inc.
10 East 40th Street, New York, NY 10019
212-689-9040

Muscular Dystrophy Association
3300 East Sunrise Drive, Tucson, AZ 85718-3208
800-572-1717
520-529-2000
520-529-5300 (Fax)
Web site: www.mdusa.org

Myasthenia gravis

Myasthenia Gravis Foundation of Greater New York
61 Gramercy Park North, Room 605, New York, NY 10010
212-533-7005

Myasthenia Gravis Foundation of America
123 West Madison, Suite 800, Chicago, IL 60602-4503
800-541-5454
312-853-0522
312-853-0523 (Fax)
Web site: www.myasthenia.org

Neurofibromatosis

The National Neurofibromatosis Foundation
95 Pine Street, 16th Floor, New York, NY, 10005
800-323-7938
212-344-6633
212-747-0004 (Fax)
Web site: www.nf.org

Pain

American Chronic Pain Association
PO Box 850, Rocklin, CA 95677-0850
916-632-0922
916-632-3208 (Fax)
Web site: www.theacpa.org

International Association for the Study of Pain
909 NE 43rd Street, Suite 306, Seattle, WA 98105-6020
206-547-6409
206-547-1703 (Fax)
Web site: www.halcyon.com/iasp

Paraplegia

See *Spinal cord injury*

Parkinson's disease

National Parkinson Foundation
1501 NW Ninth Avenue, Bob Hope Road, Miami, FL 33136
800-327-4545
305-547-6666
305-243-4403 (Fax)
Web site: www.parkinson.org

Parkinson's Disease Foundation
William Black Medical Research Building, Columbia Presbyterian Medical Center
710 West 168th Street, New York, NY 10032-9982
800-457-6676
212-923-4700
212-923-4778 (Fax)
Web site: www.pdf.org

United Parkinson's Foundation
833 West Washington Boulevard, Chicago, IL 60607
312-733-1893

Postpolio syndrome

International Polio Network
4207 Lindell Boulevard, #110, St. Louis, MO 63108-2915
314-534-0475
314-534-5070 (Fax)
Web site: www.post-polio.org

Rett syndrome

International Rett Syndrome Association
9121 Piscataway Road, Number 2B, Clinton, MD 20735
800-818-RETT
301-856-3334
301-856-3336 (Fax)
Web site: www.rettsyndrome.org

Sleep disorders

American Sleep Disorders Association
6301 Bandel Road, Suite 101, Rochester, MN 55901
507-287-6006
507-287-6008 (Fax)
Web site: www.asda.org

Spasmodic dysphonia

See *Dystonia*

Spasmodic torticollis

National Spasmodic Torticollis Association
9920 Talbert Avenue, Suite 233, Fountain Valley, CA 92708
800-HURTFUL
714-378-7838
714-378-7830 (Fax)
Web site: www.bluheronweb.com/NSTA/NSTA

Spina bifida

Spina Bifida Association of America
4590 MacArthur Boulevard, NW, Suite 250, Washington, DC, 20007-4226
800-621-3141
202-944-3285
202-944-3295 (Fax)
Web site: www.sbaa.org

Spinal cord injury

American Paralysis Association
500 Morris Avenue, Springfield, NJ 07081
800-225-0292
973-379-2690
973-912-9433 (Fax)
Web site: www.apacure.org

National Spinal Cord Injury Association
The Zalco Building, 8701 Georgia Avenue, Suite 500, Silver Spring, MD 20910
800-962-9629
301-588-6959
301-588-9414 (Fax)
Web site: www.spinalcord.org

Paralyzed Veterans of America
801 18th Street NW, Washington, DC 20006
800-424-8200
202-872-1300
Web site: www.pva.org

Stroke

American Heart Association
7272 Greenville Avenue, Dallas, TX 75231-4596
800-242-8721
214-706-1552
214-706-2139 (Fax)
Web site: www.americanheart.org

National Stroke Association
96 Inverness Drive East, Suite I, Englewood, CO 80112-5112
800-787-6537
303-649-9299
303-649-1328 (Fax)
Web site: www.stroke.org

Tourette syndrome

National Tourette Syndrome Association
42-40 Bell Boulevard, Bayside, NY 11361-2874
800-237-0717
718-224-2999
718-279-9596 (Fax)
Web site: www.tsa.mgh.harvard.edu

Tuberous sclerosis

National Tuberous Sclerosis Association
8181 Professional Place, Suite 110, Landover, MD 20785
800-225-6872
301-459-9888
301-459-0394 (Fax)
Web site: www.ntsa.org

Tremor

International Tremor Foundation
7046 West 105th Street, Overland Park, KS 66212-1803
913-341-3880

Wilson's disease

National Center for the Study of Wilson's Disease
432 West 58th Street, Suite 614, New York, NY 10019
212-523-8717
212-523-8708
Web site: www.wilsonsdiseasecenter.org

Cost of Various Tests and Treatments*

Tests and Treatments	Cost (Dollars)
Tests	
Computed tomography (CT) of head	850
CT of head with contrast	980
CT of spine without contrast	900
DNA test for:	
Fragile X	275
Huntington's disease	300
Myotonic dystrophy	275
Dystrophin Western blot (for Duchenne's muscular dystrophy)	800
Electroencephalogram (EEG)	270
With video-telemetry (per hour)	500
Electromyography (EMG)	250–750
Evoked response testing	400–500
Lumbar puncture (spinal tap)	350
Magnetic resonance imaging (MRI) of head	1,500
MRI of head with gadolinium	2,100
Nerve conduction velocity (NCV), per nerve	50
Typical cost for a study	800–1,200
Sleep studies	
Multiple sleep latency test (MSLT)	1,200
Polysomnography (PSG) for 2 nights	3,000
Positron emission tomography (PET)	3,500
Single-photon emission computed tomography (SPECT)	950
Syphilis tests	
Fluorescent treponemal antibody absorption (FTA-ABS)	35
Rapid plasma reagin (RPR)	14
Treponema microhemagglutination assay (MHA-TP)	48
Venereal Disease Research Laboratory (VDRL)	21
Treatments	
Deep brain stimulation for essential or Parkinson's tremor	25,000
Monthly wholesale cost of commonly prescribed medications:	
Aricept (donepezil 10 mg/day) for Alzheimer's disease	150
Depakote (divalproex sodium, 1500 mg/day)	40
Dilantin (phenytoin 300 mg/day) for epilepsy	30
Nelfinavir (protease inhibitor) for AIDS	600
Imitrex (sumatriptan, 50 mg pill)	12

Tests and Treatments	Cost (Dollars)
Treatments *(Continued)*	
Immunomodulator therapy for multiple sclerosis (e.g., interferon β-1b or β-1a, glatiramer)	900
Requip (ropinirole 3 mg/day) for Parkinson's disease	80
Sinemet (L-dopa/carbidopa 25/250 mg TID)	60
Viagra (sildenafil 50 mg, per pill)	10
Zidovudine (ZDV) treatment for AIDS	350
Nursing home care, annual	62,000
Penile prostheses and other treatment for erectile dysfunction	
Implants	
Inflatable	4,600
Semirigid	3,700
Injections of vasoactive medications (per erection)	10
Vacuum devices	300
Plasmapheresis (treatment for Guillain-Barré syndrome and myasthenia gravis crisis, for example)	2,500

*Approximate costs of representative tests and treatments in New York City, year 2000.

Diseases Transmitted by Chromosome Abnormalities, Mitochondria Abnormalities, and Excessive Trinucleotide Repeats

A. Chromosomes and the Diseases They Transmit

3 von Hippel-Lindau disease

4 Huntington's disease

5 Infantile and juvenile spinal muscular atrophy (Werdnig-Hoffmann and Kugelberg-Welander diseases)
   Tay-Sachs disease

6 Narcolepsy
   Spinocerebellar degeneration (Type 1)

7 Williams syndrome

9 Dystonia (early-onset primary dystonia, DYT1)
   Friedreich's ataxia
   Tuberous sclerosis (TSC1)

10 Metachromatic leukodystrophy

11 Acute intermittent porphyria
    Ataxia telangiectasia

12 Phenylketonuria
    Tuberous sclerosis

13 Wilson's disease

14 Alzheimer's disease, early onset
    Dopamine-responsive dystonia
    Porphyria variegata

15 Angelman syndrome
    Dyslexia
    Prader-Willi syndrome
    Tay-Sachs disease, GM2 gangliosidosis

16 Tuberous sclerosis (TSC2)

17 Charcot-Marie-Tooth disease
    Frontotemporal dementia
    Neurofibromatosis type 1 (NF1), peripheral, von Recklinghausen disease

18 Tourette syndrome

19   Alzheimer's disease, familial, late onset
     Apolipoprotein E (Apo-E)*
     Familial hemiplegic migraine
     Malignant hyperthermia (ryanodine receptor)
     Myotonic dystrophy

20   Creutzfeldt-Jakob, familial prion disease
     (Gerstmann-Scheinker-Strauss)

21   Alzheimer's disease, early onset familial
     Amyloid precursor protein (APP)*
     Amyotrophic lateral sclerosis (ALS), familial
     Progressive myoclonic epilepsy

22   Metachromatic leukodystrophy
     Neurofibromatosis type 2 (NF2), familial acoustic neuroma

X   Adrenoleukodystrophy
     Becker's muscular dystrophy
     Duchenne's muscular dystrophy
     Fragile X
     Lesch-Nyhan syndrome
     Mental retardation, nonspecific
     Spastic paraplegia

*Genes associated with risk factors.

B. Diseases Transmitted by Chromosomes (Number) or Mitochondria (*)

Acute intermittent porphyria (11)
Adrenoleukodystrophy (X)
Alzheimer's disease, early onset familial (14, 21)
Alzheimer's disease, late onset familial (19)
Amyloid precursor protein (APP) (21)[†]
Amyotrophic lateral sclerosis (ALS), familial (21)
Angelman syndrome (15)
Apolipoprotein E (Apo-E) (19)[†]
Ataxia telangiectasia (11)
Becker's muscular dystrophy (X)
Charcot-Marie-Tooth (17)
Creutzfeldt-Jakob, familial prion disease (20)
(Gerstmann-Schenker-Strauss)
Cytochrome c oxidase deficiency*
Dopamine-responsive dystonia (14)
Duchenne's muscular dystrophy (X)
Dyslexia (15)
Dystonia, early-onset primary dystonia, DYT1 (9)
Familial hemiplegic migraine (19)
Fragile X (X)
Friedreich's ataxia (9)
Frontotemporal dementia (17)
Huntington's disease (4)
Kugelberg-Welander disease (spinal muscular atrophy Type III) (5)
Leigh's syndrome*
Lesch-Nyhan syndrome (X)
Malignant hyperthermia (ryanodine receptor) (19)
MELAS (mitochondrial encephalomyopathy, lactic acidosis, stroke)*
Mental retardation, nonspecific (X)

MERRF (myoclonic epilepsy, ragged red fibers)*
Metachromatic leukodystrophy (10)
Myotonic muscular dystrophy (19)
Narcolepsy (6)
Neurofibromatosis NF1, peripheral, von Recklinghausen disease (17)
Neurofibromatosis NF2, familial acoustic neuroma (22)
Phenylketonuria (12)
Prader-Willi syndrome (15)
Porphyria variegata (14)
Progressive external ophthalmoplegia*
Progressive myoclonic epilepsy (21)
Spastic paraplegia (X)
Spinal muscular atrophy (5)
Spinocerebellar degeneration, Type 1 (6)
Tay-Sachs disease (5)
Tay-Sachs disease, GM2 gangliosidosis (15)
Tourette's syndrome (18)
Tuberous sclerosis (9, 16)
von Hippel-Lindau disease (3)
Werdnig-Hoffmann disease (spinal muscular atrophy Type I) (5)
Williams syndrome (7)
Wilson's disease (13)

---

*For additional and continually updated information visit www.genetests.org.
†Alzheimer's disease markers.

C. Diseases Transmitted by Mitochondria

Cytochrome c oxidase deficiency
Leigh's syndrome
MELAS (mitochondrial encephalomyopathy, lactic acidosis, stroke)
MERRF (myoclonic epilepsy, ragged red fibers)
Progressive external ophthalmoplegia

D. Diseases Transmitted by Excessive Trinucleotide Repeats

Disease	Transmission	Chromosome	Trinucleotide
Fragile X syndrome	Sex linked	X	CGG
Friedreich's ataxia	Autosomal recessive	9	GAA
Huntington's disease	Autosomal dominant	4	CAG
Myotonic dystrophy	Autosomal dominant	19	CTG
Spinocerebellar atrophies			
Type 1	Autosomal dominant	6	CAG
Type 2	Autosomal dominant	12	CAG
Type 3*	Autosomal dominant	14	CAG

---

*Machdo-Joseph disease.

Additional Review Questions

1. A 60-year-old man is brought for evaluation of dementia. On mental status testing he performs poorly on tests that are dependent on memory. In contrast, he satisfactorily answers questions that require judgment, language skills, and abstract reasoning. He has a tendency to be verbally aggressive and use profanities excessively. He has a snout and bilateral palmomental reflexes. Of the following, which condition is most likely the cause of his mental status changes?

a. Alzheimer's disease
b. Depression
c. A nonspecific dementia
d. Vascular dementia
e. None of the above

ANSWER: e. Despite his cognitive impairment and behavioral disturbances, this patient cannot be diagnosed as having dementia. Instead, he can be said to have an amnestic syndrome, in which memory is impaired exclusively. In typical cases of Alzheimer's disease and vascular dementia, memory is impaired along with other intellectual functions. In addition, vascular dementia produces physical impairments roughly in proportion to the cognitive impairment. Although Alzheimer's disease can produce an amnestic syndrome, this syndrome is a typical feature of Wernicke-Korsakoff syndrome, temporal lobe injury, and *herpes simplex* encephalitis. In some of these conditions, features of the Klüver-Bucy syndrome accompany memory impairment. Frontal release signs, except perhaps for bilateral grasp reflexes, are not diagnostically helpful, except that they indicate an organic rather than traditional psychiatric cause of mental impairment.

2. When used to alleviate excessive daytime sleepiness in narcolepsy patients, modafinil has all the following effects except which one of the following?

a. It probably acts as an α-1 adrenergic agonist.
b. It promotes wakefulness without causing excitation or nighttime insomnia.
c. It does not suppress cataplexy.
d. Stopping modafinil leads to a rebound in sleep.

ANSWER: d. Unlike stopping amphetamines and other stimulants, stopping modafinil does not lead to sleep rebound.

3. After a vigorous day of training, a 19-year-old Marine recruit suddenly develops a temperature of 103° F and then stupor. He is brought to the emergency room where he is found to have nuchal rigidity. Which three therapies or diagnostic tests should be performed as soon as possible?

a. Intravenous fluids and electrolytes
b. Oral antiepileptic drugs
c. Thiamine (50 mg IV)
d. Lumbar puncture (LP)
e. Penicillin or penicillin in combination with another antibiotic

ANSWER: a, d, e. Children and young adults brought into large groups from different geographic locations occasionally develop outbreaks of meningitis. These small epidemics typically occur in kindergartens and military recruit barracks. Most cases of acute bacterial meningitis are fatal unless treated promptly with intravenous antibiotics. In this setting, the stupor and nuchal rigidity indicate meningitis. A subarachnoid hemorrhage, which could be responsible, can be diagnosed by examination of the spinal fluid by the LP.

4. A 30-year-old man has a long history of aggressive behavior and other antisocial activities. His EEG shows an isolated, phase-reversed spike focus intermittently over the left frontal lobe. Which single statement is valid?

a. In retrospect, the behavioral disturbances were the result of partial complex seizures.
b. The EEG has absolutely no bearing on the case.

c. Specific EEG abnormalities are characteristically found in antisocial people.

d. Both the EEG and the behavior may reflect cerebral damage.

> **ANSWER:** d. The EEG indicates an area with epileptic potential in the left frontal lobe. The origin of the EEG abnormality is not necessarily a structural lesion. Nevertheless, in general, lesions in the frontal lobe as well as those in the temporal lobe can cause the partial complex seizures. However, because there are no stereotyped behavioral disturbances and the EEG shows no paroxysmal activity, most neurologists would not make the diagnosis of seizures at this time. Depending on the circumstances, further testing might be indicated.

5. An 8-year-old boy begins to have 10- to 20-second episodes of repetitive lip smacking, eyelid fluttering, and finger rubbing. During these episodes he is incoherent. Afterward he is confused and sleepy. What is the most likely diagnosis?

a. Absence (petit mal) seizures

b. Partial complex (psychomotor) seizures

c. Attention deficit disorder

d. Complex motor tics

> **ANSWER:** b. This child is having typical partial complex seizures: He has incoherence without loss of consciousness; stereotyped, simple, repetitive movements and sounds; and subsequent (postictal) confusion and somnolence. The distinction between absences and partial complex seizures in children may be difficult, but it is important. The relatively long duration and incoherence are inconsistent with complex motor tics, as well as absence (petit mal) seizures.

6. During the course of evaluation for dementia, a 68-year-old patient's CT reveals a small, calcium-containing, dense lesion without surrounding edema that arises from the right parietal convexity. It does not compress the underlying brain. Which two of the following symptoms might this lesion likely cause?

a. Dementia

b. Aphasia

c. Absence seizures

d. Partial seizures without secondary generalization

e. Partial seizures with secondary generalization

> **ANSWER:** d, e. The lesion is probably a small meningioma. Although a brain tumor, such meningiomas are common and usually innocuous. They might, however, cause seizures by irritating the underlying cortex. In this case, partial seizures arising from the parietal cortex might cause sensory symptoms on the left side of the body. Seizure activity might also undergo secondary generalization. Small meningiomas do not cause dementia. Especially in the elderly, they need not be removed.

7. Which one of the following patients is most likely to have a seizure?

a. A 65-year-old man with left Bell's palsy

b. A 70-year-old woman with a right third cranial nerve palsy and left hemiparesis

c. A 55-year-old woman with rapidly progressive paresis and sensory loss in her left arm and more so her left leg, which has hyperactive deep tendon reflexes (DTRs) and a Babinski sign

d. A 40-year-old man who, after an upper respiratory tract infection, develops ascending flaccid, areflexic weakness of both legs

> **ANSWER:** c. This patient has a lesion involving the right cerebral cortex that could cause seizures. She could have a parasagittal (parafalcine) meningioma, glioblastoma, or abscess. Patients are unlikely to have seizure if they have lesions in noncerebral cortex locations, such as the left seventh cranial nerve (a), right midbrain (b), or peripheral nerves, such as the Guillain-Barré syndrome (d).

8. Which of the following illnesses are inherited in an autosomal recessive pattern?

a. Duchenne's dystrophy

b. Hemophilia

c. Sickle cell disease

d. Phenylketonuria

e. Homocystinuria

f. Cystic fibrosis

g. Wilson's disease

h. Red-green color blindness

> **ANSWER:** c–g. Duchenne's dystrophy, hemophilia, and red-green color blindness are x-linked.

9. After a prolonged but eventually successful resuscitation from a cardiac arrest, a 70-year-old man has apathy and psychomotor retardation. He says only a few simple words. However, he repeats many long, complex phrases, and he accompanies singers on the radio. He does not have a hemiparesis or homonymous hemianopsia. What is the nature of this patient's language impairment?

a. Nonfluent aphasia
b. Fluent aphasia

c. Frontal lobe dysfunction
d. Isolation (transcortical) aphasia

ANSWER: d. Isolation (transcortical) aphasia results from isolation of the perisylvian language arc—Broca's area, the arcuate fasciculus, and Wernicke's area—from the remaining cerebral cortex. Most often, the nonlanguage cortex is destroyed by the anoxia. With the language arc remaining intact, patients are able to repeat words, phrases, and songs. However, because the language arc exists in isolation, patients are unable to integrate language with other intellectual functions. Although patients with language or other cognitive impairment may be difficult to examine, physicians should attempt to perform bedside testing for aphasia.

> **Tests for Aphasia**
> Observation of spontaneous speech
> Three formal tests
> > Comprehension
> > Naming
> > Repeating

10–15. Below are six sketches of spinal cords stained such that normal myelin is stained black and demyelinated areas remain white *(unstained)*. Crosshatching indicates Gray areas. Match the sketches with the descriptions of the clinical associations (a–f).

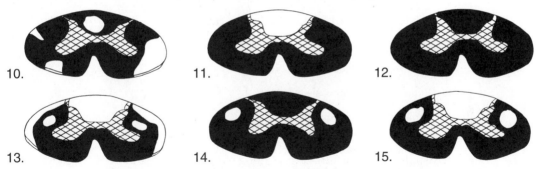

a. A 45-year-old man has had progressively severe intellectual and personality impairment for 4 years. On examination, he has loss of vibration and position sensation, absent reflexes in the legs, and a floppy-foot gait. His pupils are miotic. They constrict to closely regarded objects but not to light.
b. A 65-year-old man, who had a complete gastrectomy 4 years ago, now has dementia, hyperactive DTRs, bilateral Babinski signs, and loss of vibration sensation in the legs.
c. A 70-year-old woman has weakness of the left leg, right arm, and neck muscles. She has atrophy of many limb muscles. The physician sees fasciculations of her tongue and most atrophic muscles.
d. A 35-year-old man has optic neuritis, internuclear ophthalmoplegia, and gait impairment because of ataxia, weakness, and spasticity.
e. A 40-year-old woman and her sister have pes cavus, intention tremor of the limbs, and loss of position and vibration sensation.
f. A 70-year-old man who has schizophrenia sustains a frontal lobe gunshot wound. He takes phenytoin that leads to cerebellar dysfunction. He becomes so distraught that he becomes an alcoholic and suffers an episode of severe confusion, nystagmus, and bilateral abducens nerve palsy.

ANSWERS:

10. d. The spinal cord shows multiple areas (plaques) of demyelination (sclerosis). The patient has signs of optic nerve, brainstem, and spinal cord dysfunction. Both the clinical and pathologic information indicates multiple sclerosis (MS).
11. a. The spinal cord shows demyelination of the posterior columns. Loss of these tracts impairs position sensation and forces patients to walk with a high, uncertain,

and awkward pattern (i.e., a steppage gait). This patient has Argyll-Robertson pupils and mental abnormalities. This is a case of neurosyphilis of the brain and spinal cord (tabes dorsalis).

12. f. The spinal cord remains normal despite the cerebral injury, medication-induced cerebellar dysfunction, and Wernicke's encephalopathy.

13. e. There is degeneration of the spinocerebellar, posterior column, and corticospinal tracts. Loss of the spinocerebellar and posterior column tracts, which indicates a spinocerebellar degenerative illness, such as Friedreich's ataxia, causes intention tremor, position and vibration sense loss, and a foot deformity (pes cavus).

14. c. The spinal cord shows demyelination of the lateral corticospinal tracts and loss of the anterior horns, which contain the motor neurons. This is the typical picture of motor neuron disease, in which both the upper and lower motor neuron systems degenerate. The patient has the clinical features of amyotrophic lateral sclerosis (ALS), the most common form of motor neuron disease.

15. b. The spinal cord shows demyelination of the posterior columns and the lateral corticospinal tracts. This pattern, combined system disease, is associated with B_{12} deficiency from pernicious anemia or surgical removal of the stomach because both conditions remove intrinsic factor. Combined system disease is associated with dementia, paraparesis, hyperactive DTRs, and position and vibration sense loss. These findings are similar to those of tabes dorsalis with dementia; however, while combined-system disease causes hyperactive DTRs and Babinski signs, tabes dorsalis causes hypoactive DTRs and Argyll-Robertson pupils but neither paraparesis nor Babinski signs.

16–20. Match the visual field loss (16–20) most closely associated with each condition (a–k).

16. Left homonymous hemianopsia with macular sparing

17. Fortification scotoma

18. Central scotoma, lasting for 2 weeks

19. Bitemporal hemianopsia

20. Unilateral superior quadrantanopia

a. Retinal injury (e.g., retinal detachment or embolus from carotid artery)
b. Psychogenic disturbance
c. Migraine with aura
d. Diabetes insipidus
e. Loss of libido
f. Optic atopy
g. Amaurosis fugax
h. Internal capsule infarction
i. Aphasia
j. Occipital infarction
k. Optic or retrobulbar neuritis

ANSWERS: 16-j; 17-c; 18-k; 19-d, e, f (all associated with pituitary tumors); 20-a

21. An 80-year-old man, who is being treated for depression, has developed right-sided frontal headaches. His vision in the right eye is impaired. Temporal arteries are prominent but not especially tender. There is no papilledema, hemiparesis, or other neurologic sign. Which two conditions must be considered immediately?

a. Open-angle glaucoma
b. Metastases to the skull
c. Meningioma
d. Optic neuritis
e. Temporal arteritis
f. Narrow-angle glaucoma

ANSWER: e, f. The diagnosis of temporal arteritis should be made rapidly because, if untreated, it can cause blindness or cerebral infarction. The most commonly used diagnostic tests are the sedimentation rate and temporal artery biopsy. Likewise, untreated glaucoma (both narrow- and open-angle) can rapidly lead to blindness, but open-angle glaucoma is not associated with tenderness or pain.

22–30. Match the ocular abnormality (22–30) with the most probable cause (a–k).

22. Right third cranial nerve paresis and left hemiparesis

23. Left sixth cranial nerve paresis and right hemiparesis

24. Right Horner's syndrome, right facial hypalgesia, right limb ataxia, and left limb and trunk hypalgesia

25. Internuclear ophthalmoplegia

26. Right sixth and seventh cranial nerve paresis and left hemiparesis

27. Ptosis, facial diplegia, and ophthalmoplegia with normally reactive pupils

28. Small, irregular pupils that accommodate but do not react

29. Fever, agitated confusion, and dilated pupils

30. Stupor, miosis, and pulmonary edema

a. Neuromuscular junction impairment
b. Anticholinergic intoxication
c. Right pontine lesion
d. Left pontine lesion
e. Left midbrain lesion
f. Right midbrain lesion
g. Midline, dorsal brainstem lesion
h. Left lateral medullary lesion
i. Right lateral medullary lesion
j. Syphilis
k. Opioids

ANSWERS: 22-f, 23-d, 24-i, 25-g, 26-c, 27-a (myasthenia gravis), 28-j, 29-b (scopolamine intoxication), 30-k (heroin or methadone overdose)

31. Which three of the following are found in Alzheimer's disease but not in normal elderly individuals?

a. Loss of brain weight
b. Increase in sulci width
c. Expansion of the lateral ventricles
d. Major loss of large cortical neurons
e. Marked reduction of choline acetyltransferase in the hippocampus
f. Cerebral atrophy
g. Multiple neurofibrillary tangles
h. Senile plaques

ANSWER: d, e, g. Cerebral atrophy (a, b, c), plaques (h), neurofibrillary tangles, and granulovacuolar degeneration are found in normal brains. However, they are present in greater concentrations in Alzheimer's disease brains.

32. A 60-year-old man with dementia has a gait abnormality in which he excessively raises his legs. He seems to be climbing as he walks. His pupils are small (miotic), poorly reactive, and irregular. What is the gait abnormality?

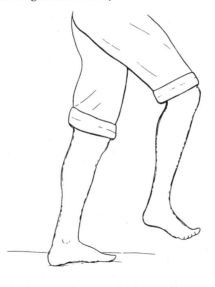

a. Gait apraxia
b. Congenital spastic paraparesis
c. Steppage gait from posterior spinal cord degeneration
d. Astasia abasia

> **ANSWER:** c. The patient has a steppage gait because he has lost position sense. He must raise his legs to avoid catching the tips of his toes when he walks and especially when he steps onto curbs. He has lost his position sense because he has tabes dorsalis and Argyll-Robertson pupils as a manifestation of tertiary syphilis. Loss of position sense from diabetic neuropathy or degenerative spinal cord diseases can also cause a steppage gait, but those diseases do not cause dementia.

33–35. Match the confabulation (33–35) with the lesion (a–c) that might produce it.

33. A blind patient "describes" clothing that an examiner is wearing. His pupils are round and reactive to light.

34. A man with recent onset of left hemiparesis claims that he cannot move his left arm and leg because he is too tired.

35. An agitated, diaphoretic middle-aged man describes bizarre occurrences and experiences visual hallucinations. When asked to repeat six digits, he seems to select random numbers.

a. Nondominant parietal lobe infarction
b. Bilateral occipital lobe infarctions
c. Hemorrhage into the limbic system

> **ANSWERS:**
>
> 33. b. In cortical blindness, some patients tend to confabulate (Anton's syndrome). Cortical blindness usually results from infarction or trauma of both occipital lobes. The pupils react normally because the optic and oculomotor nerves are unaffected.
> 34. a. Patients with hemiparesis from a nondominant hemisphere infarct often confabulate, deny, and use other defense mechanisms in ignoring their hemiparesis. Typically the right parietal lobe is the site of the lesion.
> 35. c. Patients with alcohol withdrawal can have confabulations. They may occur alone or as part of delirium tremens. However, the frequency of confabulations in Wernicke-Korsakoff syndrome is usually overestimated. Petechiae in the mamillary bodies constitute hemorrhage into the limbic system.

36. A 35-year-old man staggers into the emergency room. He is lethargic and disoriented. He has nystagmus, gait ataxia, and finger-to-nose dysmetria. Which illness is he most likely to have? What is the specific therapy?

a. Subdural hematoma
b. Cerebral infarction
c. Wernicke-Korsakoff syndrome
d. Psychogenic disturbance

> **ANSWER:** c. Thiamine 50 mg IV

37. An 11-year-old boy is admitted because of headache, nausea, and vomiting. He has had clumsiness for the 2 weeks before admission. He has papilledema, ataxia, bilateral hyperactive DTRs, and Babinski signs. Which is the most likely diagnosis?

a. MS
b. Drug abuse
c. Cerebellar tumor
d. Spinocerebellar degeneration

> **ANSWER:** c. Cerebellar astrocytomas, which are relatively common in children, block the aqueduct of Sylvius, creating obstructive hydrocephalus. The hydrocephalus increases intracranial pressure, which causes headaches, nausea, vomiting, and papilledema.

38. Which four of the following symptoms constitute the narcoleptic tetrad?

a. Inability to move on awakening (sleep paralysis)
b. Hunger or anorexia
c. Vivid dreams when falling asleep (hypnagogic hallucinations)
d. Attacks of daytime sleep (narcolepsy)
e. Night terrors (pavor nocturnus)
f. Episodic loss of muscle tone (cataplexy)
g. HLA
h. Excessive daytime sleepiness

ANSWER: a, c, d, f. The human leukocyte antigen (HLA) HLA-DQB1, which is located on chromosome 6, is detectable in more than 90% of cases of narcolepsy with cataplexy; however, it may not be detectable when cataplexy does not accompany narcolepsy. This antigen by itself does not produce the illness. Excessive daytime sleepiness is a characteristic of sleep apnea, use of several medications, and several other conditions, as well as narcolepsy.

39. An adolescent with a chronic, psychiatric disorder begins to drink large quantities of water and other fluids. After 1 week, he develops a seizure. Which three of the following conditions would most likely be responsible for the seizure?

a. Steroid abuse
b. Diabetes insipidus
c. Diabetes mellitus

d. Parkinson's disease
e. Huntington's disease
f. Psychogenic polydipsia

ANSWER: b, c. Polydipsia, whatever its cause, leads to seizures because it causes hyponatremia from "water intoxication." Alternatively, diabetes mellitus leads to hyperglycemia and secondarily hyponatremia.

40. Through which structure does CSF (cerebrospinal fluid) pass between the third and fourth ventricles?

a. Foramen of Monro
b. Lateral ventricles

c. Aqueduct of Sylvius
d. Arachnoid villa

ANSWER: c

41. A 23-year-old woman presents to a hospital with a 6-year history of progressively severe involuntary movement. She has no history of exposure to neuroleptics or any family member with similar symptoms. Her limbs, trunk, and neck continuously contort into sus-

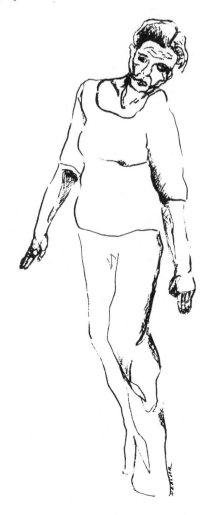

tained, twisting, and sometimes grotesque postures. Her muscles are hypertrophied. She has almost no body fat. Nevertheless, her cognitive function is normal. Of the following, which is the most likely cause of her condition?

a. Huntington's disease
b. Conversion disorder
c. Dystonia, early onset, DYT1
d. Tardive dystonia
e. Parkinson's disease
f. Cerebral palsy

> ***ANSWER:*** c. She has chronic dystonia. Her muscle hypertrophy and lack of bodily fat indicate its organic nature and chronicity. The most common causes of dystonia in young adults are early onset primary dystonia (torsion dystonia) from the DYT1 gene, tardive dystonia, Wilson's disease, the juvenile form of Huntington's disease, or, in children, dopa-responsive dystonia. Of the choices offered, the most likely is early onset dystonia from DYT1. Her physicians should inquire if her relatives are Ashkenazi Jews, which is the group that carries the DYT1 gene.

42. A 20-year-old sailor, who has a history of "glue sniffing," develops paresthesias and mild weakness in his hands and toes. Of the following, which single portion of the nervous system has been damaged?

a. Spinal cord
b. Corpus callosum
c. Peripheral nerves
d. Spinal cord
e. Neuromuscular junction

> ***ANSWER:*** c. Major components of glue, which carries a great potential for abuse, include N-hexane and other volatile hydrocarbon solvents. These substances, which are mostly lipophilic, permeate and damage the lipid-rich myelin cover of peripheral nerves. Chronic exposure causes a peripheral neuropathy.

43. Three weeks after recovering from an apparently successful repair of an anterior communicating artery aneurysm, a patient is apathetic and almost mute but not aphasic. The gait is short and hesitant. A psychiatry consultation has been solicited. Which one of the following is most likely to have complicated the aneurysm or surgery?

a. Posttraumatic stress disorder has developed.
b. Depression has developed.
c. Both anterior cerebral arteries were occluded.
d. The patient developed normal pressure hydrocephalus (NPH).
e. Dementia has developed.

> ***ANSWER:*** c. The anterior communicating arteries supply a large portion of the frontal lobes, including the medial surface of the motor cortex. Because this region controls the voluntary function of the legs and bladder, the patient should be tested for incontinence and paraparesis. Infarction of these arteries, from the aneurysm rupture or surgery, creates marked personality impairment, as well as incontinence and paraparesis. NPH sometimes develops after subarachnoid hemorrhages, but NPH patients have gait apraxia rather than paraparesis.

44. Which three of the following conditions often lead to patient's sensing "putrid smells" that the physician cannot detect?

a. Seizures that originate in the uncus
b. Sinusitis
c. Migraines
d. Seizures that originate in the parietal lobe
e. Valproic acid
f. Dental infections

> ***ANSWER:*** a, b, f. Migraines, curiously, often include visual but rarely auditory or olfactory auras. Infections in the sinuses and mouth are the most common causes of putrid smells.

45. For which conditions might an LP be indicated?

a. Subdural hematoma
b. Brain abscess
c. Brain tumor
d. Unruptured arteriovenous malformation (AVM)
e. Pseudotumor cerebri
f. MS
g. Bacterial meningitis

h. Subacute sclerosing panencephalitis
i. Viral encephalitis
j. Sexual impairment

ANSWER: e, f, g, h, i. LPs should not be done when intracranial mass lesions are suspected because CSF analysis will not be helpful and the procedure might precipitate transtentorial herniation.

46. In which part of the brain is the aqueduct of Sylvius located?

a. Cerebrum
b. Hypothalamus
c. Thalamus
d. Midbrain
e. Pons
f. Medulla

ANSWER: d

47. Which three of the following illnesses are characterized by a normal mental state despite quadriparesis and respiratory distress?

a. Guillain-Barré syndrome
b. Locked-in syndrome
c. Persistent vegetative state
d. Cervical spinal cord gunshot wound

ANSWER: a, b, d

48. An 11-year-old girl has developed twitchy, restless movements. She cannot protrude her tongue for 10 seconds. When her arms are extended, her fingers have individual flexion or extension movements. Except for irritability, her mental and emotional status is normal. Which tests would be most appropriate?

a. VDRL
b. Inquiries about oral contraceptives
c. Antistreptolysin O Titer (ALSO)
d. Pregnancy test
e. Lupus preparation

ANSWER: b, c, d, e. Chorea in adolescents may be a manifestation of rheumatic fever (Sydenham's chorea), lupus, or pregnancy (chorea gravidarum) or a reaction to oral contraceptives.

49. Which three procedures would be most helpful in determining the dominant hemisphere?

a. Positron emission tomography (PET)
b. Computed tomography (CT)
c. EEG with sphenoidal electrodes
d. Magnetic resonance imaging (MRI)
e. Intracarotid sodium amobarbital injection
f. Wada test
g. Visual evoked responses (VER)
h. Brainstem auditory evoked responses (BAER)

ANSWER: a, e, f. The Wada test is based on intracarotid amobarbital injections. Perfusion of the dominant hemisphere will induce aphasia.

50. When nonsteroidal anti-inflammatory agents are given for menstrual cramps, with which group of substance do they interfere?

a. Enkephalins
b. Endorphins
c. Prostaglandins
d. Serotonin
d. Dopamine

ANSWER: c

51. Which two statements are true regarding the dorsal raphe nucleus?

a. It contains high concentrations of endorphins.
b. Stimulating it causes pain.
c. Stimulating it produces analgesia.
d. Stimulating it produces behavioral changes.
e. Its destruction causes analgesia.
f. It contains high serotonin concentrations.

ANSWER: c, f

52. A 14-year-old boy is brought to the emergency room in a stupor. He is apneic, and his pupils are miotic. Which one of the following conditions is most likely to be the cause of this constellation of findings?

a. Brainstem stroke
b. Heroin overdose
c. Hypoglycemia

d. Postictal stupor
e. Psychogenic disturbance

ANSWER: b. Heroin overdose typically causes stupor, miosis, and apnea. It should be treated with naloxone (Narcan). Brainstem strokes may cause this constellation; however, they rarely occur in this age group. The other conditions generally cause dilated pupils but not apnea.

53–55. A 29-year-old woman has developed a tremor that is most pronounced when she writes, drinks coffee, and lights a cigarette.

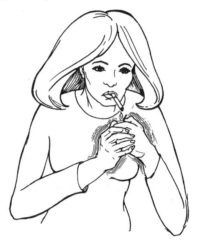

53. Which four of the following conditions can lead to such a tremor?

a. Essential tremor
b. Wilson's disease
c. Anxiety
d. Huntington's chorea

e. Athetosis
f. Benign familial tremor
g. Dystonia
h. Rett's syndrome

ANSWER: a, b, c, f. Essential tremor and benign familial tremor are probably varieties of the same condition. Wilson's disease is a rare but important condition that might be considered in young adults who develop a tremor. Anxiety can produce a tremor that is virtually indistinguishable from essential tremor: These two conditions may have a similar etiology and respond to β-adrenergic blockers.

54. Which two tests should be performed to exclude Wilson's disease when only mild tremors are evident?

a. MRI
b. SPECT
c. PET

d. Serum ceruloplasmin
e. Serum copper concentration
f. Slit-lamp examination

ANSWER: d, f

55. Which group of medications is most often effective for essential tremor?

a. Anticholinergics
b. Dopamine agonists
c. Neuroleptics

d. β-adrenergic blockers
e. Antiviral agents
f. α-adrenergic blockers

ANSWER: d

56. Of the following, which two characteristics distinguish classic neurotransmitters from endocrine hormones, such as thyroxine?

a. They or their by-products circulate in detectable quantities in the blood.
b. They are produced and stored at a site adjacent to the target organ.

c. They or their by-products are often present in detectable concentrations in the cerebrospinal fluid but not in the blood.

d. They are steroids.

ANSWER: b, c

57. *Plasticity* refers to neurons'

a. Mechanical properties
b. Ability to reorganize
c. Unchanging quality
d. Chemical properties

ANSWER: b. Plasticity means the capacity to being formed or molded. In neurologic terms, plasticity refers to the ability of the CNS to be reorganized. In general, the CNS is not plastic and reorganization does not take place. For example, the corticospinal tract always crosses. However, CNS plasticity has been postulated under certain circumstances, such as perpetuation of pain and partial recovery of some function after strokes.

58. A 28-year-old woman reports developing a gait impairment. She has a history of vigorous exercise, taking large quantities of "mega-vitamins," and avoiding red meat. She consumes no alcohol. On examination, she has marked sensory loss and absent DTRs in all limbs, but her strength is normal. Which one of the following conditions is most likely to be responsible for her symptoms?

a. Cervical spondylosis
b. Myopathy
c. Vitamin toxicity
d. Iron-deficiency anemia

ANSWER: c. Pyridoxine (vitamin B_6) in large daily doses creates a neuropathy that impairs sensation. The neuropathy is reversible after the vitamins are withdrawn. Thiamine and folate deficiency, often consequences of alcoholism, can also produce a neuropathy.

59. A 68-year-old house painter has weakness, atrophy, and areflexic DTRs in his arms. He has sensory loss in his right hand, brisk DTRs in his legs, and a right Babinski sign. Which one of the following features suggests that he has cervical spondylosis rather than ALS?

a. Hand atrophy
b. Hyperactive DTRs
c. Sensory loss
d. The Babinski sign

ANSWER: c. House painting requires prolonged neck hyperextension, which may lead to cervical spondylosis. Whatever its cause, cervical spondylosis leads to sensory and lower motor neuron loss in the arms and hands and upper motor neuron signs in the legs. Cervical spondylosis is a much more frequently occurring condition than ALS. ALS is one of the motor neuron diseases, which do not cause sensory loss.

60. Which cerebral lobes are superior to the Sylvian fissure?

a. Frontal and parietal
b. Parietal and occipital
c. Frontal and temporal
d. Parietal and temporal

ANSWER: a

61. Which cerebral lobe is inferior to the Sylvian fissure?

a. Frontal
b. Parietal
c. Occipital
d. Temporal
e. None of the above

ANSWER: d

62. As people age, what is the most common EEG change?

a. Loss of amplitude
b. Slowing of the background activity
c. Fragmentation of background
d. Episodic β activity

ANSWER: b

63. In which two ways do hypnagogic hallucinations differ from partial complex seizures?

a. Hypnagogic hallucinations are associated with flaccid, areflexic musculature.
b. Hypnagogic hallucinations often have an auditory component.
c. Hypnagogic hallucinations are associated with EEG spikes.

d. Hypnagogic hallucinations have visual, auditory, and emotional aspects.
e. Hypnagogic hallucinations are varied.

ANSWER: a, e

64. Which structure contains 80% of the brain's dopamine content?

a. Third ventricle
b. Thalamus
c. Cerebral cortex
d. Corpus striatum

ANSWER: d

65. Which condition is not associated with shortened REM latency?

a. Night terrors
b. Narcolepsy
c. Depression
d. Withdrawal from sedatives
e. Withdrawal from neuroleptics
f. Sleep deprivation

ANSWER: a

66. One week after a right cerebral infarction that caused a mild left hemiparesis, a 60-year-old man describes an intense burning sensation in the left side of his face and arm. He has a marked sensory loss to all modalities in these regions. What is the origin of the patient's symptom?

a. Parietal lobe injury
b. Brachial plexus injury
c. Lateral spinothalamic injury
d. Thalamic injury

ANSWER: d. The patient really has *thalamic pain,* which is a distressing consequence of an infarction in the thalamus. This burning sensation is attributable to deafferentation or loss of sensory input to the brain. Similar unpleasant sensations result from phantom limb and brachial plexus avulsion. Thalamic pain sometimes responds to antiepileptic drugs but generally not to analgesics. Deafferentation pain should be distinguished from neuropathic pain, in which pain results directly from nerve injury, such as postherpetic neuralgia.

67. Which two of the following tests rely on ionizing radiation?

a. CT
b. MRI
c. Isotopic brain scan
d. EEG
e. EMG
f. VER
g. BAER

ANSWER: a, c

68. In patients with the human variety of the Klüver-Bucy syndrome, which symptom is least common?

a. Oral exploration
b. Amnesia
c. Uncontrollable sexual activity
d. Placid demeanor
e. Anger

ANSWER: c. All these symptoms may be manifestations of the Klüver-Bucy syndrome in humans, as well as monkeys. Although humans may have increased sexual desire, its expression is limited to minor verbal and behavioral changes. They still abide by most social conventions. They have little or no physical aggression, homosexual activity, or sexual oral exploration. Moreover, their affect is usually bland, as with frontal lobe injury, but it may be punctuated by bursts of anger. Humans develop the Klüver-Bucy syndrome from herpes encephalitis, contusion of the temporal lobes, or multiple strokes.

69. Medical treatments occasionally produce neurologic complications. Which one of the following statements is false?

a. Human growth hormone injections given to correct short stature in children have caused Creutzfeldt-Jakob disease.
b. Smallpox vaccinations rarely cause an attack of disseminated MS-like CNS demyelination.
c. Measles vaccinations occasionally cause subacute sclerosing panencephalitis (SSPE).
d. Artificial insemination with donor semen has induced acquired immunodeficiency syndrome (AIDS).

ANSWER: c. Although elevated measles antibody titers are found in the CSF of SSPE patients (who are usually children), measles virus has not been proven to be the cause of this illness. In addition, similar elevated measles antibody titers have been detected in patients with MS. The incidence of SSPE has been markedly reduced following measles vaccination programs.

The development of Creutzfeldt-Jakob disease in children given growth hormone extracted from human pituitary glands led to the use of growth hormone synthesis by genetically engineered bacteria. Creutzfeldt-Jakob disease has also been transferred by the use of depth EEG electrodes and corneal transplantation. Smallpox vaccinations occasionally cause *postvaccinal demyelination,* a condition in which multiple areas of the CNS become demyelinated. The clinical and histologic features of postvaccinal demyelination mimic MS; however, attacks of postvaccinal demyelination are single events. This complication has been one of the major reasons that smallpox vaccinations are given sparingly. AIDS transmission has resulted from homosexual, heterosexual, and artificial semen transfer.

70. A 30-year-old woman has the sudden onset of "the worst headache of her life." She has nuchal rigidity but no lateralized signs. A CT shows blood density material in the right Sylvian fissure. Of the following, which is the best diagnostic procedure to perform?

a. LP
b. EEG
c. Isotopic brain scan
d. Cerebral arteriography

ANSWER: d. The patient probably has had a subarachnoid hemorrhage from a ruptured "berry" aneurysm. Cerebral arteriography would document the aneurysm, reveal its location and anatomy, and exclude the possibility of other sources of bleeding, such as a mycotic aneurysm or small AVM. If the resolution of MRI improves, the procedure may supplant arteriography. An LP is superfluous and possibly dangerous because, by reducing the pressure surrounding an aneurysm, it could lead to further rupture. In the presence of a large hematoma, an LP might lead to transtentorial herniation.

71. In Alzheimer's disease, which region has a pronounced neuron loss that results in an acetylcholine deficit?

a. Frontal lobe
b. Frontal and temporal lobe
c. Hippocampus
d. Nucleus basalis of Meynert

ANSWER: d. The brain has a marked loss of neurons in the hippocampus with the most striking loss occurring in the nucleus basalis of Meynert.

72. A 15-year-old waiter has episodes of feeling dizzy and dreamy that last 3 to 5 minutes. During them, he also has paresthesias in his fingertips and around his mouth. Sometimes his wrists bend, his fingers cramp together, and his foot flexes. An EEG during an episode showed slowing of the background activity and bursts of high voltage 3-Hz activity. Of the following conditions, which one is most likely to be occurring?

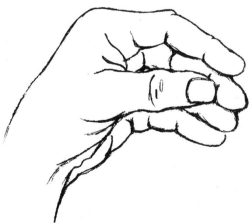

a. Partial complex seizures
b. Panic attacks
c. Petit mal (absence) seizures
d. Occupational cramps
e. Focal dystonia
f. None of the above

> **ANSWER:** f. He is probably having episodes of hyperventilation with carpopedal spasm and EEG slowing. A clinical diagnosis of hyperventilation can be confirmed if patients reproduce their symptoms by hyperventilating for 2 to 4 minutes.

73. The patient in the preceding question is asked to hyperventilate. After 90 seconds, he becomes giddy and then irrational. What is the best way to abort the test?

a. Intravenous benzodiazepine
b. Having the patient breathe into a paper bag
c. Offering reassurance
d. Inhaling oxygen

> **ANSWER:** b. He probably has developed cerebral hypoxia because of a reduction in carbon dioxide tension in the blood, which reduces cerebral blood flow. He should be asked to breathe into a paper bag to increase his carbon dioxide blood tension.

74. A 32-year-old woman is referred to a psychiatrist for postpartum depression. For the 5 months after a delivery of her fifth child, which was complicated by hemorrhage, she finds herself unable to cope with the family. She describes not having enough energy to do her share of the housework. She is unable to return to her usual occupation (dentistry). She never resumed her menses or regained her libido. She has anorexia and slight weight loss. She has a mild continual headache but no cognitive loss, visual changes, or other neurologic symptoms. Her obstetrician, internist, and a neurologic consultant find no physical signs of illness. Nevertheless, which conditions may be responsible?

a. MS
b. Lupus
c. Sheehan's syndrome
d. Pregnancy

> **ANSWER:** c. Postpartum pituitary necrosis (Sheehan's syndrome) is usually caused by deliveries complicated by hypotension. Its symptoms, which may not develop for several months to several years postpartum, include failure of lactation, scanty or no menses, sexual and generalized indifference, and being easily fatigued. Except for a subtle loss of secondary sexual characteristics, patients may have no physical abnormalities. Autoimmune diseases and hyper- or hypothyroidism may cause similar postpartum disturbances.

75. A 27-year-old man with a history of intractable seizures and violent behavior has had numerous EEGs that have shown only equivocal abnormalities. His serum phenytoin concentration has always been below the therapeutic range, despite a 500 mg/day prescription. He is suspected of abusing phenobarbital and other barbiturates, which he obtains on the basis of his diagnosis of epilepsy.

After seriously injuring a friend during a fistfight in a bar, his lawyer attributed the violence to the seizure disorder. As part of the medical-legal evaluation, an EEG was performed (see below). During the study, the patient became rigid and then had symmetric motor activity of all his limbs. Afterward, he remained unresponsive for several minutes and then became confused and amnestic. He was found to have had urinary incontinence. Evaluate the case in view of the history and EEG.

> **ANSWER:** The most prominent features of this EEG are bursts of high-voltage activity in the first and middle third of the sample. This activity is muscle artifact, which can be caused by either voluntary or involuntary muscle contraction. The diagnostic feature of this EEG is the α and β activity. This normal activity, which occurs during a pause in the muscle artifact, can be seen above and below the 1-second marker. Muscle artifact cannot distinguish between epileptic and psychogenic seizures; however, normal (α) EEG activity in the midst of apparent generalized tonic-clonic movements clearly indicates that the activity is psychogenic.
>
> Individuals with sociopathic behavior can convincingly mimic seizures. Alternatively, a patient with genuine seizures might let them become intractable by failing to

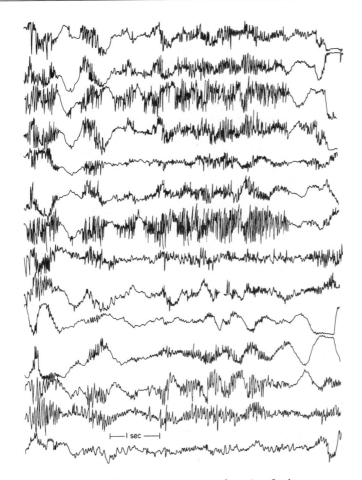

take antiepileptic drugs. The most common explanation for low serum concentrations of antiepileptic drugs is neither impaired absorption nor rapid metabolism but failure to take the prescribed dosage (i.e., noncompliance). Directed purposeful violence (aggression), as a manifestation of a seizure, is a rare phenomenon, if it exists at all. Moreover, aggression that occurs in bars is more likely to be the result of alcohol consumption than a seizure.

76. The 45-year-old woman has developed frequent blinking and involuntarily closure of her left eye (see below). The eyelid closure is forceful, lasts about 4 to 6 seconds, and is intensified by anxiety. She has no ocular abnormality, change in intellectual capacity, prior neurologic conditions, or medical illnesses. With which area is her problem associated?

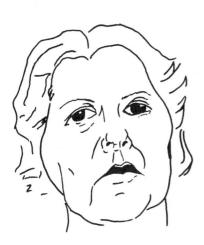
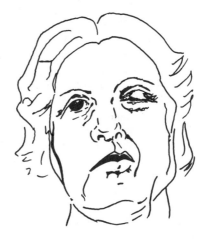

a. Corpus striatum
b. Lenticular nuclei
c. Facial nerve at the cerebellopontine angle
d. Autonomic nervous system
e. Trigeminal nerve at the cerebellopontine angle
f. Unknown regions

> *ANSWER:* c. The patient has hemifacial spasm, not blepharospasm. Note that, in addition to the closure of her left upper and lower eyelids, the muscles of the left side of her mouth contract, pull it laterally, and deepen the nasolabial fold. Hemifacial spasm, which develops in middle-aged and older individuals, is associated with an aberrant vessel compressing the facial nerve as it emerges from the brainstem. Hemifacial spasm can be treated with botulinum toxin (Botox) injections or neurosurgical decompression of the facial nerve as it exits from the brainstem at the cerebellopontine angle. Tics may involve one eye, but they are momentary. Tardive dyskinesia may cause facial movements, but it does not cause such unilateral movements. Psychogenic movement disorders are rare, and their diagnosis requires intensive investigation.

77–78. A teenage couple attempted suicide by sitting in a car with the engine running in a closed garage. They were discovered in a comatose state.

77. Three months later, the young man was alert, but bedridden, always in a flexed posture, mute, and unresponsive to stimulation. From which disorder did he suffer?

a. Dementia
b. Global aphasia
c. Persistent vegetative state
d. Depression
e. Isolation aphasia
f. Conduction aphasia
g. Multiple cerebrovascular accidents (strokes)
h. None of the above

> *ANSWER:* c. He probably had generalized cerebral cortex destruction from carbon monoxide poisoning that resulted in dementia with a decorticate (fetal) posture, that is, the persistent vegetative state.

78. Three months later, the young woman failed to recover. She could be placed in a chair. Her eyes remained open. Although she did not follow verbal requests, initiate conversation, or respond purposefully, she would repeat incessantly whatever questions or phrases that she heard from visitors, television, and nearby casual conversations. Of the choices in Question 77, from which disorder did she suffer?

> *ANSWER:* e. She sustained incomplete cortex damage that has resulted in isolation aphasia (also called "mixed transcortical aphasia"). Her injury spared the perisylvian language arc. The much larger surrounding watershed area of the cerebral cortex is especially sensitive to hypoxia. She has lost all her intellectual functions, except for a tendency—sometimes compulsion—to repeat (echolalia).

79. A 25-year-old male drug abuser, while recovering from abdominal surgery, became agitated, severely anxious, irrational, and diaphoretic. When he had persistent postoperative pain, despite moderate doses of various opioids, he was given pentazocine. A psychiatric consultation is requested. While a full investigation is being undertaken, which one of the following medications would be most appropriate?

a. A major tranquilizer
b. Methadone
c. Alcohol
d. Phenobarbital
e. Steroids
f. Benadryl
g. Pentazocine
h. Butorphanol

> *ANSWER:* b. Pentazocine (Talwin), butorphanol (Stadol), and other mixed opioid agonist-antagonist preparations can precipitate withdrawal in opioid addicts. (Being aware

of their vulnerability, opioid addicts often claim, with some justification, that they are allergic to these preparations.) Methadone or other opioids will abort the withdrawal symptoms and provide analgesia.

80. A 28-year-old nurse, who has previously been healthy, is hospitalized for the sudden onset of generalized muscle weakness. An internist diagnoses hypokalemic myopathy. What are four causes of hypokalemic myopathy that develops in young and middle-aged adults?

a. Adrenal insufficiency
b. Pernicious anemia
c. Diuretic use or abuse
d. Vomiting
e. Diarrhea from laxative use or abuse
f. Steroid use
g. Excessive vitamin use

ANSWER: c, d, e, f. Hypokalemic myopathy in previously healthy young adults may be iatrogenic, a sign of underlying illness, or self-induced. Hypokalemia is especially likely to be self-induced by health care workers who surreptitiously take diuretics. Steroids may cause weakness by a direct muscle injury (steroid myopathy) or indirectly by depleting serum potassium (hypokalemic myopathy). Weakness is an occasional paradoxical result of bodybuilders using steroids.

81. Which two of the following statements concerning prions are true?

a. They contain RNA.
b. They contain reverse transcriptase.
c. They are infective agents.
d. They may be the cause of Creutzfeldt-Jakob disease.
e. They are identifiable in cerebral biopsy tissue of Alzheimer's disease patients.

ANSWER: c, d. Prions are protein-containing infective agents that contain neither DNA nor RNA. They are believed to cause Creutzfeldt-Jakob disease. Prions can be identified in cerebral biopsies of patients with Creutzfeldt-Jakob but not Alzheimer's disease. The human immunodeficiency virus (HIV) is an RNA virus that contains reverse transcriptase.

82–88. Match the clinical description of patients with mental status changes and the appropriate CT.

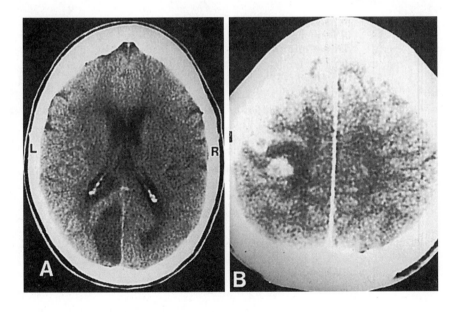

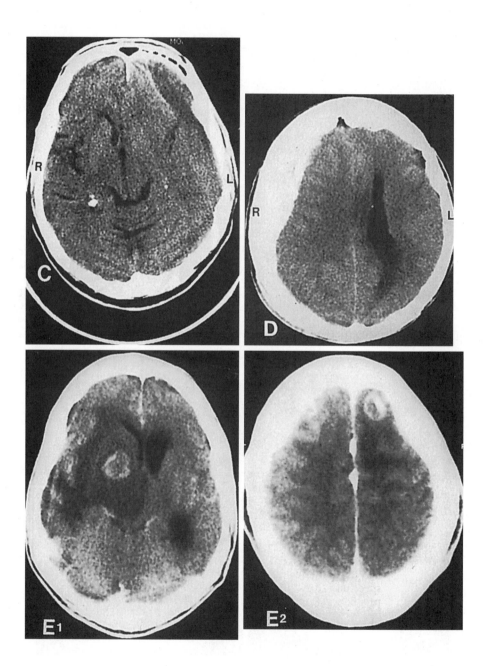

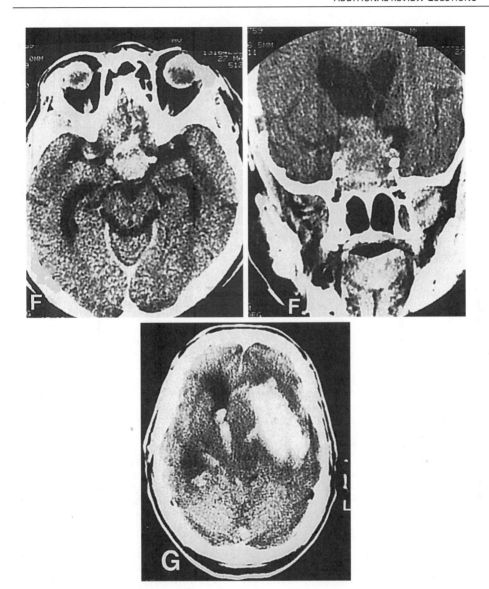

82. A 23-year-old woman, who had just delivered a baby boy 5 days earlier, had the sequential development of personality changes, agitation, garbled speech, seizures, and right hemiparesis. She had had an uneventful pregnancy. She did not use alcohol, tobacco, or drugs, but her boyfriend is a former drug addict.

83. A 45-year-old man was placed in restraints and given neuroleptics for agitated behavior. Later in the night, although the patient is stuporous, he screams about a headache. Examination reveals papilledema and a mild left hemiparesis that the patient, in his obtundation, seems to ignore.

84. A 65-year-old man has found that for several weeks he has had difficulty reading newspapers and books. Although his memory and other aspects of his general intellect are intact, he stumbles, almost incoherently, when reading. Nevertheless, he can repeat phrases, comprehend spoken statements, and even transcribe entire sentences.

85. An 80-year-old man has malaise, mild frontal headaches, and progressively severe cognitive impairment with prominent anomias. Otherwise, he has no abnormalities on neurologic or general medical examination. Routine laboratory tests, including a sedimentation rate, are normal.

86. A 50-year-old architect is unable to complete his work. When he relates his history, he seems inattentive, but his cognitive capacity is grossly normal. However, he cannot make simple drawings.

87. A 38-year-old woman, who has been infertile, has the onset of headaches and bitemporal hemianopsia.

88. A 55-year-old hypertensive man has the sudden onset of a severe headache, aphasia, and right hemiparesis.

ANSWERS:

82. e. The two CTs show two circular lesions that are each enhanced by contrast infusion. The use of contrast infusion can be surmised by the fact that the falx, a thick, linear vascular structure, is white (seen more clearly on E2 than E1). The conventional representation consists of placing "L" or "R" notations on the appropriate side of the scan. A large lesion, surrounded by extensive edema, is deep in the left cerebral hemisphere (Scan E1). Another is in the right frontal lobe (E2). In the lower cut (E1), the anterior and occipital horns of the left lateral ventricle are compressed, and midline structures are shifted to the right. In the higher cut, a shift is not possible because the falx forms a rigid barrier. The lesions, being multiple masses and enhanced by contrast, are indicative of toxoplasmosis, bacterial abscesses, and metastatic tumors. Because her sexual partner is a drug addict, her most likely diagnosis is an AIDS-induced cerebral toxoplasmosis.

83. d. Before looking at the image of the brain, note that this CT follows the convention: The CT portrays the brain with the left and right sides reversed. It shows that a thick white border overlies the right side of the brain. In addition, the right lateral ventricle is obliterated by compression. Bone, fresh blood, and calcium are denser than brain tissue and therefore portrayed as white on a CT. The patient has an acute subdural hematoma compressing the right cerebral hemisphere.

84. a. This CT shows a relatively large, dark, semicircular area, adjacent to the posterior falx, in the left occipital lobe. Its lucency and pattern indicate that it is an infarction of the posterior cerebral artery. The patient has the interesting and important neuropsychologic condition, *alexia without agraphia* or inability to read with preserved ability to write. Alexia without agraphia, which is a *disconnection syndrome,* usually results from damage to the left occipital lobe and posterior corpus callosum.

85. c. This CT shows an abnormality overlying the left frontal lobe that has a white rim in its anterior portion. The mixed black and gray intensities indicate that its density is less than that of the brain. Cerebrospinal fluid, edema fluid, aged blood, and necrotic brain—all portrayed as black on the CT—are the most common hypodense tissues. The frontal horn of the left lateral ventricle is compressed, and the left frontal lobe is shifted slightly to the right. This CT indicates a chronic subdural hematoma. The symptoms of chronic subdural hematomas are usually a dull headache and cognitive impairment, including exacerbations of age-related language impairment, such as anomias. Although subdural hematomas are typically produced by trauma, the injury is often so trivial that patients often do not recall it. Because chronic subdural hematomas are slowly evolving, they do not cause papilledema or prominent lateralized signs. Subdural hematomas are a commonly occurring, correctable cause of dementia.

86. b. The CT shows a lesion located in the posterior portion of the right cerebral hemisphere that has a white center and fragments of a white ring surrounding it. The white falx indicates infusion of contrast material. The lesion is probably a tumor or other mass. Lesions in the nondominant parietal lobe, whatever their etiology, produce constructional apraxia, hemi-inattention, anosognosia, and, according to some neurologists, impaired emotional communication. This patient's presenting symptom is probably a manifestation of constructional apraxia. Because symptoms of right hemisphere lesions are often accompanied by anosognosia, patients may ignore them or describe them only in imprecise terms.

87. f. *Left,* This axial, contrast-enhanced CT reveals a circular radiodense lesion in the midline, just anterior to the midbrain. *Right,* In this coronal view, the lesion can be seen to be arising from the sella and growing into the hypothalamus. The lateral ventricles are pushed aside and dilated, which suggests that blockage of the third ventricle has caused hydrocephalus. The white, upside-down, wishbone-shaped structure in the posterior portion of the axial CT is the normal venous drainage. In adults,

pituitary lesions are usually adenomas that cause endocrine disturbances, including elevated prolactin concentrations, headaches, and, when large, bitemporal hemianopsia. Craniopharyngiomas and meningiomas in that location are uncommon.

88. g. This CT reveals a large intracerebral hemorrhage with blood that has extended into the ventricle in the left side of the brain (the right side of the picture). Hypertensive cerebral hemorrhages, such as this one, usually occur in the putamen, thalamus, pons, or cerebellum.

89–90. A physician is called to see a colleague who has developed severe headache, nausea, and vomiting. The colleague is known to be hypertensive and seriously depressed. She finds that he is stuporous and diaphoretic with nuchal rigidity and bilateral Babinski signs. His blood pressure is 210/130 mm Hg. Bottles of chlorpromazine, isocarboxazid, propranolol, meperidine, and hydrochlorothiazide are in the medicine chest.

89. What are the two most likely diagnoses?

a. Medication interaction
b. Meningitis
c. Intracranial hemorrhage
d. None of the above

ANSWER: a, c. The patient has classic signs of an intracranial hemorrhage: headache, stupor, nausea, vomiting, and nuchal rigidity. The origin could have been a hypertensive cerebral hemorrhage that was not prevented by the antihypertensive medications. Alternatively, the etiology could have been a drug-induced hemorrhage from the isocarboxazid (Marplan). That medication, like tranylcypromine (Parnate), phenelzine (Nardil), and others, is a monamine oxidase (MAO) inhibitor. Meperidine (Demerol) and dextromethorphan will cause similar, potentially fatal interactions. MAO inhibitors cause acute, severe hypertension if certain foods, such as aged cheese, or medications are ingested. Sometimes depressed people purposefully take prohibited foods in suicide attempts.

90. If the problem is caused by an MAO inhibitor, which of the following medications should be given?

a. Meperidine
b. Chlorpromazine
c. Propranolol
d. Hydrochlorothiazide
e. Phentolamine
f. Dibenzoxazepine

ANSWER: e. The most specific treatment for a hypertensive reaction to an MAO inhibitor is the α-adrenergic blocking agent, phentolamine (Regitine), at a dose of 5 mg given slowly intravenously. Of the medications that are usually readily available, propranolol or chlorpromazine would be most helpful. Although the headache may be agonizingly severe, meperidine (Demerol) is contraindicated.

91. Which structure connects the hippocampus and the hypothalamus?

a. Corpus callosum
b. Cingulate gyrus
c. Fornix
d. None of the above

ANSWER: c. The fornix connects the hippocampus with the mamillary bodies, which are an extension of the hypothalamus. The mamillary bodies communicate through the mamillothalamic tract with the anterior nucleus of the thalamus.

92. After extraction from a high-speed motor vehicle accident (MVA), the driver was stuporous and had facial contusions. After regaining consciousness, he was noted to have paresis of his right arm and leg, which also had decreased position sensation. The left arm and leg had decreased sensation to pin prick. He had a right-sided Babinski sign. The paresis persisted even though he fully regained consciousness and had no language, ocular, or visual impairment. Where would the lesion have to be located to explain the paresis?

a. Frontal lobe
b. Brainstem
c. Cervical spinal cord
d. Lumbar spinal cord

ANSWER: c. He has a hemitransection of the cervical spinal cord. The cervical spinal cord is vulnerable because, when the forehead strikes the wheel or dashboard, the head and neck snap backward (hyperextended). In general, drivers involved in a high-speed MVA, especially if they display behavioral abnormalities, should be evaluated for drug and alcohol use.

93. Which statement concerning the cerebellum is false?

a. MS frequently involves the cerebellum.
b. Lesions in the cerebellum may cause scanning speech.
c. In adults, strokes and tumors involve the cerebellum less often than the cerebrum.
d. A lesion in a cerebellar hemisphere causes contralateral limb ataxia.

ANSWER: d. A lesion in a cerebellar hemisphere causes *ipsilateral* limb ataxia. Possibly because the cerebellum receives only about 10% of the brain's blood supply, about 10% of strokes and tumors involve the cerebellum.

94. Which sign is not found with the others?

a. Fasciculations
b. Spasticity
c. Babinski signs
d. Clonus

ANSWER: a. Fasciculations are a manifestation of lower motor neuron injury. In contrast, spasticity, Babinski signs, and clonus are all manifestations of upper motor neuron injury.

95. In Parkinson's disease, which tract undergoes degeneration? What is the function, origin, and destination of each tract?

a. Nigrostriatal
b. Geniculocalcarine
c. Spinothalamic
d. Corticospinal

ANSWER: a. The nigrostriatal tract, which undergoes degeneration in Parkinson's disease, originates in the substantia nigra and terminates in the striatum (caudate and putamen). The geniculocalcarine tract conveys the visual pathways from the lateral geniculate bodies to the calcarine cortex of the occipital lobes. The spinothalamic tract conveys pain pathways from the dorsal horn of the spinal cord to the contralateral thalamus. (Crossing shortly after it originates, the spinothalamic tract ascends in the spinal cord contralateral to the side of its origin.) The corticospinal tract originates in the motor strips of the cerebrum and descends, after crossing in the medulla, in the spinal cord to the contralateral anterior horn cells of the spinal cord. It conveys voluntary motor system signals.

96. Of the following substances, which one is most likely to produce seizures during an acute intoxication?

a. Cocaine
b. Phencyclidine (PCP)
c. Δ9–TCH
d. Heroin
e. Valium
f. Amphetamine
g. Alcohol
h. Morphine

ANSWER: a. Cocaine, whether smoked, inhaled, injected, or swallowed, readily causes seizures. Almost one-half of the cases of cocaine-induced seizures occur in first-time users. Phencyclidine (PCP) and amphetamine cause seizures less frequently. Heroin and other opioids usually do not cause seizures, except from hypoxia, massive overdose, or contaminants. Benzodiazepines and alcohol rarely cause seizures during an intoxication; however, withdrawal from these substances regularly produces seizures that are sometimes intractable (i.e., status epilepticus). The active agent in marijuana, Δ9-TCH, actually has a mild antiepileptic drug effect.

97. Which two of the substances listed in Question 96 are associated with seizures after several days of abstinence?

ANSWER: e, g

98. Which one of the substances listed in Question 96 is most likely to cause a stroke?

ANSWER: a. Cocaine often causes cerebral hemorrhages and bland infarctions. Cocaine-induced strokes are likely to present with seizures. Amphetamine produces similar mental changes but less often strokes or seizures.

99. A 19-year-old college student was brought to the emergency room because of physical and mental agitation, vivid hallucinations, and combative behavior after using marijuana. Although she had often previously used marijuana, she had never developed such a reaction.

She was hypertensive, oblivious to a laceration, and kept her eyes wide open. She made repetitive, purposeless kissing movements. Which of the substances listed in Question 96 is probably responsible?

    ANSWER: b. Somebody probably laced her marijuana with phencyclidine (PCP).

100. Which are two effects of the normal gamma-aminobutyric acid (GABA)-induced influx of chloride ions?

a. Neurons are inhibited.
b. Neurons are excited.
c. The resting potential is made more negative.
d. The resting potential is made more positive.
e. NMDA receptors are activated.

    ANSWER: a, c. The normal resting potential is –70 mV. An influx of chloride ion (Cl⁻), which makes the resting potential more negative, inhibits neuron activity.

101. In the initial treatment of a depressed Parkinson's disease patient who is already being treated with L-dopa and selegiline, which medication is contraindicated?

a. Fluoxetine
b. Tricyclic antidepressants
c. MAO inhibitors
d. Amoxapine
e. All of the above

    ANSWER: e. None of these medications should be given in this situation. Amoxapine, an older, unique antidepressant, has dopamine-blocking activity that will exacerbate Parkinson's disease. Selegiline is a monoamine oxidase inhibitor that might cause a toxic reaction with fluoxetine and tricyclic antidepressants. Thus, in most cases, selegiline will have to be discontinued. ECT (electroconvulsive therapy) is safe and effective in Parkinson's disease patients. Psychotherapy, support groups, and physical and occupational therapy may be helpful; however, depression induced by Parkinson's disease almost always requires medications.

102. Insert the proper enzyme (a–d) into the synthetic steps (1–4) for epinephrine synthesis.

    Tyrosine —1→ DOPA —2→ Dopamine —3→ Norepinephrine —4→ Epinephrine

a. DOPA decarboxylase
b. Phenylethanolamine *N*-methyl-transferase
c. Dopamine β-hydroxylase
d. Tyrosine hydroxylase

    ANSWER: 1-d, 2-a, 3-c, 4-b. Tyrosine —tyrosine hydroxylase→ DOPA —DOPA decarboxylase→ Dopamine —dopamine β-hydroxylase→ Norepinephrine —phenylethanolamine *N*-methyl-transferase→ Epinephrine

103. In Question 102, which is the rate-limiting enzyme?

    ANSWER: d. Tyrosine hydroxylase

104. A 23-year-old man has a history of schizophrenia for which he has been receiving dopamine-blocking neuroleptics. He has also been an intravenous drug abuser. He comes to the emergency room because he has developed involuntary spasmodic muscle contractions in his left arm. He has a deep skin infection in his left forearm. His examination is otherwise normal. What conditions may be responsible?

a. Localized neuroleptic-induced dystonia
b. Partial status epilepticus
c. Conscious attempt to secure drugs
d. A reaction to a toxin elaborated by an infection

    ANSWER: d. The localized form of tetanus occurs in individuals, especially drug addicts, who have partial immunity from distant or ineffective immunizations. The generalized form of tetanus, which develops in individuals who were not immunized, causes the muscles of the entire body to have contractions and the jaw to close forcefully (trismus).

105. Which mental disturbance is least frequently a component of Alzheimer's disease?

a. Delusions
b. Suicide ideation
c. Hallucinations
d. Anxiety

ANSWER: b. With the onset of dementia, Alzheimer's disease patients typically develop anxiety. Delusions and hallucinations are manifestations of moderate-to-severe dementia. Remarkably few Alzheimer's disease patients have suicidal ideation.

106. Which three of the following conditions are associated with spasticity?

a. MS that affects only the spinal cord
b. Parkinson's disease
c. Cerebellar degeneration
d. Poliomyelitis
e. HTLV-1 myelitis
f. Myotonic dystrophy
g. Neuroleptic-induced parkinsonism
h. Middle cerebral artery occlusion

ANSWER: a, e, h. Spasticity is increased muscle tone resulting in an increased resistance to stretching. It is a sign of injury to the upper motor neurons of the corticospinal tract, which can occur in the cerebrum, brainstem, or spinal cord. Spasticity is characteristic of MS affecting the brain or the spinal cord, HTLV-1 myelitis (spinal cord infection), and strokes. In contrast, muscle rigidity, which is an inflexibility of muscle, is a sign of basal ganglia disorders, such as naturally occurring or neuroleptic-induced parkinsonism. Cerebellar degeneration leads to muscle hypotonia. Poliomyelitis is an infection of the lower motor neurons that leads to muscle flaccidity and atrophy. Myotonic dystrophy induces myotonia, which is delayed muscle relaxation after a contraction or after percussion.

107. In the preceding question, which three choices are associated with clonus?

ANSWER: a, e, h. Clonus, like spasticity, is a manifestation of injury to the upper motor neurons of the corticospinal tract.

108. Which of the following structures represents the beginning of the lower motor neuron?

a. Spinal cord
b. Cauda equina
c. Anterior horn cells of the spinal cord
d. Neuromuscular junction
e. Corticospinal tract
f. Cervical-medullary junction

ANSWER: c. The corticospinal tract, which contains the upper motor neurons, terminates on the anterior horn cells of the spinal cord to synapse with the lower motor neuron.

109. Onto which of the following structures do the corticobulbar fibers terminate?

a. Anterior horns cells of the spinal cord
b. Cranial nerve nuclei I to XII
c. Certain cranial nerve nuclei
d. Autonomic nervous system pathways

ANSWER: c. The corticobulbar tract, which is analogous to the corticospinal tract, conveys motor information to the motor nuclei of the brainstem. It contains upper motor neurons and innervates nuclei of cranial nerves that have motor function but not those that are sensory, such as the olfactory, optic, and acoustic nerves.

110. Microscopic examination of brains with Alzheimer's disease will almost always reveal all except which two of the following structures?

a. Neurofibrillary tangles
b. Senile plaques
c. Loss of neurons
d. Prions
e. Lewy bodies
f. Amyloid

ANSWER: d, e. Prions, protein-containing infectious agents that have no nucleic acid, are found in Creutzfeldt-Jakob's disease. Lewy bodies, intracytoplasmic eosinophilic inclusions, are characteristically found in Parkinson's disease in the substantia nigra. They are also found in the cerebral cortex in Lewy body disease.

111. Which one of the following conditions is not characterized by neurofibrillary tangles?

a. Alzheimer's disease
b. Down's syndrome
c. Dementia pugilistica
d. Huntington's disease

ANSWER: d. Neurofibrillary tangles are paired helical filaments that are associated with amyloid plaques and neuron loss. They are closely associated with Alzheimer's disease where they correlate with the severity of the dementia. In addition, they are found in several other conditions that cause dementia, such as Down's syndrome, and to a limited extent in normal individuals older than 65 years. In other words, neurofibrillary tangles are not pathognomic of Alzheimer's disease.

112. Which structure forms the roof of lateral ventricles? The fourth ventricle?

a. Caudate nuclei
b. Corpus callosum
c. Pons
d. Medulla
e. Cerebellum

ANSWER: b and e. The corpus callosum forms the roof of the lateral ventricles, and the cerebellum forms the roof of the fourth ventricle.

113. Match the structures (1–10) with their location (a–e).

1. Oculomotor
2. Trochlear
3. Abducens
4. Trigeminal motor
5. Vagus motor
6. Hypoglossal
7. Locus ceruleus
8. Substantia nigra
9. Red nucleus
10. Facial nerve

a. Midbrain
b. Pons
c. Medulla
d. Cerebral hemisphere
e. Cerebellum

ANSWERS: 1-a, 2-a, 3-b, 4-b, 5-c, 6-c, 7-b, 8-a, 9-a, 10-b

114. A veteran sustained a gunshot wound that transected the thoracic spinal cord 10 years before death. This is a sketch of an upper level of his cervical spinal cord. It has been treated with a stain that blackens normal myelin. Identify the demyelinated tracts.

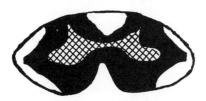

ANSWER: The salient feature is that certain ascending tracts, which are sensory, are unstained and presumably demyelinated because of the spinal cord injury. The spinothalamic tract, which is anterolateral, and the spinocerebellar tract, which is posterior-lateral and also peripheral, are both mostly unstained. The medial portion of the posterior column, the fasciculus gracilis, is also unstained. In contrast, the lateral segment of the posterior column, which consists of the fasciculus cuneatus, is stained. The difference occurs because the f. gracilis originates in the legs and was interrupted by the gunshot wound. Thus, it is unstained; however, the f. cuneatus remained undamaged and its myelin is normally stained. This man's deficits included paraplegia, incontinence, and loss of all sensory modalities in his trunk below the umbilicus and in his legs.

115. Which substance is absent in biopsies of voluntary muscles of Duchenne's dystrophy patients?

a. Dystrophin
b. Acetylcholine
c. Ion channels
d. Insulin

ANSWER: a

116. A patient who has sustained a left cerebral embolus has left-right confusion, finger agnosia, and agraphia. Which other neuropsychologic abnormality is expectable?

a. Alexia
b. Dementia

c. Acalculia
d. Amnesia

ANSWER: c. Gerstmann's syndrome, which is usually caused by a dominant parietal lobe lesion, consists of left-right confusion, finger agnosia, agraphia, and acalculia; however, all four components are rarely present, and each may be incomplete (e.g., dysgraphia and dyscalculia).

117. In the limbic system, which tract conveys impulses between the hippocampus and the mamillary bodies?

a. Mamillothalamic tract
b. Cingulate gyrus

c. Fornix
d. None of the above

ANSWER: c. The sequence in the limbic system is hippocampus and adjacent amygdala; fornix; mamillary bodies; mamillothalamic tract; anterior nucleus of the thalamus; cingulate gyrus.

118. Which chromosome contains the gene for β-amyloid?

a. 4
b. 14

c. 21
d. X

ANSWER: c. Chromosome 21 contains the gene for β-amyloid and is triplicated in most cases of Down's syndrome (trisomy 21).

119. At birth, a male infant is found to have a delicate saclike protrusion at the base of his spine. His legs have flaccid, areflexic paraplegia, and urine dribbles continually from his penis, which never has erections. What condition is present?

a. Cerebral diplegia
b. Meningomyelocele
c. Dandy-Walker malformation

d. Arnold-Chiari malformation
e. Spina bifida

ANSWER: b. The baby most likely has a meningomyelocele. This congenital abnormality consists of a deformed spinal cord or cauda equina protruding through an incompletely closed spinal canal. It causes paraplegia with bladder, bowel, and sexual dysfunction. Meningomyeloceles have been attributed to maternal exposure to environmental toxins, such as potato blight, and medications, including (in rare instances) valproic acid and carbamazepine. The abnormality, which may be detected in utero, might be prevented with folic acid and other vitamins during pregnancy.

120. Which two of the following clinical features distinguish ALS from cervical spondylosis?

a. Weakness of the arms
b. Atrophy of the arms
c. Hyperactive DTRs in the legs
d. Fasciculations in the tongue
e. Sensory loss in the fingers and hands

ANSWER: d, e. Sensory loss in the fingers and hands would be present in cervical spondylosis but not ALS. Fasciculations are found in both conditions, but tongue fasciculations are found only in ALS.

121. Which of the following is not a feature of ataxia-telangiectasia?

a. Deficiency in IgA and IgE
b. Autosomal dominant inheritance
c. Onset of ataxia in childhood
d. Dilated vessels on the conjunctiva
e. Death from sinus or respiratory infection

ANSWER: b. Ataxia-telangiectasia is a neurocutaneous disorder that is inherited in an autosomal recessive pattern. Children with this disorder have telangiectasia of conjunctival blood vessels, ataxia, and potentially fatal IgA and IgE deficiencies. They may also have cognitive impairment.

122. Which tests are most important in assessing language function?

a. Calculating serial sevens, reading, comprehending
b. Reading, repeating, and complex tasks
c. Naming objects, following requests, and repeating
d. Recalling six digits, reading, and naming common objects

ANSWER: c. Abnormalities in naming objects, following requests, or repeating indicate aphasia. Calculating serial sevens relies on several cognitive functions, including attention, memory, and arithmetic. Performing complex tasks is a measure of apraxia. Recalling six digits might be a test of either memory or merely repeating.

123. Which two of the following areas of the brain are most vulnerable to chronic alcoholism?

a. Cerebellar hemispheres
b. Optic nerves
c. Cerebellar vermis
d. Corpus callosum
e. Mammillary bodies

ANSWER: c, e. Although each of these areas may be damaged, cerebellar vermis atrophy is a frequently occurring sign of chronic alcoholism. Cerebellar vermis atrophy causes gait ataxia. Repeated bouts of alcohol consumption lead to damage of the mammillary bodies and other areas of the limbic system.

124. A 66-year-old hypertensive businesswoman had the sudden painless onset of left-sided hemiparesis. She remains fully alert, comfortable, oriented, and with good memory and judgment. In addition, she has right-sided ptosis, the right pupil is dilated, and the right eye is laterally deviated. Which of the following events probably developed?

a. Periaqueductal petechial hemorrhages
b. Subdural hematoma with herniation
c. Midbrain arterial thrombosis
d. Cerebral hemorrhage

ANSWER: c. She sustained a midbrain arterial thrombosis that damaged her third cranial nerve and adjacent corticospinal tract (Weber's syndrome). Because midbrain, pons, and medulla lesions are distant from the cerebrum, her cognitive functions are almost always preserved. Periaqueductal petechial hemorrhages are indicative of Wernicke's encephalopathy, a condition in which patients have memory impairment, nystagmus, and ataxia, as well as oculomotor paresis. Subdural hematoma with herniation causes brainstem compression that leads to stupor if not coma and to decerebrate posturing. A cerebral hemorrhage could cause a third cranial nerve palsy only by its mass effect herniating downward to compress the nerve and necessarily the brainstem. Moreover, a cerebral hemorrhage would usually cause stupor, confusion, and headache.

125. What is the most caudal extent of the central nervous system (CNS)?

a. Foramen magnum
b. Occipital-cervical junction
c. Thoraco-lumbar junction
d. Sacrum
e. Neuromuscular junction

ANSWER: c. The CNS terminates at the junction of vertebrae T12–L1. At this point, the spinal cord terminates by forming the cauda equina.

126. Which of the following EEG patterns most clearly indicates that a patient might have epilepsy?

a. Theta waves
b. Sharp waves
c. K complexes
d. Spindles
e. Vertex sharp waves
f. Spikes-and-wave complexes

ANSWER: f. Spikes-and-wave complexes at 3-Hz are indicative of petit mal (absence) epilepsy. Theta waves, which are merely slow waves, are found when people are sleepy, in normal people older than 65 years, in metabolic disturbances, and as a sign of a structural lesion. Sharp waves only signify an underlying area with an epileptic potential. K complexes, spindles, and vertex sharp waves are all EEG patterns found in normal sleep.

127. Which condition will be most reliably detected or excluded by a routine EEG?

a. Partial complex seizures
b. Persistent vegetative state
c. Metabolic encephalopathy
d. Anterior cerebral infarction
e. Cerebellar hematoma
f. Narcolepsy

ANSWER: c. The EEG is sensitive to metabolic aberrations, as occurs in hepatic encephalopathy and drug use. A routine EEG may not capture partial complex seizures, and interictal patterns are inconsistent. The persistent vegetative state, although leading to EEG slowing and disorganization, is not associated with a particular pattern. Structural lesions cannot be identified or excluded reliably by an EEG. A multiple sleep latency test (MSLT) or polysomnogram (PSG) is helpful in diagnosing narcolepsy.

128. Which four of the following are more characteristic of sleep terrors than nightmares?

a. Occur in deep NREM sleep
b. Are actually frightening dreams
c. Are associated with sleepwalking
d. Follow a partial awakening
e. Have contents that are often recalled on awakening
f. Are accompanied by sweating and tachycardia
g. Are associated with epileptiform EEG activity

ANSWER: a, c, d, f. Sleep terrors are a variety of parasomnia, but nightmares are dreams with a frightening content. Seizures often develop during sleep, and sometimes they arise exclusively during sleep.

129. Which two of the following are said to induce tics?

a. Methylphenidate
b. Anticholinergics
c. Encephalitis
d. Seizures

ANSWER: a, c. Although reports have described tics developing in children treated with methylphenidate (Ritalin) and other stimulants for attention deficit hyperactivity disorder, the number of cases is minute, and a causal relationship remains unproven. In contrast, tics as well as Parkinson's disease have routinely followed encephalitis.

130. On several occasions, a 21-year-old college student has been unable to rise from bed upon awakening in the morning. He becomes terrified, and twice he found himself having visual hallucinations. He is otherwise in good mental and physical health. Which of the following conditions is the most likely cause of these symptoms?

a. Incipient psychosis
b. A paroxysm of spikes and waves from the mesial temporal cortex
c. An intrusion or persistence of REM sleep into wakefulness
d. Cerebral artery vasospasm

ANSWER: c. He is probably having sleep paralysis and sleep hallucinations. Although other aspects of narcolepsy should be sought, sleep deprivation and alcohol abuse should be considered.

131. During withdrawal from chronic cocaine use, a patient describes having vivid, frightening dreams. Which is the most likely explanation for his dreams?

a. Emergence of psychosis
b. Drug-seeking behavior
c. Nocturnal seizures
d. REM rebound

ANSWER: d. Marijuana and cocaine, as well as numerous medicines, suppress REM sleep. During withdrawal from chronic use, there is a compensatory increase in REM sleep (i.e., REM rebound).

132. Six weeks after a cardiac arrest with asystole, a 48-year-old man opens his eyes. However, he is mute and unresponsive to verbal and gestured requests. Although he breathes normally, he has flexion of his limbs, cannot eat or swallow food that is placed in his mouth, and is incontinent of urine. An EEG shows slow, low-voltage, disorganized activity. An additional month passes and he does not improve. What are his mental status, cognitive capacity, and prognosis?

> *ANSWER:* He is in a persistent vegetative state. He has no cognitive capacity. His prognosis for a functional recovery is less than one in a thousand. If specified by a living will, withdrawal of mechanical supports may be appropriate.

133. At 6 months after a stroke in which his basilar artery was occluded, a 75-year-old retired merchant seaman remains quadriplegic, mute, unable to follow verbal or gestured requests, and unable to breathe, eat, or swallow. However, through eyelid blinks, he can communicate using Morse code, which he had used in the Navy. An EEG often shows 10-Hz activity over the occipital area. What condition is present, and what is his cognitive capacity? How does he compare to the prior patient?

> *ANSWER:* In contrast to the prior case, this man has intact cognitive capacity. He has the locked-in syndrome, in which the base of the pons and medulla are damaged, injuring breathing and swallowing brainstem centers and cutting off communication between the brain and the spinal cord.

134. Match the cell type (a–f) with its function (1–6).

a. Microglia
b. Astrocytes
c. Oligodendrocytes
d. Schwann cells
e. Ependymal cells
f. Neurons

1. Form the myelin in the central nervous system
2. Serve a chemical and physical supportive role for neurons
3. Act as phagocytes
4. Form the myelin in the peripheral nervous system
5. Line the ventricles
6. Basic element of the nervous system

> *ANSWERS:* a-3, b-2, c-1, d-4, e-5, f-6

135. Of the following, which is the most common cause of chronic, malignant pain being "refractory"?

a. Failure to use tricyclic antidepressants in conjunction with analgesics
b. Administering doses of opioids that suppress respirations
c. Undertreatment with opioids
d. Patients having personality disorders

> *ANSWER:* c. Undertreatment, especially failure to prescribe opioids, is probably the most common physician deficiency in controlling malignant pain. Generous doses of opioids are clearly indicated in most forms of acute and chronic, malignant pain. They may also be indicated in some forms of chronic benign pain.

136. Which of the following is the most common cause of coma in the United States?

a. Cerebral hemorrhage
b. Subarachnoid hemorrhage
c. Seizures
d. Drug overdose
e. Subdural hematoma

> *ANSWER:* d. Drug overdose, not cerebral mass lesions, is the most common cause of coma in the United States.

137. Which of the following neurologic infections is caused by a spirochete?

a. AIDS encephalitis
b. Meningococcal meningitis
c. *Herpes simplex* encephalitis
d. Lyme disease

> *ANSWER:* d. Lyme disease, which is an infection by spirochete *Borrelia burgdorferi*, can cause a meningitis, encephalitis, facial nerve injury (which mimics Bell's palsy), or a polyneuropathy.

138. Which three of the following individuals might have an EEG showing electrocerebral silence?

a. A 10-year-old boy who drowned in an icy pond
b. A 60-year-old man who took a massive overdose of barbiturates

c. A 55-year-old woman with the locked-in syndrome

d. A 65-year-old man with profound Alzheimer's disease dementia

e. A 17-year-old boy with massive head trauma from a motor vehicle accident

f. A 79-year-old man in a persistent vegetative state

ANSWER: a, b, e. EEG electrocerebral silence, a "flat" EEG in the vernacular, is associated with brain death. Head trauma, when the victim is a candidate to be an organ donor, is the most common circumstance when an EEG is performed to confirm a clinical diagnosis of brain death. On the other hand, an EEG showing electrocerebral silence cannot be interpreted as confirming brain death in either individuals who have hypothermia, such as occurs in children who have drowned in icy ponds, or anyone who has taken a barbiturate overdose. Although these individuals often have no clinical sign of brain activity and have EEGs with electrocerebral silence, they often make a full recovery.

139. Which three of the following are effects of caffeine?

a. Headaches

b. Bradycardia

c. Prolonged sleep latency

d. Sleep fragmentation

e. Urinary retention

f. Tremor

ANSWER: c, d, f. Although one of the world's most widely consumed drugs, caffeine impairs sleep, induces diuresis, provokes a tremor in susceptible individuals, and causes tachycardia, palpitations, and other cardiac disturbances. Its mental effects mimic anxiety. Missing a customary morning coffee produces the most common cause of morning headache, caffeine-withdrawal headache.

140. Which three of the following headaches occur predominantly in the morning?

a. Muscle contraction headaches

b. Sleep apnea

c. Brain tumors at their onset

d. Chronic obstructive lung disease

e. Sleeping in a warm room with no fresh air

f. Trigeminal neuralgia

ANSWER: b, c, d, e. Increased carbon dioxide blood levels from pulmonary dysfunction or absence of circulating air leads to painful cerebral vasodilation. At their onset, brain tumors cause increased intracranial pressure only when the patient is recumbent.

141. Insert the proper substrates (a–e) into the synthesis and metabolism of dopamine (1–5).

1 $\xrightarrow{\text{tyrosine hydroxylase}}$ 2 $\xrightarrow{\text{DOPA decarboxylase}}$ 3 $\xrightarrow{\text{dopamine } \beta\text{-hydroxylase}}$
4 $\xrightarrow{\text{phenylethanolamine } N\text{-methyl-transferase}}$ 5

a. Dopamine

b. Epinephrine

c. DOPA

d. Norepinephrine

e. Tyrosine

ANSWER: 1-e, 2-c, 3-a, 4-d, 5-b. Tyrosine $\xrightarrow{\text{tyrosine hydroxylase}}$ DOPA $\xrightarrow{\text{DOPA decarboxylase}}$ Dopamine $\xrightarrow{\text{dopamine } \beta\text{-hydroxylase}}$ Norepinephrine $\xrightarrow{\text{phenylethanolamine } N\text{-methyl-transferase}}$ Epinephrine

142. Which tract conveys information between the mamillary bodies and the thalamus?

ANSWER: The mamillothalamic tract connects the mamillary bodies with the anterior nucleus of the thalamus.

143. Complete the indolamine pathway.

Tryptophan $\xrightarrow{\text{tryptophan hydroxylase}}$ 5-_____ $\xrightarrow{\text{amino acid decarboxylase}}$
5-_____ $\rightarrow$ 5-_____

ANSWER: Tryptophan $\xrightarrow{\text{tryptophan hydroxylase}}$ 5-hydroxytryptophan $\xrightarrow{\text{amino acid decarboxylase}}$ 5-hydroxytryptamine (serotonin) $\rightarrow$ 5-HIAA

144. A neurologist examined a 70-year-old man who sustained a right cerebral infarction resulting in left hemiplegia. As the neurologist was washing her hands at a bedside sink, the patient pointed to his left arm and asked her, "Doc! Did you forget your arm?" What disturbance probably gave rise to that question?

a. Inappropriate humor
b. Dementia
c. Anosognosia
d. A psychogenic disturbance

ANSWER: c. Patients with nondominant hemisphere lesions, unable to comprehend their left hemiplegia, often disown their body parts and assign them to others. Patients with anosognosia commonly use projection and other defense mechanisms.

145. Which of the following statements regarding flumazenil is true?

a. It enhances the actions of benzodiazepines.
b. It produces panic attacks in all individuals.
c. It blocks the actions of benzodiazepines.
d. It produces anxiety in normal individuals.

ANSWER: c. Flumazenil blocks the actions of benzodiazepines. It is used to reverse benzodiazepine overdose and in some cases of hepatic encephalopathy, which may result in part from benzodiazepine-like false neurotransmitters. It has no effect in most individuals but precipitates panic attacks in susceptible individuals.

146. During which period of gestation is the neural tube formed?

a. First trimester
b. Second trimester
c. Third trimester
d. Variable time
e. At the moment of conception

ANSWER: a. During the third and fourth weeks of gestation, the dorsal ectoderm invaginates to form a closed, midline neural tube that eventually gives rise to the spinal cord and other elements of the CNS. This is an intricate maneuver that is susceptible to disruption by medications, including antiepileptic drugs, and toxins. Improper neural tube formation leads to neural tube defects, such as the Arnold-Chiari malformation, spina bifida, and meningomyelocele.

147. Match the medication category (1–5) with its potential adverse reaction or side effects (a–e).

1. β-blocker
2. Phenytoin
3. Caffeine
4. Anticholinergics
5. SSRIs with MAO inhibitors

a. Agitation, myoclonus, fever, diarrhea
b. Blurred vision, urinary difficulty, forgetfulness
c. Palpitations, tachycardia, anxiety
d. Exfoliative dermatitis, especially at mucocutaneous borders
e. Bradycardia, orthostatic hypotension, fatigue

ANSWERS: 1-e, 2-d (Stevens-Johnson syndrome), 3-c (caffeinism), 4-b, 5-a (serotonin syndrome)

148. Which characteristic distinguishes dementia and toxic-metabolic encephalopathy?

a. Permanence
b. Development only in adults
c. Development only in individuals with normal intelligence
d. Inattention
e. Being alert
f. Disorientation

ANSWER: e. Depending on the etiology, both dementia and toxic-metabolic encephalopathy, which is also called delirium, can be reversed. Dementia and toxic-metabolic encephalopathy develop in children, young adults, and individuals who are mentally retarded. Both dementia and toxic-metabolic encephalopathy share many clinical features, including inattention and disorientation. However, patients with toxic-metabolic encephalopathy are typically lethargic or stuporous, although sometimes they are overly vigilant and characteristically have a fluctuating level of consciousness. In contrast, individuals with dementia are alert. Complicating this distinction, patients with dementia are much more susceptible to toxic-metabolic encephalopathy than normal individuals. When patients with Alzheimer's disease develop pneumonia, for example, they often manifest a confusing combination of changes in their behavior, thought, and mood.

149. With which condition is long-standing methysergide (Sansert) treatment associated?

a. Retroperitoneal fibrosis
b. Liver function abnormalities
c. Neural tube closure defects
d. Insomnia

ANSWER: a

150. A 19-year-old female college student, who seemed to have developed a chronic, non-infectious hepatitis the preceding year, begins to have a subtle decline in her grades, dysarthria, tremor, and depression. Except for abnormal liver function tests, routine laboratory testing and also CT, MRI, CSF, and EEG reveal no abnormalities. Which test should be ordered next?

a. HIV
b. HTLV-1
c. Mononucleosis spot test
d. Antistreptolysin O titer
e. Serum ceruloplasmin
f. MS evaluation

ANSWER: e. This patient has hepatic dysfunction, cognitive impairment, depression, tremor, and dysarthria. The patient may have Wilson's disease (hepatolenticular degeneration), in which case the sooner the diagnosis is made and the sooner treatment is instituted, the better the prognosis. A low serum concentration of ceruloplasmin, the copper-carrying serum protein, is indicative of Wilson's disease. This illness, which is transmitted as an autosomal recessive condition, may affect only the liver, but when it has neurologic complications, a Kayser-Fleischer ring may be found on a slit-lamp examination of the cornea. Other causes of hepatic dysfunction and mental changes include mononucleosis, alcoholism, and other substance abuse. MS is unlikely in view of the progressive course, early onset of cognitive impairment, and normal MRI.

151. Match the spinal cord tract (a–d) with its function (1–5).

a. Pyramidal
b. Spinothalamic
c. Fasciculus gracilis
d. Spinocerebellar

1. Ascends from the spinal cord to the cerebellum
2. Descends to innervate the anterior horn cells
3. Ascends to provide pain sensation
4. Transmits position sense from the upper extremities
5. Transmits position sense from the lower extremities

ANSWERS: a-2, b-3, c-5, d-1

152. Which five characteristics indicate that facial weakness is more likely due to a seventh cranial nerve lesion than a cerebral lesion?

a. Only flattening of the nasolabial fold
b. Loss or alteration of taste sensation
c. Inability to close the eyelid muscles and to smile on the same side of the face.
d. Hyperacusis or tinnitus ipsilateral to the facial weakness
e. Aphasia
f. Mastoid pain
g. Pain in the mastoid area before the facial weakness

ANSWER: b, c, d, f, g. Weakness of upper as well as lower facial muscles and the disruption of hearing and taste sensations characterize a cranial nerve VII injury. When the nerve is inflamed, pain is referred to the mastoid region.

153. A 35-year-old woman who has difficulty describing her symptoms seems to have, several times yearly, a several-hour episode of monocular visual obscuration followed by a throbbing, generalized headache. A general medical and neurologic evaluation and CTs with and without contrast infusion are normal. Which one of the following conditions is most likely?

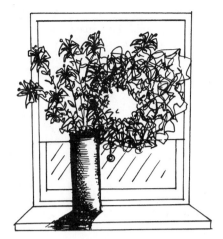

a. Migraine without aura (common migraine)
b. Transient ischemic attacks (TIA) from basilar artery stenosis
c. Migraine with aura (classic migraine)
d. Transient ischemic attacks (TIA) from carotid artery stenosis
e. An AVM
f. MS
g. Tension headaches

> *ANSWER:* c. Transient monocular visual disturbances that result from TIAs of the carotid artery (amaurosis fugax) usually last for less than 20 minutes, are unaccompanied by headache, and either resolve or progress to a stroke after a few episodes. Basilar artery TIAs may cause bilateral visual changes accompanied by vertigo and ataxia but usually not headaches or numerous recurrences. MS may cause episodes of unilateral visual loss and pain in or around the eye (optic neuritis), but the symptoms have a duration of several days to weeks and usually are accompanied by other neurologic deficits. AVMs may cause repeated bouts of an homonymous hemianopsia and headache, but they are almost always evident on CTs with contrast. Migraine with aura (classic migraine) but not migraine without aura (common migraines) includes visual auras. Often patients have mild forms of migraine with aura that are unrecognized because they do not experience dramatic visual hallucinations or they have prostrating headaches accompanied by nausea and vomiting. Tensions headaches are frequently episodic, but they are not associated with monocular visual symptoms.

154. Which two are common side effects of dopamine precursor or agonist treatment for Parkinson's disease?

a. Dyskinesias
b. Vivid dreams
c. Neuroleptic malignant syndrome
d. Seizures
e. Elevated serum prolactin concentration

> *ANSWER:* a, b. Excessive dopamine activity causes dyskinesias and vivid dreams. Neuroleptic malignant syndrome has occurred only in rare cases after the abrupt withdrawal of medications that enhance dopamine activity. Dopamine precursors and agonists do not cause seizures. They suppress serum prolactin concentrations.

155. A 17-year-old woman had been found at birth to have phenylketonuria (PKU) and was treated successfully with a strict phenylalanine-free diet. However, as a teenager, she frequently deviated from her diet, engaged in antisocial behavior, and recently conceived. Her boyfriend, who is the father, is not a carrier of PKU. Which of the following statements regarding the fetus is false?

a. If the fetus is male, he will almost certainly be a heterozygote for PKU and carry the gene.
b. In affected individuals, the blood tyrosine level is low and phenylalanine levels elevated.
c. Although the mother may sustain brain damage by her deviation from the diet, the fetus, which has normal metabolic enzymes, will be unharmed.
d. PKU infants are normal at birth.

ANSWER: c. Because PKU is an autosomal recessive disorder, the mother carries two abnormal genes, but the father has none. Both male and female offspring will be heterozygote. Even though the fetus is heterozygote, the affected mother's excessive phenylalanine intake can overwhelm the fetus' metabolic capacity and produce excessive concentrations of phenylalanine and its metabolic products, which are toxic to the brain. In other words, PKU women must strictly adhere to the diet when they are pregnant.

156. Which five varieties of tremor may be suppressed with β-blocker medication?

a. Essential
b. Performance anxiety
c. Resting
d. Lithium-induced
e. Benign
f. Cerebellar
g. Hyperthyroid
h. Psychogenic

ANSWER: a, b, d, e, g, h. β-blockers suppress the tremor associated with excessive autonomic nervous system activity that may result from anxiety, medications, or genetic factors. The resting tremor in as many as 10% of Parkinson's disease patients responds somewhat to β-blockers.

157. Match the lesion (a–g) with the movement disorder (1–6).

a. Atrophy of the caudate nuclei heads
b. Lewy bodies
c. Depigmentation of the substantia nigra
d. Infarction of the contralateral subthalamic nucleus
e. Compression of the seventh cranial nerve by an aberrant vessel
f. Depigmentation of the locus ceruleus
g. DYT1 gene

1. Parkinson's disease
2. Huntington's disease
3. Early onset primary (torsion) dystonia
4. Hemifacial spasm
5. Meige's syndrome
6. Hemiballismus

ANSWERS: a-2, b-1, c-1, d-6, e-4, f-1, g-3

158. Several days after an automobile accident, in which he sustained a whiplash injury, a 16-year-old boy begins to notice progressively worsening neck pain and weakness in his fingers. He has loss of pin sensation in a shawl pattern over his shoulder, upper arms, and hands but intact joint position and vibration sensation. DTRs in his arms are diminished, but those in his legs are brisk. Plantar reflexes are equivocal. Which of the following processes may be developing?

a. Worsening of the whiplash symptoms
b. Development of a herniated cervical intervertebral disk
c. Bleeding into the center of the spinal cord
d. Emergence of poststress symptoms

ANSWER: c. Hematomyelia, bleeding into the center of the spinal cord, which usually occurs in the cervical portion of the spinal cord, may follow neck injuries from motor vehicle, trampoline, horseback riding, or diving accidents. Hematomyelia forms a lesion similar to a syringomyelia (syrinx), in which the crossing fibers of the lateral spinothalamic tract are stretched and the anterior horn cells are compressed—impairing pin and temperature sensation and also lower motor neuron function. In addition, the corticospinal tracts are mildly compressed, which causes long tract motor signs in the legs. The congenital, nontraumatic variety of this disorder, syringomyelia, develops more insidiously, but the findings are similar.

159. Four months after delivering a healthy child, a 29-year-old woman has constant fatigue and bitemporal headaches. She is experiencing amenorrhea and galactorrhea. What is the most likely cause of her chronic fatigue?

a. Chronic Epstein-Barr virus (EBV) infection
b. Lyme disease
c. Secondary adrenal insufficiency

d. Excessive daytime sleepiness
e. Myasthenia gravis
f. Medication side effect
g. Drug or alcohol abuse
h. Infectious mononucleosis

ANSWER: c. All these conditions purportedly cause chronic fatigue syndrome. One well-recognized syndrome—postpartum fatigue, headaches, amenorrhea, and galactorrhea—is associated with pituitary adenomas (Chiari-Frommel syndrome). Another cause of excessive postpartum fatigue is pituitary infarction after a delivery complicated by profound hypotension (Sheehan's syndrome). In both cases, pituitary damage leads to (secondary) adrenal insufficiency.

160. In the preceding question, which visual field abnormality is associated with her condition?

a. Homonymous hemianopsia
b. Bitemporal hemianopsia or superior quadrantanopia
c. Binasal hemianopsia or superior quadrantanopia
d. None of the above

ANSWER: b. Bitemporal hemianopsia or superior quadrantanopia is associated with pituitary lesions that compress the overlying optic chiasm.

161. Which two of the following features are more commonly found in Alzheimer's disease than vascular dementia?

a. Depression
b. Motor impairments
c. Behavioral disturbances
d. Dysarthria and gait impairment
e. Wandering
f. Pseudobulbar palsy

ANSWER: c, e. Behavioral disturbances, hallucinations, agitation, wandering, and delusions are found more frequently in Alzheimer's patients. In contrast, vascular dementia more commonly causes depression (especially severe depression), gait impairment, dysarthria and other signs of pseudobulbar palsy, and unilateral or bilateral spastic paresis.

162. A 40-year-old man was struck on the back of his head with a baseball bat. He sustained a skull fracture and was rendered comatose for 2 days. When he became conversant, he confabulated about visitors and often wrongly identified people. He seemed to have marked visual impairment, but he denied it. His pupils were round and reactive. Funduscopy revealed no abnormalities. Extraocular movements were normal. What is the nature of his visual impairment?

a. Retinal detachments
b. Ocular trauma
c. Ocular blindness
d. Cortical blindness
e. Anosognosia

ANSWER: d. He has sustained cortical blindness because of trauma to the visual cortex in the occipital lobes. In cortical blindness, the eyes, optic nerves, and oculomotor nerves—which form the light reflex arc—are spared. His denial of blindness and tendency to confabulate about questions that depend on sight (Anton's syndrome) is a variety of anosognosia that usually follows sudden loss of vision. Anton's syndrome may result from occlusion of both posterior cerebral arteries, usually from an embolus that lodges at the tip of the basilar artery, which causes infarction of both occipital lobes.

163. Match the system (a–d) with the associated structures (1–4).

a. Cholinergic
b. Serotonergic
c. Noradrenergic (norepinephrine-containing)
d. Dopaminergic

1. Nucleus basalis of Meynert
2. Dorsal raphe nucleus
3. Locus ceruleus
4. Mesolimbic and mesocortical tracts

ANSWERS: a-1, b-2, c-3, d-4

164. What is the cardinal feature of conduction aphasia?

a. Patients cannot name objects.
b. Patients cannot follow simple requests.
c. Patients cannot repeat.
d. Patients have diffuse cognitive impairment.

> **ANSWER:** c. In conduction aphasia, a lesion interrupts the perisylvian language arc and severs the connection between Wernicke's and Broca's areas. Thus, patients cannot repeat what they hear.

165. Which one of the following conditions is not a disconnection syndrome?

a. Alexia without agraphia
b. Conduction aphasia
c. Split-brain syndrome
d. Gerstmann's syndrome
e. Ideomotor apraxia

> **ANSWER:** d. All conditions except Gerstmann's syndrome are disconnection syndromes. Another distinction is that all the conditions except for the split-brain syndrome usually result from dominant hemisphere lesions.

166. Which part of the body is most commonly involved in tardive akathisia?

a. Head
b. Arms
c. Legs
d. Trunk

> **ANSWER:** c. In tardive akathisia, the legs are involved most frequently and most severely, but the trunk, head, neck, and arms may also be involved. When akathisia is extensive, it resembles chorea.

167. Which are the two most common movements in tardive akathisia?

a. Walking or marching in place
b. Tremor of legs
c. Crossing or rapidly adducting and abducting the legs
d. Periodic flexion at the hip and ankle, especially when asleep

> **ANSWER:** a, c.

168. What treatable neurologic illness that might be confused with tardive dystonia often develops in young adults and causes personality change, dystonia, or both?

a. Athetosis
b. Cerebral palsy
c. Wilson's disease
d. SSPE

> **ANSWER:** c. The diagnostic tests would be determination of the serum ceruloplasmin and a slit-lamp examination of the eye. In Wilson's disease, the serum ceruloplasmin is low or absent. If the disease affects the brain, an ophthalmologist can usually detect Kayser-Fleischer rings in the cornea on a slit-lamp examination. The potential mental disturbances include personality changes, depression, dementia, and psychosis.

169. A 48-year-old waiter develops tremor at rest, rigidity, and bradykinesia. Otherwise her neurologic examination reveals no abnormalities. What is the best initial treatment of her condition?

a. Providing the missing enzyme
b. Giving the deficient neurotransmitter
c. Transplanting cells that synthesize the deficient neurotransmitter
d. Providing precursors that cross the blood-brain barrier for the deficient neurotransmitter

> **ANSWER:** d. Despite her relatively young age, she probably has Parkinson's disease. Restoring dopamine would correct her symptoms and also provide a therapeutic trial. Although dopamine is the deficient neurotransmitter, orally administered dopamine does not penetrate the blood-brain barrier. L-dopa, its precursor, crosses the blood-brain barrier and, by the action of dopa-decarboxylase, is metabolized to the active neurotransmitter, dopamine. Transplanting cells and ablative neurosurgical procedures have not been perfected and are yet not indicated in the initial stages of the illness.

170. By which pathway do almost all lung cancers spread to the brain parenchyma?

a. Hematogenous dissemination
b. Lymphatic spread
c. CSF seeding
d. Bony extension

ANSWER: a. The brain does not have a lymphatic supply.

171. A 55-year-old woman and her twin brother, who live hundreds of miles apart, have each developed insomnia that has not responded to several medications. An examination of each of them reveals inattentiveness and mild confusion, labile hypertension and tachycardia, and myoclonus. MRIs show atrophy of the thalamus. Which illness has developed?

a. A prion disease
b. Alzheimer's disease
c. Lewy body disease
d. Vascular dementia
e. Manic-depressive illness

ANSWER: a. They probably have developed fatal familial insomnia. This genetic susceptibility to prions causes refractory insomnia, cognitive and personality changes, autonomic and endocrine system hyperactivity, and motor changes, including myoclonus. Fatal familial insomnia is similar to Creutzfeldt-Jakob disease because of the average age of onset (approximately 50 years), cognitive impairment, myoclonus, and cerebral cortical spongiform changes.

172. What is the lowermost level of the body at which upper motor neurons are found?

a. Foramen magnum
b. Medulla
c. Beginning of the spinal cord
d. First lumbar vertebrae (L1)

ANSWER: d. The spinal cord contains upper motor neurons, which are carried in the corticospinal tract. Because the spinal cord terminates at L1 by giving rise to the cauda equina, the L1 level is the lowermost extent of upper motor neurons and the CNS.

173. A patient was prescribed a tricyclic antidepressant for diabetic neuropathy. Shortly after taking it, he developed abdominal distention and other symptoms and signs of intestinal obstruction. CT of the abdomen showed a paralytic ileus but no mass lesion or focal obstruction. What would be the best medication to correct the problem?

a. Neostigmine
b. ACh
c. Milk of magnesia
d. Cascara

ANSWER: a. The patient has developed pseudoobstruction from the anticholinergic side effects of the tricyclic antidepressant. Neostigmine, an acetylcholinesterase (AChE) inhibitor, will restore ACh activity and bowel motility.

174. Of the following, which is the most significant risk factor for strokes?

a. Type A personality
b. Race
c. Hypertension
d. Obesity

ANSWER: c. Of the numerous risk factors for strokes, hypertension and advanced age are the two greatest. Other risk factors, including obesity, diabetes, race, and elevated cholesterol levels, are so closely associated with each other and hypertension that their individual effect is difficult to assess. Psychological factors carry no significant risk.

175. A 50-year-old person has noticed diplopia on looking to the left. The right pupil is poorly reactive to light and larger than the left. There is right-sided ptosis. Which injury is most likely to have occurred?

a. Left sixth cranial nerve palsy
b. Right third cranial nerve palsy
c. Right transtentorial herniation
d. Left third cranial nerve palsy
e. Left transtentorial herniation
f. Myasthenia-induced paresis

ANSWER: b. Although diplopia on left lateral gaze might be attributable to either a left sixth or right third cranial nerve palsy, in this case the other signs of a third cranial nerve palsy indicate that the right third cranial nerve is responsible. Patients with herniation are stuporous or comatose: They are not alert enough to be able to express any symptom, except perhaps headache. Myasthenia does not affect the pupil.

176. With which other finding is tremor on intention most closely associated?

a. Dysdiadochokinesia
b. Rigidity
c. Bradykinesia
d. Ataxia of gait
e. Tremor at rest

ANSWER: a. Tremor on intention and other limb coordination problems, such as dysdiadochokinesia (impaired rapid alternating movements), are associated with cerebellar hemisphere injury. Tremor at rest is a manifestation of Parkinson's disease. Ataxia of gait is related to injury of the midline cerebellum (vermis) or the entire cerebellum.

177. Which feature is common to partial complex and petit mal (absence) seizures?

a. 3-Hz spike-and-wave EEG activity
b. Auras
c. Automatisms
d. Postictal confusion

ANSWER: c. Both conditions may induce repetitive, purposeless activities, such as lip-smacking movements. Thus, on clinical grounds alone, partial complex and absences may be confused.

178. Which of the following medications does not lower the seizure threshold?

a. Maprotiline (Ludiomil)
b. Diazepam (Valium)
c. Clomipramine (Anafranil)
d. Chlorpromazine (Thorazine)

ANSWER: b

179. Which of the following is not a side effect of antiepileptic drugs?

a. Allergic reactions
b. Liver or bone marrow toxicity
c. Gastrointestinal disturbances
d. Teratogenicity
e. Potentiating oral contraceptives

ANSWER: e. Phenytoin and possibly carbamazepine can interfere with oral contraceptives.

180. Videotaped monitoring of seizure patients is useful in determining which of the following?

a. The variety or frequency of the seizures
b. The presence of psychogenic seizures
c. The site of the origin of seizures
d. Correlation of seizures with antiepileptic drug blood levels
e. All of the above

ANSWER: e

181. The presence of Todd's hemiparesis after a generalized tonic-clonic seizure indicates that the patient probably has which of the following type of epilepsy?

a. Absence
b. Partial with secondary generalization
c. Primary generalized tonic-clonic
d. Partial elementary

ANSWER: b. Hemiparesis for as long as 24 hours after a seizure (Todd's paresis) suggests a cortical origin and temporary dysfunction of the adjacent motor area. Todd's paresis is often found with seizures induced by strokes or tumors.

182. Which of the following medications inhibits HIV reverse transcriptase?

a. Trimethoprim-sulfamethoxazole (Bactrim, Septra, and others)
b. Pyrimethamine (Daraprim)
c. Ganciclovir (Cytovene)
d. Zidovudine (Retrovir)
e. Pentamidine

ANSWER: d. Previously known as AZT and often given when HIV infection is first detected, zidovudine has increased median survival after diagnosis. Side effects include myopathy, headache, fatigue, malaise, and confusion. Trimethoprim-sulfamethoxazole and pentamidine are each effective for *Pneumocystis carinii* pneumonia (PCP). Pyrimethamine (Daraprim) is the treatment of choice for cerebral toxoplasmosis. Ganciclovir (Cytovene) is useful for cytomegalovirus (CMV) infections, especially CMV retinitis and colitis.

183. Which of the following infections is not a common complication of AIDS?

a. Pneumococcal meningitis
b. Mycobacterium tuberculosis
c. Mycobacterium avian complex
d. Syphilis
e. Mucosal candidiasis (oral thrush)

ANSWER: a. Because their cellular immunity is impaired, AIDS patients are particularly vulnerable to syphilis, tuberculosis, and fungal infections. However, their antibody-producing ability is relatively preserved and they can fight bacterial infections.

184. Which of the following areas of the brain is most susceptible to anoxia?

a. Medulla
b. Wernicke's area
c. Globus pallidus
d. Hippocampus

ANSWER: d. Although the entire cerebral cortex is sensitive, the hippocampus is exquisitely sensitive. The globus pallidus is damaged not only with anoxia but also with carbon monoxide poisoning.

185. Which two features would indicate that seizures were partial complex rather than petit mal?

a. Impaired consciousness
b. Fluttering eyelids
c. Symptoms that might constitute an aura
d. Childhood onset
e. Duration of 5 seconds
f. Tendency toward retrograde amnesia, personality change, or sleep after the seizure

ANSWER: c, f (see Table 10–4)

186. Which of the following are found in Alzheimer's disease?

a. Neuron loss in nucleus basalis of Meynert
b. Amyloid surrounded by abnormal neurites
c. Paired helical filaments within neurons
d. Loss of synapses
e. Lewy bodies in the cortex
f. All of the above

ANSWER: f. Amyloid surrounded by abnormal neurites, plaques, and paired helical filaments (neurofibrillary tangles) are characteristic of Alzheimer's disease. However, they are also found in people with Down's syndrome and dementia pugilistica. Lewy bodies, which are characteristic of Parkinson's disease, are found in the cerebral cortex in about 20% of the brains of Alzheimer's patients.

187. When botulinum toxin treatment is administered for focal dystonias, such as spasmodic torticollis, what is its mechanism of action?

a. Like curare, botulinum blocks acetylcholine neuromuscular receptors.
b. Botulinum impairs acetylcholine presynaptic release at the neuromuscular junction.
c. Botulinum depletes dopamine.
d. Like pyridostigmine (Mestinon), botulinum enhances acetylcholine activity.
e. Like nerve gas, botulinum creates a depolarization of the postsynaptic acetylcholine receptor site.
f. Acetylcholine strength is increased because its re-uptake is blocked by botulinum.

ANSWER: b. Botulinum inhibits dystonic muscle contractions by impairing acetylcholine release from the presynaptic neuron at the neuromuscular junction. Although botulinum may cause some weakness, the dystonia is greatly reduced. Curare and many nerve gases block the acetylcholine neuromuscular receptors, and in this way they can induce lethal paralysis. In contrast to the activity of dopamine and many other neurotransmitters whose action is partly terminated by re-uptake, acetylcholine activity is terminated entirely by cholinesterase metabolism.

188. Match the area of the nervous system (a–i) with its location (1–4).

a. Anterior horn cells
b. Corpus callosum
c. Locus ceruleus
d. Bulb
e. Vermis

f. Cranial nerve nuclei for swallowing
g. Origin of phrenic nerve
h. Heschl's gyrus
i. Hippocampus

1. Cerebrum
2. Cerebellum

3. Brainstem
4. Spinal cord

ANSWERS: a-4, b-1, c-3, d-3, e-2, f-3, g-4, h-1, i-1

189. Match the brainstem region (a–l) with its location (1–5).

a. Cranial nerve nucleus that innervates the jaw muscles
b. Cranial nerves that move eyes medial
c. Trochlear nerve
d. Cranial nerves that move eyes laterally
e. Beginning of the nigrostriatal tract
f. Cranial nerves that innervate the tongue muscles
g. Cranial nerves that govern speech and swallowing
h. Thalamus
i. Hypothalamus
j. Locus ceruleus
k. Crossing of the pyramids
l. Cranial nerve that innervates the upper and lower face muscles

1. Diencephalon
2. Midbrain
3. Pons
4. Medulla
5. None of the above

ANSWERS: a-3, b-2, c-2, d-3, e-2, f-4, g-4, h-1, i-1, j-3, k-4, l-3

190. Which two statements concerning syphilis or neurosyphilis are true?

a. In an appropriate clinical setting, a positive CSF-VDRL test confirms the diagnosis of neurosyphilis.
b. A dramatic increase in the incidence of syphilis has occurred in conjunction with the AIDS epidemic.
c. A negative CSF-VDRL test is strong evidence against a diagnosis of neurosyphilis.
d. A positive serum VDRL or RPR at a dilution of 1:2 is strong evidence of syphilis.

ANSWER: a, b. A large proportion of patients with neurosyphilis—40% in one study—have a negative CSF-VDRL. On the other hand, a positive CSF-VDRL is strong evidence that a patient has neurosyphilis. False-positive serum results, which are generally 1:4 or less, are attributable to other infection, rheumatologic diseases, drug addiction, and changes in serum proteins found with old age. False-negative serum results may be found when the disease is "burnt out," the infectious activity is low, or in rare cases when the antibody concentration is so great that a visible reaction is prevented (prozone inhibition).

191. Match the skin lesions (a–k) with its associated neurologic disorders (1–11).

a. Adenoma sebaceum (angiofibromas)
b. Kaposi's sarcoma
c. Vaginal chancre
d. Congenital facial angioma in the distribution of the first division trigeminal nerve
e. Acute eruption of vesicles in the distribution of the first division trigeminal nerve
f. Café au lait spots
g. Protuberance of skin and soft tissue at the base of the spine
h. Erythema migrans
i. Anesthetic, depigmented patches on the coolest regions of the face and body
j. Dermatitis, diarrhea, and dementia
k. White lines across the nails (Mees' lines)

1. Possible later development of Treponema in the CNS
2. Round growths in the brain that cause dementia and seizures
3. Intracerebral angioma that causes seizures but usually not bleeding
4. Development of encephalitis and cerebral lymphoma
5. Neurofibromas
6. Lancinating pain in the distribution of the skin lesion
7. Impotence
8. Pellagra
9. Lyme disease
10. Leprosy
11. Arsenic poisoning

ANSWERS: a-2, b-4, c-1, d-3, e-6, f-5, g-7, h-9, i-10, j-8, k-11

192. Identify the structures (1–6) on this MRI of a normal brain.

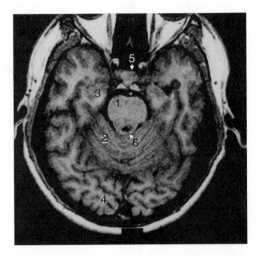

a. Origin of most partial complex seizures
b. Third ventricle
c. Fourth ventricle
d. Midbrain
e. Pons
f. Medulla
g. Origin of ACTH
h. Visual cortex
i. Governs coordination

ANSWERS: 1-e, 2-i (cerebellum), 3-a (mesial temporal lobe), 4-h (occipital cortex), 5-g (pituitary gland), 6-c (upper portion of the fourth ventricle)

193. Regarding the MRI in the preceding question, which view of the brain is portrayed?

a. Axial
b. Lateral
c. Coronal
d. Sagittal

ANSWER: a. This view is the traditional axial or transaxial image.

194. Match the neurotransmitter (a–d) with the area of the brain where it is formed (1–4).

a. Norepinephrine
b. Dopamine
c. Serotonin
d. Acetylcholine

1. Nucleus basalis of Meynert, which is inferior to the globus pallidus in the basal forebrain.
2. Raphe nucleus, which runs diffusely in the brainstem
3. Substantia nigra in the midbrain
4. Locus ceruleus, which is in the pons

ANSWERS: a-4, b-3, c-2, d-1

195. Which two of the following are associated with meningomyeloceles?

a. Mental retardation
b. Hydrocephalus
c. Neurofibromatosis
d. Intravenous drug abuse

ANSWER: a, b. Meningomyeloceles, which are lower neural tube closure defects, are associated with abnormalities of the upper end of the neural tube, particularly hydrocephalus and mental retardation.

196. About 10 days after beginning treatment with phenytoin, a 10-year-old child develops blisterlike lesions on the skin, eyes, mouth, and other mucous surfaces. Which condition is most likely?

a. Meningococcal meningitis
b. Child abuse

c. Allergy
d. Seizure associated trauma

ANSWER: c. The child has developed the Stevens-Johnson syndrome, which is a rare, life-threatening, allergic reaction. It has a predilection for mucous surfaces.

197. Which antiepileptic drug has a chemical structure that most closely resembles a tricyclic antidepressant?

a. Phenytoin
b. Phenobarbital

c. Carbamazepine
d. Valproic acid

ANSWER: c. Carbamazepine closely resembles imipramine.

198. Which is the best study in attempting to locate mesial temporal sclerosis?

a. CT
b. MRI

c. EEG
d. Routine x-rays

ANSWER: b. MRI provides better resolution than CT. Also, with the MRI, the skull does not create artifacts that might obscure structures mostly surrounded by the skull.

199. Which cell transmits congenital illnesses attributable to mitochondria defects?

a. The egg and the sperm in equal proportion
b. The egg exclusively
c. The sperm exclusively
d. The amniotic fluid

ANSWER: b. All the mitochondria in the embryo derive from the egg. Mitochondria in the sperm are contained in the tail, which drops off as the head penetrates the egg.

200. A neurologist performs a test on a 35-year-old man who had developed gait impairment. The test consists of asking him to stand with his feet together and his eyes open and then closed. With his eyes open, the patient was stable, but when his eyes were closed, the patient began to topple. To avoid falling, he separated his feet to catch himself. Damage in which two regions of the nervous system would most likely cause this test result?

a. Peripheral nervous system
b. Cerebellum
c. Posterior columns of the spinal cord

d. Labyrinthine system
e. Corticospinal tracts

ANSWER: a, c. The neurologist has subjected the patient to the Romberg test, in which a positive (abnormal) result consists of inability to stand erect with closed eyes. The underlying theory is that joint position sensation is normally conveyed through peripheral nerves to the posterior columns of the spinal cord to the brain. An intact system permits continual sensory monitoring and compensatory motor adjustments. Patients with cerebellar or labyrinthine disease would not be affected by their eyes being open or closed. Romberg tests are positive in peripheral neuropathies, such as diabetic neuropathy, and CNS diseases that have a predilection to affect the posterior columns of the spinal cord, such as MS and tabes dorsalis.

201. Identify the structures (a–f) on this MRI of a normal brain.

a. Single-headed white arrow
b. Double-headed white arrow
c. Relatively dark bandlike structure descending diagonally from single-headed black arrow
d. Cerebral lobe above the double-headed white arrow
e. Cerebral lobe below the double-headed white arrow
f. Area of the double-headed black arrow

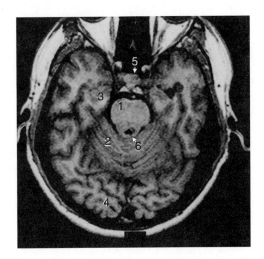

1. Frontal lobe
2. Temporal lobe
3. Parietal lobe
4. Occipital lobe
5. Caudate nucleus
6. Globus pallidus
7. Putamen
8. Internal capsule
9. General area of the nucleus basalis Meynert
10. Falx
11. Sylvian fissure

ANSWERS:

a-5. The head of the caudate nucleus constitutes the lateral border of the lateral ventricle.

b-11. The Sylvian fissure, which extends to the parietal lobe, separates the frontal from the temporal lobes.

c-8. The internal capsule, which contains the corticospinal and corticobulbar tracts, descends medially from the cerebral cortex to the brainstem.

d-1.

e-2.

f-9. The nucleus basalis of Meynert is difficult to visualize, but it is in the median forebrain bundle near the hypothalamus.

202. Regarding the MRI in the preceding question, which view of the brain is portrayed?

a. Axial
b. Transaxial
c. Coronal
d. Sagittal

ANSWER: c

203. Of the following, which is the most common form of inherited mental retardation?

a. Alzheimer's disease
b. Rett's syndrome
c. Trisomy 18
d. Fragile X syndrome
e. Turner's syndrome
f. Trisomy 21

ANSWER: d. Of the choices, the fragile X syndrome is the most common cause of inherited mental retardation. It sometimes has features of autism. The fragile X syndrome causes retardation in one boy in 1,000 to 1,500. These boys tend to have a long, thin face, large ears, and large testes. In 1 girl in 2,000 to 2,500, the fragile X syndrome causes retardation that is milder. The condition has no specific clinical features but may now be diagnosed by DNA analysis that demonstrates excessive trinucleotide repeats on the X chromosome. Trisomy 21 (Down's syndrome) is technically a genetic but not an inherited condition because neither parent carries the genetic abnormality nor is affected with the disorder. The incidence of Down's syndrome births is falling because of prenatal testing.

204. Why is carbidopa administered along with L-dopa in the treatment of Parkinson's disease?

   a. Carbidopa is a decarboxylase inhibitor that retards the metabolism of CNS L-dopa.
   b. Carbidopa maximizes the nigrostriatal L-dopa concentration.
   c. Carbidopa is a monoamine oxidase inhibitor.
   d. Carbidopa is a dopa agonist.

> ***ANSWER:*** b. Carbidopa is a decarboxylase inhibitor that is administered in fixed combinations with L-dopa (Sinemet). Because carbidopa does not cross the blood-brain barrier, it retards only systemic L-dopa metabolism and maximizes nigrostriatal L-dopa concentration. Because smaller doses of L-dopa are effective when administered with carbidopa, the cost is less and patients have fewer L-dopa side effects.

205. A neurologist is asked to evaluate a 68-year-old woman who has begun to have problems walking and performing her activities of daily living. As part of the examination, the neurologist asks the patient to remain in place while she pulls her backward by the shoulders. On one test, the patient involuntarily takes at least six steps backward. On another test, she seems to fall backward "en bloc" (see the figure below). What is the significance of the patient's reaction?

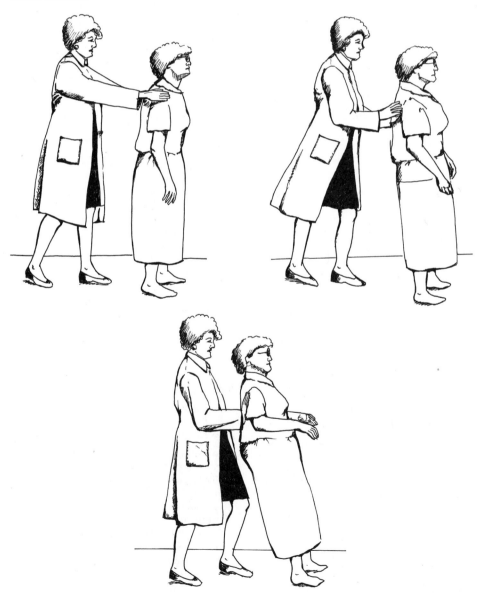

a. She has paresis of all her limbs, as though she had bilateral cerebral infarctions.
b. She has lost cerebellar function.
c. She has impaired postural reflexes.
d. Although the CNS may be normal, the labyrinthine system has been damaged.

> **ANSWER:** c. She first had retropulsion and then a positive pull test, which are both manifestations of basal ganglia dysfunction impairing postural reflexes. The pull test (pictured above) is positive in both Parkinson's disease and use of dopamine-blocking neuroleptics.

206. Match the treatment of Parkinson's disease (a–d) with its mechanism of action (1–4).

a. Pergolide
b. L-dopa

c. Selegiline
d. Bromocriptine

1. A dopamine precursor
2. A dopamine agonist

3. A monoamine oxidase A inhibitor
4. A monoamine oxidase B inhibitor

> **ANSWERS:** a-2, b-1, c-4, d-2

207. With which condition(s) is violent (directed, aggressive) behavior associated?

a. Epilepsy, all forms
b. Partial complex seizures
c. Episodic dyscontrol syndrome

d. Mental retardation
e. Males with the genotype XYY

> **ANSWER:** c

208. A 68-year-old man who had been in good health experienced a 20-minute episode of aphasia and right hemiparesis 2 days before an evaluation. He has a bruit over the right carotid artery, but otherwise he has normal general and neurologic examinations. An EEG, MRI of the head, and routine blood tests are normal. An angiogram discloses 50% stenosis of the left common carotid artery at its bifurcation. Which is the best course of treatment?

a. Investigate the right carotid artery.
b. Suggest a daily aspirin.
c. Refer him for left carotid surgery.
d. Continue to follow him but add no treatment.

> **ANSWER:** b. Recent, large studies indicate that in patients who have had a TIA (symptomatic patients), carotid endarterectomy was preferable to aspirin in reducing strokes when carotid stenosis was at least 70%. Because carotid bruits often are detectable over a nonstenotic carotid artery, they should not necessarily be taken as a sign of underlying carotid stenosis. Carotid bruits may be due to blood turbulence from minor atherosclerotic changes or greater blood flow through a normal artery because its counterpart is stenotic. They can also result from stenosis of the external carotid artery.

209. In Alzheimer's disease, with which pathologic feature is dementia most closely associated?

a. Cerebral atrophy
b. Senile plaques

c. Neurofibrillary tangles
d. Pick bodies

> **ANSWER:** c. Although the initial studies indicated that plaques were the abnormality most closely associated with dementia, recent work indicates that the tangles are even more closely associated. Cerebral atrophy is an age-related change.

210. Which is the most commonly occurring brainstem infarction?

a. Midbrain infarction
b. Pontine infarction

c. Lateral medullary syndrome
d. Medial medullary syndrome

> **ANSWER:** c

211. Which of the following conditions does a positive response to the Tensilon (edrophonium) test indicate?

a. Muscular dystrophy
b. Myasthenia gravis

c. Myotonic dystrophy
d. None of the above

ANSWER: b. Tensilon (edrophonium) is a cholinesterase inhibitor that prolongs the effectiveness of acetylcholine at the neuromuscular junction. This test temporarily reverses ocular and facial weakness in an individual with myasthenia gravis.

212. Which two of the following neurotransmitters project from the brainstem to the spinal cord?

a. Norepinephrine
b. Dopamine
c. Serotonin

ANSWER: a, c. Projections of norepinephrine and serotonin extend the length of the spinal cord. Dopamine tracts may be extensive, but they are confined to the brain.

213. Which of the following neurotransmitters is not a catecholamine?

a. Norepinephrine
b. Dopamine
c. Serotonin
d. Epinephrine

ANSWER: c. Serotonin is an indole, which is a five-member ring containing nitrogen joined to a benzene (six-member) ring. Catecholamines have a benzene ring with two hydroxyl groups and one amine group.

214. Which of the neurotransmitters in the preceding question is not derived from tyrosine?

ANSWER: c. Serotonin is derived from tryptophan. The others are derived from tyrosine.

215. Which EEG pattern does benzodiazepines induce?

a. α
b. β
c. θ
d. Δ

ANSWER: b. Benzodiazepines induce β activity. It is a characteristic change that may indicate surreptitious benzodiazepine use.

216. Where does the corticospinal tract cross as it descends?

a. Internal capsule
b. Base of the pons
c. Pyramids
d. Anterior horns cells

ANSWER: c. The crossing of the corticospinal tracts in the pyramids gives rise to their alternative name, pyramidal tracts.

217. In right-handed individuals, which artery supplies Broca's area and the adjacent corticospinal tract?

a. Anterior cerebral
b. Middle cerebral
c. Posterior cerebral
d. Basilar

ANSWER: b. The left middle cerebral artery supplies these areas and also the underlying internal capsule.

218. Which group of illnesses are *all* suggested by the presence of spasticity, hyperactive DTRs, and Babinski signs?

a. Poliomyelitis, strokes, spinal cord trauma
b. Bell's palsy, strokes, psychogenic disturbances
c. Spinal cord trauma, strokes, congenital cerebral injuries
d. Brainstem infarction, cerebellar infarction, spinal cord infarction
e. Parkinson's disease, generalized dystonia, cerebellar infarction

ANSWER: c. These signs indicate upper motor neuron injury, which would be found in central nervous system diseases that injure the corticospinal (pyramidal) tract. They would not be found in disease of the (1) peripheral nerves, (2) cranial nerves outside the brainstem (including Bell's palsy), (3) cerebellum, or (4) extrapyramidal system (including Parkinson's disease).

219. Patients with which group of illnesses usually have muscles that are paretic, atrophic, and areflexic?

a. Poliomyelitis, diabetic peripheral neuropathy, traumatic brachial plexus injury
b. ALS, brainstem infarction, psychogenic disturbance
c. Spinal cord trauma, strokes, congenital cerebral injuries
d. Brainstem infarction, cerebellar infarction, spinal cord infarction
e. Parkinson's disease, strokes, cerebellar infarction
f. Guillain-Barré syndrome, MS, and uremic neuropathy

ANSWER: a. These signs indicate lower motor neuron injury, which includes diseases of the anterior horn cell (e.g., poliomyelitis), peripheral nerves, and their plexuses.

220. A 73-year-old woman has had the sudden onset of the following signs: right-sided limb ataxia, dysarthria, lack of facial sensation on the right face and left side of the body, and a right-sided Horner's syndrome. To which side will the palate deviate when she attempts to say "ah"?

a. Right
b. Left

c. Both
d. Neither

ANSWER: b. She has a right-sided lateral medullary syndrome. The lesion encompasses the right nucleus ambiguus, which leads to paresis of the right palate. Right-sided paresis causes the palate to deviate to the left when the palatal muscles contract.

221. Which is the most characteristic change in Huntington's disease?

a. D_2 dopamine receptors are hypoactive.
b. D_2 dopamine receptors are hyperactive.
c. ACh receptors are reduced in the nucleus basalis of Meynert.
d. Gamma-aminobutyric acid (GABA) concentrations are reduced to less than 50% of normal in the corpus striatum.

ANSWER: d. GABA concentrations are reduced to less than 50% of normal in the caudate nuclei, which is one of the major components of the corpus striatum. In Alzheimer's disease, ACh receptors are reduced in the nucleus basalis of Meynert.

222. Of the following, which two tests provide the most reliable confirmation of the clinical diagnosis of MS when it is in a quiescent state?

a. MRI of the head
b. VERs
c. CSF studies for oligoclonal bands
d. CSF studies for myelin basic protein
e. CT of the head

ANSWER: a, c. The multiplicity of tests indicates that no single test is definitive. Moreover, most may be abnormal in non-MS demyelinating conditions, chronic CNS infections, and inflammatory diseases. The MRI portrays plaques as hyperintense white patches, which may be enhanced with gadolinium infusion. Oligoclonal bands in the CSF are also a reliable marker. Although large doses of contrast and delayed studies increase the sensitivity of CT, it is still insensitive to many cerebral lesions and unable to detect lesions in the optic nerves and the spinal cord. The CSF myelin basic protein concentration may be elevated in an acute attack of MS, but other inflammatory conditions and infectious illnesses may also elevate its concentration. When MS is quiescent, the concentration of CSF myelin basic protein is usually normal.

223. Which of the following descriptions best characterize the MRI changes of MS?

a. Multiple, white areas scattered in the cerebrum
b. Conversion of the cerebral hemisphere white matter to gray
c. Loss of the myelin signal throughout the corpus callosum
d. Periventricular, high-intensity abnormalities

ANSWER: d. The MRI shows large, white, hyperintense lesions in the periventricular region. It may also reveal lesions in the optic nerve or spinal cord. Bright, small, or punctate intracerebral lesions may result from cerebrovascular disease. Because their etiology is not established, they are called "unidentified bright objects or UBOs."

224. When is MS most likely to be exacerbated?

a. During pregnancy
b. During times of stress
c. In adolescence
d. After trauma
e. During the first 3 postpartum months

ANSWER: e. Although pregnancy is associated with some protection, the first 3 postpartum months are associated with MS exacerbations. The other factors are unproven precipitants of MS exacerbations.

225. When contemplating having a second child, a young mother who had developed MS during the postpartum period of her first delivery inquires about the effect of a second or third pregnancy on her MS. What is the current thinking?

a. Deliveries are almost always more complicated when the mother has MS.
b. MS worsens in a stepwise pattern with each succeeding pregnancy.
c. The number of pregnancies has little or no effect on the ultimate outcome of MS.
d. Her offspring, compared to the general population, will have an increased risk of developing MS.
e. Fetal malformations are more common than in the general population.

ANSWER: c, d

226. Which MS features are associated with cognitive impairment?

a. Paraparesis and blindness
b. Chronicity of the illness
c. Enlarged cerebral ventricles
d. Corpus callosum atrophy
e. Area and volume of cerebral plaques visualized by MRI
f. Decreased glucose metabolism on positron emission tomography

ANSWER: All

227. After being comatose for 2 weeks after an attempted strangulation, a 35-year-old woman babbles incoherently. She seems to repeat conversations that take place around her. Although weak, she can eat, sit, and watch television. Although she does not seem to see the television, she repeats the dialogue. She does not respond to visual stimulation. Her pupils are equal and reactive to light. Which is the best description of her condition?

a. Coma
b. Psychosis
c. Vegetative state
d. Locked-in syndrome
e. Isolation aphasia, dementia, and cortical blindness from watershed infarctions
f. None of the above

ANSWER: e. She has isolation aphasia because of her ability only to repeat. She also has cortical blindness because she cannot see, but her pupil function is spared. She is not comatose because she has interaction with her environment and possesses verbal and motor activity. In the vegetative state and the locked-in syndrome, patients cannot vocalize, eat, or sit.

228. Which of the following are characteristics of the *N*-methyl-D-aspartate receptor?

a. It is usually called the NMDA receptor.
b. It regulates calcium channels.
c. Excitatory neurotransmitters, such as glutamate, bind onto this receptor.
d. Overstimulation of the receptor leads to cell death by calcium flooding.
e. The NMDA receptor may be excitotoxic in strokes, epilepsy, and Huntington's disease.

ANSWER: All

229. Which of the following are not characteristics of the carpal tunnel syndrome?

a. It results from compression of the median nerve at the wrist.
b. Tinel's sign indicates carpal tunnel syndrome.
c. Repetitive stress injury causes the carpal tunnel syndrome.

d. It results in pain and weakness of the forearm extensor and supinator muscles.
e. It is typically worse at night.

> *ANSWER:* d. Carpal tunnel syndrome results from compression of the median nerve at the wrist. It may be caused by trauma, fluid retention, pregnancy, repetitive stress, and acromegaly. Tinel's sign is indicative of the disorder. In contrast, tennis elbow consists of pain and weakness of the forearm extensor and supinator muscles. It results from bursitis, muscle swelling, or entrapment of branches of the radial nerve. The most common cause of tennis elbow is occupational injury, not tennis.

230. What is the pattern of innervation of the anal and urinary bladder sphincters?

a. An internal sphincter is innervated by the peripheral nervous system, and an external sphincter is innervated by the autonomic nervous system.
b. An internal sphincter is innervated by the autonomic nervous system, and an external sphincter is innervated by the peripheral nervous system.
c. An internal sphincter is innervated by the central nervous system, and an external sphincter is innervated by the autonomic nervous system.
d. An internal sphincter is innervated by the peripheral nervous system, and an external sphincter is innervated by the central nervous system.

> *ANSWER:* b. In both sites, the internal sphincter is more powerful than the external sphincter.

231. A 49-year-old man being treated for alcohol withdrawal seizures became progressively more stuporous. Which three conditions might be considered?

a. Hypoglycemia
b. Antiepileptic drug intoxication
c. Bleeding from the small intracranial veins
d. Alcoholic stupor
e. All of the above

> *ANSWER:* a, b, c. Chronic alcoholism leads to cirrhosis that depletes stored glycogen. Unless glucose is supplied continuously, patients may develop hypoglycemia that causes seizures, as well as stupor. Inadvertent excessive treatment with antiepileptic drugs is relatively common, especially if a cirrhotic liver cannot metabolize medications. Bleeding from cerebral small veins, which characteristically leads to a subdural hematoma, is common in alcoholics because they have head trauma and impaired coagulation ability. Another possibility in alcoholic patients is that hepatic encephalopathy has developed.

232. Through which structure is CSF normally absorbed?

a. Spinal cord
b. Inner surface of the lateral ventricles
c. Choroid plexus
d. Arachnoid membrane
e. Cerebral hemisphere tissue

> *ANSWER:* d. CSF is normally formed in the choroid plexus and absorbed through the arachnoid layer of the meninges, predominantly at the base of the brain. When infection (as in meningitis) or blood (a subarachnoid hemorrhage) inflames the arachnoid membrane, CSF absorption is impaired and communicating or normal pressure hydrocephalus may develop. In those conditions, CSF may be absorbed through the ventricles.

233. A 75-year-old woman after vigorous hair washing at her local beauty parlor develops vertigo, nausea, and diplopia. She has ataxia when she begins to walk. A CT shows no abnormalities. What is the most likely cause of her disturbance?

a. Cerebral infarction
b. Brainstem ischemia
c. A chemical in the hair wash
d. Labyrinthitis

> *ANSWER:* b. She probably has had hyperextension (excessive backward bending) of her neck that crimped her vertebral arteries and precipitated a small infarction in the vertebrobasilar distribution. People who have osteophytes that press against the vertebral arteries as they pass upward through the cervical spine are apt to interrupt the vertebral blood flow if their neck is bent backward (hyperextended). Brainstem infarctions usually cannot be detected by CTs because of artifact generated by the surrounding skull.

234. A 35-year-old psychiatrist in her last trimester of pregnancy has painful tingling in most of her hands and all of her fingers. She also finds that small objects seem to drop from her fingers. The symptoms are worse in the late afternoon and early morning hours. She has no objective abnormalities. Percussion of the wrist re-creates the paresthesias. What is the cause of her problem?

a. Entrapment of the median nerve in each wrist
b. Peripheral neuropathy
c. Cervical spondylosis
d. Guillain-Barré syndrome
e. Lyme disease

ANSWER: a. She has bilateral carpal tunnel syndrome, that is, median nerve compression or entrapment at the wrist. The usual distribution of the median nerve is the palmar surface of the thumb, adjacent two fingers, and the lateral portion of the palm, but many people with carpal tunnel syndrome have sensory disturbances that do not strictly conform to the textbook's map. Paresthesias in the median nerve distribution produced by tapping the flexor surface of the wrist—Tinel's sign—are virtually pathognomonic. This disorder usually results from fluid accumulation in the carpal tunnel, as occurs during pregnancy, before menses, and after trauma to the wrist, including "repetitive stress injuries" (e.g., typing on a keyboard, wrist exercising, and sometimes excessive driving). Nerve conduction velocity studies that demonstrate slowing across the flexor surface of the wrist confirm the diagnosis. Her carpal tunnel syndrome will probably resolve after delivery. Most patients respond to wrist splints, diuretics, or change in activities. Individuals who do not respond to these conservative measures may benefit from steroid injections into the carpal tunnel or surgery.

235. A 19-year-old student at a small New England college develops ascending, flaccid, and areflexic weakness of her legs, trunk, and then arms. When she develops ocular, facial, and pharyngeal weakness, she is intubated for ventilator support. During periods of agitation, she was found to be hypoxic. Which of the following conditions is the most likely cause of her paralysis?

a. MS
b. Conversion disorder
c. Poliomyelitis
d. Guillain-Barré syndrome
e. Herniated cervical intervertebral disk

ANSWER: d. She most likely has Guillain-Barré syndrome (also called "acute inflammatory demyelinating polyradiculoneuropathy [AIDP]") because of the extensive peripheral neuropathy. Poliomyelitis is asymmetric and does not involve ocular motility. Many infectious illnesses—*Campylobacter jejuni* infection, mononucleosis, Lyme disease, AIDS, hepatitis—can produce the Guillain-Barré syndrome, but no particular agent is identified in most cases. The mental changes result from hypoxia rather than direct cerebral involvement.

236. Which three of the following statements about CNS and PNS myelin are true?

a. The same cells produce CNS and PNS myelin.
b. Oligodendrocytes are to Schwann cells as the CNS is to the PNS.
c. They insulate electrochemical transmissions.
d. They are usually affected by the same illness.
e. The optic nerves are covered by CNS myelin.

ANSWER: b, c, e

237. Which conditions might an HIV infection produce?

a. Dementia
b. Myelopathy
c. Guillain-Barré syndrome
d. Myopathy

ANSWER: All

238. Which structure connects the hippocampus to the mamillary bodies?

a. Cingulate gyrus
b. Mamillothalamic tract
c. Fornix
d. Amygdala

ANSWER: c

239. Following vigorous treatment with dopamine-blocking antipsychotic agents for a recurrence of schizophrenia with psychotic behavior, a 29-year-old man lapses into stupor. He is found to have a temperature of 104° F, tachycardia, and axial and appendicular rigidity. Which one of the following strategies would be least appropriate?

a. Treatment with dopamine agonists, such as bromocriptine
b. Administration of intravenous fluids
c. Excluding infectious causes of fever, particularly meningitis
d. Administration of muscle relaxants, such as dantrolene
e. Administration of dopamine precursors, such as L-dopa with carbidopa
f. Halting further administration of antipsychotic agents

> *ANSWER:* e. Although other causes could be considered, the patient probably has developed the neuroleptic malignant syndrome. The standard treatments aim to the dopamine depletion, dehydration, fever, and muscle rigidity.

240. Which of the following statements are true regarding acetylcholine?

a. It is a neurotransmitter at the neuromuscular junction.
b. It is a neurotransmitter in the CNS.
c. Like GABA, acetylcholine is an inhibitory neurotransmitter.
d. Acetylcholine is deactivated as much by re-uptake as metabolism.

> *ANSWER:* a, b

241. Which condition is characterized by absence of dystrophin on a muscle biopsy?

a. Myotonic dystrophy
b. Becker's dystrophy
c. Duchenne's dystrophy
d. Diabetic neuropathy

> *ANSWER:* c. Absence of dystrophin, the normal muscle cell membrane protein, is virtually diagnostic of Duchenne's dystrophy. In Becker's dystrophy, the variant of Duchenne's dystrophy, dystrophin is reduced or abnormal. In the dystrophin test, muscle biopsies are tested for dystrophin to distinguish among these conditions and exclude others that might mimic them.

242. Against which site are antibodies directed in myasthenia gravis?

a. ACh nicotinic postsynaptic receptors
b. ACh muscarinic postsynaptic receptors
c. ACh quanta
d. AChE

> *ANSWER:* a

243. If an EEG shows "K complexes," in which state of consciousness is the patient?

a. Coma
b. Deep sleep
c. Light sleep
d. Dreaming
e. Alert
f. In a metabolic encephalopathy
g. Beset by a generalized seizure
h. Beset by a partial complex seizure
i. Pretending to be unresponsive
j. Sedated by medications or drugs

> *ANSWER:* c. K complexes are indicative of Stage 2 NREM sleep, which is relatively light sleep.

244. Which two conditions are associated with quadriparesis?

a. Hypokalemia
b. REM activity
c. Hyponatremia
d. Cocaine

> *ANSWER:* a, b. Hypokalemic periodic paralysis, cataplexy, and REM periods during normal sleep cause episodic areflexic quadriparesis. Hyponatremia, when severe, causes stupor and seizures but not quadriparesis.

245. Regarding mitochondrial DNA (mtDNA), which statement(s) are true?

a. Ragged red fibers are virtually pathognomonic of an mtDNA abnormality.
b. An individual's mtDNA is inherited exclusively from the mother.
c. mtDNA is not inherited in the chromosomes.

d. mtDNA abnormalities are not inherited in a classic Mendelian pattern.

e. Abnormalities often produce combinations of myopathies, lactic acidosis, and progressively severe encephalopathies.

f. All of the above.

ANSWER: f

246. Which of the following is/are true regarding dystrophin?

a. Dystrophin is located in the muscle cell's surface membrane.

b. Dystrophin is absent in Duchenne's dystrophy.

c. Dystrophin is absent in myotonic dystrophy.

d. Dystrophin absence is a reliable marker of Duchenne's dystrophy that can be detected with a commercially available test.

e. Dystrophin is abnormal in Becker's dystrophy, which results from the same gene as Duchenne's dystrophy.

f. Dystrophin is abnormal in myotonic dystrophy, which results from the same gene as Duchenne's dystrophy.

ANSWER: a, b, d, e

247. Which are genetic characteristics of myotonic dystrophy?

a. Females as well as males are susceptible to the illness.

b. mtDNA might be affected.

c. In successive generations, the disease appears at a younger age because of anticipation.

d. In successive generations, the disease is more severe because of anticipation.

e. Like other dominantly inherited nervous system disorders—Huntington's disease, early onset primary (torsion) dystonia, tuberous sclerosis, and neurofibromatosis—myotonic dystrophy is not associated with storage of a particular metabolic product.

ANSWER: a, c, d, e

248–252. What is the mechanism of action of the following poisons?

248. Poison gases

249. Tetanus

250. Botulism

251. Cyanide

252. Carbon monoxide

a. Blocks the release of glycine, an inhibitory neurotransmitter

b. Poisons the respiratory energy pathway

c. Interferes with the oxygen-carrying capacity of hemoglobin

d. Inactivates acetylcholinesterase (AChE), which causes excessive ACh activity

e. Blocks the release of acetylcholine from the presynaptic membrane of the neuromuscular junction

f. Blocks the release of acetylcholine from the presynaptic membranes in the brainstem

ANSWERS: 248-d, 249-a, 250-e, 251-b, 252-c

253–258. Match the lifestyle (253–258) with its consequences (a–e).

253. Steroid injections for body building

254. Deer hunting in Connecticut

255. Using tryptophan-containing products as a hypnotic

256. Alcoholism

257. Eating undercooked game.

258. Excessive pyridoxine (vitamin B_6) consumption

a. Myositis

b. Eosinophilia-myalgia syndrome

c. Upper and lower facial nerve paresis
d. Hypertrophied muscles, excessive facial hair, amenorrhea
e. Peripheral neuropathy

ANSWERS:

253. d

254. c or e, a. Tics in Connecticut are vectors for Lyme disease. Undercooked venison may contain *Trichinella.*

255. b. Tryptophan has been contaminated by substances that cause eosinophilia and myalgia.

256. e. Alcoholism, probably through the associated nutritional deficiency, causes peripheral neuropathy.

257. a. *Trichinella* causes trichinosis.

258. e. Taking excessive pyridoxine (vitamin B_6) causes a peripheral neuropathy.

259. A 24-year-old man, who has a history of substance abuse, is brought to the emergency room after his parents found him standing in the local high school football field dressed only in short pants at midnight in the middle of the winter. He was oblivious to the freezing temperature and snow flurries. Although standing with his eyes open, he was mute and unresponsive to his parents' questions and requests. In the emergency room, he has hypertension and tachycardia. He remains totally uncommunicative. He drools and stares at his parents and physicians. He has intermittent nystagmus in all directions. His muscle tone is so great that it makes him rigid. Which one of the following substances is most likely to have caused his condition?

a. Alcohol   c. Methamphetamine
b. Cocaine   d. Phencyclidine (PCP)

ANSWER: d. His abnormal behavior and mental status, chiefly the "wide awake coma," in combination with the nystagmus and muscle rigidity, is characteristic of PCP intoxication. Wernicke-Korsakoff syndrome causes nystagmus but not muscle rigidity.

260. A 25-year-old right-handed patient underwent a commissurotomy for intractable seizures. It was successful, but he describes not being able to express himself fully. Which is the most likely explanation?

a. Aphasia is a complication of the procedure.
b. Commissurotomy patients lose cognitive function.
c. Emotions generated in the left hemisphere are not as readily verbalized as those generated in the right hemisphere.
d. Emotions generated in the right hemisphere are not as readily verbalized as those generated in the left hemisphere.

ANSWER: d

261. Of the following illnesses, which four are most likely to be affecting this kindred?

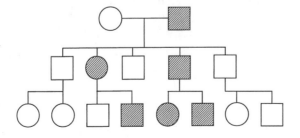

a. Duchenne's muscular dystrophy
b. Myotonic dystrophy
c. Hemophilia
d. Sickle cell disease
e. Wilson's disease
f. Huntington's disease
g. Alzheimer's disease
h. Early onset primary (torsion) DYT1 dystonia

ANSWER: b, f, g, h. As in the standard portrayal of genetic information, females are represented by circles, males by squares, and affected individuals by shaded forms. In this and subsequent questions, paternity is assured, parents are unrelated by blood, and parents who are not pictured are free of the illness. This kindred illustrates an autosomal dominant disease that has affected males and females. Myotonic dystrophy and Huntington's disease are classic autosomal dominant disorders. Early onset primary (torsion) dystonia is inherited as an autosomal illness but the penetrance is only 30% to 40%. Alzheimer's disease is usually a sporadic illness, but many families are affected by an autosomal dominant inheritance. A recessive disorder, such as sickle cell disease, is unlikely because the female in generation 1 and two spouses in generation 2 (not represented) would each have to be a carrier.

262. The individual in this kindred developed a genetic illness that was fatal in childhood. Which two of the illnesses listed in Question 261 might have been responsible?

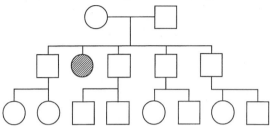

ANSWER: d, e. Her illness was autosomal recessive because neither parent had been affected. Because the patient was a girl, she could not have had Duchenne's muscular dystrophy or hemophilia, which are both x-linked recessive illnesses.

263. In this kindred, what is the chance that, if the woman in generation 2 were to have another son, he would have the illness that has affected his two older brothers?

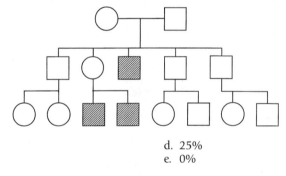

a. 100%
b. 75%
c. 50%

d. 25%
e. 0%

ANSWER: c. The illness is an x-linked disorder because the only family members with the illness are male. The woman with two affected sons has one normal and one abnormal gene. Only 50% of her future sons will inherit an abnormal gene.

264. Of the illnesses listed in Question 261, which one is most likely to have affected the three individuals in Question 263?

ANSWER: a. Duchenne's muscular dystrophy

265. In this kindred, five individuals are affected by a genetic illness that became fatal at the ages designated by the numerals. Of these illnesses, which one is most likely to be responsible?

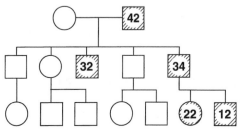

a. Duchenne's muscular dystrophy
b. Myotonic dystrophy
c. Hemophilia
d. Sickle cell disease
e. Wilson's disease
f. Huntington's disease
g. Alzheimer's disease
h. Early onset primary (torsion) dystonia

ANSWER: f. The illness is an autosomal dominant disorder that becomes apparent and fatal at a relatively young age. Although myotonic dystrophy and early onset primary (torsion) DYT1 dystonia become apparent in children and young adults, neither is usually fatal at that time. Familial Alzheimer's disease becomes apparent before sporadically developing cases but usually not until at least late middle age.

266. In Question 265, the disease becomes apparent at a younger age in successive generations. In which illnesses listed in Question 261 is that pattern characteristic?

ANSWER: b, f. The tendency of individuals in successive generations to show signs of a genetic illness at a younger age, termed *anticipation*, is attributable to the instability of abnormal DNA. The phenomenon is clearer in males than females. Anticipation is a characteristic of myotonic dystrophy, Huntington's disease, and other illnesses associated with trinucleotide repeats.

267. Which two forms of communication are based, like speech and hearing, in the dominant hemisphere's perisylvian language arc?

a. Reading and writing
b. Melody for most people
c. American Sign Language
d. Cursing
e. Prosody
f. Body language

ANSWER: a, c

268. Which of the following is a disconnection syndrome?

a. Nonfluent aphasia
b. Conduction aphasia
c. Fluent aphasia
d. Isolation aphasia
e. Dementia
f. Global aphasia

ANSWER: b. Disconnection syndromes generally refer to neuropsychologic disorders in which connections between the primary neuropsychologic centers are severed, but the centers themselves are intact and capable of functioning. Conduction aphasia consists of the separation of Wernicke's and Broca's areas. Other disconnection syndromes are the split-brain syndrome and alexia without agraphia.

269. Which two of the following arteries perfuse Broca's area?

a. Anterior cerebral artery
b. Middle cerebral artery
c. Posterior cerebral artery
d. Internal carotid artery system

ANSWER: b, d

270. What is the common neurologic term for the zone of cerebral cortex between branches of the major cerebral arteries?

a. Watershed area (border zone)
b. Limbic system
c. Cornea
d. Arcuate fasciculus

ANSWER: a

271. Which condition is caused by hypoperfusion of the watershed area?

a. Alexia without agraphia
b. Fluent aphasia
c. Hemiparesis
d. Isolation aphasia

ANSWER: d. The perisylvian language arc is well-perfused by relatively large branches of the middle cerebral artery. The more distal cortical regions, the watershed areas, have a tenuous blood supply from distal branches of the anterior, middle, and posterior cerebral arteries. With hypotension, the watershed areas often receive insufficient blood supply and develop ischemia; however, the language arc generally continues to receive an adequate supply. When the perisylvian language arc survives but the outlying cortex is damaged, language function is isolated. It will be devoid of cognitive input, and the patient will be able only to perform repetition.

272. Which cerebral artery perfuses the cerebral motor cortex for the contralateral leg?

a. Anterior cerebral artery
b. Middle cerebral artery
c. Posterior cerebral artery

ANSWER: a

273. After a CVA, in which the main symptom was left-sided sensory loss, a patient's left hand had involuntary or unconscious movements. The patient alternated between describing the hand in derogatory terms, being oblivious to it, and ascribing the hand to his roommate. When the patient became hallucinatory and paranoid, a psychiatry consultation was requested. Which condition is the most likely explanation?

a. Hemiballismus
b. Alien hand syndrome
c. Dementia
d. Aphasia
e. Anosognosia
f. Post-CVA psychosis

ANSWER: b. The alien hand syndrome, which may be a component of the nondominant parietal lobe syndrome, is the perceptual disorder that the hand is independent of them or particularly that it acts under another person's control. Anosognosia and other symptoms of nondominant parietal lobe damage may accompany these delusions. Patients often employ defense mechanisms in response to their problem, but sometimes they become irrational and agitated.

274. Which of the following apraxias is most closely associated with dementia and incontinence?

a. Ideational
b. Dressing
c. Ideomotor
d. Buccofacial
e. Oral
f. Gait

ANSWER: f. In normal pressure hydrocephalus (NPH), patients have gait apraxia, urinary incontinence, and dementia. The apraxia is the most characteristic feature. It is also the feature most readily responsive to treatment by insertion of a ventriculoperitoneal shunt.

275. A 40-year-old woman had migraine headaches as a teenager, but they were replaced by tension headaches once she married and had two children. During the past 5 years, the headaches evolved into a pattern of dull, symmetric, nonthrobbing pain present throughout every day. She has come to rely on prescription medications but not opioids. However, when the headaches flare up, which is about once a month, she visits an emergency room, where physicians give her opioid injections. Further evaluation reveals no underlying neurologic or serious psychiatric disorder. How should this problem be classified?

a. Chronic daily headaches
b. Tension headaches
c. Status migrainous
d. Obsessive-compulsive disorder

ANSWER: a. This woman has a distinct entity, chronic daily headache (CDH), which typically evolves from migraine and superimposed tension headaches. Its key feature is usually medication abuse or at least daily use of analgesic or vasoconstrictor medications. Occasionally patients are addicted to opioids, sedatives, or anxiolytics. In some patients, depression leads to CDH, but in many others, depression results from it. Patients with CDH also take medication to avoid "rebound" headaches and withdrawal symptoms. CDH is a major diagnostic problem because patients request medication for their headaches, but the symptom is medication-induced.

276. Patients often perceive migraine pain in or behind their eye (i.e., in the periorbital or retro-orbital location) even though the abnormality is in the meninges or extracranial vessels. What accounts for this discrepancy?

a. Intraocular pressure rises during migraines.
b. Changes that occur in the ocular circulation produce pain.
c. The trigeminal nerve innervates the meninges and the pain is referred.
d. Nerve receptors for pain in the brain misperceive the location of pain.
e. None of the above

ANSWER: c. The trigeminal nerve innervates the meninges, as well as the eye and its orbit. The brain itself has no pain receptors. Thus, neurosurgeons can operate on the brain without using anesthesia, and the patient can remain awake during certain neurosurgical procedures. In migraines and cluster headaches, pain is referred to the eye, which is supplied by the first division of the trigeminal nerve.

277. A despondent farm worker impulsively ingests a nearby, common organophosphorous insecticide poison. He becomes confused, dysarthric, and ataxic. He has bradycardia, miosis, excessive salivation, sweating, and muscle weakness with fasciculations. Which of the following is the best antidote?

a. Atropine
b. Neostigmine

c. Physostigmine
d. None of the above

ANSWER: a. The farm worker poisoned himself with an acetylcholinesterase (AChE) inhibitor, which is the active ingredient of common organophosphorous insecticide poisons. He has thus developed acetylcholine (cholinergic) toxicity, which is characterized by miosis, bradycardia, and fasciculations. The antidote to the CNS effects must be an anticholinergic medication, typically atropine, which crosses the blood-brain barrier. Often other medications, such as pralidoxime, must be administered to reverse the excessive acetylcholine (cholinergic toxicity) at the neuromuscular junction.

278. After a self-prepared meal, a novice plant lover develops excitation, restlessness, euphoria, dilated pupils, an uncomfortable dry mouth, and an intense thirst. Which of the following would be the best antidote?

a. Atropine
b. Neostigmine

c. Physostigmine
d. None of the above

ANSWER: c. This question is the counterpart of the preceding question. This patient has atropine poisoning, which is characterized by excitement, dry mouth, and dilated pupils. The excessive anticholinergic activity must be counteracted by an acetylcholinesterase (AChE) inhibitor that crosses the blood-brain barrier. A general rule is that atropine and physostigmine counteract each other.

279. Which two of the following statements are true regarding saccades?

a. Their speed is about 30°/s.
b. Their speed is rapid and can reach 700°/s.
c. They are governed by supranuclear centers.
d. Abnormalities in saccades characterize the onset of Alzheimer's disease.

ANSWER: b, c. Saccades, the high-velocity conjugate gaze movements, are generated by cerebral conjugate gaze centers. Abnormal saccades are one of the first physical findings in Huntington's disease and are also found in schizophrenia.

280. Which one of the following statements is false regarding pursuit eye movements?

a. They are the smooth, steady tracking movements used to follow moving objects.
b. They are abnormal in Huntington's disease.
c. They are governed by supranuclear centers.
d. They are abnormal in many patients with schizophrenia.

ANSWER: c. Pursuits, the relatively slow, smooth conjugate gaze movements, are generated mostly by the pontine conjugate gaze centers. They are abnormal slow and irregular in schizophrenia and, to a lesser extent, in affective disorders, as well as in basal ganglia disorders.

281. In which four conditions might combinations of unilateral miosis, ptosis, and anhidrosis be found?

a. Pancoast tumors
b. Cluster headache
c. Migraine with aura

d. Lateral medullary syndrome
e. Midbrain infarction
f. Chiropractic neck manipulation

ANSWER: a, b, d, f. Horner's syndrome, which consists of ptosis, miosis (small pupil), and anhidrosis (lack of sweating), results from injury to the sympathetic supply of the face and eye. The combination of miosis and ptosis, usually without the anhidrosis, is a classic sign of cluster headaches. Vigorous chiropractic neck manipulation may lead to dissection of the vertebral artery, which causes posterior inferior cerebellar artery (PICA) occlusion and the lateral medullary (Wallenberg) syndrome. Those conditions also cause most or all of the signs of Horner's syndrome. Pancoast tumors produce all the elements of Horner's syndrome because these tumors invade sympathetic ganglia in the chest. In contrast, parasympathetic innervation of the pupil is carried along with the third cranial nerve, which originates in the midbrain. Migraines and midbrain infarctions may impair parasympathetic innervation and cause dilation of the pupil.

282. To which four vision-impairing conditions are the elderly particularly susceptible?

a. Cataracts
b. Glaucoma
c. Strabismus
d. Amblyopia ex anopia

e. Macular degeneration
f. Temporal arteritis
g. Psychogenic visual loss

ANSWER: a, b, e, f. Strabismus is congenital extraocular muscle weakness. If uncorrected, the affected eye will become blind from disuse (i.e., amblyopia ex anopia).

283. A neurologic examination of a 75-year-old man shows no abnormality of cognitive or physical function except for impairment of vibration sensation in both great toes. Pain and temperature sensations are preserved. Ankle DTRs are absent. Plantar reflexes are flexor. Which is the most likely explanation for the findings?

a. Combined system disease
b. Alzheimer's disease
c. MS

d. Diabetes
e. None of the above

ANSWER: e. He probably has age-related peripheral nervous system changes, which consist first of loss of DTRs and sense of vibration. Combined system disease and MS, which are CNS diseases, cause spasticity and Babinski signs (extensor plantar reflexes). Diabetic neuropathy, which develops several years after the onset of the illness, is associated with early loss of pain and temperature.

284. A 14-year-old boy with pronounced mental retardation has repetitive, stereotyped movements. He has a large forehead, large lobulated ears, and macro-orchidism. His sister is reportedly physically normal but slow in school. His mother, who is 43 years old, is planning on remarrying and conceiving. Which two of the following statements is true?

a. The boy probably has the fragile X chromosome.
b. Because her son's condition is rare, the mother's next pregnancy has no greater risk than for other women of her age.
c. The sister probably is, as the mother says, merely a mediocre student and does not need to be evaluated further.
d. Because she is 43 years old, further evaluation is indicated for future pregnancies.

ANSWER: a, d. The boy has the fragile X syndrome, which is an inherited disorder transmitted by a faulty X chromosome. This syndrome, the most frequent causes of inherited mental retardation, accounts for about 10% of all cases of mental retardation. As if the disorder were transmitted as an incompletely recessive sex-linked trait, fragile X occurs in a modified form—mild mental retardation—in girls.

This mother must be concerned. Because she is 43 years old, she might have a child with Down's syndrome (trisomy 21). Down's syndrome is not considered inherited "on a technicality": an affected child did not receive the condition from an affected parent. Down's syndrome causes mental retardation and, in the fifth and sixth decades, an Alzheimer-like dementia. The mother must also be concerned because the fragile X syndrome is inherited, and future conceptions are in danger of this disease, as well as Down's syndrome. A different father will not reduce the risk of fragile X syndrome because the mother is the carrier of the defective gene.

As a general rule, when genetic conditions cause mental retardation, they are apparent early and are accompanied by physical abnormalities.

The younger sister must also be evaluated. She could have a modified form of the fragile X syndrome and thus herself be a carrier. In any case, she ought to be evaluated for her poor school performance.

Another general rule is that pregnant women over 40 years old should have amniocentesis to detect Down's syndrome, fragile X, and numerous other conditions. Also, the mother should undergo screening that is more extensive because she has one child with mental retardation.

285. A 17-year-old boy has numerous light brown, flat "birthmarks," which are each larger than 3 cm by 1 cm, and axillary "freckles." He inquires about some nodules that have been developing on his arms and face. Which two statements concerning these new lesions are true?

a. They represent von Recklinghausen's disease or neurofibromatosis.
b. They are closely associated with bilateral acoustic neuromas.
c. His siblings and parents ought to be examined because one of them is likely to have the same condition.
d. They are adenoma sebaceum (angiofibromas), which is the cutaneous manifestation of tuberous sclerosis.

ANSWER: a, c. He has von Recklinghausen's disease or neurofibromatosis type 1 (NF1), which is a common inherited neurocutaneous disturbance characterized by a triad of six or more café au lait spots and nodules (neurofibromas) on peripheral nerves that become apparent in adults. NF1 patients tend to develop meningiomas. About 50% of them acquire the disorder through inheritance. The other 50% apparently acquire it by mutation.

In contrast, a different disorder, previously also called von Recklinghausen's disease and now called neurofibromatosis type 2 (NF2), causes bilateral acoustic neuromas and sometimes several café au lait spots. NF1 and NF2 are transmitted on different autosomal chromosomes: NF1 is transmitted on chromosome 17 and NF2 on 22.

Tuberous sclerosis is a completely different inherited neurocutaneous disorder. It consists of a combination of nodules on the malar surface of the face and tubers in the brain that cause seizures and mental deterioration. Depending on the family, tuberous sclerosis is transmitted on chromosome 9 or 11. Tuberous sclerosis and NF1 provide the clinician with an excellent opportunity to make a diagnosis by inspection.

286. A 68-year-old man was brought to the emergency room after he called his wife to say that he had become lost while visiting his customers in neighboring towns. Because he was agitated, a psychiatrist was asked to consult. She calmed him and then determined that his primary problem was memory impairment for recent events, such as where he had traveled and with whom had he visited. He retained basic, personal knowledge, such as his name, telephone number, and even his social security number. She also established that he was aware of his impairment and that he had no physical neurologic deficits. Results of a head CT and the routine blood tests were normal. By the end of several hours, the problem cleared. Which of the following conditions is the least likely diagnosis?

a. Transient global amnesia (TGA)   c. Psychogenic amnesia
b. Partial complex seizure   d. An anticholinergic medication

ANSWER: c. The cardinal feature of this several-hour episode of amnesia is the preservation of personal, deeply seated ("overlearned") information. He most likely had a TGA. As in this case, TGA causes amnesia, particularly for recently acquired information, which contradicts the implication that the amnesia encompasses all memory tasks (i.e., despite its name, the amnesia in TGA is not really *global*). Partial complex seizures and medications with anticholinergic side effects are reasonable alternative explanations; however, these conditions generally cause a clouding of the sensorium. The least likely possibility is psychogenic amnesia, sometimes called a fugue state, because it is associated with the patients who are unable to recall their name, home address, spouse's name, and other overlearned information. Patients with psychogenic amnesia usually have a global deficit.

287. A 4-year-old girl's parents notice that she has begun to lose her beautiful voice and charming conversational ability. Moreover, she has developed a habit of playing repetitively with her hands. She seems to be washing them or clapping for hours at a time. The physician fails to keep her attention. Although he finds the child's eyes to be blue, her hair blond, and her head circumference relatively smaller compared to her height and age than he previously recorded, he diagnoses autism and refers her to a psychiatrist. Which disorder may be misdiagnosed, in this setting, as autism?

a. Down's syndrome   d. Rett's syndrome
b. PKU deficiency   e. Nonspecific mental retardation
c. Mental retardation

ANSWER: d. The child probably has Rett's syndrome. This condition is diagnosed on clinical criteria: young girls with acquired microcephaly who lose their verbal abilities and begin to perform repetitive, purposeless hand movements (stereotypies). It is a cause of autistic behavior. Its manifestations are often present, in retrospect, by age 2 years; however, the diagnosis is usually not made until age 5 years. If it had been untreated, PKU would have caused severe mental retardation in infancy.

288. Which of the following statements are true regarding REM (rapid eye movement) latency?

a. REM latency is normally 90 to 120 minutes.
b. REM latency can be determined by a polysomnogram (PSG), but the standard test is the multiple sleep latency test (MSLT), which is performed during the day.
c. REM periods with latencies shorter than 5 to 10 minutes are often considered to be sleep onset REM periods (SOREMPs).
d. REM latency is dependent on sleep latency.
e. Sleep latency is dependent on REM latency.
f. Alcohol-induced sleep is associated with SOREMPs.
g. Restless leg syndrome is associated with SOREMPs.
h. Alcohol and hypnotic withdrawal is associated with SOREMPs.
i. Depression is associated with SOREMPs.
j. Narcolepsy is associated with SOREMPs.
k. Sleep apnea is associated with SOREMPs.
l. Sleep deprivation is associated with SOREMPs.

ANSWER: a, b, c, h, i, j, k, l

289. A 17-year-old high school student begins to fall asleep in class. Despite being warned to get more sleep at night, she continues to fall asleep not only in class but also during more stimulating activities, such as watching football games. A complete evaluation shows that she is otherwise in good health. After being assured that she does get at least 6 hours of sleep a night, what should be the physician's next steps?

a. Delaying the sleep phase
b. Additional blood tests
c. PSG (polysomnography) or MSLT (multiple sleep latency test)
d. EEG

ANSWER: b, then c. Teenagers vary between being excessively sleepy and never being willing to go to bed. Although they often normally have excessive daytime sleepiness (EDS), sleeping in class and during exciting events is abnormal. If she seems to sleep 6 to 8 hours at night, her physician should consider common causes of EDS in teenagers: depression, mononucleosis and other medical illnesses, and drug and alcohol use. Then narcolepsy and sleep apnea should be considered. She should have HLA typing because narcolepsy is closely associated with HLA-DQB1. The PSG and particularly the MSLT will reveal SOREMPs in narcolepsy. The EEG is not suitable for detecting the onset of sleep or the presence of REM.

Narcolepsy is often overlooked in teenagers despite its onset before age 25 in 90% of cases. Only after several years do patients with narcolepsy develop the dramatic cataplexy. Overall, only 10% of patients with narcolepsy have the complete narcolepsy-cataplexy tetrad: narcolepsy, cataplexy, sleep paralysis, and sleep hallucinations.

Delayed sleep phase syndrome, which does cause EDS and can occur in teenagers, is associated with a full, restful 6 to 8 hours of sleep but at the "wrong" time. Patients remain awake until late at night and, if possible, sleep late into the next day. Because this teenager had at least 6 hours of sleep, she should have been rested.

290. A 77-year-old man developed EDS at age 75 years. He takes no medications, does not use alcohol, and is in good health. During the night, his wife reports, he has violent movements of his whole body. She does not know if her husband has restful sleep, but her own sleep is not. Which one of the following should be the next step?

a. Delaying the sleep phase
b. Additional blood tests
c. PSG
d. EMG
e. MSLT

ANSWER: c. People with potentially injurious movements during sleep should be tested with a PSG. An MSLT is unnecessary because narcolepsy is unlikely in view of the lack of daytime naps. Several disorders cause nocturnal movements in 77-year-old individuals: periodic limb movements, restless leg syndrome, sleep apnea, seizures, and REM sleep disorder. All these conditions interrupt sleep—the bed partner's as well as the patient's—and cause EDS.

291. Which four effects can be attributed to benzodiazepines?

a. Increase in total sleep time of 10%
b. Increase in total sleep time of 33%
c. Increase in total sleep time of 67% or more
d. Reduced sleep fragmentation
e. Increase in slow-wave NREM sleep
f. Hip fractures from an increased tendency to fall
g. Weight gain
h. Lowered seizure threshold
i. Anterograde amnesia

ANSWER: a, d, f, i

292. From which structures do most subdural hematomas arise?

a. Lacerated middle meningeal arteries
b. Ripped bridging veins
c. Lacerated great vein of Galen
d. Aneurysms of the middle or anterior cerebral arteries

ANSWER: b. Meningeal arterial bleeding leads to epidural hematomas. Aneurysms lead to bleeding that is predominantly subarachnoid. Venous bleeding, which is often so slow that it may be called oozing, leads to subdural hematomas.

293. Which three of the following are closely associated with spastic cerebral palsy?

a. Necrotic areas in the white matter around the ventricles, *periventricular leukomalacia*
b. Kernicterus
c. Detection by neonatal ultrasound examination
d. Foreshortened, spastic limbs
e. Thalidomide

ANSWER: a, c, d. Kernicterus is associated with basal ganglia bilirubin staining. Thalidomide causes congenital limb deformity (phocomelia).

294. Which one of the following is most closely associated with neonatal periventricular leukomalacia?

a. Athetosis
b. Spastic cerebral palsy, all varieties
c. Spastic diplegia
d. MS

ANSWER: c. Neonatal periventricular white matter necrosis leads to spastic diplegia. MS and sometimes vascular dementia cause periventricular white matter changes, but these are conditions that affect adults.

295. One hour after a grilled tuna fish dinner in a fancy Chicago restaurant, a 29-year-old previously healthy physician feels "very sick" and has profound nausea and vomiting. She has beet-red skin and hypotension, but a temperature of only 100°F. The episode begins to subside after 2 hours. In addition to general supportive measures, which of the following is the best treatment?

a. Antibiotics
b. Antidiarrhea medication
c. Antihistamines
d. Antiparasitic medications

ANSWER: c. Even when eaten raw, tuna fish and most other deep water fish are usually safe. However, if these fish are not refrigerated, bacteria in their gut and gills may proliferate and produce histidine. The histidine, which resists cooking, is transformed into histamine in the human intestine. As in this case, victims develop *histamine poisoning* that responds to antihistamine injections. In other circumstances, people who eat any fish, especially freshwater fish, can become infested with parasites. However, routine cooking usually eliminates that threat. Uncooked shellfish harbor hepatitis virus. Barracuda and grouper fish are often contaminated with toxins that are heat-sensitive. Antidiarrheal medications for these fish poisons are ineffective and counteract the body's natural protective reaction to expel toxins.

296. Which one of the following is incorrect regarding the Glasgow Coma Scale (GCS)?

a. It measures only three clinical parameters: eye opening, verbal response, and motor response.
b. A high score indicates a greater depth of coma.
c. GCS scores can be correlated with posttraumatic amnesia.
d. GCS scores cannot be correlated with posttraumatic headaches.

> **ANSWER:** b. GCS scores range from 3 to 15. Patients with low scores are less responsive, have deeper coma, and are more likely to die. If they survive, they have longer posttraumatic amnesia. Notably, GCS scores cannot be correlated with posttraumatic headaches or whiplash injury.

297. Which one of the following statements is false regarding the relationship of alcohol to head trauma?

a. Alcohol is a frequent contributory factor in motor vehicle, diving, and other accidents that result in head trauma.
b. Alcohol withdrawal may complicate recovery from posttraumatic coma.
c. Alcohol use in patients surviving major head trauma increases the incidence of seizures.
d. Alcohol is a good sedative and minor tranquilizer in patients who have survived minor head trauma.
e. Patients who survive head trauma who use alcohol are particularly prone to violence, as occurs in the episodic dyscontrol syndrome.

> **ANSWER:** d. Alcohol is neither a good sedative nor minor tranquilizer in patients who have survived head trauma. It induces insomnia, irritability, and excessive daytime sleepiness. Excessive alcohol use, which occurs in many head trauma patients, impairs memory and judgment. Posttraumatic insomnia and anxiety may require specific medications, possibly antidepressants, and, for a stress disorder, psychotherapy. Patients with prolonged anxiety and insomnia should be investigated for cognitive impairment.

298. When confronted with patients who have sustained acute multiple trauma, emergency medical attention is often exclusively directed at head injuries. During their examinations and transportation, an unstable cervical spine can lead to spinal cord injury. Which of the following are complications of cervical spine injury?

a. Respiratory failure
b. Quadriplegia or paraplegia
c. Herniated intervertebral disks
d. Urinary retention
e. Carotid artery dissection
f. All of the above

> **ANSWER:** f. Acute cervical spinal cord injury is sometimes overshadowed by head injury. Facial and scalp lacerations, which bleed profusely, are compelling and distracting. Manipulation of the head and neck can be disastrous. Combined head and neck injuries occur in motor vehicle accidents in which the face or forehead strikes the windshield and the neck snaps backward. This type of injury also occurs in diving accidents in which people strike their head in a shallow pool and compress their cervical spine.

299. A 22-year-old Marine, who survived a penetrating frontal lobe shrapnel injury, has episodes of violent, aggressive, destructive behavior. These episodes occur when he drinks only one or two beers and are precipitated by little provocation. A careful neurologic examination reveals hyperreflexia on the left side and a Babinski sign on the right. His MRI shows bilateral frontal lucencies. An EEG shows intermittent sharp waves that are phased reversed in the left temporal lobe and intermittent slowing when he is drowsy. Which one of the following should a consultant psychiatrist first recommend?

a. Further neurologic evaluation
b. Psychotherapy
c. Use of an antiepileptic drug
d. Use of a minor or major tranquilizer
e. None of the above

ANSWER: a. He probably has episodic dyscontrol syndrome, which is violent behavior—often with aggression (directed violence)—that typically follows congenital or acquired head trauma. Patients often have abnormal reflexes and minor, nonspecific EEG abnormalities. Although antiepileptic drugs may ameliorate the outbursts, the disorder is not epilepsy. In his case, the sharp waves on the EEG might indicate seizures apart from the violence. He should undergo EEG-TV monitoring that would determine if he has seizures, but the episodes of violence are probably not ictal events. In addition, he should undergo neuropsychologic tests, which might reveal cognitive deficits.

300. A 68-year-old woman loses her accuracy in her relatively complicated assembly-line job. Her family brings her for evaluation for depression and dementia. Soon after the interview begins, she becomes upset and attempts to put on her robe. However, she tries to put both hands through the left sleeve. She becomes confused and frustrated. Then she puts the robe on backward. Finally, she is perplexed as to how to extricate herself. Which condition is she displaying?

a. Dementia
b. Apraxia
c. Dressing apraxia
d. Left-right confusion
e. Neglect
f. Anosognosia
g. Inattention

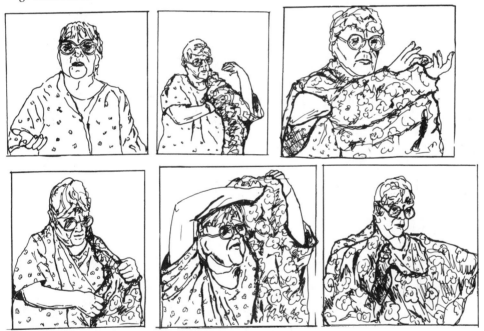

ANSWER: c. Dressing apraxia is a dramatic manifestation of nondominant hemisphere injury, such as a tumor (as in this case), with the parietal lobe being the primary site of involvement. Dressing apraxia is an inability to clothe oneself caused by a combination of visual-spatial impairment, somatotopagnosia, and motor apraxia. Like other apraxias, dressing apraxia is more than inattention, visual loss, or lack of sensation on one side of the body. Patients with dressing apraxia are befuddled or stymied when attempting to put on a coat, shirt, or hospital robe. Unlike patients with anosognosia, those with dressing apraxia are aware of their problem and are frustrated.

Examiners wishing to demonstrate the phenomenon might ask patients to dress in a hospital robe with one sleeve turned inside-out. Even when warned about the sleeve's being reversed, patients will be unable to dress. Not appreciating the problem or being unable to solve it, they tend to change the normal sleeve into an abnormal sleeve, reverse any of their corrections, put both arms through the same sleeve, or drastically misalign the two sides. (The patient's MRI is reproduced in Figure 20–19.)

301. Which three of the following tumors originate from glial cells?

a. Astrocytomas
b. Glioblastoma multiforme
c. Oligodendrogliomas
d. Lymphomas
e. Meningiomas

ANSWER: a, b, c

302. A 31-year-old right-handed waiter has had partial complex seizures since he was 16 years old. His seizures have been refractory to antiepileptic drugs, except in intoxicating doses. They prevent him from working, traveling, or entering relationships. CCTV documented that his seizures originate in a right-sided temporal lobe focus. MRI showed atrophy of the right hippocampus. PET could not be performed. Which of the following is probably the best therapy?

a. Partial right temporal lobectomy
b. A commissurotomy
c. Adding an antidepressant
d. None of the above

ANSWER: a. Surgery that removes the focus has been a major medical advance that, in skilled hands, benefits about 75% of selected epilepsy patients. PET is unnecessary. A preoperative Wada test is used to determine if the proposed surgery will lead to aphasia. A commissurotomy, which should block the spread of seizures through the corpus callosum, has limited usefulness.

303. Which statement regarding EEG changes that follow ECT is false?

a. Unilateral ECT is associated with predominantly unilateral β activity.
b. Bilateral ECT induces generalized theta and delta activity.
c. Greater post-ECT slowing is associated with greater antidepressant effect.
d. Greater post-ECT slowing is associated with greater amnesia.

ANSWER: a. Unilateral ECT is associated with unilateral EEG slowing (theta and delta activity).

304. What portion of the skull lies immediately medial and anterior to the mesial surface of the temporal lobe?

a. The temporal bone
b. The occiput
c. The sphenoid wing
d. The petrous pyramid
e. The nasopharynx

ANSWER: c. The mesial surface of the temporal lobe is immediately adjacent to the sphenoid wing. Insertion of nasopharyngeal EEG electrodes places them as close as possible to the mesial surface of the temporal lobe. Scalp EEG electrodes, which are placed over the temporal bones, overly the temporal lobe's lateral surface.

305. Match the area of the CNS (a–h) with the following structures (1–8).

1. Amygdala
2. Angular gyrus
3. Nucleus basalis of Meynert
4. Olfactory nerves
5. Broca's area
6. Medial longitudinal fasciculus
7. Uncus
8. Thalamus

a. Frontal lobe
b. Parietal lobe
c. Occipital lobe
d. Temporal lobe
e. Deep in the cerebrum
f. Cerebellum
g. In the dorsal, medial portion of the pons and midbrain
h. Diencephalon

ANSWERS: 1-d, 2-b, 3-e, 4-a, 5-a, 6-g, 7-d, 8-h

306. Which structure is immediately medial and superior to the hypothalamus?

a. Thalamus
b. Corpus of Luysii
c. Corpus callosum
d. Third ventricle

ANSWER: d

307. A 10-year-old boy has had three seizures during the previous 4 years. All have occurred during sleep at night and have consisted of facial paresthesias, abnormal sensations in his right arm, and speech arrest. His neurologic examination, routine laboratory testing, and an MRI are all normal. An EEG performed during sleep shows centrotemporal spikes. Which two of the following statements regarding the boy are true?

a. He has rolandic epilepsy.
b. He has a sleep disorder, not a seizure disorder.
c. As an adult, he is likely to develop epilepsy.
d. This condition will probably disappear by the time he is 21 years old.

ANSWER: a, d. He has rolandic epilepsy, which is an inherited seizure disorder peculiar to children that is readily responsive to antiepileptic drugs.

308. When a 60-year-old man, who was being evaluated for dementia, was asked to copy the sequence of figures on the top row, he reproduced the sequence on the bottom.

□ □ ○ □ □ ○ □ ○
□ □ ○ □ □ □ □ □

When he realized his error, he crumpled the paper, grasped it tightly, laughed uncontrollably, and then urinated. Which of the following conclusions can most reliably be drawn from his copying and behavior problems?

a. He has apraxia for figure copying, which is indicative of nondominant parietal lobe dysfunction.
b. He has dementia, but the problems are nonspecific.
c. These problems are indicative of the subcortical dementias.
d. They are typical of frontotemporal dementia.

ANSWER: d. The patient perseverated. He could not "switch sets" from drawing squares to circles. Then he demonstrated labile, impetuous behavior, possibly a grasp reflex, and loss of inhibition (the laughing and urinating). These are all signs of frontal lobe impairment.

309. In which condition would the results of evoked potentials be least helpful?

a. Depression
b. Psychogenic blindness
c. MS
d. Optic neuritis
e. Deafness in uncooperative patients
f. Auditory capacity in autistic children

ANSWER: a. Brainstem auditory evoked responses (BAERS), visual evoked responses (VERs), and somatosensory evoked responses can provide an objective measurement of the function of the auditory, visual, and sensory systems.

310. Which two statements are true regarding the relationship of interictal violence to epilepsy?

a. Violent behavior is no more prevalent among patients with partial complex seizures than other seizures.
b. The consensus among neurologists is that epilepsy does not cause crime. Instead, epilepsy, head trauma, and other brain injuries lead to conditions, such as poor impulse control and lower socioeconomic status, that predispose people to crime.
c. Interictal violence is associated with childhood onset seizures.
d. Interictal violence can be reduced with benzodiazepines.

ANSWER: a, b

311. In which two patients might brain biopsies reveal Lewy bodies?

a. A 78-year-old person who had encephalitis as a young adult, with tremor, rigidity, and bradykinesia
b. A 70-year-old person who presents with 6 months of dementia, rigidity, and bradykinesia
c. A 40-year-old retired boxer with slurred speech, festinating gait, mild dementia, and resting tremor
d. A 30-year-old former intravenous drug abuser with tremor, rigidity, and bradykinesia

ANSWER: a, b. Lewy bodies are found in the substantia nigra in Parkinson's disease, especially in the postencephalitic variety (Patient *a*). They are also found in diffuse Lewy body disease, which causes dementia and mild parkinsonism (Patient *b*). However, they are not found in dementia pugilistica (Patient *c*) or MPTP-induced parkinsonism (Patient *d*).

312. Called to evaluate a 63-year-old man who demands to be released from the oncology service of a general hospital, a psychiatrist finds the patient to be relatively calm, oriented, and aware that he has "a melanoma that will be fatal in the near future." Physical examination and laboratory tests reveal no major abnormalities; however, the patient seems to fall to his left and is inattentive to friends and family who stand on his left side. Before making a determination about whether the patient is competent, which of the following tests should the psychiatrist request?

a. Serum calcium determination
b. EEG
c. Mini-Mental Status Examination
d. CT or MRI of the brain
e. Liver function tests

ANSWER: d. Melanomas tend to spread widely by blood-borne dissemination. Although the patient seems to be making a rational decision, an element of anosognosia might be present in view of his left-sided inattention and motor difficulties. A CT or MRI would be the best test to detect a metastasis in the nondominant parietal lobe. Whether or not a lesion were present, the psychiatrist would have to judge whether his degree of anosognosia rendered him incompetent.

313. A 67-year-old woman, who has just been admitted with the sudden onset of left-hemiparesis, was asked to bisect a line. Which is the most likely result?

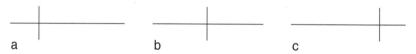

a b c

ANSWER: c. She undoubtedly sustained an extensive right cerebral insult, most likely a stroke. Patients with this perceptual disorder do not appreciate the leftward extent of the horizontal line. They are also likely to be unaware of their left hemiparesis, that is, have anosognosia.

314. Which is the single most commonly occurring risk factor for falls in the elderly?

a. Transient ischemic attacks
b. Use of sedatives or hypnotics
c. Cardiac arrhythmias
d. Alzheimer's disease

ANSWER: b

315. A psychiatrist is asked to see a 25-year-old methadone-maintenance patient hospitalized after his first seizure. The patient has developed agitated, belligerent behavior. A CT performed 3 days before showed a single small, ring-enhancing lesion in the right frontal lobe. He was given phenytoin and antitoxoplasmosis medications. Methadone was continued. Of the following, which is the most likely cause of his behavior?

a. Cerebral toxoplasmosis
b. AIDS dementia
c. Phenytoin-enhanced hepatic metabolism
d. Antitoxoplasmosis medications

ANSWER: c. Phenytoin induces hepatic enzymes that metabolize other medications, including methadone. Thus, instituting phenytoin in methadone patients precipitates withdrawal. Individuals in methadone-maintenance programs are often HIV positive because of prior or concomitant intravenous drug abuse. Many of them have AIDS. This patient may have cerebral toxoplasmosis, but a single small lesion in the right frontal lobe is unlikely to be the cause of his behavioral disturbances.

316. Which three are characteristics of neurosyphilis in AIDS patients?

a. Neurosyphilis is likely to be accompanied by ocular involvement.
b. The diagnosis may be obscured by negative serologic tests.

c. Treatment with penicillin may be deleterious.
d. Neurosyphilis occurs rarely in AIDS patients.
e. The usual doses of penicillin may be inadequate.

ANSWER: a, b, e

317. Which two are the greatest risk factors for dementia in AIDS patients?

a. The CD4 count below 1,000 cells/mm^3
b. Being HIV positive
c. Anemia
d. Depression
e. Weight loss

ANSWER: c, e. Dementia is usually a relatively late manifestation of AIDS. It occurs when immunodeficiency is pronounced and anemia and systemic symptoms have developed. A low CD4 count is an early manifestation of AIDS and long precedes dementia in almost all cases. Only a pronounced CD4 depletion, typically below 200 cells/mm^3, is a risk factor for AIDS dementia.

318. Although the distinction's value has been questioned, many neurologist continue to divide dementia into cortical and subcortical varieties. Which of the following illnesses are considered examples of cortical (c) or subcortical (sc) dementia?

a. AIDS dementia
b. Alzheimer's disease
c. Huntington's disease
d. Normal pressure hydrocephalus
e. Parkinson's disease
f. Frontotemporal dementia, including Pick's disease

ANSWERS: a-sc, b-c, c-sc, d-sc, e-sc, f-c. The distinction is arbitrary and fallible because several of these illnesses have overlapping features. The dementia in both AIDS and Huntington's disease, for example, has cortical as well as subcortical features.

319. Which one of the following statements concerning hallucinations in Alzheimer's disease is false?

a. Hallucinations are mostly visual but are sometimes auditory or olfactory.
b. They are associated with a rapid decline in cognitive function.
c. They have little prognostic value.
d. They are associated with clearly abnormal EEGs.

ANSWER: c. They are clearly indicative of a poor prognosis.

320. If a man is 45 years old, in which decade of life is he?

a. Third
b. Fourth
c. Fifth
d. Sixth

ANSWER: c. The man has entered his fifth decade. This nomenclature is often a source of confusion.

321. Which statement most closely describes the gate control theory of pain control?

a. Descending pathways inhibit pain.
b. Endogenous opioids suppress pain.
c. Activity of large-diameter, heavily myelinated fibers inhibit pain transmission by small, sparsely myelinated fibers.
d. Substance P and serotonin, carefully balanced, regulate pain transmission.

ANSWER: c

322. Which one of the following statements is true regarding the periaqueductal gray matter?

a. Stimulation of the periaqueductal gray matter produces analgesia by liberating endogenous opioids.
b. Hemorrhage into the periaqueductal gray matter is associated with thiamine deficiency.

c. The periaqueductal gray matter surrounds the aqueduct of Sylvius, which is the passage for CSF between the third and fourth ventricles.
d. The periaqueductal gray matter is in the midbrain.
e. All of the above

ANSWER: e

323. Which is not a characteristic of enkephalins?

a. They are peptides.
b. They are neurotransmitters.
c. Naloxone inhibits enkephalins.
d. Serotonin inhibits enkephalins.

ANSWER: d

324. Which of the following substances serves as the neurotransmitter for pain?

a. Enkephalins
b. Serotonin
c. Substance P
d. Endogenous opioids

ANSWER: c

325. In regard to their analgesic strength, nonsteroidal anti-inflammatory drugs (NSAIDs) can be as potent analgesics as opioids. In which other ways are NSAIDs similar to opioids?

a. They are addictive.
b. They produce greater analgesia with increasingly higher doses.
c. They promote tolerance to the analgesia.
d. Most cause gastrointestinal bleeding.
e. None of the above

ANSWER: e. Unlike opioids, NSAIDs are not addictive and do not induce tolerance. In addition, at a certain dose, their analgesic effect reaches a maximum "ceiling effect." Increased doses do not produce additional analgesia. Moreover, additional medication will expose patients to side effects, particularly gastrointestinal bleeding.

326. What is the primary mechanism of action of NSAIDs?

a. They inhibit prostaglandin synthesis.
b. They enhance serotonin activity.
c. They enhance opioid activity.
d. They cause opioid-like psychological side effects.
e. All of the above

ANSWER: a

327. Which two of the following features are included in a syndrome in 3- to 6-year-old girls that mimics autism?

a. Stereotypical hand wringing movements
b. Acquired microcephaly
c. Low-set, large ears
d. Fair skin and eczema
e. Simian palm crease
f. Seizures

ANSWER: a, b. Rett's syndrome, which has prominent autistic features, is characterized by repetitive hand movements and acquired microcephaly in young girls. Boys with mental retardation caused by fragile X syndrome have large, low-set ears and large testicles. The simian palm crease is a characteristic of trisomy 21. Fair skin and eczema are manifestations of PKU.

328. A first-grade boy runs with his left hand fisted. When asked to walk on the sides of his feet, the left thumb tends to flex toward the palm, as though he were starting to make a fist. Which three other stigmata of neurologic injury can be expected?

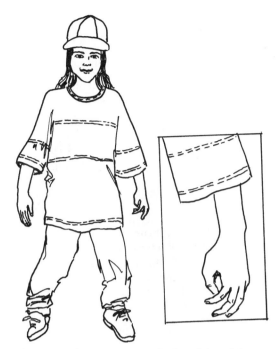

a. Hyperactive DTRs in the left arm
b. Mental retardation
c. Clumsy movements with the left arm

d. Spasticity of the arm
e. Hypoactive DTRs in the left arm
f. Athetosis

ANSWER: a, c, d. He is displaying a "cortical thumb." This sign usually indicates congenital corticospinal tract injury that, in turn, would also cause hyperactive DTRs, spasticity, and clumsiness. In cases of unilateral involvement, the affected thumb, fingers, or entire arm may be smaller than the unaffected counterpart. A unilateral cortical thumb and other soft signs suggest (contralateral) congenital cerebral injury; however, when they occur bilaterally, they have less significance. Adults may develop a cortical thumb after a cerebral infarction or traumatic injury.

329. Which are four advantages of nonsteroidal anti-inflammatory drugs (NSAIDs) over opioids?

a. NSAIDs do not create tolerance.
b. Additional NSAIDs produce greater analgesia, that is, they have no ceiling effect.
c. Patients develop no withdrawal symptoms when NSAIDs are stopped.
d. NSAIDs can be as effective as opioids.
e. NSAIDs have virtually no psychological side effects.
f. NSAIDs produce gastric irritation much less frequently than opioids.

ANSWER: a, c, d, e

330. In which two regions do peripheral nerves carrying pain sensation synapse with ascending spinal cord tracts?

a. Sympathetic nervous system
b. In the spinal cord

c. Lateral spinothalamic tract
d. Substantia gelatinosa

ANSWER: b, d. PNS fibers enter the spinal cord and synapse with the lateral spinothalamic tract in the substantia gelatinosa. The spinothalamic tract crosses the spinal cord and ascends to the thalamus, where it undergoes another synapse.

331. Match the speech pattern (a–c) with the disorder (1–3).

a. Strained and strangled
b. Hypophonic and monotonous
c. Scanning

1. MS affecting the cerebellum
2. Parkinson's disease
3. Spasmodic dysphonia

ANSWERS: a-3, b-2, c-1

332. Which four statements are true concerning reflex sympathetic dystrophy?

a. The disorder is mediated, at least in part, by the sympathetic nervous system.
b. Dry, shiny, and scaly skin is a characteristic.
c. Because the pain is increased by touch, patients protect their affected limb.
d. Sympathetic blockage will provide temporary relief in many cases.
e. The pain is confined to the injured nerves' dermatomes.
f. Antiepileptic drugs provide a cure and diagnostic confirmation.

ANSWER: a, b, c, d

333. Why is succinylcholine used in conjunction with ECT?

a. It makes the brain more susceptible to the beneficial effects of ECT because it lowers the seizure threshold.
b. It paralyzes muscles by binding to the neuromuscular junction ACh receptors.
c. It reduces subsequent amnesia.
d. It is given to enhance ECT effect, but its usefulness has never been established.
e. It reduces oral secretions that the patient could aspirate.
f. It interferes with cerebral ACh and induces amnesia for the event.

ANSWER: b. Succinylcholine blocks the neuromuscular junction. It paralyzes muscles and prevents massive muscle contractions that can cause fractures and other bodily injuries. Succinylcholine does not cross the blood-brain barrier and thus does not affect the seizure threshold or memory pathways. Atropine is administered to reduce secretions.

334. A 32-year-old woman is brought to the emergency room by her family, who have not seen her in 3 years. The psychiatrist and neurologist find that she has slow and disordered thinking, word-finding difficulties, bilateral weakness and spasticity (but left-sided more than right-sided), and dysarthria and dysphagia. A noncontrast CT of the head and CSF analysis reveal no abnormalities, but an MRI shows numerous, large abnormal areas in the cerebral white matter. Which disorder need not be considered?

a. Toxoplasmosis
b. Adrenoleukodystrophy
c. Toluene (volatile substance) abuse
d. Progressive multifocal leukoencephalopathy (PML)
e. MS

ANSWER: b. The patient's signs—aphasia, pseudobulbar palsy, bilateral corticospinal tract signs, and possibly dementia—indicate diffuse cerebral injury. All the disorders could eventually cause these signs. Also, except for toxoplasmosis, all are demyelinating diseases that can be detected by MRI but not CT. The least likely possibility is adrenoleukodystrophy: It develops only in boys because it is a sex-linked genetic disorder. Because toxoplasmosis and PML are complications of AIDS, she should have an HIV test, as well as a routine evaluation.

335. To which parts of the brain do the letters (A–E) refer?

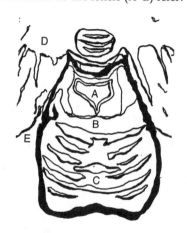

1. Lateral ventricle
2. Third ventricle
3. Aqueduct of Sylvius
4. Fourth ventricle
5. Midbrain
6. Pons
7. Medulla
8. Cerebellum
9. Cerebrum
10. Corticospinal tracts
11. Cerebellar tracts
12. Bulbar cranial nerves
13. Oculomotor cranial nerves
14. Cerebellopontine angle cranial nerves

ANSWERS: The sketch shows the pons (B = 6), which is the bulky portion of the brainstem, and the inferior aspect of the cerebellum (D = 8). The fourth ventricle (A = 4) is located in the uppermost portion of the pons. Corticospinal and cerebellar tracts (C = 10 and 11) cross through the base of the pons. Cranial nerves 5, 7, and 8 (E = 14) emerge from the cerebellopontine angle. The pons also contains the locus ceruleus (Fig. 21–2) and cranial nerve 6 (Figs. 2–9 and 4–10).

336. Which four clinical features are characteristics of frontotemporal dementia but not Alzheimer's disease?

a. Dementia
b. Familial tendency
c. Oral exploration
d. Personality disturbances
e. Age-proportional incidence
f. Disinhibition
g. Language disturbances
h. Impaired spatial orientation

ANSWER: c, d, f, and g. Although the clinical features of frontotemporal dementia and Alzheimer's diseases overlap, frontotemporal dementia is more apt to cause pronounced behavioral and personality disturbances, including elements of the Klüver-Bucy syndrome and lack of inhibition (disinhibition) but preserved spatial orientation.

337. Which one of the following MRI abnormalities is most closely associated with chronic schizophrenia that has been resistant to treatment?

a. Cerebellar atrophy
b. Corpus callosum atrophy
c. Symmetry of the planum temporale
d. Enlargement of the lateral ventricles

ANSWER: d. Schizophrenic patients with chronic, progressive deterioration resistant to treatment have large lateral ventricles accompanied by a large third ventricle and cerebral cortical atrophy. In addition, the amygdala and hippocampus are decreased in volume and the planum temporale is unlikely to show the normal symmetry.

338. Which visual field cut is associated with alexia without agraphia?

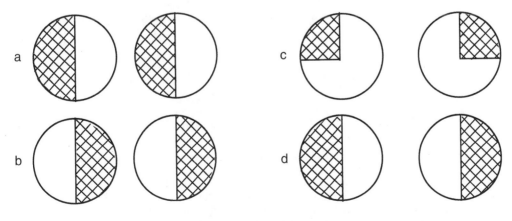

ANSWER: b. A right homonymous hemianopsia is associated with alexia without agraphia. In fact, a right homonymous hemianopsia is virtually a prerequisite for the condition.

339. Which one of the following results from sequential mental status tests indicates Alzheimer's disease?

a. A precipitous decline over 6 months
b. A decline over 6 months and then a plateau for 3 years
c. A borderline score in a well-educated individual
d. An uneven decline interrupted by several plateaus lasting 12 to 18 months

ANSWER: d. A precipitous decline suggests a rapidly progressive illness, such as Creutzfeldt-Jakob's disease, AIDS, or a glioblastoma. A plateau of more than 2 years is unusual for Alzheimer's disease. A borderline score in well-educated individuals is a common diagnostic dilemma. Such individuals might not have been very intelligent in the first place; they could have developed other problems, such as alcoholism; or they could have developed depression (pseudodementia) rather than dementia. An uneven decline, including some plateaus, is typical of Alzheimer's disease.

340. Match the view (a–c) with its common description (1–3).

a. Transaxial
b. Coronal
c. Sagittal

1. Front-to-back or head-on
2. Top-down view
3. Side view

ANSWERS: a-2, b-1, c-3

341. Numerous soldiers were exposed to Agent Orange during the Vietnam War. Which of the following neurologic problems have been found in rigorous scientific studies to be attributable to Agent Orange exposure?

a. Brain tumors
b. Peripheral neuropathy
c. Cognitive impairment
d. Neuropsychologic deficits
e. None of the above

ANSWER: e. No evidence has linked Agent Orange exposure to these neurologic problems.

342. In which two regions of the brain are pathologic changes most pronounced in Alzheimer's disease?

a. Primary motor cortex
b. Occipital cortex
c. Association areas, such as the parietal-temporal junction
d. Olfactory lobe
e. Limbic system, especially the hippocampus

ANSWER: c, e. These regions are especially atrophic and contain high concentrations of plaques and tangles.

343. Which three of the following medications elevate the serum prolactin concentration?

a. Thorazine
b. Bromocriptine
c. Haloperidol
d. Clozapine
e. Pergolide
f. L-dopa
g. Risperidone

ANSWER: a, c, g. Dopamine and dopamine agonists inhibit the release of prolactin by acting of the tubero-infundibular tract. In contrast, dopamine-blocking neuroleptics trigger prolactin release and produce elevated serum concentrations. Prolactin concentration is also elevated for about 20 minutes after most generalized and partial complex seizures. Prolactinomas, a common pituitary adenoma, secrete prolactin. Bromocriptine can suppress prolactinomas and obviate surgery.

344. Which two of the following nuclei constitute the corpus striatum?

a. Caudate
b. Putamen
c. Globus pallidus
d. Subthalamic
e. Substantia nigra

ANSWER: a, b

345. In hepatolenticular degeneration, to which two structures does "lenticular" refer?

a. Caudate
b. Putamen
c. Globus pallidus
d. Subthalamic
e. Substantia nigra
f. Corticospinal tract
g. Thalamus
h. The liver
i. The cornea

ANSWER: b, c. Being adjacent and forming a pie-shaped or lenslike structure, the putamen and globus pallidus form the lenticular nuclei. In hepatolenticular degeneration (Wilson's disease), copper deposits damage these basal ganglia, the liver, and other organs. Deposits in the cornea form the characteristic Kayser-Fleischer rings.

346. Which one of the following is not characteristic of apolipoprotein E (Apo-E)?

a. Apo-E is cholesterol-carrying protein produced in the liver and brain.
b. Apo-E binds amyloid.
c. Apo-E is encoded on chromosome 19 in three isoforms: Apo-E2, Apo-E3, and Apo-E4.
d. Apo-E is a risk factor for strokes.

ANSWER: d. Being homozygote for an Apo-E allele, Apo-E4, is associated with a markedly increased incidence of Alzheimer's disease.

347. Which three structures are depigmented in Parkinson's disease?

a. Substantia nigra
b. Locus ceruleus
c. Dorsal motor nuclei
d. Anterior thalamic nuclei
e. Lewy bodies

ANSWER: a, b, c

348. A family brings their 72-year-old patriarch for the evaluation of dementia that has developed along with mild rigidity and bradykinesia during the past several months. His course has been particularly troubled by visual hallucinations. What might the brain show?

a. Plaques and tangles in the hippocampus
b. Lewy bodies in the cerebral cortex
c. Lewy bodies in the substantia nigra
d. Atrophy of the head of the caudate

ANSWER: b. He probably has diffuse Lewy body disease. Lewy bodies in the substantia nigra are characteristic of Parkinson's disease, which does not cause dementia at its onset. Alzheimer's disease causes plaques and tangles in the cerebral cortex and especially the hippocampus, but it usually does not present with either pyramidal or extrapyramidal signs. Huntington's disease characteristically causes atrophy of the head of the caudate nuclei.

349. In the treatment of Parkinson's disease, which dopamine receptors do dopamine agonists stimulate?

a. D_1
b. D_2
c. Both
d. Neither

ANSWER: b. All commercially available dopamine agonists stimulate D_2. They may either stimulate or inhibit D_1.

350. In a pallidotomy for treatment of Parkinson's disease, in which structure is the lesion placed?

a. The putamen
b. The basal ganglia medial to the putamen
c. The corpus striatum

d. The substantia nigra
e. The thalamus

> *ANSWER:* b. The globus pallidus is medial to the putamen. Lesions placed in the globus pallidus markedly reduce rigidity and bradykinesia in the contralateral limbs. Lesions placed in the thalamus reduce tremor but have much less effect on the other symptoms, which are usually more incapacitating.

351. A 50-year-old architect's hand forms a painful cramp several minutes after he starts to work. Early in his career, he would develop similar cramps only after many hours of non-stop work. Which condition forces his hand into this position?

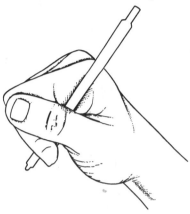

a. Psychogenic disturbance
b. Age-related disturbance
c. Motor neuron disease

d. Focal dystonia
e. Exercised-induced cramp

> *ANSWER:* d. He has developed writer's cramp, which is an occupational cramp. This disorder is a focal dystonia, not a psychologic reaction. After several decades, musicians, writers, architects, and other workers who use their hands in a repetitive fashion sometimes develop work-related focal dystonias. His writer's cramp might respond to botulinum toxin injected into the muscles that go into spasm.

352. A 60-year-old man has been developing involuntary contractions of all the facial muscles. The contractions, which begin around the eyes, are bilateral and symmetric. They accumulate to have a duration of several seconds and prevent him from seeing. He remains conscious during the contractions. His jaw, tongue, and ocular muscles are unaffected. Which type of illness is the most likely cause?

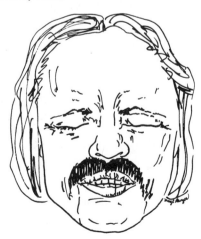

a. Seizure disorder
b. Iatrogenic illness

c. Cranial dystonia
d. Psychogenic condition

ANSWER: c. He has Meige's syndrome, which is a cranial dystonia that is more extensive than blepharospasm. Most individuals with cranial dystonias have no history of psychiatric illness or exposure to neuroleptics. When tardive dyskinesia involves facial muscles, it usually involves the tongue and jaw muscles. Meige's syndrome and blepharospasm respond to botulinum injections, but the tongue cannot be readily injected because, if it were weakened, it might fall back and occlude the airway.

353. Which five illnesses result from trinucleotide repeats?

a. Huntington's disease
b. Spinocerebellar atrophy
c. Wilson's disease
d. Dystonia

e. Fragile X syndrome
f. Duchenne's muscular dystrophy
g. Myotonic dystrophy
h. Friedreich's ataxia

ANSWER: a, b, e, g, h. Excessive repeats of three nucleotide bases in the DNA create those illnesses. Moreover, the instability of trinucleotide repeats causes the symptoms and signs to appear in younger family members in successive generations (anticipation).

354. In which three ways does the DNA in the juvenile and adult varieties of Huntington's disease differ?

a. Unlike the DNA in the adult variety, the DNA in the juvenile variety typically has more than 60 trinucleotide repeats.
b. The juvenile variety has a greater tendency toward anticipation in successive generations.
c. The juvenile variety usually results from the father's unstable, abnormal DNA.
d. The juvenile variety tends to cause rigidity rather than chorea.
e. The juvenile variety affects girls more often than boys.

ANSWER: a, c, d

355. Which nuclei are most atrophied in Huntington's disease?

a. Lenticular nuclei
b. Corpus striatum

c. Subthalamic nuclei
d. Mamillary bodies

ANSWER: b. Atrophy of the head of the caudate nuclei is characteristic of Huntington's disease.

356. A 33-year-old man with AIDS develops vision impairment, confusion, and word-finding difficulties. His MRI is shown below. Which process is causing his symptoms?

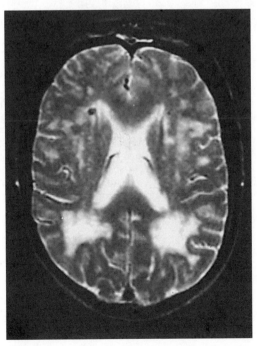

a. HIV encephalitis
b. MS
c. Toxoplasmosis
d. Progressive multifocal leukoencephalopathy (PML)
e. Lymphoma

> **ANSWER:** d. The MRI shows two large, hyperintense lesions in the white matter of the occipital lobes. Similar, scattered lesions are located in the dominant hemisphere (on the right side of the MRI). The occipital lesions have caused the visual difficulties. The dominant hemisphere lesions have caused the language problems.
>
> Unlike most intracerebral mass lesions, PML regions are not surrounded by edema and do not exert a mass effect, such as a shift of midline structures or compression of adjacent ventricles. HIV encephalitis does not cause discrete lesions. Although MS attacks white matter, its lesions are typically periventricular. Toxoplasmosis, a common complication of AIDS, causes multiple mass lesions that are not restricted to the white matter. Cerebral lymphomas in AIDS patients are usually large, single mass lesions.

357. A 60-year-old man, who had been in excellent health, develops apathy, inattention, and a flattened affect during a 3-week vacation. His MRI is shown. Which is the most likely diagnosis?

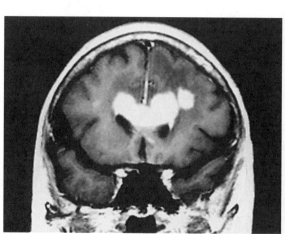 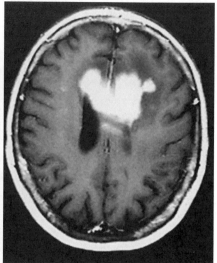

a. A frontal lobe glioblastoma
b. MS
c. Lymphoma
d. Progressive multifocal leukoencephalopathy (PML)

> **ANSWER:** a. The MRI view on the left is coronal, and the right is transaxial or axial. The patient's symptoms are manifestations of frontal lobe dysfunction. The MRI study shows a hyperintense lesion in both frontal lobes that spreads through the corpus callosum in a "butterfly" pattern. The clinical features and MRI indicate that he is harboring a frontal lobe butterfly glioblastoma, which is a relatively common tumor in this age group. His age and lack of risk factors virtually exclude MS, lymphoma, and PML. Metastatic carcinoma is a possibility, but metastases are usually multiple, surrounded by edema, and do not spread through the corpus callosum.

358. With which neurotransmitter alteration is Huntington's disease most closely associated?

a. Increased GABA
b. Decreased GABA
c. Decreased NMDA
d. Increased ACh
e. Decreased ACh

> **ANSWER:** b. In Huntington's disease, GABA is markedly decreased. ACh is also decreased, but less severely than GABA. In contrast, the NMDA receptor has increased activity.

359. A psychiatrist is called to evaluate the mental capacity of a 75-year-old man who is mute, frail, thin, and immobile in bed. His trunk is flexed and his arms spastic and flexed. His hands are clasped shut. His legs are also flexed and spastic. The skin overlying his hips and sacrum show signs of early decubiti. Of the following, which illness is most likely to be present?

a. A dominant hemisphere infarction
b. Guillain-Barré syndrome
c. Alzheimer's disease
d. Depression

ANSWER: c. He has decorticate posture from an extensive, severe cerebral disease, such as multi-infarct or vascular dementia, Creutzfeldt-Jacob disease, and Alzheimer's disease or other degenerative illness. The spasticity indicates upper motor neuron disease. Guillain-Barré syndrome, in contrast, would cause atrophy and flaccidity. Depression can lead to decorticate posture, but not spasticity or decubiti.

360. Which three of the following findings indicate a deliberate head injury in an infant?

a. Retinal hemorrhages
b. Discrepancy between history and contusions
c. An Arnold-Chiari defect
d. CT or MRI showing dural hemorrhages of varying ages
e. Absence of the corpus callosum
f. Subconjunctival hemorrhages

ANSWER: a, b, d. Blood of varying ages in the face, retinae, subdural spaces, and brain of an infant indicates deliberate trauma (i.e, the "shaken baby syndrome"). Absence of the corpus callosum and Arnold-Chiari defects are congenital malformations. Subconjunctival hemorrhages usually result from minimal, accidental trauma or from minor illnesses.

361. Which three of the following involuntary movements are typically preceded by an urge to move?

a. Periodic limb movements
b. Restless leg syndrome
c. Stereotypies
d. Akathisia
e. Chorea
f. Tics

ANSWER: b, d, f

362. Which two conditions typically produce brief, random, involuntary movements accompanied by motor impersistence that develop over several days in a 10-year-old child?

a. Tourette's syndrome
b. Lyme disease
c. Mononucleosis
d. Sydenham's chorea
e. Neuroleptic-induced dystonia
f. Withdrawal emergent dyskinesia

ANSWER: d, f. The child has chorea, which indicates Sydenham's chorea or withdrawal emergent dyskinesia. Tourette's syndrome evolves slowly and produces stereotyped tics. Neuroleptic-induced dystonia usually produces extension of the head and neck (retrocollis) and is rare in children. Lyme disease and mononucleosis, which both occur in children, do not regularly produce chorea.

363. Which one of the following children is most apt to have a mitochondria disorder?

a. A 10-year-old boy who develops dystonia of one foot that begins to spread to the ipsilateral hand
b. An 8-year-old boy who has had a head toss intermittently for 2 years and then develops an intermittent cough for which there is no pulmonary explanation
c. A 6-year-old girl who develops polyuria and polydipsia
d. An 11-year-old autistic girl
e. A 9-year-old boy with mild mental retardation
f. A 9-year-old boy who is short and mildly mentally retarded and has repeated hospitalizations for lactic acidosis

ANSWER: f. The lactic acidosis indicates a systemic metabolic impairment. Curiously, it occurs on an intermittent basis.

364. Deficiency of which one of the following vitamins causes CNS demyelination?

a. Niacin

b. Pyridoxine (vitamin B$_6$)

c. B$_{12}$

d. Citric acid (vitamin C)

ANSWER: c. B$_{12}$ deficiency causes demyelination in the posterior tracts of the spinal cord, cerebrum, and other areas of the CNS. It also causes a peripheral neuropathy. Niacin deficiency causes pellagra. Pyridoxine deficiency causes a neuropathy and seizures. Citric acid deficiency causes scurvy.

365. A 64-year-old man, with the recent onset of dementia, has marked behavioral disturbances, kisses the examiner, and has impaired language comprehension, repetition, and naming. He can copy complicated mechanical drawings but often incorporates erotic sketches in them. He has no hemiparesis or other overt neurologic deficits. He suddenly dies of a myocardial infarction. Which two features will examination of the brain probably reveal?

a. Ventricular dilation

b. Caudate lobe atrophy

c. Severe generalized atrophy

d. Atrophy predominantly of the frontal and temporal lobes

e. Intraneuronal argentophilic inclusions

f. Plaques and tangles

g. Spirochetes

h. None of the above

ANSWER: d, e. In view of the prominent behavioral and personality changes, disinhibition, and aphasia, the most likely diagnosis is frontotemporal dementia. This is an inheritable illness that includes the condition formerly known as Pick's disease. Cases associated with silver-staining (argentophilic) inclusions in the neurons are a subgroup of frontotemporal dementia termed Pick's disease.

366. An 18-year-old suburban high school student, with newly developing social and academic difficulties, begins to have rapid, involuntary facial movements and a continual cough. The neurologist finds an otherwise normal neurologic examination, including cognitive function, MRI, EEG, HIV, serum ceruloplasmin, Lyme titer, and syphilis tests. She concludes that the patient has no primary neurologic illness and refers him for a psychiatry consultation. During the course of a psychiatric evaluation, which three other tests should be performed as soon as possible?

a. A complete family history

b. IQ and other academic-psychologic testing

c. Therapeutic trial of haloperidol

d. Testing for MS

e. Other testing

ANSWER: a, b, e. The neurologist is "half right." The development of tics occurs before age 13 years in 90% of patients. Therefore, the development of tics—vocal or respiratory as well as motor—in a teenager should prompt evaluation for use of cocaine and other stimulants. MS does not usually cause movement disorders because it is a white matter disease. (The basal ganglia are composed of gray matter.) Huntington's disease and Sydenham's chorea would be unlikely in this situation.

367. Which two features are present in the involuntary neck movements of tardive dystonia but absent in idiopathic spasmodic torticollis?

a. Response to botulinum injections

b. Movements being predominantly retrocollis

c. Hypertrophy of the neck muscles

d. Accompanying oral-buccal-lingual movements

ANSWER: b, d. Both varieties of involuntary neck movements respond to botulinum toxin, but neither responds consistently to anticholinergic or other oral medications. Tardive dystonia is usually accompanied by other tardive dyskinesias.

368. Which one of the following substances has an unpaired electron?

a. Monoamines

b. Free radicals

c. Dopamine

d. Choline acetyl transferase (ChAT)

ANSWER: b. Free radicals are unstable atoms or molecules because they contain a single, unpaired electron. They seize electrons from adjacent atoms or molecules, which oxidizes them. Methylphenylpyridinium (MPP^+), which is the metabolic product of MPTP, is the best-known example of a free radical.

369. Which one of the following does not occur during sleep?

a. Periodic leg movements
b. Restless leg syndrome
c. Parkinson's disease tremor
d. Apnea
e. Palatal myoclonus
f. Generalized seizures
g. Partial seizures
h. Migraines

ANSWER: c

370. A 19-year-old student developed progressively severe intellectual impairment during the preceding year. Examination reveals a resting tremor, dysarthria, and rigidity. The cornea has a brown-green discoloration in its periphery. Liver function tests are abnormal. Which of the following is most likely to be found on further evaluation?

a. Trinucleotide repeats
b. Atrophy of the caudate nucleus
c. History of drug abuse
d. Decreased concentration of the serum protein that transports copper

ANSWER: d. He has Wilson's disease. His serum would contain insufficient ceruloplasmin, the copper-carrying protein. Trinucleotide repeats and atrophy of the caudate nucleus indicate Huntington's disease. Although not the case in this patient, drug abuse should be considered in progressive cognitive impairment in teenagers and young adults.

371. A 35-year-old alcoholic man with mild, chronic cirrhosis is brought to the emergency room because of agitation and belligerent behavior. Examination reveals disorientation, slurred speech, and asterixis. He has no nystagmus, extraocular paresis, pupillary abnormality, or lateralized signs. Laboratory data include the following: mildly abnormal liver function tests, 26% hematocrit, and blood in the stool. Which condition is the most likely cause of his behavioral disturbances and confusion?

a. Wernicke's encephalopathy
b. Alcohol-induced hypoglycemia
c. Hepatic encephalopathy
d. Subdural hematoma
e. Delirium tremens (DTs)

ANSWER: c. Hepatic encephalopathy from gastrointestinal bleeding is the most likely cause. People with cirrhosis or other causes of hepatic insufficiency will develop encephalopathy when gastrointestinal bleeding results from esophageal varices or gastric ulceration. Sometimes encephalopathy will follow a high-protein meal. In both cases, the protein breaks down in the intestine to form ammonia or other toxins. Mental changes and asterixis often occur, as in this case, before liver function tests become markedly abnormal. Psychotropic medications that require hepatic metabolism should be avoided or used sparingly in patients with hepatic insufficiency.

Physicians should consider Wernicke's encephalopathy, alcohol-induced hypoglycemia, and subdural hematomas in alcoholics with mental changes. Even without particular indications of these diagnoses, treatment might include intravenous thiamine and, after blood tests are drawn, intravenous glucose.

372. Regarding nicotinic and muscarinic ACh receptors, which statement is false?

a. Neuromuscular junctions rely on nicotinic receptors.
b. Atropine and scopolamine block muscarinic receptors.
c. Nicotinic receptors are blocked by curare.
d. The CNS has both ACh receptors, but those in the cortex are predominantly nicotinic.

ANSWER: d. ACh receptors in the cortex are predominantly muscarinic. Administering atropine or scopolamine will produce an Alzheimer-like memory impairment.

373. Following cocaine use that led to small bilateral temporal-parietal hemorrhages, a 28-year-old man has visual difficulties. He has a left homonymous hemianopsia but 20/25 visual acuity bilaterally. His problem is that he cannot name similar items unless he can "experience" them. For example, he cannot identify a dog and cat unless he can feel or smell them. Also, he cannot distinguish between a pen and pencil unless he writes with each. Similarly, unless the patient speaks with his family members, he cannot identify them. Otherwise, he has no problems on language testing: He can name and state the use of all objects that he touches, repeat long and complicated phrases, and follow two- and three-step requests. Which is the best description of his visual impairment?

a. Cortical blindness
b. Aphasia
c. Hemi-inattention
d. Visual agnosia
e. A psychogenic disturbance
f. Toxic-metabolic encephalopathy

ANSWER: d. A perceptual problem, visual agnosia, prevents him from identifying similar objects despite knowing their name and use. He also has prosopagnosia, a variety of visual agnosia, in which he cannot identify familiar faces. These conditions probably result from lesions, as in his case, that are anterior to the occipital visual cortex and impair its communication with the parietal association areas. He does not have blindness because his visual acuity is 20/25; aphasia because he passed the aphasia tests; hemi-inattention because he brings the objects into his consciousness through tactile routes; or toxic-metabolic encephalopathy because he remained alert enough to complete the testing.

374. In the cholinergic system in Alzheimer's disease, which receptor shows the greatest impairment of binding?

a. Muscarinic, presynaptic
b. Muscarinic, postsynaptic
c. Nicotinic, presynaptic
d. Nicotinic, postsynaptic

ANSWER: a. The presynaptic muscarinic receptor has the greatest reduction in ACh binding.

375. Which three conditions result from reduced presynaptic ACh release?

a. Lambert-Eaton syndrome
b. Myasthenia gravis
c. Botulism
d. Tetanus
e. Insecticide poisoning
f. Botulinum treatment

ANSWER: a, c, f. Lambert-Eaton syndrome is a remote effect of cancer involving the neuromuscular junction. It causes rapid fatigability because of depleted ACh stores or slowed ACh packet release. Similarly, botulism and botulinum toxin injections impair ACh release. In contrast, myasthenia gravis results from defective ACh postsynaptic receptors. Anticholinesterase insecticides cause paralyzing, continual postsynaptic receptor stimulation. Tetanus results from loss of normal spinal cord inhibition.

376. After a several-day bout of cocaine and other drug use, a 33-year-old woman presents with hyperactivity of the hands and feet and an inability to sit still. Her gait is jerky, and she cannot stand "at attention." Her thinking is bizarre, and she describes a "need" to move. Of the following, which one is the most likely cause of her movements?

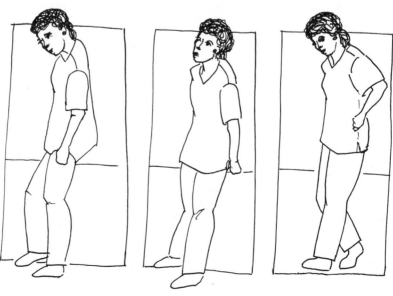

a. Drug-induced psychosis
b. Akathisia
c. Sydenham's chorea
d. Excessive dopamine activity
e. Alcohol withdrawal

ANSWER: d. Although each of these conditions can cause chorea or similar hyperactivity with prominent leg movements, her use of cocaine strongly suggests that she is experiencing "crack dancing." Her chorea presumably results from cocaine increasing dopamine and other neurotransmitter activity. These movements subside spontaneously over 1 to 3 days. Until then, they may be treated with small doses of dopamine-blocking neuroleptics.

377. With which receptor does glutamate bind to create neurotoxic reactions?

a. NMDA
b. Muscarinic ACh
c. Nicotinic ACh
d. Dopamine
e. Glutamate
f. None of the above

ANSWER: a. Glutamate-NMDA interactions are neurotoxic in Huntington's disease and possibly other neurologic illnesses, such as epilepsy and strokes.

378. Which are the four pigmented nuclei?

a. Locus ceruleus
b. Oculomotor
c. Dorsal motor X
d. Trigeminal motor
e. Substantia nigra
f. Nucleus basalis of Meynert
g. Red nucleus
h. Abducens

ANSWER: a, c, e, g. The four pigmented nuclei are one *red* (red nucleus, Fig. 4–8), one *blue* (locus ceruleus [copper sulfate-like], Fig. 21–2), and two *black* nuclei (substantia nigra, Figs. 4–8 and 18–2, and dorsal motor X, Fig. 5–10).

379. A 45-year-old man is brought to the emergency room where he is initially belligerent and then stuporous. He is jaundiced, anemic, and has signs of a recent gastrointestinal hemorrhage superimposed on chronic cirrhosis. A neurologic examination shows asterixis and bilateral Babinski signs but equal pupils and no hemiparesis. A CT of the head was normal. What would an EEG most likely reveal?

a. α activity
b. Electrocerebral silence
c. Triphasic waves
d. 3-Hz spike-and-wave activity

ANSWER: c. The patient has hepatic encephalopathy in which the EEG typically contains triphasic waves. EEG α activity is found in normal, alert individuals who have their eyes closed. They must be free of anxiety and not concentrating. Electrocerebral silence is found in brain death. 3-Hz spike-and-wave activity is a characteristic of absence seizures.

380. A 60-year-old man with Parkinson's disease was under treatment with deprenyl and L-dopa-carbidopa. When depression developed, SSRI treatment was initiated. Two days later, he began to be agitated, confused, febrile (temperature 100° F), diaphoretic, rigid, tremulous, and have myoclonus. His CPK was 120. Which syndrome has probably developed?

a. Dopamine intoxication
b. Neuroleptic malignant syndrome
c. Serotonin syndrome
d. None of the above

ANSWER: c. The serotonin syndrome is characterized by mental status changes, autonomic disturbances, and muscle abnormalities. It follows the administration of various medications that increase serotonin activity to toxic levels. It is a rare condition whose features are similar to neuroleptic malignant syndrome, but its fever and CPK elevations are not as great. It has been described following administration of SSRIs; MAO inhibitors, including deprenyl; other antidepressants, including the heterocyclics and tricyclics; and the serotoninergic migraine medication, sumatriptan.

381. Which one of the following illnesses is caused by an RNA-containing infectious agent?

a. Creutzfeldt-Jakob disease
b. Bovine spongiform encephalopathy
c. Fatal familial insomnia
d. AIDS-dementia

ANSWER: d. HIV, which is an RNA retrovirus, causes AIDS-dementia. The other conditions are caused by prions, which contain neither RNA nor DNA.

382. A 76-year-old woman survived a nondominant cerebral hemisphere stroke but has a residual left hemiparesis and sensory impairment. She sometimes finds that at night her left hand moves about and touches her left leg or trunk. She jolts upright, fearful that the hand, which is not hers, is groping at her. Similarly, during the daytime, she jokes that the hand feels like her late husband's. What is the most likely explanation?

a. Narcolepsy, with hallucinations
b. Panic attacks
c. Nocturnal epilepsy
d. Alien hand syndrome
e. A delusion
f. None of the above

ANSWER: d. In the alien hand syndrome, which typically follows a nondominant hemisphere stroke, a patient's hand retains some rudimentary motor and sensory functions. Patients feel that their hand is physically and psychologically detached. Moreover, its movements are governed by someone else (the alien).

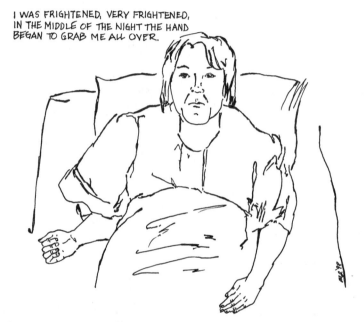

383–390. In assigning a value to a biologic test for a disease, what will be the effect of the following changes (383–390) on the test's sensitivity and specificity (a–i)?

a. Sensitivity and specificity will both increase.
b. Sensitivity and specificity will both decrease.
c. Sensitivity and specificity will remain unchanged.
d. Sensitivity will increase and specificity will decrease.
e. Sensitivity will decrease and specificity will increase.
f. Sensitivity will increase.
g. Sensitivity will decrease.
h. Specificity will increase
i. Specificity will decrease.

383. Technical changes in the test that increase false-negative results.

384. Technical changes that increase true-positive results.

385. Using the test on a population in which the disease is less prevalent.

386. Technical changes that increase false-positive results.

387. Technical changes that increase true-negative results.

388. Lowering the cutoff point of the test results so that both true and false-positive results increase.

389. Changing the cutoff point of the test results so that both true and false-negative results increase.

390. Testing for a disease in which individuals with and without the disease can be more readily identified.

ANSWERS: 383-g, 384-f, 385-c, 386-i, 387-h, 388-d, 389-e, 390-a

Sensitivity is defined by the proportion of true-positive results. It equals true-positives / true-positives + false-negatives. This formula is equivalent to true-positives / all positives. A highly sensitive test will detect almost all individuals with a disease; however, depending on its sensitivity, the test may also incorrectly identify individuals who do not actually have the disease.

Specificity is defined by the proportion of valid *negative* results. It equals true-negatives / (true-negatives + false-positives). Specificity increases either when true-negatives increase or false-positives decrease, but it is not directly proportional to true positives. In other words, if a highly specific test is positive, the patient is highly likely to have the illness; however, a negative result may not exclude it.

Tests proposed for Alzheimer's disease must be highly specific and sensitive because the clinical diagnosis is approximately 90% accurate.

391. Which of the following antiepileptic medications (AEDs) inhibit the hepatic cytochrome P-450 oxidases.

a. Valproate (valproic acid/divalproex) (Depakote)
b. Carbamazepine (Tegretol)
c. Phenytoin (Dilantin)
d. Gabapentin (Neurontin)

ANSWER: a. Valproate is the only commonly used AED that inhibits the P-450 enzyme system. Carbamazepine, phenytoin, and phenobarbital all induce the enzyme system. Thus, these AEDs reduce the effectiveness of oral contraceptives and other medications. Gabapentin, lamotrigine, and vigabatrin have little or no effect on the enzyme system.

392. Of the following MRI abnormalities associated with MS, which is most closely associated with cognitive impairment?

a. Total lesion area or volume
b. Enlarged cerebral ventricles
c. Corpus callosum atrophy
d. Periventricular white matter demyelination

ANSWER: a. In MS, cognitive impairment is more closely associated with total lesion area or volume visualized on MRI ("the lesion load") than other MRI abnormalities. It is also associated with physical disability, duration of the illness, and cerebral hypometabolism, portrayed on PET.

393. During the evaluation of a 66-year-old man for the onset of dementia, the physician asked the patient to copy a sequence of four sets, each of three squares followed by a circle. After completing one set, the patient copied only the squares. When he was unable to complete the task, he shouted, cursed, and broke the pencil. An MRI showed generalized cerebral atrophy, especially in the frontal lobes. Of the following, which is the most likely underlying pathology?

a. Plaques and tangles
b. Spirochetes in gummas
c. Intraneuronal argentophilic inclusions
d. Intraneuronal eosinophilic intracytoplasmic inclusions

ANSWER: c. As in Question 308, the patient had perseveration, easy frustration, emotional outburst, decrease in verbal output, and lack of inhibition. Those symptoms suggest frontal lobe dysfunction. The underlying problem could be either vascular dementia or, more likely, frontotemporal dementia. Many cases of frontotemporal dementia, which are labeled Pick's disease, are characterized by intraneuronal argentophilic inclusions. Spirochetes in gummas are a sign of neurosyphilis. Intraneuronal eosinophilic intracytoplasmic inclusions are Lewy bodies, which are a sign of diffuse Lewy body disease.

394. A 17-year-old boy brought to the emergency room after a verbal fight with his parents appears to have quadriparesis and blindness. However, his motor tone, DTRs, plantar reflexes, and cranial nerves are intact. His pupils are 4 mm, round, and reactive to light. In addition, when rotating a drum with vertical stripes in front of him, his eyes repetitively follow the stripes and then snap back, but again follow the stripes. What is the implication of his ocular movements?

a. He has ingested PCP or related toxin.
b. He should be given thiamine.
c. His opticokinetic nystagmus is intact.
d. He has sustained a traumatic injury to his occipital lobe.

ANSWER: c. He has intact opticokinetic nystagmus, which is a normal irresistible ocular motility reflex. It indicates that his visual and ocular motility pathways are intact. Its presence in someone who seems to be blind generally indicates that the "visual loss" is on a psychogenic basis.

395. Depression following strokes is closely associated with all of the following except which condition?

a. Marked gait impairment
b. Nonfluency and word finding difficulties
c. Impaired memory and judgment
d. Suicide ideation
e. Pseudobulbar palsy

ANSWER: d. Poststroke depression is closely associated with physical, language, cognitive deficits, and pseudobulbar palsy. Its manifestations often include insomnia, weight loss, ruminations, and sadness. However, ideas of worthlessness and suicide occur in only about 10% of patients with poststroke depression.

396. Which statement is true concerning Angelman's syndrome?

a. Angelman's syndrome occurs exclusively in girls.
b. Children with Angelman's syndrome have imprinted behavior, as described by Konrad Lorenz.
c. Angelman's syndrome's phenotype is determined by genetic imprinting.
d. An Angelman's syndrome boy is likely to have a sister with Prader-Willi syndrome.

ANSWER: c. In Angelman's syndrome and its counterpart, Prader-Willi syndrome, the condition's phenotype depends on which parent passed on the defective gene (genetic imprinting). Konrad Lorenz described behavioral imprinting among social animals, which is a quite different phenomenon. His theories won him a Nobel Prize in 1973.

397. Which one of the following statements is true regarding adults with ADHD?

a. Although stimulants may be effective therapy in children with ADHD, they are usually ineffective in adults with ADHD.
b. Most cases of childhood ADHD persist in adults.
c. Adults with ADHD usually benefit from phenobarbital.
d. ADHD adults are liable to develop antisocial personality disorder.

ANSWER: d. Stimulants are effective in adult as well as childhood ADHD. Only about 15% of children with ADHD grow into adults with ADHD. Phenobarbital and other sedatives are apt to cause paradoxical hyperactivity in ADHD children and adults. ADHD adults are liable to develop antisocial personality disorder, substance abuse, and other problems.

398. Which change in second messenger characterizes dopamine D_1 receptors?

a. Adenyl cyclase
b. Acetyl choline
c. COMT
d. NMDA

ANSWER: a. Increased activity of dopamine D_1 receptors increases AMP production through increased adenyl cyclase.

399. Match the sign (a–f) with its closest implication (1–6).

a. Babinski
b. Lhermitte
c. Romberg
d. Tinel
e. Lasègue's
f. Hoover

1. Irritation of a lumbar nerve root
2. Spinal cord posterior column impairment
3. Corticospinal tract injury
4. Cervical spinal cord irritation
5. Psychogenic leg paresis
6. Compression of the median nerve

ANSWER: a-3, b-4, c-2, d-6, e-1, f-5

400. In assessing a highly accomplished physician for dementia, in the absence of prior neuropsychologic testing, which of the following is the *least* reliable indication of cognitive decline?

a. Results of a current neuropsychologic battery
b. Scores obtained on a current Scholastic Achievement Test (SAT) compared to those in high school
c. Comparison of current to high school mathematical ability
d. Job performance, regardless of the results on the neuropsychological tests

ANSWER: c. Mathematical ability is an isolated cognitive function that does not reflect overall cognitive capacity. Even in highly successful, intellectual individuals, it may not have been well developed during childhood. Also, with lack of use, mathematical skills atrophy. In contrast, vocabulary and reading skills, which are deeply ingrained ("overlearned"), are highly resistant to cognitive impairment.

401. Which medication produces the lowest relapse rate in chronic alcoholics?

a. Naltrexone
b. Disulfiram
c. SSRIs
d. Lithium

ANSWER: a

402. A 10-year-old boy has increasingly greater behavioral and academic difficulties for 6 months. The neurologist finds clumsiness, Babinski signs, and inability to walk "in tandem" (one foot in front of the other [heel-to-toe walking]). The MRI showed extensive cerebral demyelination with surrounding inflammation. In retrospect, an older brother had the same illness but died of adrenal failure before it was diagnosed. Which one of the following statements is incorrect?

a. The patient's urine will contain metachromatic granules.
b. Adrenal replacement therapy will correct the adrenal insufficiency but not the neurologic deterioration.
c. This condition can mimic MS; however, it typically occurs in children, leads to death in approximately 5 years, and is characterized by adrenal failure.
d. This condition results from defective peroxisomes.

ANSWER: a. He and his brother have had adrenoleukodystrophy (ALD), which is a sex-linked leukodystrophy that begins in childhood. ALD typically presents with behavioral, emotional, and cognitive difficulties. Soon afterward corticospinal tract and cerebellar signs develop and predominate. At the same time, the adrenal glands fail. ALD results from the accumulation of very long chain fatty acids because of defective peroxisomes, which are intracellular organelles.

Metachromatic granules in the urine indicate metachromatic leukodystrophy (MLD). This illness is another CNS demyelinating disease that usually presents in childhood. However, unlike ALD, MLD symptoms may not appear until victims are young adults, it is inherited in an autosomal recessive pattern, and it does not cause adrenal insufficiency.

403. In normal sexual arousal, what is the role of nitric oxide?

a. It leads to vasoconstriction.
b. It promotes the production of cGMP-phosphodiesterase.
c. It promotes cGMP activity.
d. It leads to amnesia.

ANSWER: c. Nitric oxide promotes cyclic guanylate cyclase monophosphate (cGMP) activity, which leads to vasodilation. The vasodilation leads to genital engorgement.

404. What is the mechanism of action of sildenafil (Viagra)?

a. It increases cGMP activity.
b. It enhances cGMP-phosphodiesterase.
c. It promotes the production of cyclic guanylate cyclase monophosphate (cGMP).
d. It provokes the release of nitric oxide (NO).

ANSWER: a. Sildenafil (Viagra) increases cGMP activity by inhibiting its metabolic enzyme (cGMP-phosphodiesterase).

405. With which phenomenon does the day's lowest body temperature coincide?

a. Intense REM sleep
b. Intense slow-wave sleep
c. Sleep onset
d. 12 noon
e. 4:00 PM

ANSWER: a. When REM activity is most likely to be present, in the early morning, the body's temperature reaches its daily low point.

406. A 40-year-old woman developed burning and prickly sensations in her feet when trying to fall asleep. She had less pronounced symptoms during the daytime. The sensations caused her, she felt, to have irregular movements of her legs and feet. They compelled her to pace around her bedroom for one hour before being able to sleep. Once asleep, she had regular dorsiflexion of her feet and ankles. General medical, neurologic, and psychiatric evaluations revealed no serious abnormalities. Which test should be performed next?

a. PSG
b. MRI
c. EEG
d. Routine blood chemistry and complete blood count
e. MSLT
f. None of the above

ANSWER: d. She has restless leg syndrome. As in her case, it is associated with periodic leg movements. She does not have akathisia. Causes of restless leg syndrome include diabetic and uremic polyneuropathy, iron deficiency, and pregnancy—conditions that should be detectable on a general medical examination or routine blood tests.

407. Which of the following statements concerning melatonin is false?

a. Tryptophan is the amino acid from which melatonin is synthesized.
b. Its primary metabolic product is serotonin.
c. Selective serotonin re-uptake inhibitors can increase plasma serotonin concentration.
d. Tryptophan deficiency reduces melatonin plasma concentration.
e. Melatonin is an indolamine.

ANSWER: b. Melatonin is synthesized through the following synthetic pathway: tryptophan $\rightarrow$ serotonin $\rightarrow$ N-acetyl-serotonin $\rightarrow$ melatonin.

408. Which of the following statements concerning melatonin is false?

a. The suprachiasmatic nucleus of the hypothalamus contains receptors for melatonin.
b. Melatonin is synthesized and secreted from the pineal gland during darkness.
c. Bright light enhances melatonin synthesis and secretion.
d. Melatonin is probably the method by which light-dark cycles regulate circadian hormonal secretion.

ANSWER: c. Bright light suppresses melatonin synthesis and secretion. Darkness enhances melatonin synthesis and secretion from the pineal gland. Melatonin receptors on the suprachiasmatic nucleus probably allow melatonin to influence circadian hormone rhythm and the sleep-wake cycle.

409. A 26-year-old woman consults a neurologist for headaches that began to develop 6 weeks before the visit. She had no history of trauma, infections, or risk factors for AIDS. She had irregular menses. She was obese. She had florid papilledema and bilateral abducens nerve palsies. She was fully alert and able to ambulate. She has no ataxia. Of the following, which should be the next diagnostic step?

a. Perform tests for AIDS
b. Obtain a head CT or MRI
c. Perform an LP, which will be therapeutic as well as diagnostic
d. None of the above

ANSWER: b. She probably has pseudotumor cerebri in view of her age, obesity, menstrual irregularity, and absence of focal findings. Before performing an LP, she should have either a CT or MRI to exclude tumor, obstructive hydrocephalus, and other causes of increased intracranial pressure.

410. In the preceding question, what is a CT most likely to reveal?

a. Normal brain and ventricles
b. Dilated ventricles
c. Small or "slitlike" ventricles
d. Transtentorial herniation

ANSWER: c. As if the brain were simply swollen from its interstitial edema, the ventricles are compressed in pseudotumor cerebri. The cerebral swelling also stretches and impairs the sixth cranial nerves, which produces the abducens nerve palsies.

411. What is the effect of dopamine stimulating D_2 receptors?

a. The interaction stimulates adenyl cyclase activity.
b. The interaction inhibits adenyl cyclase activity.
c. The interaction has no effect on adenyl cyclase activity.

ANSWER: b. Dopamine–D_1 receptor interaction stimulates adenyl cyclase activity, but dopamine–D_2 receptor interaction inhibits adenyl cyclase activity.

412. A 6-year-old boy begins to have inward turning of his left foot that is most pronounced after school is finished at 3:00 PM. One trick that he shows his parents—he has no friends—is that if he walks backward, his foot assumes a normal position. The boy's pediatrician conceded that the boy probably had sustained a subtle congenital cerebral injury ("cerebral palsy"). When the neurologist evaluated the boy at 4:00 PM, his legs had intermittent, sustained, inward turning of both legs and rotation of the lower trunk. DTRs were normal. The next morning, the neurologist saw no such movements. Which of the following will be least productive?

a. Inquire as to the ethnicity, as well as the health, of the boy's parents and grandparents.
b. Prescribe a therapeutic trial of L-dopa.
c. Restrict phenylalanine-containing foods.
d. Check for the DYT1 gene.
e. Determine the serum ceruloplasmin concentration.

ANSWER: c. Phenylketonuria (PKU), which would be treated by restricting phenylalanine-containing foods, becomes apparent in infancy and is characterized by mental retardation but not dystonia. The diurnal fluctuation of dystonia in children indicates dopamine-responsive dystonia (DRD). Other affected family members should be sought. Tricks that temporarily abolish dystonia—walking backward, skipping, dancing, or applying pressure to the involved limb—confirm a diagnosis of dystonia. Other causes of dystonia in childhood include early onset primary dystonia, which is found predominantly in Ashkenazic Jews and identified by the DYT1 gene, and Wilson's disease. None of them produce a diurnal fluctuation.

413. Which term is applied to cell death that is programmed, sequential, and energy requiring?

a. Necrosis
b. Apoptosis
c. Anoxia
d. None of the above

ANSWER: b

414. Which one of the following is not a characteristic of apoptosis?

a. It is the mechanism of cell death in Huntington's disease and ALS.
b. In Huntington's disease, inflammatory cells surround dying cells.
c. Some organs, such as the thymus gland, mature through apoptosis.
d. Apoptosis is often referred to as "programmed cell death."
e. Apoptosis requires energy.

ANSWER: b. Apoptosis, which is the mechanism of cell death in Huntington's disease, does not produce an inflammatory response to cell death. In contrast to apoptosis, necrosis elicits a prominent inflammatory response.

415. Which of the following statements concerning the tissue oxidation is false?

a. Hydrogen peroxide is a free radical and an oxidant.
b. Free radicals are oxidants.
c. Oxidants have one or more unpaired electrons and seek to acquire electrons.
d. Oxidation is fatal to tissue.
e. Normal cellular metabolism produces oxidants that are detoxified by mitochondria.

ANSWER: a. Hydrogen peroxide is an oxidant but not a free radical. According to the oxidative stress theory of Parkinson's disease, oxidants are incompletely removed by defective mitochondria. The ensuing tissue oxidation destroys basal ganglia.

416. Which of the following characteristics is responsible for paramagnetic agents, such as gadolinium, being able to increase the signal of cerebral lesions during MRI studies?

a. They cross the intact as well as the permeable blood-brain barrier.
b. They attenuate ionizing radiation.
c. They alter the time for protons to resume their alignment after RF signals have been applied.
d. They release photons.

ANSWER: c. Paramagnetic agents used in MRI do not cross the intact blood-brain barrier. When tumors, abscesses, and other lesions disrupt the barrier, these agents penetrate into the surrounding brain. Paramagnetic agents alter the time for protons to resume their alignment in magnetic fields. CT depends on ionizing radiation. Radioligands used in PET and SPECT release photons.

417. Which of the following statements regarding radioligands in PET and SPECT is true?

a. These radioligands have a half-life that typically exceeds 7 days.
b. In PET, the radioligands release positrons, which interact with electrons. The reaction annihilates both particles. Their masses are converted into two photons.
c. In PET, radioligands produce an anatomic image that has the same resolution as CT.
d. PET radioligands are specific enough to diagnose Alzheimer's disease.

ANSWER: b. PET produces a relatively gross anatomic image. It can suggest Alzheimer's disease and frontotemporal dementia but not with the specificity required by a clinician.

418. A 33-year-old man with MS has paraparesis and a left-sided visual impairment. He finds that the neurologist's red tie appears maroon when he uses only his left eye but is its true red color when he uses only his right eye. Which is the most likely explanation for his visual perception problem?

a. He has color blindness.
b. The MS has affected his occipital cortex.
c. He has a persistent ocular migraine.
d. He has color desaturation.
e. He has developed a psychogenic disturbance.

ANSWER: d. He has color desaturation, which is a common manifestation of optic neuritis. Color blindness, especially the red-green variety, is a sex-linked genetic disorder that affects both eyes and is apparent from childhood. MS can affect the occipital cortex, but lesions there would cause hemianopsia and not affect color perception in this manner. Ocular migraines can cause a unilateral scotoma but not color perception impairments.

419. PET and SPECT use ligands that produce photons. Which of the following does not describe the general composition of ligands?

a. Organic molecules bound to a radioisotope
b. Organic molecules bound to a central metal ion, such as hemoglobin
c. Organic molecules bound to an inorganic molecule
d. Organic molecules bound to a tracer element

ANSWER: c

420. This is the MRI of a 23-year-old man who had noticed that he had been losing hearing ability in his left ear for one year. The MRI was performed during infusion of gadolinium. Where is the lesion located?

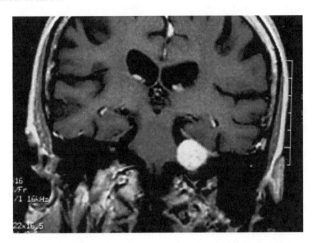

a. Lateral to the pons
b. In the pons

c. In the temporal lobe
d. None of the above

ANSWER: a. The lesion arises from the acoustic nerve, which can be seen as a bright streak above and medial to the lesion. The lesion is located in the cerebellopontine angle.

421. The man described in the previous question undergoes surgery. Most of the lesion is removed. Facial strength and most of his hearing is preserved. What is the most likely histology of the lesion?

a. Glioblastoma
b. Medulloblastoma

c. Neuroma
d. Meningioma

ANSWER: c. He most likely has an acoustic neuroma. A meningoma is possible but less likely, mostly because of his relatively young age. Glioblastomas and medulloblastomas are intra-axial.

422. The man described in the previous two questions recovers from surgery. He is found to have no abnormalities except for two or three small café au lait spots. He is well for several years, but then the hearing in his right ear begins to fail. An MRI shows a lesion on the right side similar to the initial one. What is the most likely underlying diagnosis?

a. Toxoplasmosis
b. Neurofibromatosis
c. Metastatic carcinoma
d. A mitochondrial disorder

ANSWER: b. Bilateral acoustic neuromas indicate that he has the "central type" of neurofibromatosis (NF2), which is inherited on chromosome 22 in an autosomal dominant pattern. Unlike the more common "peripheral" variety of neurofibromatosis (NF1), NF2 produces few neurofibromas or café au lait spots.

423. Which of the following abnormalities is least likely to be found in a 66-year-old man with hypertension who suddenly developed left hemiparesis 2 days before the examination?

a. Inability to recognize sadness in the face of family members
b. Inability to draw a simple house
c. Flattened affect in his speech and facial expression
d. Tendency to use nonsensical or incorrect words

ANSWER: d. He has sustained a nondominant stroke, which would cause flattened speech, lack of emotion, and aprosody. He would also have constructional apraxia, which would impair his ability to copy or draw simple figures, such as a clock or a small house. However, he would not make paraphasic errors, which is a manifestation of aphasia.

424. An 85-year-old retired millionaire is brought to the hospital by his lifelong butler. The patient, who had a 10-year history of Parkinson's disease complicated by dementia, had had a seizure. His psychiatrist has been prescribing haloperidol at bedtime because of nocturnal hallucinations, delusions, screaming, and a tendency to wander, but that antipsychotic and several others did not control his bizarre thinking or abnormal behavior. A CT showed a small acute and larger chronic subdural hematoma. After neurosurgeons drained the subdural hematomas, the patient returned to his usual state. One month later, the patient was readmitted with a fracture-dislocation of his cervical spine and quadriparesis. What is the most likely cause of the repeated hospitalizations?

a. Falls due to the wandering
b. Other forms of trauma
c. Adverse reactions to medications
d. Age-related deterioration

ANSWER: a or b. The first admission probably resulted from a combination of acute traumatic bleeding superimposed on a chronic subdural hematoma. The second admission was due to a fall or deliberate trauma in which there was hyperextension of the head and neck. In patients with dementia who sustain multiple trauma, elder abuse should be suspected.

425. A 73-year-old woman was admitted to the hospital immediately after the sudden onset of left-sided hemiparesis. Within 2 hours, a head CT was normal. The neurologists infused tissue plasminogen activator (tPA). During the next 3 days, she became agitated and belligerent. She accused the staff of keeping her in the hospital even though nothing was wrong with her. What is the most likely cause of her feeling that "nothing is wrong"?

a. The tPA has caused a delirium.
b. A new stroke developed on the third day of hospitalization.
c. Anosognosia became manifest.
d. She has developed dementia.

ANSWER: c. The thrombolytic agent, tPA, has some potential side effects, such as intracerebral bleeding, but delirium is not one of them. Patients with anosognosia often do not appreciate their situation and reject assistance and medical regimens.

426. As part of a reevaluation because of the patient in the preceding question, this CT was obtained on the fifth hospital day. What does it reveal?

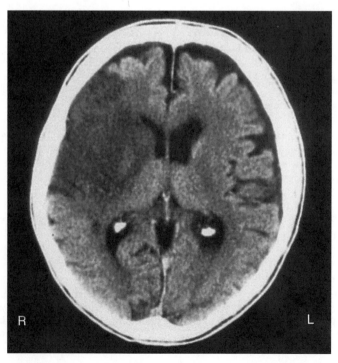

a. A right middle cerebral artery stroke
b. A right cerebral tumor
c. A left middle cerebral artery stroke
d. Occlusion of the right internal carotid artery
e. Occlusion of the left internal carotid artery

ANSWER: a. In keeping with the convention, this CT displays the patient's right side on the left: note the markings. It shows a classic pattern of a middle cerebral artery stoke due to occlusion of the artery. The tPA failed to dissolve the clot. The middle cerebral artery region is darker than the normal brain because it is necrotic; it has been deprived of relatively radiodense blood. CTs performed within the first day or two after a stroke are often normal because necrosis has not as yet developed. In this scan, the right anterior horn of the lateral ventricle is compressed by stroke-induced swelling. In contrast, the regions supplied by the anterior and posterior cerebral arteries are spared. The lesion is not a tumor because the initial CT would have been abnormal; the mass effect on this CT would have been greater, and the lesion does not contain any sign of a mass lesion.

427. During the previous 8 years, a 35-year-old woman has had progressively severe gait impairment, dysarthria, and then cognitive impairment. Her general medical evaluation and routine blood tests were normal. Her neurologic examination revealed signs of dementia, pseudobulbar palsy, optic atrophy, corticospinal tract impairment, and cerebellar dysfunction. A CT showed only mild cerebral atrophy. Based on her MRI, which portion of the nervous system has been affected?

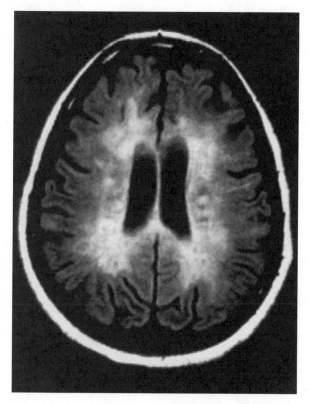

a. The gray matter
b. CNS myelin

c. All parts of the CNS
d. The ventricular system

ANSWER: b. The MRI shows confluent regions of demyelination surrounding the lateral ventricles. There is cerebral atrophy. As this case illustrates, MRI is superior to CT in detecting white matter abnormalities.

428. In regard to the patient in the previous question, which of the following illnesses would be least likely to have caused her neurologic problems?

a. MS

c. PML

b. Adrenoleukodystrophy

d. Toluene abuse

ANSWER: b. Each of these conditions causes demyelination, which can produce such symptoms. However, adrenoleukodystrophy is a sex-link disorder that would usually appear in male infants and children. When adrenoleukodystrophy affects young men, it causes mania, dementia, and gait impairment accompanied by signs of adrenal insufficiency. Death usually ensues within 2 years after such symptoms appear. The pattern of periventricular demyelination is typical of MS.

429. A 25-year-old woman has a pupil that is abnormally large and slightly irregular. The pupil remains large when a light is shown into it and has almost no constriction with accommodation. She has no ptosis and no paresis of any extraocular muscle. A dilute solution of pilocarpine, which would not affect a normal pupil, is applied to the eye. The pupil promptly constricts to a normal size. What is the etiology of her pupil's enlargement?

a. Sympathetic denervation
b. Parasympathetic denervation
c. Self-induced anisocoria
d. Argyll-Robertson

ANSWER: b. She has an Adie's pupil, which is sometimes called a "tonic pupil." It is a benign condition that results from parasympathetic denervation. Because of loss of parasympathetic innervation, the affected pupil responds unusually rapidly and forcefully to cholinergic agents. In contrast, pupils with sympathetic denervation, such as Horner's syndrome and Argyll-Robertson pupils, are small.

430. Which of the following statements regarding the actions of serotonin receptors in migraines is false?

a. Sumatriptan (Imitrex) is a 5-HT_{1D} agonist.
b. Sumatriptan-5-HT_{1D} receptor interactions produce vasoconstriction.
c. Dihydroergotamine (DHE), which is also a vasoconstrictor, produces the same effect as the triptans.
d. Methysergide (Sansert) is a 5-HT_2 antagonist.

ANSWER: c. Both the triptans and DHE produce cerebral vasoconstriction and alleviate the headache; however, the triptans, but not DHE, alleviate migraine's autonomic nervous system symptoms.

431. In which condition would elevated levels of creatine phosphokinase (CPK) be unexpected?

a. In a person found unconscious after 2 days
b. Immediately following a neuroleptic-induced dystonic reaction
c. After an episode of status epilepticus
d. With use of atypical antipsychotics
e. With use of typical antipsychotics

ANSWER: d

432. Which is the phenotype of untreated infants with congenital absence of phenylalanine hydroxylase?

a. Mental retardation, deafness, and epilepsy
b. Episodes of encephalopathy and lactic acidosis
c. Mental retardation, self-mutilation, hyperuricemia, and spasticity
d. Mental retardation, eczema, and fair complexion
e. Rigidity, dystonia, and gait impairment that occur in the late afternoon

ANSWER: d. Infants with congenital absence of phenylalanine hydroxylase have phenylketonuria (PKU), which causes mental retardation, eczema, and lack of pigment in the hair and eyes. Mental retardation, deafness, and epilepsy suggest a congenital rubella infection. Episodic encephalopathy and lactic acidosis suggests a mitochondrial DNA disorder. The combination of mental retardation, self-mutilation, hyperuricemia, and spasticity indicates Lesch-Nyhan syndrome. Rigidity, dystonia, and gait impairment that occur in the late afternoon indicate dopamine-responsive dystonia.

433. In which chromosome is amyloid precursor protein (APP) encoded?

a. 4
b. 17
c. 21
d. X
e. O

ANSWER: c

434. A 60-year-old woman reports having had several episodes, each lasting several days, of incapacitating dizziness. The dizziness develops suddenly and is associated with nausea but not tinnitus or hearing loss. The physician determined that the dizziness is actually vertigo and that it is present only when her head changes position. During the examination, when she is supine, with her head and neck hyperextended and her head rotated 45° to the right, she develops vertigo and nystagmus. The rest of her neurologic examination, formal hearing tests, and an MRI scan of her brain are normal. Which is the best treatment?

a. Neurosurgery for an acoustic neuroma
b. Canalith repositioning maneuvers
c. ASA for basilar artery TIAs
d. An SSRI for panic attacks

ANSWER: b. The maneuver that led to nystagmus (the Dix-Hallpike Test) indicates that she has benign position vertigo. Its cause has been unexplained until recently, when evidence has been presented that it results from debris in a semicircular canal (otoliths). Canalith repositioning consists of the physician's hyperextending and then rotating the patient's head, which moves the otoliths from the semicircular canal to the utricle.

435. Which of the following antidepressants is least likely to cause sexual dysfunction?

a. Fluvoxamine
b. Fluoxetine
c. Bupropion
d. Trazodone
e. Paroxetine

ANSWER: c. Bupropion, unlike the SSRIs, inhibits dopamine re-uptake. Trazodone can induce priapism.

436. During the past year, a 10-year-old boy has developed a progressively severe gait impairment, in which his left foot turns inward when he walks. The movement does not occur when he walks backward or sleeps. His neurologic examination, including cognitive function, is otherwise normal. A serum ceruloplasmin, MRI of his head, EEG, and routine studies were normal. A trial of L-dopa produced no benefit. Which statement is correct?

a. The gait abnormality's pattern, with a normal evaluation, is indicative of a psychogenic disturbance.
b. He probably has Sydenham's chorea.
c. His ethnicity is paramount.
d. He should have an immediate orthopedic evaluation.
e. He should have an MRI of the spine.

ANSWER: c. A gait impairment that is abolished by walking backward, skipping, dancing, or running might be due to a psychogenic disturbance; however, it more likely represents a "trick" that individuals with dystonia unconsciously employ to suppress or circumvent an involuntary movement. He should be evaluated for the onset of early onset dystonia, which is due to the DYT1 gene and is almost always confined to Ashkenazi (Eastern European) Jews. Dystonia is one of the most frequently misdiagnosed conditions: Especially at its onset, patients with dystonia are often said to have a conversion disorder. The course is too long for Sydenham's chorea.

437. Match each of the descriptions (a–n) with the region (1–13).

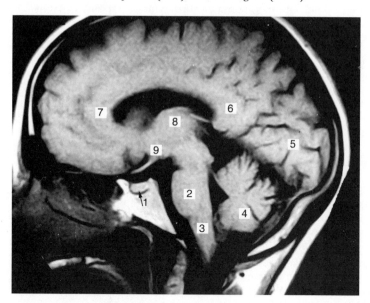

a. Structure where the optic nerves' nasal fibers cross
b. Cortex where the optic tract terminates
c. Structure that secretes ACTH
d. Structure where face and body pain tracts synapse
e. Structure where the fasciculus gracilis and f. cuneatus terminate
f. When patients have alexia without agraphia, this structure is damaged
g. Contains nuclei for cranial nerves VI, VII, and VIII
h. Contains the dorsal raphe nuclei
i. Structure injured when patients have crossed hypalgesia and Horner's syndrome ipsilateral to facial numbness
j. Structure contains caudal raphe nuclei
k. Structure contains the locus ceruleus
l. Its midline region is the vermis
m. The site of the crossing of the fibers conveying position and vibration sensation
n. Derives from the Greek, *knee,* as in *genuflect,* to bend at the knee in worship

ANSWERS:

1-c. The *pituitary gland* secretes ACTH and other hormones. Note that it is inferior to the optic nerves and chiasm.

2-g, k. The *pons* not only contains the nuclei for cranial nerves VI, VII, and VIII but also the motor division and most of the sensory divisions of cranial nerve V. The dorsal raphe nuclei, which gives rise to serotonin-generating neurons, are based primarily in the pons but extend into the midbrain. In addition, the pons contains the locus ceruleus, which gives rise to norepinephrine-generating neurons.

3-i, j, m. When patients have crossed hypalgesia and Horner's syndrome ipsilateral to facial numbness, they probably have infarctions in the *medulla* causing the lateral medullary syndrome. The medulla also contains the caudal raphe nuclei, which gives rise to serotonin-generating neurons. Tracts from the caudal raphe nuclei descend into the spinal cord to promote analgesia. Ascending sensory tracts for position and vibration (fasciculus gracilis and f. cuneatus) cross (decussate) in the medial lemniscus, which is located in the medulla.

4-l. The vermis is the inferior, medial structure of the *cerebellum.* In alcoholics, it characteristically undergoes atrophy.

5-b. The optic (the geniculocalcarine) tract terminates in the visual cortex of the *occipital lobe.*

6-f. Tracts conveying written language information from the right occipital lobe to the language centers in the dominant, left cerebral hemisphere must pass through the *splenium of the corpus callosum.*

7-n.

8-d, e. Tracts that convey pain from the face and body—the trigeminal nerve's sensory divisions and the spinothalamic tract, respectively—synapse in the *thalamus*. From there, sensation is widely disbursed to the cerebral cortex, reticular activating system, limbic system, and other areas. The f. gracilis and f. cuneatus, which convey proprioception from the lower and upper extremities, respectively, also terminate in the thalamus. Those sensations are also conveyed to the cortex, particularly the post-central gyrus.

9-a. The optic nerves' nasal fibers cross at the *optic chiasm*. An optic nerve can be seen anterior and inferior to the hypothalamus.

438–440. A 63-year-old man was sent for psychiatric consultation for inappropriate behavior. The psychiatrist, finding that the patient had headaches, cognitive impairment, and a mild left-hemiparesis, requested an MRI.

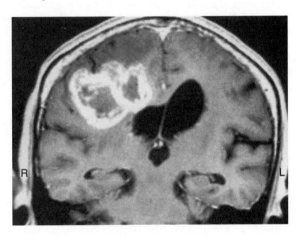

438. Which view has been displayed?

a. Transaxial
b. Axial
c. Sagittal

d. Coronal
e. None of the above

ANSWER: d.

439. In which region of the brain is the lesion localized?

a. Right frontal-parietal
b. Left frontal-parietal
c. Right temporal

d. Left temporal
e. Right occipital
f. Left occipital

ANSWER: a. The lesion is in the right cerebral hemisphere (note the letters superimposed on the lateral portion of the skull). It is above and lateral to the lateral ventricle and well above the Sylvian fissure, which separates the temporal lobe from the overlying frontal and temporal lobes.

440. Based on the MRI, which of the following is the most likely etiology?

a. Hemorrhagic stroke
b. Thrombotic stroke
c. Meningioma
d. Glioblastoma multiforme
e. MS
f. PML

ANSWER: d. The lesion is most likely a glioblastoma multiforme because it is a multi-lobulated mass that arises from the white matter. It compresses the adjacent lateral ventricle and shifts midline structures. MS plaques and PML, which also arise from the white matter, do not create mass effect. Strokes usually conform to the distribution of cerebral arteries and do not cause mass effect.

441. How is the antiepileptic effect of divalproex and topiramate conveyed?

a. They increase CNS glutamine concentration.
b. They decrease CNS glutamine concentration.
c. They increase CNS glutamate concentration.
d. They decrease CNS glutamate concentration.
e. They increase CNS GABA concentration.
f. They decrease CNS GABA concentration.

ANSWER: e. Divalproex, topiramate, gabapentin, and vigabatrin increase CNS concentration or activity of the inhibitory neurotransmitter GABA.

442. A psychiatrist is called to evaluate a 13-year-old girl who, after receiving successful treatment for status epilepticus, remains withdrawn, depressed, and amnestic for all events that occurred during the several weeks before the episodes. She had no history of seizures, drug abuse, or other neurologic problem; however, she had had multiple recent admissions for abdominal pain, a spiral humerus fracture, and headaches. The EEG was normal, but the CT showed a linear, nondepressed skull fracture. Her phenytoin level was in the therapeutic range. Her routine blood tests and toxicology screens were all unremarkable. Which would be the best course of action for the psychiatrist?

a. Use a tricyclic antidepressant
b. Use a SSRI
c. Change her antiepileptic drug
d. Stop all antiepileptic drugs
e. None of the above

ANSWER: e. In view of the spiral limb fracture, as well as the skull fracture, child abuse should be suspected. Sexual abuse as well as physical abuse is common in children with pseudoseizures.

443. During the previous 2 years, this 7-year-old boy has been developing a progressively severe gait impairment that is most pronounced in the afternoon and evening. During those periods of the day, physicians find that he has a positive pull test and rigidity in all his limbs. When he awakes in the morning, his gait is entirely normal. He has had no cognitive decline, behavioral disturbances, or personality change. There is no family history of this disorder or any other neurologic illness. Which of the following is the most likely cause of his gait impairment?

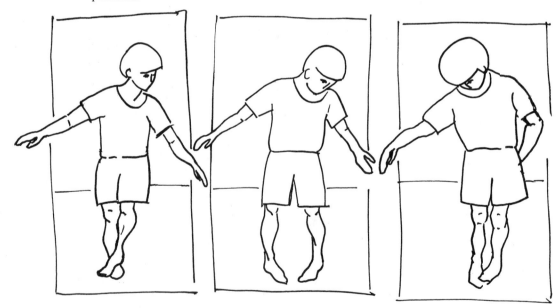

a. Dopa-responsive dystonia
b. DYT1 dystonia
c. Adrenoleukodystrophy
d. Athetotic cerebral palsy
e. Wilson's disease
f. Huntington's disease

ANSWER: a. This boy has involuntary movements of all his limbs (as pictured) and a positive pull test, which signifies basal ganglia pathology. Of all the illnesses, only dopa-responsive dystonia has a diurnal fluctuation. Nevertheless, each of these ill-nesses can appear in childhood and present with gait impairment. Subtle clinical dif-ferences can separate some of them. Adrenoleukodystrophy causes spasticity rather than involuntary movements in boys. Athetotic cerebral palsy appears by age 4. The childhood variant of Huntington's disease causes rigidity and, almost simultaneously, cognitive or personality changes. The duration of the illness, as well as the diurnal fluc-tuation, excludes Sydenham's chorea.

444. Which is the best test for the patient described in Question 443?

a. MRI
b. Serum ceruloplasmin
c. Small doses of L-dopa
d. Genetic testing
e. None of the above

ANSWER: c. Administering small doses of L-dopa to patients suspected of having dopamine-responsive dystonia serves as a reliable therapeutic trial. In addition, be-cause the manifestations of these illnesses are similar and a delay in diagnosis may lead to irreversible brain damage, children presenting with such a movement disorder should undergo MRI, serum ceruloplasmin determination, and, in many cases, genetic testing.

445. A 60-year-old man, who was recently placed in a nursing home, requested a psychi-atric consultation because he began to experience episodes of visual hallucinations. A typical hallucination consisted of multiple glowing lamps in the left visual field that were reproduc-tions of a table lamp located in the right side of his room. The most remarkable aspect of the hallucinations, he explained, were that they occurred entirely in his left visual field, which had been rendered blind by a stroke the previous year. The stroke had also caused left-sided sensory loss and mild hemiparesis. Another remarkable aspect of the hallucinations were that they consisted of single or multiple replications of objects that he had recently seen in his in-tact right visual field. The episodes lasted for only several minutes and occurred once or twice daily. During them, he remained fully alert but mesmerized. At almost all other times, he was despondent, discouraged about his health, and unable to sleep restfully. Of the following, which will be the most likely treatment?

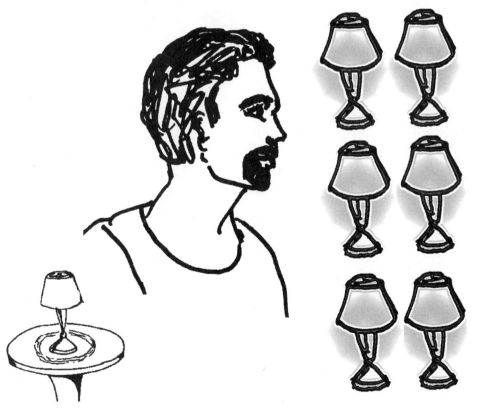

a. Tricyclic antidepressant
b. SSRI
c. Antiepileptic drug
d. Psychotherapy
e. Removal of one of his medications

ANSWER: c. The patient is experiencing palinopsia. This disorder, which is also called "visual perseveration," consists of recurrent images within an area of visual loss. These visual hallucinations typically occur in a left homonymous hemianopsia. They are usually duplications of individuals or objects in the intact right visual field. Although palinopsia has resulted from depression, LSD and other toxins, and metabolic aberrations, most cases result from recurrent partial seizures from right occipital strokes, neoplasms, or other lesions. When strokes lead to depression, the lesion is usually situated in the frontal lobes (left more often than right) or deeper structures but usually not an occipital lobe.

Index

Note: Page numbers in *italics* refer to illustrations; page numbers followed by t refer to tables.

KAUFMAN

ISBN 0-7216-8995-7

90038

9 780721 689951